THE SHOULDER AND THE OVERHEAD ATHLETE

THE SHOULDER AND THE OVERHEAD ATHLETE

FIRST EDITION

Editors

SUMANT G. KRISHNAN, MD

*Clinical Assistant Professor of Orthopaedic Surgery
University of Texas Southwestern Medical Center;
Attending Orthopaedic Surgeon
Shoulder Service, W.B. Carrell Memorial Clinic;
Assistant Team Physician
Dallas Cowboys, Dallas Stars, and Southern Methodist University
Dallas, Texas*

RICHARD J. HAWKINS, MD

*Clinical Professor of Orthopaedic Surgery
University of Colorado Health Sciences Center;
Attending Orthopaedic Surgeon
Steadman Hawkins Clinic;
Head Team Physician
Denver Broncos and Colorado Rockies
Vail, Colorado*

RUSSELL F. WARREN, MD

*Professor of Orthopaedic Surgery
Weill Medical College of Cornell University;
Surgeon-in-Chief, Emeritus, and Attending Orthopedic Surgeon
Hospital for Special Surgery;
Head Team Physician
New York Giants
New York, New York*

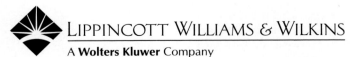

LIPPINCOTT WILLIAMS & WILKINS
A **Wolters Kluwer** Company
Philadelphia • Baltimore • New York • London
Buenos Aires • Hong Kong • Sydney • Tokyo

Acquisitions Editor: Robert A. Hurley
Developmental Editor: Michelle M. LaPlante
Production Editor: Rakesh Rampertab
Manufacturing Manager: Colin Warnock
Cover Designer: Christine Jenny
Compositor: Lippincott Williams & Wilkins Desktop Division
Printer: Edwards Brothers, Inc.

© 2004 by LIPPINCOTT WILLIAMS & WILKINS
530 Walnut Street
Philadelphia, PA 19106 USA
LWW.com

Printed in the USA

Library of Congress Cataloging-in-Publication Data
0-7817-4614-0

Care has been taken to confirm the accuracy of the information presented and to describe generally accepted practices. However, the authors, editors, and publisher are not responsible for errors or omissions or for any consequences from application of the information in this book and make no warranty, expressed or implied, with respect to the currency, completeness, or accuracy of the contents of the publication. Application of this information in a particular situation remains the professional responsibility of the practitioner.

The authors, editors, and publisher have exerted every effort to ensure that drug selection and dosage set forth in this text are in accordance with current recommendations and practice at the time of publication. However, in view of ongoing research, changes in government regulations, and the constant flow of information relating to drug therapy and drug reactions, the reader is urged to check the package insert for each drug for any change in indications and dosage and for added warnings and precautions. This is particularly important when the recommended agent is a new or infrequently employed drug.

Some drugs and medical devices presented in this publication have Food and Drug Administration (FDA) clearance for limited use in restricted research settings. It is the responsibility of the health care provider to ascertain the FDA status of each drug or device planned for use in their clinical practice.

10 9 8 7 6 5 4 3 2 1

We dedicate this book to all of the athletes who teach us about the complexities and challenges of the shoulder and who remind us how much we enjoy caring for them.

CONTENTS

Contributing Authors ix
Foreword xi
Preface xiii
Acknowledgments xv

SECTION I. GENERAL PRINCIPLES

1. The Overhead Athlete—Challenges and Decision-Making 3
   Richard J. Hawkins and Sumant G. Krishnan

2. Shoulder Anatomy and Biomechanics During Overhead Motions 10
   James E. Tibone, Rick B. Cunningham, and Patrick J. McMahon

3. Clinical Examination of the Overhead Athlete: The "Differential-Directed" Approach 23
   John M. Tokish, Sumant G. Krishnan, and Richard J. Hawkins

4. Imaging of the Overhead Athlete 50
   Charles P. Ho and Eric D. Smith

5. The Assessment of Outcomes for the Treatment of the Overhead Athlete 65
   John E. Kuhn

6. Resistance Training and Core Strengthening 82
   Donald A. Chu, Christine Boyd, and Andrea Hammer

7. Specific Exercises for the Throwing Shoulder 95
   Kevin E. Wilk and Michael M. Reinold

8. Interval Program and Its Implication for the Throwing Athlete 117
   Michael W. Allen and Sumant G. Krishnan

SECTION II. LESIONS OF THE OVERHEAD SHOULDER

9. Internal Impingement 125
   James R. Andrews and Patrick J. Casey

10. Surgical Treatment of Partial Thickness Rotator Cuff Tears 135
    John E. Conway and Steven B. Singleton

11. Subacromial Impingement and Full Thickness Rotator Cuff Tears in Overhead Athletes 146
    Champ L. Baker, Andrew L. Whaley, and Mark Baker

12. Unidirectional Anterior Instability 163
    Russell F. Warren and William D. Prickett

13. Unidirectional Posterior Instability 177
    Thomas A. Joseph and Sumant G. Krishnan

14. Multidirectional Instability 186
    Gary Misamore, Peter Sallay, and Brent Johnson

15. Disorders of the Biceps Tendon 196
    David W. Altchek and Brian R. Wolf

16. Acromioclavicular Joint Disorders 209
    Mark S. Schickendantz and Richard B. Jones

17. Scapulothoracic Problems in Overhead Athletes 222
    W. Ben Kibler and John Mcmullen

18. Fractures 236
    Sumant G. Krishnan, Robert J. Nowinski, and Wayne Z. Burkhead

19. Neurologic and Vascular Lesions 267
    Louis U. Bigliani, Walter G. Stanwood, and William N. Levine

20. Disorders in Pediatric Athletes 284
    Mininder S. Kocher and James O'Holleran

SECTION III. SPORT-SPECIFIC SHOULDER INJURIES AND MANAGEMENT IN OVERHEAD ATHLETES

21. Baseball 301
    James R. Andrews and Christopher G. Mazoué

22. Football 318
    Russell F. Warren, Bryan T. Kelly, Ronnie P. Barnes, and John W. Powell

23. Tennis 340
    David W. Altchek and Daniel E. Weiland

24. Swimming 349
    Scott A. Rodeo

Appendix 363
Index 369

CONTRIBUTING AUTHORS

Michael W. Allen, PT, ATC, CSCS   Director of Physical Therapy, Steadman Hawkins Denver Clinic, Englewood, Colorado; Physical Therapist, Colorado Rockies, Denver, Colorado

David W. Altchek, MD   Associate Attending Orthopaedic Surgeon, Sports Medicine and Shoulder Service, The Hospital for Special Surgery; Consultant, United States Tennis Association, New York, New York

James R. Andrews, MD   Orthopaedic Surgeon, Alabama Sports Medicine and Orthopaedic Center; Consultant, Washington Redskins, Birmingham, Alabama

Champ L. Baker, Jr, MD   Associate Clinical Professor, Department of Orthopaedic Surgery, Medical College of Georgia; Attending Physician, The Hughston Clinic, PC, Augusta, Georgia

Mark Baker, PT   Director of Rehabilitation, The Hughston Clinic; Physical Therapist, Columbus Cottonmouths Hockey Team, Columbus, Georgia

Ronnie P. Barnes, MS, ATC   Head Athletic Trainer, New York Giants, New York, New York

Louis U. Bigliani, MD   Chief, Center for Shoulder, Elbow & Sports Medicine, Department of Orthopaedic Surgery, Columbia-Presbyterian Medical Center, New York, New York

Christine Boyd, MD   Sports Medicine Fellow, Department of Sports Medicine, Stanford University, Stanford, California

Wayne Z. Burkhead, MD   Attending Orthopaedic Surgeon, Shoulder Service, W.B. Carrell Memorial Clinic, Dallas, Texas

Patrick J. Casey, MD   Alabama Sports Medicine and Orthopaedic Center, Birmingham, Alabama

Donald A. Chu, PT, PhD, ATC   Director, Performance Enhancement, Stanford Athletics, Arrillaga Family Sports Center, Stanford, California

John E. Conway, MD   Chief, Department of Orthopedics, Harris methodist Forth Worth Hospital; Head Team Physician, Texas Rangers Baseball Club, Forth Worth, Texas

Rick B. Cunningham, MD   Department of Orthopaedic Surgery, University of Pittsburgh, Pittsburg, Pennsylvania

Andrea Hammer, MD   Stanford Athletics, Arrillaga Family Sports Center, Stanford, California

Richard J. Hawkins, MD   Clinical Professor of Orthopaedic Surgery, University of Colorado Health Sciences Center; Attending Orthopaedic Surgeon, Steadman Hawkins Clinic; Head Team Physician, Denver Broncos and Colorado Rockies, Vail, Colorado

Charles P. Ho, MD, PhD   Director, National Orthopaedic Imaging Associates, California Advanced Imaging, Atherton, California

Brent Johnson, MD   Department of Orthopaedic Surgery, Indiana University, Indianapolis, Indiana

Richard B. Jones, MD   Director, Mountain Sports Health, Mountain Orthopedic Associates, Clyde, North Carolina

Thomas A. Joseph, MD   Clinical associate, Section of Sports Medicine and Shoulder Surgery, The Orthopaedic Center, Canfield, Ohio

Bryan T. Kelly, MD   Sports Medicine and Shoulder Service, Hospital for Special Surgery, New York, New York

W. Ben Kibler, MD   Medical Director, Sports Medicine Center, Lexington Clinic; Team Physician, Lexington Legends, Lexington, Kentucky

Mininder S. Kocher, MD, MPH   Attending Orthopaedic Surgeon, Department of Orthopaedic Surgery, Children's Hospital Boston, Boston, Massachusetts; Team Physician, Laswell College, Newton, Massachusetts

Sumant G. Krishnan, MD, Clinical Assistant Professor of Orthopaedic Surgery, University of Texas Southwestern Medical Center; Attending Orthopaedic Surgeon, Shoulder Service, W.B. Carrell Memorial Clinic; Assistant Team Physician, Dallas Cowboys, Dallas Stars, and Southern Methodist University, Dallas, Texas

John E. Kuhn, MD   Chief, Shoulder Surgery, Vanderbilt Sports Medicine; Team Physician, Vanderbilt University Athletic Department, Nashville, Tennessee

William N. Levine, MD   Assistant Professor, Center for Shoulder, Elbow, and Sports Medicine, Department of Orthopaedic Surgery, Columbia-Presbyterian Medical Center, New York, New York

Christopher G. Mazoué, MD   Alabama Sports Medicine Institute, Birmingham, Alabama

Patrick J. McMahon, MD   Assistant Professor, Department of Orthopedic Surgery, University of Pittsburgh, Pittsburgh, Pennsylvania

John Mcmullen, MS, ATC   Sports Medicine Center, Lexington Clinic, Lexington, Kentucky

Gary Misamore, MD   Clinical Associate Professor, Department of Orthopaedic Surgery, Indiana University; Team Physician, Butler University and Indianapolis Colts, Indianapolis, Indiana

Robert J. Nowinski, DO   Clinical Assistant Professor, Department of Orthopedic Surgery, Ohio University College of Osteopathic Medicine, Athens, Ohio

James O'Holleran, MD   Division of Sports Medicine, Department of Orthopaedic Surgery, Children's Hospital, Harvard Medical School, Boston, Massachusetts

John W. Powell, PhD, ATC   Director, Graduate Athletic Training Program, Michigan State University; Athletic Trainer, Michigan State University Athletic Teams, East Lansing, Michigan

William D. Prickett, MD   Sports Medicine and Shoulder Service, Hospital of Special Surgery, New York, New York

Michael M. Reinold, DPT, ATC   Coordinator of Rehabilitative Research and Clinical Education, Healthsouth Sports Medicine and Rehabilitation Center, American Sports Medicine Institute, Birmingham, Alabama; Tampa Bay Devil Rays Major league, Baseball Club, St. Petersburg, Florida

Scott A. Rodeo, MD   Associate Professor, Sports Medicine and Shoulder Service, Hospital for Special Surgery, New York, New York; Associate Team Physician, New York Giants, New York, New York

Peter Sallay, MD   Department of Orthopedic Surgery, Indiana University, Indianapolis, Indiana

Mark S. Schickendantz, MD   Clinic Instructor, Department of Orthopedic Surgery, Cleveland Clinic; Director of Orthopedic Services, Cleveland Indians Baseball Club, Cleveland, Ohio

Steven B. Singleton, MD   Orthopaedic Surgeon, Ben Hogan Center/Harris Methodist Forth Worth, Fort Worth, Texas

Eric D. Smith, MD   National Orthopedic Imaging Associates, California Advanced Imaging, Atherton, California

Walter G. Stanwood, MD   Center for Shoulder, Elbow & Sports Medicine, Columbia-Presbyterian Medical Center, New York, New York

James E. Tibone, MD   Clinical Professor, Department of Orthopaedic Surgery, University of Southern California; Team Physician, University of Southern California, Los Angeles, California

John M. Tokish, MD   Staff Orthopedic Surgeon, United States Air Force Academy Hospital; Team Physician, Falcon Football, United States Air Force Academy, Colorado Springs, Colorado

Russell F. Warren, MD   Professor of Orthopaedic Surgery, Weill Medical College of Cornell University; Surgeon-in-Chief, Emeritus, and Attending Orthopedic Surgeon, Hospital for Special Surgery; Head Team Physician, New York Giants, New York, New York

Daniel E. Weiland, MD   Orthopedic Resident, Hospital for Special Surgery, New York, New York

Andrew L. Whaley, MD   Fellow in Sports Medicine, The Hughston Clinic, PC, Columbus, Georgia

Kevin E. Wilk, PT   Adjunct Associate Professor, Division in Physical Therapy, Marquette University, Milwaukee, Wisconsin; Rehabilitation Consultant, Tampa Bay Devil Rays Baseball Club, Tampa Bay, Florida

Brian R. Wolf, MD   Assistant Professor, Department of Orthopaedic and Rehabilitation, University of Iowa Hospitals and Clinics; Co-Team Physician, University of Iowa Athletics, Iowa City, Iowa

FOREWORD

It is an honor to be asked to write the foreword for this text on *The Shoulder and the Overhead Athlete*. The editors have done a great job in gathering the experts, and the contributors are to be congratulated on bringing us up-to-date scientifically and clinically, so that we can treat the overhead athlete optimally.

Sometimes, when we see words in print, we believe it to be the gospel—the end-all-to-be-all. Yet, the practice of medicine is fluid. I'm not certain there will ever be a "final word" on the clinical practice of shoulder injuries in the athlete. One of the main benefits of this book is that it brings us to the next level in our query for perfection. This book is a "work in progress."

To illustrate how much has been learned about the shoulder over the past few decades, I'd like to share with you a committee meeting in the 1960s. At this committee meeting, a group of us "experts" decided to put together a course on the shoulder. After hours of discussion, it was decided that we did not know enough for a whole course on just the shoulder. In order to fill in the course, we needed to expand it to cover the shoulder, elbow, and spine. So here we are forty years later, and we could fill many courses with the content of care of the shoulder, and indeed this book provides us with excellent information on just one single group of shoulder patients.

One of the strengths of this book is that it takes into consideration areas that we are just beginning to focus: prevention and rehabilitation. It is but one human body upon which many disciplines practice: coaches, physicians, trainers, strength and conditioning specialists, and therapists just to name a few. We will each be given opportunities to work with multiple disciplines. May we approach those people knowing that each of us contributes a uniqueness to the care of the athlete. Each of these disciplines is as important as knowing what surgery to perform. True excellence will only be attained with integration of all those disciplines.

When reading this book, we will want to keep all of this in mind: medicine and surgery as a "work in progress" and the multiple disciplines directed to the care of the overhead athlete. It is this mind-set that will return our athletes to the field with 100% of their abilities.

Frank W. Jobe, MD
Kerlan-Jobe Orthopaedic Clinic
Centinela Hospital Medical Center

PREFACE

Knowledge is of two kinds: we know a subject ourselves, or we know where we can find information about it.
—Samuel Johnson

Almost ten years have passed since the last publication dedicated to shoulder injuries in athletes. During any meeting on shoulder pathology, there is usually a session dedicated to the difference in each type of shoulder injury with regard to athletes versus other patients. Shoulder injuries in athletes hold a separate place in both discussion and management. Furthermore, shoulder injuries in *overhead* athletes represent yet another subset that is spoken of distinctly and with specific diagnostic and therapeutic challenges when compared to other patients. We decided to attempt to gather each of those separate "discussions" in one place, one forum, and one compilation.

Too often texts of this nature are dichotomously dedicated either to orthopaedic surgeons or to nonsurgical practitioners without attempting to integrate the two. We have attempted to bridge this gap because shoulder injuries in overhead athletes should be managed with a multidisciplinary approach: the majority of these patients are treated nonsurgically. In addition, prevention of the injury in the first place holds the highest promise for allowing each of these athletes to reach their full potential. Orthopaedic surgeons, physical therapists, athletic trainers, and anyone who cares for athletes participating in sports with overhead maneuvers hopefully understand this "team" concept.

The writings should read as a personal "round-table" discussion with the renowned experts in each of their fields. The ideas discussed here are neither dogma nor "the rule"—they are the ideas born from the continual and evolving understanding of this very complex grouping of shoulder patients. The text is divided into sections dedicated to each problem that would be encountered in the care of all overhead athletes—from adolescent pitchers, to high-school swimmers, to professional tennis players. The first eight chapters are devoted to a general understanding, diagnosis, rehabilitation, and prevention of injury. The next group of chapters focuses on specific disorders, from diagnosis to surgical treatment to return to play. The last section identifies and manages some of the more common sport-specific shoulder injuries that make up yet another separate subsection in this complicated group of athletes.

It is our sincere hope that everyone who cares for overhead athletes—be they any athlete such as a baseball player, football quarterback, swimmer, tennis player, handball or volleyball player, javelin thrower, professional or amateur, adult or child, male or female—will seek out this book and our collective "work in progress." The more we begin to understand, the more our thinking "evolves," and we continue to be enlightened in the process...that is the most important purpose of this book. Please join us on this adventure.

Sumant G. Krishnan, MD
Richard J. Hawkins, MD
Russell F. Warren, MD

ACKNOWLEDGMENTS

This book could not have been completed without the timely and thorough contributions from each author. These recognized experts have many demands placed upon them on a daily basis, yet each found a way to adhere to our strict and short deadline for publication. Each also provided what we feel is exceptionally written work that reads with a personal flair.

The editorial and publication team at Lippincott Williams & Wilkins (Jim Merritt, Michelle M. LaPlante, Robert A. Hurley, and Rakesh Rampertab) produced this book from start to finish in a fraction of the time a text of this magnitude requires. Their attention to detail is borne out by the quality of this publication.

Our respective staffs continue to amaze us with their abilities to coordinate the various and sundry tasks and appointments that have allowed us to collaborate on this extensive project. They are too numerous to name individually, but each continues to be essential to our work.

Last, but certainly not least, this work would not have been possible without the unwavering support and understanding of our immediate families—Kim and Sophie (SGK), Susan (RJH), and Laurie (RFW). They tolerated the late nights and personal sacrifices that become necessary in bringing a project like this to fruition.

We thank you with all of our hearts.

Sumant
Rich
Russ

THE SHOULDER AND THE OVERHEAD ATHLETE

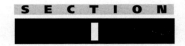

SECTION

I

GENERAL PRINCIPLES

1

THE OVERHEAD ATHLETE— CHALLENGES AND DECISION-MAKING

RICHARD J. HAWKINS
SUMANT G. KRISHNAN

INTRODUCTION

From an orthopedic and therapy point of view, it has been some time since we have had an updated book on the overhead athlete's shoulder. The changes in the past 10 years have been significant in this arena. Our understanding of the rehabilitation and injury prevention aspect of shoulder problems in the overhead athlete has dramatically improved. Biomechanical studies and a better understanding of the many processes that occur have contributed to better understanding of the function of the athlete's shoulder. Better appreciation of SLAP (superior labrum anterior-to-posterior) lesions, internal impingement, the relationship between excess translation and instability, and cuff pathology have advanced over the past decade. Ten years ago, we knew little about SLAP lesions and internal impingement and, therefore, had limited understanding of how to treat them. With the development of arthroscopic surgery, we can now fix SLAP lesions, debride internal impingement lesions, and address excess translation effects by applying suturing or radiofrequency heat.

From a surgical and rehabilitative perspective, there are several factors to consider in determining how the overhead athlete's shoulder may differ from that of the average patient. For example, what is the definition of an athlete? Obviously, Roger Clemens qualifies, but what about the rest of us? Many of us like to consider ourselves athletes and perhaps we are such, functioning at very different levels and within a varied group of endeavors. Regardless of the definition of an athlete, when we consider the athlete's shoulder and how it differs, we need to analyze it from different viewpoints.

These viewpoints relate to the level of participation, the sport and position played, the intensity of involvement, the motivation, and the age of the athlete (Fig. 1-1). For these athletes, we need to consider whether they are recreational, amateurs, or professionals. There are financial implications at the professional level. Once athletes are properly identi-

fied according to participation level and type of activity, we then need to consider whether they are unique in their diagnoses and pathologies and whether their treatment, therefore, should vary from that of the normal population. This is likely the case. When analyzing the outcome of treatment for an athlete, should the measurements be tailored to the patient's athletic profile?

Levels of participation progress through competition at youth, recreational, high school, college, professional, and international levels. All sports could be related to the athlete's shoulder, but the sports that cause shoulder problems in particular relate to the overhead nature of such sports as baseball, tennis, swimming, volleyball, and javelin throwing. Other sports such as football, soccer, and basketball may also be related to shoulder injury, but in the first group of sports, the injury is likely overuse-related, whereas in the second group, the injury is likely traumatic. For example, a baseball pitcher who throws many pitches in a game may have tendinosis, whereas an outfielder who falls on an outstretched arm may have a dislocated shoulder.

Athletes have a strong desire to participate. The higher the level at which an athlete participates, frequently the higher the motivation and the greater the desire for normalcy. This influences the need for early and appropriate diagnosis and aggressive treatment programs along with

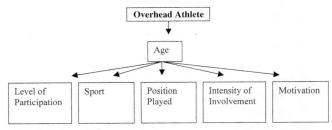

FIGURE 1-1. Analysis of shoulder problems in the overhead athlete first involves an assessment of the various reasons that the athlete's shoulder differs from that of the general population.

appropriate injury prevention programs. Athletes may be disabled by problems that may not affect the average sedentary individual. Frequently, the higher the demand for participation in these athletes, the greater the potential for injury. Many professional baseball pitchers find themselves on the injury disabled list because of shoulder problems.

It is unusual to see problems in very young children who participate in athletic endeavors, even those who pitch a lot of baseballs. Progressing through the years, athletes develop problems with overuse and tendinosis and may end up as a masters athlete in the older age group with a complete-thickness rotator cuff tear, which is unheard of in youth.

DIAGNOSTIC IMPLICATIONS

Problems and diagnoses in the athlete's shoulder may differ from those in the general population. At the same time, athletes may have exactly the same problem as occurs in the general population, particularly when trauma is involved. If a patient, whether an athlete or not, is involved in a motor vehicle accident, he or she may sustain an acute dislocation of the shoulder. This injury can also occur in the football lineman who tackles someone. It is important, particularly in the overuse situation, to keep in mind that athletes do have different problems and different diagnoses. For example, the professional baseball pitcher who presents with shoulder pain often demonstrates excess anterior translation and internal impingement. Conversely, the 45-year-old nonathlete workman who presents with shoulder pain almost never has a diagnosis of anterior shoulder instability. It is much more common for this patient to have impingement degenerative cuff disease. Volleyball players are frequently subject to suprascapular nerve problems. Hockey players commonly get their shoulders jammed into the boards, resulting in acromioclavicular dislocations. Consequently, diagnoses may vary, depending on the sport and other features. In overhead athletes, it is important to keep in mind the implications of an acute injury versus a chronic overuse situation.

Diagnosing the Problem

Depending on the level of participation and time of season, among other factors, diagnosis may need to be established "yesterday." In some circumstances, there is time enough for "Mother Nature" to take her course, allowing the diagnosis to evolve and become clear on its own. At the professional level, however, we are quick to establish a diagnosis, exposing the athlete immediately to x-ray studies, magnetic resonance imaging (MRI), and whatever else is needed to aid in establishing the diagnosis, so that appropriate, effective, and efficient treatment can be instituted quickly. At the Little League level, however, we often allow some time for these diagnoses to become evident. In the Little Leaguer, the

approach is less aggressive with regard to using diagnostic testing toward establishing an immediate diagnosis, so as to avoid compromising the health of the patient.

Clinical Examination

After a fracture, acromioclavicular dislocation, or acute dislocation of the glenohumeral joint, the clinical examination is fairly straightforward. Patients present with a painful shoulder with limited range of motion. In many overhead athletes who present with shoulder pain due to overuse, the physical findings vary, but frequently consist of limitation of internal rotation and crossed-arm adduction, scapular dysfunction, weakness in certain ranges (e.g., external rotation), and instability findings (e.g., excess translation, positive relocation testing, and often signs of impingement). Many overhead athletes, such as throwers, have excess external rotation. This constellation of physical examination signs is frequently found in the high-profile overhead athlete, such as the professional baseball pitcher, but it is rarely found in the general population (1).

Instability and Translation

In the overhead athlete's shoulder, it is critical to understand the relationship between translational measurements and instability. Instability is *a loss of control of the ball in the socket that produces symptoms.* These symptoms are usually of "looseness" or "coming out" and those described as *instability-related.* The difficulty occurs when pain is the only symptom occurring in a shoulder that has excess translation, which may or may not be interpreted as translation or be labeled as "instability." It is common for overhead athletes to have excess translation, and recent appreciation of different pathologies such as internal impingement and SLAP lesions may bear some relationship to this excess translation. These patients may have no symptoms or signs of instability other than this excess translation, complicating the diagnosis. Many patients have considerable physiologic translation of the ball in the socket and yet have no symptoms of instability. It remains unknown whether excess translation can create a tendinosis problem through stretching of the joint capsule and tendons, or whether excess work of these same structures will cause pain. When performing translational testing on patients who complain of instability, particularly when they are awake, it is important to ask them if the testing reproduces the instability complex by reinforcing the symptoms and direction of displacement of the unstable shoulder. In assessing for translation in a patient who has perceived instability, we translate the shoulder posteriorly and describe how far it goes. For example, it may just move up the face of the glenoid, it may perch on the glenoid rim, or it may go over the rim. We then go through the following sequence of questions with the patient:

1. Do you feel your shoulder go out and come back in with my testing?
2. Is that the sensation you feel when your shoulder comes out?
3. Does it go in that direction?

If these questions are all answered in the affirmative, the diagnosis, or at least partial diagnosis, of posterior instability would be established.

Recent literature suggests that throwers with excess translation may not function biomechanically at their maximum capacity. In the presence of a SLAP lesion or internal impingement, a stabilizing procedure may be performed, more to address the excess translation than to address the possibility of instability. This may directly address the goal of making the shoulder more sound biomechanically.

There is a fine line between diagnosing excess translation and instability, particularly in patients with pain. Under these circumstances, it may be conjecture, at best, to say these patients have instability. Research work, particularly by Harryman and Matsen, has shown that translation does not equal instability (2). Certain symptoms more clearly represent instability, such as when a patient complains of the "shoulder coming out," "shoulder is loose" or there is "catching and clunking." The shoulder can, in the face of excess translation particularly with reproduction of those symptoms, clearly represent instability. It is common in patients who have a tendency toward multidirectional or posterior instability to reflect equal translational findings in both shoulders. Yet one is symptomatic, and the other is not.

Physical Signs

Over the past 10 years, many new physical examination signs have been described that aid in the diagnosis of shoulder problems in the athlete (1). Many signs suggest a SLAP lesion (3). These include the active compression test or O'Brien's test, the moving valgus test of O'Driscoll, Kibler's anterior slide test, Andrews' clunk test, and the biceps load test, among others. Bicipital signs are often present with SLAP lesions, as are impingement signs. These overlapping signs often make the accuracy of the tests unpredictable. Gerber described the lift-off test, demonstrating subscapularis insufficiency (4). Recent publications have demonstrated the belly-press test as indicative of upper subscapularis problems and the lift-off test as more indicative of lower or entire subscapularis insufficiency (5). These are just a few of the newer tests that have evolved and are described in later chapters.

In the past when we performed forward elevation of the shoulder, we looked at active and passive motion with stressing at the extremes, trying to elicit pain. Currently, with that same maneuver, we combine impingement signs, crossed-arm stressing for acromioclavicular pathology, and SLAP and biceps signs, with the intention of converging on an accurate diagnosis. Chapter 3 on physical examination in the athlete is a more "differential-directed" approach; that is, "going for the money" with these various tests while favoring a particular underlying diagnosis. We must also, as Chapter 3 indicates, understand a comprehensive and organized approach to physical examination without sacrificing completeness during the differential-directed approach.

Imaging

Imaging in the athlete's shoulder is often essential to aid in diagnosis and in directing treatment. We are blessed with very experienced musculoskeletal MRI sports medicine radiologists. The experience of the reader as well as the different sequences obtained aid in establishing the appropriate diagnosis. Some radiologists prefer gadolinium contrast to enhance accuracy of some studies, such as those for labral tears. X-ray, ultrasound, and other modalities also have their respective roles.

Injections

Injections can also aid in diagnosis. In an athlete for whom we are trying to distinguish intraarticular pathology (e.g., SLAP, internal impingement) from subacromial pathology, we often perform an intraarticular injection, especially if we believe that is "where the money is." Subacromial, acromioclavicular, and biceps injections are also performed to aid in sorting out the predominant pain generator. These injections may also be therapeutic when combined with steroids.

The diagnostic injection procedure itself may provide valuable clues for diagnosis. Such factors are discussed in Chapter 3:

1. Who did the injection?
2. Where was the numbing medicine inserted; for example, into the subacromial space?
3. Did the physician examine the athlete after the injection in the office?
4. Did the athlete and the physician come to a conclusion as to whether immediate relief was obtained regarding signs?
5. How much relief was obtained? 0%, 25%, 50%, 75%, more than 90%?
6. Did the injection provide a therapeutic effect?

It would be helpful for drawing diagnostic conclusions to pinpoint any of these particular factors as a contributor to that therapeutic effect. For example, if a patient 2 months after a subacromial injection obtained 100% relief, it would be reasonable to draw a connection between the site of injection and pain relief.

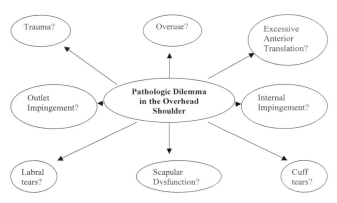

FIGURE 1-2. Pathologic dilemma in the overhead athlete.

PATHOLOGIC DILEMMA IN THE OVERHEAD ATHLETE

The pathologic findings in the overhead athlete relate to the diagnosis. These athletes can have the same pathology as that in the general population, such as occurs in an acute anterior dislocation of the shoulder with a Bankart lesion or in a rotator cuff tear of a degenerative nature as seen in the older individual. In the overuse situation, there is often eccentric overload, undersurface rotator cuff irritation, subtle anterior instability, and biomechanical scapular dysfunction.

A dilemma exists with the many pathologies that can occur in the throwing shoulder of the overhead athlete, particularly in high-level pitchers in baseball (Fig. 1-2). When dealing with athletes at this level, it is not uncommon to arthroscope the shoulder and observe classic impingement with subacromial scarring and undersurface rotator cuff tearing. These athletes may also have internal impingement with posterior cuff and superior labral degeneration. If they also have SLAP lesions and excess anterior translation, there may be labral degeneration anteriorly. All of these pathologies can occur in the throwing shoulder, and it is important to appreciate this as a dilemma. These pathologies are addressed under Surgical Aspects.

TREATMENT ASPECTS

Rehabilitation and Prevention

Because of their desire, many high-performance athletes gear their rehabilitation program toward performance enhancement as well as injury prevention. To achieve these goals, the focus is on eccentric control of the glenohumeral muscles, a stable and efficient scapular platform, elimination of tight posterior capsular structures, and appropriate muscle balance. Velocity and power in performance of an overhead activity come through the kinetic chain from the ground up. The shoulder itself provides only a nominal amount of power for velocity in overhead activities. Never-

theless, the fine-tuning and eccentric control necessary in the glenohumeral joints is important to overhead performance and injury prevention.

Frequently, the injured athlete desires an aggressive rehabilitation program to return him or her to normal; therefore, the program must address all biomechanical abnormalities. If the athlete has pain from overuse, then the principles applied in the prevention and performance enhancement arena can be applied in treating the injury.

As one attempts to control the glenohumeral and scapulothoracic articulations, it is important to remember that strength and coordination of the lower extremities and torso are critical. In professional college and high school athletes, many undergo an injury prevention and performance enhancement program related to the shoulder and other parts of the body. Once the injury occurs, the deficiencies are appropriately addressed.

In this textbook, each section deals with the appropriate postoperative rehabilitation for the surgeries performed. Also addressed are core strengthening, weight training, and preventive exercises for overhead athletes.

Postoperatively, patients pass through various phases: initial passive motion is followed by active motion with terminal stretch, and finally resistive exercises and functional exercises in preparation for return to play. In general, there are two types of postoperative rehabilitation programs: The first relates to those shoulder surgeries that do not require extensive time for tissue healing because nothing is "fixed" during the surgery. Typically, this might consist of debridement of the labrum, debridement of internal impingement, arthroscopic subacromial decompression, bursectomy, or debridement of the rotator cuff. In these procedures, the athlete can proceed quickly through the phases of rehabilitation, which usually consist of initial passive, then active terminal stretching, followed by resistance and strengthening. The rate at which these athletes pass through the program under these circumstances is related to pain and motion. For the throwing athlete, we usually err on the side of caution, being conservative before allowing the athlete to return into an overhead program.

The second type of postoperative rehabilitation program involves procedures that require time for tissue healing, usually because of a repair of some sort. These may include a SLAP stabilizing procedure or a Bankart operation (plus or minus the use of heat to augment that repair). However, we cannot truncate the healing process regardless of whether these procedures are performed arthroscopically or openly. Healing takes time, and these time parameters have been established over the years.

In these two examples, an athlete with a simple labral debridement may return to throwing in 3 or 4 weeks, whereas an athlete who undergoes arthroscopic stabilization procedure augmented by heat in addition to a SLAP repair may not be allowed to return to throwing for 4 or 5 months, and to competition at 8 or 9 months.

Various sections of this book emphasize different aspects of rehabilitation. When asked where they obtain their velocity, most athletes will point to the core of their body—the trunk and upper thighs. They appreciate that the shoulder, elbow, and extremity are for fine-tuning and control, whereas some of the more experienced throwers understand that rehabilitation can be for injury prevention.

Often, the scapula is abnormal in the overhead athlete, particularly in patients who have instability, such as multidirectional or posterior instability. However, scapular dyskinesia may be no less common in those who have impingement, rotator cuff pathology, or SLAP pathology. In Chapter 3 the examination features of scapular abnormalities are analyzed; in Chapters 6 and 7, the need to obtain a stable scapular platform is emphasized.

Implications of Treatment

Treatment of an athlete's shoulder should differ little from treatment of the normal patient population. However, there are ramifications that vary. Age alone is an important consideration. For example, a Little League pitcher versus a professional baseball pitcher not only would have a different diagnosis but often a different treatment program.

Within the athletic arena, there is a push for aggressive treatment to allow a rapid return to activity. This is the desire of most athletes. There are aspects that have an effect on the treatment programs (e.g., whether an athlete is a professional or an amateur, young versus old, and his or her role within the team makeup). There are financial considerations, particularly at the professional level. The athlete's desire, particularly at a higher level, sometimes is not paralleled in the average individual. Finally, parental, coaching, and administrative pressures can also influence treatment.

Return to Play

Return to play in the overhead athlete must be tempered based on many variables such as age, level of participation, motivational factors, and timing in the sports season. As physicians, therapists, and trainers, we must not compromise the health of our patients in urging them to return to play before they are ready. For example, a high school athlete with a mild lingering neurologic injury from a burner would be advised to sit out of sports until the injury resolves; professional athletes, on the other hand, often insist that they are able to participate—and they do participate, sometimes against our better judgment.

At the professional level, it is important to explain to the athlete the risks involved with certain pathologies in their return to play. Many professional athletes understanding the pathology and risks make a decision to participate. For example, a professional football player who sustains a small rotator cuff tear at the beginning of the season and insists on playing must be informed of the probability of enlarging that tear with the possibility of compromising his career.

Communication

Communication at all levels of participation with overhead athletes is challenging. As physicians, therapists, and trainers, we have a responsibility to address concerns and problems with our athletes. Over the years, we have found that an efficient way of handling communication, particularly at the professional and college level, is through the head trainer and sometimes with discussions with head coaches. It is important for the physicians, therapists, and training staff to agree on a plan and to present this plan in a unified way to the athlete. Any mode of action that exposes the athlete to surgery must be carefully evaluated, discussed, and agreed upon before being discussed with the athlete. The higher the level of the athlete, the more "skittish" he or she becomes when certain phrases are expressed without clear explanation. Keep in mind that we have a responsibility to these athletes to treat them as our patients. We need to be careful about unfair coercion by coaches and others regarding treatment.

SURGICAL ASPECTS

The dilemma of diagnoses with a multitude of physical signs and the dilemma of a multitude of pathologies that present in the overhead shoulder pose challenges regarding surgical decisions. Seemingly, the higher the level of sports participation, the more varied and extensive the diagnoses that can be present at any one time. For example, it is not uncommon to take a professional pitcher to the operating room to examine his shoulder and note that he has excess anterior translation, nor is it uncommon to arthroscope his shoulder and notice that he has a subacromial bone spur with scarring in the subacromial bursa. We might also find undersurface cuff tearing, a type 2 SLAP lesion, and internal impingement of the shoulder. Hopefully, we would have understood the influence of physical examination to support what is the most problematic of these pathologies, in addition to selective diagnostic injections which help us understand better the source of pain. Sometimes the surgery is extensive, and other times we pick out and deal with what is clearly in our mind the one pathology causing a problem. This can be a most difficult decision in the athlete's shoulder. As our good friend Dr. James (Jimmy) Andrews taught us, we do not want to be too extensive with our surgeries and be known as the doctor that ended an athlete's career ("primum non nocerum"). The greater the experience with such problems leads to the better the judgment of "what to do" and "what not to do." In the face of all these pathologies, it is appropriate that we only do the correct amount of surgery.

The surgical goals in the athlete's shoulder are not only to return the athlete to good function but, even greater, to allow performance at the expected and desired level. Frequently, the outcomes after major reconstructions of the shoulder are guarded, particularly in the athlete's functional outcome. Thus it is possible that, in the athlete's shoulder, the less surgery performed, the better. The expectation of these athletes for performance constantly challenges us to design appropriate surgical procedures without compromising athletic function.

If we consider shoulder instability, for example, operations such as the Putti-Platt, Bristow, and Magnuson-Stack have not stood the test of time for high performance in the overhead athlete. The principles now are geared toward lesser surgery and less violation of tissue planes, for example, performing a capsulolabral reconstruction through a subscapular split or addressing instability arthroscopically (Fig. 1-3).

Sometimes with a myriad of physical signs and potential pathologies, it is difficult to know what to do surgically, and eventual surgery may be decided by exclusion. If we are unsure about what to do, we may proceed to the operating room and by exclusion perform the appropriate procedure. Examination under anesthesia for translation and arthroscopy to analyze pathology may lead us to the right procedure. For example, an athlete with shoulder pain and an unknown diagnosis may reveal a significant superior labrum anterior to posterior (SLAP) lesion with an otherwise normal presentation. Therefore, we would perform a SLAP repair (Fig. 1-4). Alternatively, a patient may have subacromial scarring and degeneration of the coracoacro-

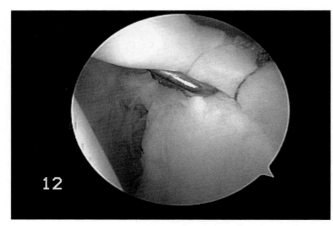

FIGURE 1-4. Superior labrum anterior to posterior (SLAP) repair. Arthroscopic view of probe testing completed repair.

mial ligament without showing any sign of excess anterior translation, negative intraarticular examination or SLAP, or internal impingement and biceps pathology. In that case, we would perform subacromial decompression.

EVALUATION AND OUTCOME ANALYSIS

Should we evaluate the athlete's shoulder the same as we do shoulders of nonathletic individuals? It is probable that we need to have a different evaluation system, looking sometimes at similar but occasionally different parameters. For example, endurance performance in an athlete is critical to the return to desired function. We have been working with the American Shoulder and Elbow Surgeons and the American Orthopaedic Society for Sports Medicine to develop an athlete's evaluation form. Outcome analysis for the treatment of the overhead athlete is discussed in depth in Chapter 5.

Therefore, it appears necessary in the athlete to have a separate system to measure outcome of the various treatment programs, whether they are operative or nonoperative. The primary goal of the athlete is to return to the previous level of participation or to enhance the performance, allowing him or her to achieve the desired level. Endurance is something that is particularly difficult to measure in these athletes and relates to their ability to participate and perform at a high level. If a scoring system was applied, it would heavily weight performance and return to activity. There are many scoring systems available for shoulder problems such as the UCLA, the HSS, the ASES, the Rowe score, and the modified Neer system, among others. None of these are geared toward the specific needs and goals of the athlete and frequently fall short of appropriate outcome assessment.

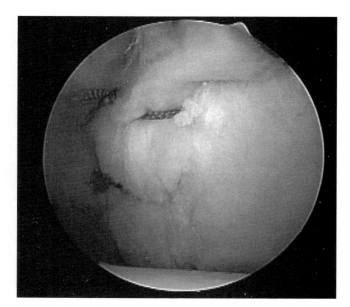

FIGURE 1-3. Arthroscopic posterior and posterosuperior labral repair.

CONCLUSION

The treatment of the overhead athlete's shoulder often has one singular focus: return to play at the same or higher level of performance. Often, many pathologies coexist in the overhead shoulder. Determining which of these entities is responsible for the pain, instability, or decreased function remains the art of the treatment of the overhead athlete. Nonoperative means must be exhausted before considering operative management—especially because most nonstructural lesions in the overhead shoulder can be successfully eliminated with rehabilitation.

Communication is essential between the physician, therapist, trainer, coach, management, and (of course) the athlete. Return to play is determined not only by the injury present but also by the attitude of the athlete, training staff, and management. In this respect, the shoulder in the overhead athlete at all levels of competition (from Little League to Olympic volleyball) represents a diagnostic and thera-peutic dilemma that must be analyzed systematically and treated comprehensively.

REFERENCES

1. Krishnan SG, Hawkins RJ, and Bokor DJ. Clinical evaluation of shoulder problems. In: Rockwood CA, Matsen FA, eds. *The shoulder,* 3rd ed. Philadelphia: WB Saunders, 2004.
2. Matsen FA, Thomas SC, Rockwood CA, et al. Glenohumeral instability. In Rockwood CA, Matsen FA, eds. *The shoulder,* 2nd ed. Philadelphia: WB Saunders, 1998:611–754.
3. Snyder SJ, Karzel RP, Del Pizzo W, et al. SLAP lesions of the shoulder. *Arthroscopy* 1990;6:274–279.
4. Gerber C, Krushell RJ. Isolated rupture of the tendon of the subscapularis muscle. Clinical features in 16 cases. *J Bone Joint Surg* 1991;73:389–394.
5. Tokish JM, Decker M, Ellis H, et al. The belly press test for the physical examination of the subscapularis muscle: electromyographic validation and comparison to the lift-off test. Presented at the American Shoulder and Elbow Surgeons 3rd Biennial Open Meeting, Orlando, Florida, 2002.

2

SHOULDER ANATOMY AND BIOMECHANICS DURING OVERHEAD MOTIONS

**JAMES E. TIBONE
RICK B. CUNNINGHAM
PATRICK J. MCMAHON**

INTRODUCTION

The goal in treating the overhead athlete is to eliminate pain and enable return to sports. Current knowledge of shoulder anatomy, biomechanics, and pathoanatomy has dramatically improved treatment of injuries in the overhead athlete. Full function is possible after treatment of common shoulder maladies, such as acromioclavicular joint osteoarthritis (1) and glenohumeral joint instability (2,3).

An enormous range of shoulder mobility is necessary in order to place one's hand in the many positions demanded by tasks of everyday life. Simple shoulder motions necessitate coordinated actions at four separate articulations. Compared with other diarthrodial joints, there is little inherent bony stability in the glenohumeral joint. Instead, we rely on soft tissues to adequately restrain the shoulder while enabling a full range of motion. When these same soft tissue structures are injured, there can be a significant loss of function. This is especially true when the physiologic limits of the tissues are exceeded or impaired. This situation is less common in the general population, but it is a frequent finding in individuals who participate in competitive overhead athletics. In this population, the athlete repetitively demands the extremes of shoulder range of motion, which maximally stresses both the static and dynamic shoulder restraints, often leading to injury.

In this chapter, the anatomy and biomechanics of the shoulder in the overhead athlete are described. The stages of the throwing motion, including electromyographic (EMG) data, are reviewed for both the normal and the injured shoulder. Baseball pitching is explored in some detail, but swimming and tennis are also considered.

ANATOMY AND BIOMECHANICS: NORMAL AND PATHOLOGIC

Before reviewing shoulder anatomy and biomechanics as they apply to the overhead athlete, some definition of terms is necessary. Even though the term *shoulder* is often used in reference to the glenohumeral joint, normal shoulder function requires coordinated motion at four articulations: sternoclavicular, acromioclavicular, glenohumeral, and scapulothoracic. Furthermore, the shoulder is composed of 30 muscles, three bones (humerus, clavicle, and scapula), and the upper thorax. In this chapter, shoulder motion refers to the complex interaction of all these structures.

The actions between the humerus and the glenoid are described as follows. Small linear movements that take place between articular surfaces are *translations*. These translations can be in the anteroposterior, superoinferior, and mediolateral directions. When translation is excessive, there is increased *laxity,* and when this laxity becomes symptomatic, there is *instability*. In normal shoulders, motion is composed of small glenohumeral translations and large angular rotations between the humerus and the scapula (4,5). The rotation may be internal-external, adduction-abduction in the scapular plane, and adduction-abduction in the horizontal plane.

Overview of Anatomy Relevant to Throwing and Overhead Athletics

Glenohumeral Anatomy and Motion

The rotator cuff is composed of four muscles: the supraspinatus, subscapularis, infraspinatus, and teres minor. The supraspinatus has its origin on the posterosuperior scapula, superior to the scapular spine. It passes under the acromion, through the supraspinatus outlet, and inserts on the greater tuberosity. The supraspinatus is active during the entire arc of scapular plane abduction. Intratendinous strain increases as the shoulder is abducted from 15 to 60 degrees (6). Paralysis of the suprascapular nerve results in an approximately 50% loss of abduction torque (7). Simulated supraspinatus retraction in a cadaveric study involving one third, two thirds, and the entire tendon resulted in losses of torque measuring 19%, 36%, and 58% respectively (8). Overuse activity has been thought to be a major contributing factor in the development of supraspinatus tendinopathy. A recent animal study supports this theory, demonstrating an increase in cellularity, a loss of normal collagen fiber organization, and a lower modulus of elasticity and maximum stress to failure (9).

The infraspinatus and teres minor muscles originate on the posterior scapula, inferior to the scapular spine, and insert on the posterior aspect of the greater tuberosity. Their tendinous insertions are not separate from each other or the supraspinatus tendon. In this way, the rotator cuff tendon differs morphologically from a typical tendon. It consists of an interdigitating confluence of collagen bundles from all of the rotator cuff muscles, forming a hood or aponeurosis over the humeral head (10). The infraspinatus and teres minor act together to externally rotate and extend the humerus. Together, these muscles contribute approximately 80% of the external rotation strength with the arm in an adducted position.

The subscapularis muscle arises from the anterior scapula and is the only muscle to insert on the lesser tuberosity. It acts to internally rotate and flex the humerus. The tendinous insertion of the subscapularis is continuous with lateral aspect of the anterior capsule; therefore, these two structures have been considered responsible for providing anterior glenohumeral stability (11,12).

The orientation of the shoulder muscles to the glenohumeral joint is such that the joint reaction force has a large component that acts perpendicular to the glenoid fossa (13) to compress the concave humeral head into the glenoid fossa. Labeled "concavity-compression" by Lippett and co-workers (14), this maintains anterior joint stability over a large range of shoulder motion (13–15). Likewise, simulated inactivity of the supraspinatus and subscapularis muscles yielded an 18% and 17% decrease, respectively, in the force needed to dislocate the joint (16). Glenohumeral joint compression through muscle contraction was also found to be responsible for resisting inferior translation of the humeral head; ligament tension and negative intraarticular pressure were less important (17). With traumatic instability, there is increased translation in functionally important arm positions, and dynamic stabilizers are often able to re-center the humeral head. However, in atraumatic instability, the head remains decentralized despite muscle activity (18).

The deltoid is the largest shoulder girdle muscle, and it envelops the proximal humerus. It has a tripennate origin at the clavicle, acromion, and scapular spine and inserts at the deltoid tubercle on the lateral aspect of the humeral shaft. The three muscle bellies of the deltoid have different functions. The anterior portion is primarily a forward flexor and abductor of the glenohumeral joint; the middle portion is an abductor; and the posterior portion extends the humerus. The middle and posterior heads provide more glenohumeral compression and less shear than does the anterior head of the deltoid (19). The deltoid is active throughout the entire arc of glenohumeral abduction. Paralysis of the axillary nerve results in a 50% loss of abduction torque (7). The deltoid muscle can fully abduct the glenohumeral joint with the supraspinatus muscle inactive.

The humeral head is approximately one third of a sphere, with the diameter being an average of 45 mm. The glenoid has a 35-mm vertical diameter and a 25-mm horizontal diameter (20–26). Relative to the plane of the scapula, the glenoid is angled superiorly and posteriorly approximately 5 degrees (5,25). This glenoid orientation offers little bony restraint to inferior instability with the arm at the side. The anterosuperior aspect of the glenoid is the area of maximum contact stresses in the normal shoulder (27).

The proximal humerus is made up of four anatomic parts: the articular surface, the greater tuberosity, the lesser tuberosity, and the diaphyseal shaft. The humeral head is angulated medially 45 degrees to the long axis of the humeral shaft, and on average it is retroverted 20–25 degrees relative to the transcondylar axis of the distal humerus (26). However, a study of asymptomatic college baseball players found that mean humeral retroversion was 36.6 degrees in the dominant extremity and 26 degrees in the nondominant extremity. This adaptive change in proximal humeral anatomy may account for the loss of internal rotation and gains in external rotation seen in pitchers' dominant extremity more than would alterations in the soft tissues (28).

Between the two tuberosities is the intertubercular groove, in which lies the tendon of the long head of the biceps brachii. This tendon is held in place by the coracohumeral ligament, superior glenohumeral ligament, and the transverse humeral ligament. During abduction of the glenohumeral joint, the proximal humerus slides on the tendon of the long head of the biceps brachii. If the tendon ruptures, translation of the humeral head is increased (29). An EMG study suggests that, in a patient with traumatic unilateral anterior instability, the biceps muscle plays an active compensatory role in stabilizing the shoulder when it is in an abducted and externally rotated position (30).

Soslowsky and co-workers (31) used stereophotogrammetry to demonstrate that the radius of curvature of the humeral head and the glenoid are not statistically different. Additionally, they showed that together both surfaces approximate the surface of a sphere. However, this point is controversial, and others believe that the surfaces are not conforming and that the contact between them is variable (32,33).

In the glenohumeral joint, three different types of motion may occur: spinning, sliding, and rolling (33). *Spinning* occurs when the contact point on the glenoid remains the same while the humeral head contact point is changing. *Sliding* is pure translation of the humeral head on the articular surface of the glenoid. At the extremes of motion, and certainly in unstable joints, glenohumeral sliding occurs. In this circumstance, the contact point on the glenoid is moving, while that for the humerus remains the same. The third type of action, *rolling*, may also occur at the glenohumeral joint. Rolling is a combination of humeral head sliding and spinning relative to the glenoid such that the contact point changes on both the glenoid and the humeral head (33).

Capsuloligamentous and Labral Anatomy

Although originally disputed, it is now agreed that glenohumeral ligaments are consistently present, although some variation in their insertion sites has been described. The superior glenohumeral ligament (SGHL) arises at the supraglenoid tubercle just anterior to the long head of the biceps brachii (Fig. 2-1). If the glenoid has the markings of a clock with the 12 o'clock position superiorly and the 3 o'clock position anteriorly, then the origin of the SGHL would correspond to the area from the 12 o'clock to the 2 o'clock positions. The SGHL runs inferiorly and laterally to

insert on the humerus, just superior to the lesser tuberosity. The SGHL along with the coracohumeral ligament is part of the rotator interval.

The middle glenohumeral ligament (MGHL) usually arises from the neck of the glenoid just inferior to the origin of the SGHL. The MGHL may also originate with the SGHL, with the SGHL and long biceps tendon, or with the long biceps tendon with an absent SGHL (34). Its fibers blend in with the subscapularis tendon before inserting on the lesser tuberosity. The presence of the MGHL is the most variable (35). In a magnetic resonance imaging (MRI) study of asymptomatic volunteers, it was found in only 79% of patients (36).

The inferior glenohumeral ligament (IGHL) is a complex structure. The IGHL has an anterior and a posterior band, with an axillary pouch between the two bands (37). In abduction and external rotation, the anterior band fans out, and the posterior band becomes cordlike. Likewise, with internal rotation, the posterior band fans out, and the anterior band appears cordlike. The posterior band originates between the 7 o'clock and 9 o'clock position from the glenoid. With the arm at the side, both the anterior and posterior bands pass through a 90-degree arc and insert on the humerus.

The anterior band of the IGHL arises between the 2 o'clock and the 4 o'clock position on the glenoid. In most people, the anterior band of the IGHL has its origin from

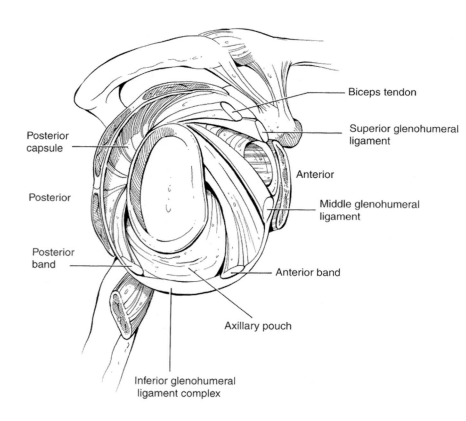

Posterior capsule

Posterior

Posterior band

Biceps tendon

Superior glenohumeral ligament

Anterior

Middle glenohumeral ligament

Anterior band

Axillary pouch

Inferior glenohumeral ligament complex

FIGURE 2-1. Capsuloligamentous anatomy viewed from the side with the humeral head removed. The biceps tendon and the superior and middle glenohumeral ligaments are labeled. The inferior glenohumeral ligament complex consists of an anterior and posterior band with an interposed axillary pouch. The posterior capsule is the tissue located above the posterior band. (From O'Brien SJ, et al. The anatomy and histology of the inferior glenohumeral ligament complex of the shoulder. *Am J Sports Med* 1990;18:449–456, with permission.)

the labrum with some fibers extending to the glenoid neck; however, in some shoulders, the anterior band has its origin solely on the glenoid neck (38). In a cadaveric study simulating the late cocking phase of throwing, it was found that cutting the entire IGHL resulted in the greatest increase in external rotation; however, this increase in external rotation was not significantly different from sectioning the coracohumeral ligament. Furthermore, cutting the anterior band of the IGHL alone caused little increase in external rotation (39). In a cadaveric study simulating a first time anterior shoulder dislocation and Bankart lesion, it was found that there was little unrecoverable stretching of the IGHL (40). However, with repetitive loading of the inferior glenohumeral ligament, the ligament becomes lax with an unrecoverable increase in length of the ligament (41).

The labrum is located along the periphery of the glenoid and is the site of attachment of the capsuloligamentous structures and the long head of the biceps brachii tendon. Huber and Putz (42) showed that the tendon fibers of the long head of the biceps continued posteriorly as periarticular fiber bundles, thereby constituting the "labrum" in the posterior superior quadrant. The remaining labrum is composed of dense fibrous connective tissue with a small fibrocartilaginous transition zone at the anterior inferior attachment of the osseous glenoid rim (38,43,44). Several investigators have suggested that the labrum may act as a load-bearing structure for the humeral head and serve to increase the surface area of the glenoid (31,32). Howell and Galinat (45) showed that the labrum deepened the glenoid socket by nearly 50%. Lippett and co-workers have shown that removal of the labrum decreases the joint's stability to shear stress by 20% (14). However, a recent cadaveric study found that the average contribution of the labrum to glenohumeral stability through concavity compression was only 10% (46).

Scapulothoracic Anatomy and Motion

The scapulothoracic muscles include the trapezius (upper, middle, and lower portions), levator scapulae, serratus anterior, pectoralis minor, and rhomboids. Postural support is provided by the levator scapulae and the upper trapezius. The middle trapezius and rhomboids retract the scapula, whereas the serratus anterior protracts the scapula. Upward rotation of the scapula is accomplished by the trapezius and serratus anterior. The upper trapezius and levator scapulae can also elevate the scapula. These muscles position the scapula on the thoracic cage in order to allow for maximum shoulder motion and stability.

Motion between the scapula and the thorax—the scapulothoracic articulation—is an integral part of normal shoulder function. Other than muscular attachments, the scapula is supported only by the acromioclavicular joint and the coracoclavicular ligaments. Because of this, the scapula is able to move in many directions. The relative motion of the scapulothoracic articulation and glenohumeral joint during abduction is termed the scapulothoracic rhythm. In the first 30 degrees of abduction, glenohumeral motion is greater than scapulothoracic motion by up to a 7:1 ratio (5,47). However, this ratio changes with the speed at which the arm is abducted; at high speeds, glenohumeral motion is more dominant than at slower speeds of abduction (48). Beyond 30 degrees, both joints contribute equally to shoulder abduction (5,47). Thus, over the entire arc of abduction, more motion occurs at the glenohumeral joint than the scapulothoracic joint. The overall mean ratio of glenohumeral to scapulothoracic motion is approximately 1.7:1 (49).

Normal scapular motion consists of substantial rotations around 3 axes, not simply upward rotation. In the resting position, the superior edge of the scapular spine is rotated anteriorly from the frontal plane a mean of 31 degrees (50). With the initiation of abduction, the scapula can translate medially or laterally, or in rare instances, oscillate on the chest wall (26). As the shoulder abducts, the scapula rotates not only in the plane of abduction, but also in a plane perpendicular to it. The superior edge of the scapula rotates anteriorly about 6 degrees during the first 90 degrees of shoulder abduction. Beyond 90 degrees, 16 degrees of posterior scapular rotation occurs (51).

Acromioclavicular and Sternoclavicular Anatomy and Motion

The sternoclavicular joint is stabilized by four ligaments and an intraarticular disk. The interclavicular ligament provides restraint to superior joint motion and is taut when the shoulder is at the side (52). Anterior and posterior motion is prevented by anterior and posterior capsular structures (5). The posterior capsule is the most important restraint for anterior and posterior translation of the sternoclavicular joint. The anterior capsule is a secondary restraint to anterior translation (53). Inferiorly, the joint is stabilized by the costoclavicular ligaments, which run obliquely and laterally from the first rib to the clavicle. The costoclavicular and interclavicular ligaments have little effect on anterior or posterior translation of the sternoclavicular joint (53).

At the acromioclavicular joint, superior motion of the distal clavicle is prevented by the coracoclavicular ligaments: the conoid and the trapezoid. The acromioclavicular capsule is the primary restraint to anterior and posterior motion, with the acromioclavicular ligament being a superior thickening of the capsule.

During shoulder abduction, the clavicle rotates approximately 30 degrees superiorly in the coronal plane. The clavicle also rotates anteriorly approximately 10 degrees as the shoulder is abducted from 0 to 40 degrees. There is an additional 15 degrees of anterior rotation of the clavicle when the shoulder is abducted from 130 to 180 degrees (26). The large axial rotations initially reported by Inman and colleagues (26) have since been questioned. By placing pins in the clavicle and the acromion, Rockwood and Green (52). have shown that the clavicle rotates axially less than 10 degrees over the entire arc of shoulder abduction. This finding is supported by the clinical observation that fixing the clavicle to the scapula does not significantly limit shoulder motion.

Stages of Pitching and Throwing Motion, Including Electromyographic Data

Overhead throwing is a total body activity. It is an elaborate, synchronous progression of body movements that starts in the legs and trunk, proceeds to the upper extremities, and concludes in the rapid propulsion of the ball. However, the temporal onset of muscular torques in the upper extremity is not in a strictly proximal-to-distal progression (54).

The effectiveness of a thrower is determined by various factors, including velocity, accuracy, spin production, and endurance. Synchrony of muscular contractions and neurologic control throughout the body are essential to produce an effective throwing motion. Effectiveness also necessitates repetitive throwing at a level that maximally stresses the physiologic limits of the shoulder. A delicate balance exists between mobility and stability of the joints of the upper extremities while throwing, and maintenance of this fragile balance is paramount. Small aberrations in the mechanisms that control stability have a significant and cumulative effect on upper extremity function and increase the risk of crossing the fine line between maximal throwing effectiveness and injury.

Sporting activities that involve the overhead throwing mechanism include baseball, softball, tennis, and swimming. The biomechanics of throwing has been most studied in baseball (55–62). Although the mechanics of throwing seem to differ slightly between player positions, the motions are similar. Most throwing studies have concentrated on the pitcher because the motion is more constant, the collection of EMG data is easier, and pitchers frequently injure their shoulder. From a virtual standstill, a professional pitcher accelerates a 142-g baseball to a release velocity of more than 90 mph in just 50 msec. Tremendous tensile, compressive, and rotational forces must be created and dissipated in the shoulder. A detailed description of the throwing motion helps clarify how this is done.

The Normal Shoulder

The baseball pitch is divided into five stages (Fig. 2-2): stage I is the wind-up, stage II is early cocking, stage III is late cocking, stage IV is acceleration, stage V is follow-through or deceleration. Stage V can be divided into early and late parts.

In stage I, the pitcher stands facing the batter with the shoulders parallel to the rubber. The pivot foot (right for right-handed throwers) is positioned on the rubber. In the wind-up stage, the body mechanics are individual. In general, wind-up begins with the stride foot (left for right-handers) coiling backward, away from home plate, and the arms swinging overhead. At this time, the position of the fingers on the ball is finalized and the pitcher conceals this from the batter using the glove. The pivot foot rotates on the rubber as weight is transferred to it. Stage I concludes with the ball leaving the glove hand and the body balanced on the pivot foot. The EMG activity of the shoulder girdle and upper extremities is low during the wind-up, which reflects a lack of critical events related to performance or to injury potential.

Cocking is divided into early (stage II) and late (stage III) stages. Early cocking (stage II) starts with pivot leg extension that propels forward the stride leg, nondominant upper extremity, and trunk. The gluteus maximus of the pivot leg is important in providing this propulsion. Temporarily, the dominant upper extremity lags behind the rest of the body. The trapezius and the serratus anterior muscles form a force couple to upwardly rotate and protract the scapula. This scapula motion is essential to place the glenoid in a stable position for the abducting and rotating humeral head. If the scapula is not positioned correctly, impingement can occur (63). However, Weiser and colleagues (64) found that repetitive or chronic protraction of the scapula may result in excessive strain and, ultimately, insufficiency in the anterior band of the inferior glenohumeral ligament.

The deltoid and supraspinatus muscles act in synergy to abduct the humerus. Saha (65) described the glenohumeral muscles as both *drivers* and *steerers*. In this scenario, the deltoid is the driver of the motion, and the supraspinatus is the steerer that fine-tunes the position of the humeral head in the glenoid. The remainder of the rotator cuff muscles have less activity during this phase (63), indicating the importance of the supraspinatus in functioning with the deltoid in humeral abduction during this stage. The early cocking stage is terminated as the stride foot contacts the ground.

Late cocking (stage III) begins with rapid forward motion of the trunk (56). The dominant shoulder rotates forward. Abduction of the humerus is maintained and external rotation increases from 46 to 170 degrees (66). Muscle forces are needed to overcome the inertia and gravity that act on the shoulder in horizontal abduction, external rotation, and adduction. Static and dynamic restraints combine to stabilize the shoulder against these forces. In this position, the primary static anterior stabilizer of the glenohumeral joint is the anterior band of the inferior glenohumeral ligament (20). The subscapularis also acts as a barrier to anterior translation, together with the pectoralis major and the latissimus dorsi. These mus-

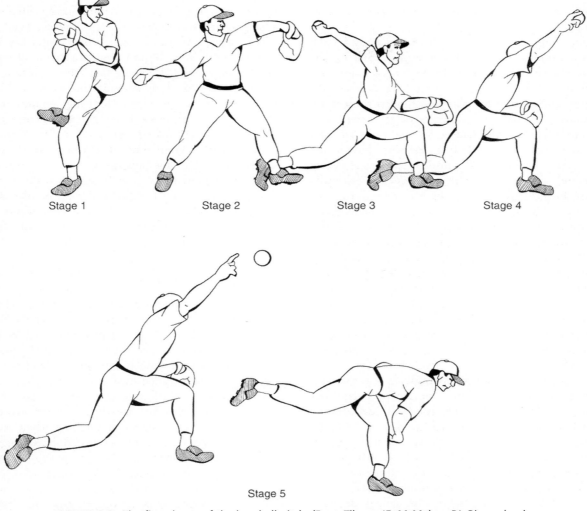

Stage 1   Stage 2   Stage 3   Stage 4

Stage 5

FIGURE 2-2. The five phases of the baseball pitch. (From Tibone JE, McMahon PJ. Biomechanics and pathologic lesions in the overhead athlete. In: Iannotti JP, Williams GR Jr, eds. *Disorders of the shoulder: diagnosis and management.* Philadelphia: Lippincott Williams & Wilkins, 1999, with permission.)

cles act as a dynamic sling to augment the inferior gleno-humeral ligament (63). Although supraspinatus and deltoid activity diminishes as the humerus ceases to abduct, the other rotator cuff muscles increase in activity and help stabilize the humeral head (63). During late cocking, the infraspinatus and teres minor actively externally rotate the humerus. They also act as check reins to anterior subluxation.

Although there is no further abduction of the shoulder during late cocking, the scapulothoracic muscles continue to be active to produce a stable platform for the humeral head and to enhance maximal humeral external rotation (63). The middle portion of the trapezius, rhomboids, and levator scapulae are all key in providing scapular stabilization. The serratus anterior is also important in opposing

retraction and stabilizing the scapula. Sometimes symptoms of anterior instability of the glenohumeral joint are experienced during this stage because of an imbalance of the scapula-stabilizing mechanisms (59).

Stage IV or the acceleration stage begins with maximal shoulder external rotation and terminates with ball release. The humerus internally rotates approximately 100 degrees in one-half second (66). The humeral internal rotation torque is 14,000 inch-pounds, with an angular velocity of 6,100 degrees/sec (56,58,67). The acceleration of the arm is coincident with the deceleration of the rest of the body, producing efficient transfer of energy to the upper extremity and ball (56). A large glenohumeral joint compressive force (860 N) occurs, which has a stabilizing effect. Synchronous muscular contraction about the glenohumeral joint and scapulothoracic articulation provides both stability and rapid motion of the upper extremity.

Shoulder angular velocity is imparted mainly by the lower extremities and trunk, but it is increased by the actions of the latissimus dorsi and pectoralis major. The latissimus dorsi has even higher activity than the pectoralis major (63), and it is anatomically positioned to generate large torques (68). These two muscles are important contributors to ball velocity, evidenced by a clinical study that reported that they are the only two muscles to have a positive correlation between peak torque in isokinetic testing and pitching velocity (69). The subscapularis, especially the upper portion, also has very high activity during the acceleration stage and functions with the pectoralis major and latissimus dorsi (63). Whereas the pectoralis major and the latissimus dorsi are the primary propellers of the arm, the subscapularis acts to position the humeral head precisely in the glenoid. This coordinated function of the subscapularis with the latissimus dorsi has been observed in other overhead athletics as well (61,70). Teres minor activity is also high, with the muscle acting as a check rein to anterior instability. Athletes may note symptoms during the acceleration stage of throwing, typically from anterior instability.

Stage V is deceleration or follow-through. It is the most taxing stage of throwing because the kinetic energy not transferred to the ball must be absorbed by the decelerating arm and body. Deceleration is estimated to be 500,000 degrees/sec^2. at the shoulder, with an external rotation torque of approximately 15,000 inch-pounds at the humerus (56,62). This stage begins with ball release. It can be divided into early and late stages; some authors separate stage V into deceleration and follow-through. In deceleration, the trunk and dominant lower extremity rotate forward. The shoulder continues to adduct and internally rotate to 30 degrees. In general, deceleration of the upper extremity is accomplished by simultaneous contraction of opposing muscles around the shoulder (63). The trapezius, serratus anterior, and rhomboids all demonstrate high or very high activity. The deltoid is active, especially the posterior and middle portions, which are positioned to oppose the motion of the upper extremity. The teres minor has the highest activity of all the glenohumeral muscles, providing a posterior stabilizing check rein. Injury to the posterior glenohumeral joint stabilizers commonly become apparent during this stage.

Late follow-through is a noncritical stage, with all of the shoulder muscles exhibiting decreasing activity (63). All of the kinetic energy has been dissipated, and the trunk is beginning to extend, allowing the pitcher to field the position.

In summary, the entire throwing motion takes less than 2 seconds, with the final three stages taking less than half a second to complete (71). The kinematics of throwing different types of pitches is not significantly different (72). There are appreciable changes seen in professional pitchers when considering throws made in early and late innings, with decreases in maximum external rotation of the shoulder, knee angle at ball release, ball velocity, maximum distraction force at both the shoulder and elbow, and horizontal adduction torque (73). Throwing requires the rapid transmission of immense forces throughout the shoulder. The peak force has been estimated to be 27,000 inch-pounds, which is four times that seen in the leg during a soccer kick (56). This puts the shoulder at great risk for injury. Young pitchers should be cautioned about throwing breaking pitches and limitations should be placed on the number of pitches they throw, because both of these factors have been associated with an increased risk of elbow and shoulder pain (74).

The Injured Shoulder

Shoulder pain is relatively common amongst elite overhead throwing athletes. Barnes and colleagues (75) found that 56% of the college and professional level baseball players who were seen in their clinic had shoulder pain. The injured shoulder exhibits alterations from the normal muscle activity outlined earlier. For example, Glousman and co-workers (57) found that elite pitchers with anterior shoulder instability had decreased serratus anterior EMG activity in all stages of pitching when compared with normal. In fact, all muscles tested showed significant EMG differences between the two groups of pitchers, except for the middle deltoid. The biceps and supraspinatus muscles had more activity in the unstable shoulders. This was thought to be a compensatory mechanism to help stabilize the humeral head against the glenoid fossa. In addition, the infraspinatus showed increased activity during the late cocking phase of the pitching motion in those with instability.

Alterations from normal serratus anterior muscle function are meaningful because they indicate an abnormality in the coordinated rotation of the scapula on the thorax or the scapulothoracic rhythm. Because of the rapidity of upper extremity motion during throwing, observation of scapular motion is nearly impossible. However, even during isolated shoulder abduction, EMG activity in the serratus anterior muscle in the athlete with anterior joint instability is diminished when compared with normal (76). Normal scapulothoracic rhythm has been extensively studied (5,25,26,47,77), and these studies indicate that the normal scapulothoracic rhythm with anterior joint instability has been altered, possibly resulting in scapular lag. This can result in hyperangulation increasing contact between the rotator cuff and superior labrum and thereby cause internal impingement.

Stages of Swimming Motion, Including Electromyographic Data

The shoulder is a vulnerable joint in the swimmer. Ninety percent of the propulsive force in swimming comes from the upper extremity (78,79). Most other sports (e.g., running, bicycling, golfing, pitching, or batting) require the feet to push into the ground (or bicycle pedal), which initiates the propulsive or ground reaction force. In swimming, there is no such force. In swimming, the athlete must pull the body over the arm. Another unique aspect of swimming is upper extremity endurance. Competitive athletes may swim 10,000 to 14,000 meters (6 to 8 miles) a day, 6 or 7 days a week. Distance swimmers may double that distance. This distance equates to 16,000 shoulder revolutions per week, or approximately 2500 revolutions per day. Many of these revolutions are done in sequence, without any rest for the muscles. Although a golfer swings, they then walk and rest the shoulder. The continuous shoulder movement seen in swimming can cause injury from repetitive microtrauma resulting in "swimmer's shoulder." Adding to the complexity of these mechanical characteristics of swimming is the fact that the shoulder is relatively unstable. When putting together the training distances, unique propulsive demands, and inherent shoulder laxity, the risk of injury is understandably high. Shoulder problems are reported in 66% of swimmers, whereas only 57% of professional pitchers, 44% of collegiate volleyball players, and 29% of collegiate javelin throwers report shoulder injuries (80). When comparing collegiate level female soccer players and swimmers, glenohumeral translation for the swimmers was significantly greater than that seen in the soccer players (81).

The swimming strokes can be divided into pull-through and recovery phases (82). In the freestyle stroke the pull-through phase is subdivided into hand entry, mid-pull-through, and end of pull-through (Fig. 2-3). During hand entry, the shoulder is internally rotated and abducted, and the body roll begins. Body roll reaches a maximum of 40 to 60 degrees from horizontal. In mid-pull-through, the shoulder is abducted 90 degrees and is in neutral rotation. With the end of pull-through, the humerus is internally rotated and fully adducted as the body returns to horizontal.

The recovery phase is subdivided into elbow lift, midrecovery, and hand entry. In elbow lift, the shoulder begins to abduct and externally rotate. The body roll begins in the opposite direction from pull-through. In midrecovery, the shoulder is abducted 90 degrees and externally rotated beyond neutral. Body roll reaches a maximum of 40 to 60 degrees in the opposite direction. Breathing occurs by turning the head to the side. In hand entry, the shoulder is externally rotated and maximally abducted, and the body is returned to neutral roll.

In the backstroke at hand entry, the shoulder is externally rotated and abducted as body roll begins from neutral position. In mid-pull-through, the shoulder is abducted 90 degrees in neutral rotation with maximum body roll. At the end of pull-through, the shoulder is internally rotated and adducted, and there is no body roll. In the recovery phase of the backstroke, there is hand lift, rather than elbow lift. In hand lift, the shoulder begins with abduction and external rotation, and the body roll allows the arm to clear the water. In midrecovery, the shoulder is 90 degrees abducted and body roll is maximal.

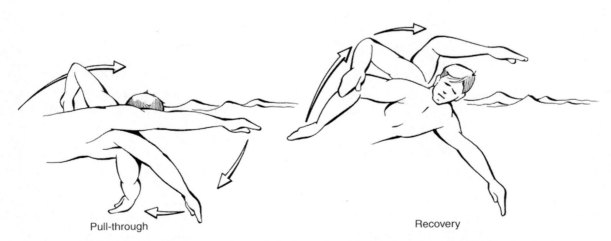

Pull-through

Recovery

FIGURE 2-3. The pull-through phase of the freestyle stroke can be subdivided into hand entry, mid pull-through, and end of pull-through. The recovery phase can be subdivided into elbow lift, mid recovery, and hand entry. (From Tibone JE, McMahon PJ. Biomechanics and pathologic lesions in the overhead athlete. In: Iannotti JP, Williams GR Jr, eds. *Disorders of the shoulder: diagnosis and management.* Philadelphia: Lippincott Williams & Wilkins, 1999, with permission.)

In the butterfly stroke, the pull-through phase is the same as in freestyle, but there is absence of body roll in all stages. To avoid shoulder flexion or extension, the hands are spread apart at the mid-pull-through stage. The recovery phase is again similar to that in freestyle, with an absence of body roll. Body lift allows both arms to clear the water. Shoulder flexion and extension do not occur.

The EMG indicates the rotator cuff is important during swimming (70,83). Supraspinatus, infraspinatus, and middle deltoid activity dominate the recovery phase as they abduct and externally rotate the extremity in preparation for a new pull-through. This position, similar to the cocking phase of throwing, places the shoulder at risk for subacromial impingement (84). The serratus anterior also has an important function during recovery. It allows the acromion to rotate clear of the abducting humerus and provides a stable glenoid base on which the humeral head can rotate. The serratus anterior works at nearly maximal levels to accomplish this. Significantly decreased EMG activity of the serratus anterior muscle was found in swimmers with shoulder pain. During the pulling stage of the freestyle stroke, there was significantly less activity in the serratus anterior in subjects with a painful shoulder when compared with normal (85). The serratus anterior demonstrates similar findings during the pull-through stage of the butterfly stroke in subjects with a painful shoulder (86). If this muscle becomes fatigued during the course of a number of cycles, scapular rotation may not coincide with humeral abduction. As a result, external (outlet) impingement syndrome may develop.

The biceps brachii muscle exhibits erratic activity during all of the different swimming strokes. It acts primarily at the elbow, which is similar to its role in pitching. The latissimus dorsi and pectoralis major are propulsive muscles, with a resulting action similar to that seen during the acceleration phase of throwing.

In summary, particular attention must be paid to conditioning the rotator cuff and serratus anterior muscles to decrease the common problem of swimmer's shoulder and outlet impingement syndrome. Exercises must concentrate specifically on increasing the endurance of the serratus anterior muscle.

The Stages of Tennis Motion, Including Electromyographic Data

The tennis serve can be divided into the same stages of muscle activity as a baseball pitch. Deltoid function is low during cocking compared with pitching because trunk rotation contributes to shoulder abduction. The acceleration and follow-through stages of a tennis serve demonstrate muscle patterns and activity that are similar to those observed in throwing a baseball. As with pitching, a tennis serve generates high angular momentum with 75% of it being concentrated in the racket arm near impact (87). Because the motions for serving the tennis ball are similar to those for pitching, tennis players may benefit from the same conditioning program as that outlined for pitchers. Likewise, emphasis should be placed on rehabilitating the rotator cuff and serratus anterior muscles.

The ground strokes, both forehand and backhand, can be divided into three stages (Fig. 2-4). In stage I, racquet preparation begins with shoulder turn and ends with the initiation of weight transfer to the front foot. Stage II is acceleration and

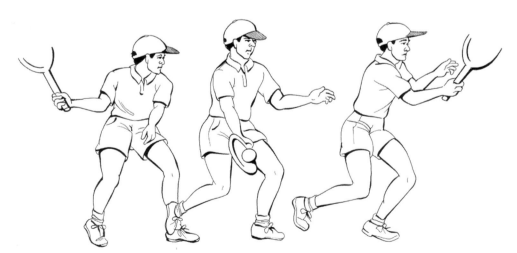

FIGURE 2-4. The ground strokes of tennis, both forehand and backhand, can be divided into three stages: racquet preparation, acceleration, and follow-through. (From Tibone JE, McMahon PJ. Biomechanics and pathologic lesions in the overhead athlete. In: Iannotti JP, Williams GR Jr, eds. *Disorders of the shoulder: diagnosis and management.* Philadelphia: Lippincott Williams & Wilkins, 1999, with permission.)

begins with weight transfer to the front foot accompanied by forward racquet movement and culminates in ball impact. Stage III is follow-through and begins at ball impact and ends with completion of the stroke. The forehand ground stroke reveals a relatively passive wind-up sequence. Trunk rotation provides some of the force for shoulder motion. In follow-through, there is a marked decrease in activity among the accelerating muscles and a concomitant increase in the external rotators responsible for deceleration. The backhand ground stroke is similar in concept, but opposite in muscle activity, to the forehand. Follow-through demonstrates deceleration with increased activity of the internal rotators.

BIOMECHANICS OF INJURIES COMMON IN OVERHEAD ATHLETES

Instability

Soft tissues, including the capsulolabral structures, are vital to guide and limit shoulder motion. The Bankart lesion that occurs after anterior glenohumeral dislocation (88,89) is an injury of the anteroinferior capsulolabral structures. It includes the glenoid insertion site of the anterior band of the IGHL, which is important in preventing anterior joint dislocation (20).

Simulation of a Bankart lesion in prior biomechanical studies demonstrated anterior glenohumeral subluxation but not dislocation (90,91). This testing was done in the apprehension position of horizontal abduction and external rotation. A force external to the glenohumeral joint was applied to the humeral head and translation of the humeral head was measured. The findings confirmed that the IGHL is the primary static restraint to anterior glenohumeral instability (20,92). After repair of the IGHL, normal translation of the joint was restored (91). A critical size of glenoid rim defect was thought to result in instability *in vivo* (93). Biomechanical study found the humeral head translated with significantly less force when the width of the osseous defect was greater than 20% of the glenoid width (average width, 6.8 mm) (94).

Another method of study was to test the joint in tension to determine the biomechanical properties of the anteroinferior capsulolabral complex. Large failure loads resulted (95), and the anteroinferior capsulolabrum was the initial structure to fail (96). Stretching of the anteroinferior capsulolabrum occurred (97), but only a small amount was permanent (98,99). Stretching occurred along the length of the involved soft tissues regardless of the failure mode (40).

SLAP Lesions

Lesions involving the superior labrum and the origin of the tendon of the long head of the biceps brachii (or biceps anchor) can cause shoulder pain and instability. In the overhead throwing athlete, the pain may be disabling, especially when symptoms have been present for a prolonged period of time. These lesions were initially reported as tearing of the anterosuperior labrum from the glenoid and attributed to traction from the biceps tendon (100) because the elbow was decelerated during the follow-through phase of throwing. However, Tibone and co-workers recently demonstrated that the etiology of SLAP lesions may be due to posterior capsular contracture, which prevents the humerus from gaining full external rotation and thereby forces the head posterosuperior on the glenoid (101). Snyder and co-workers (85). later coined the acronym "SLAP" to represent lesions of the "superior labrum from anterior-to-posterior." Four types of SLAP lesions were described based on injury to not only the superior labrum but also the biceps anchor (85). The most common (accounting for more than half) was a type II SLAP lesion in which the superior labrum and the biceps anchor were avulsed from the glenoid. Pain was thought to result from the detached labrum being interposed in the joint. The overhead athlete would sometimes also describe sensations of joint instability with this lesion. Even though classification of SLAP lesions was later expanded to include additional types (102, 103), the type II SLAP lesion remains the most commonly reported.

Biomechanical studies found that simulated type II SLAP lesions result in increased glenohumeral translations in both the anteroposterior and superoinferior directions (104). Translations were increased regardless of whether the type II SLAP lesion was completely detached or elevated in a periosteal sleeve (105). Likewise, the torsional rigidity of the shoulder was diminished after simulation of a type II SLAP lesion, and strain in the inferior glenohumeral ligament increased (106). Even though repair of a type II SLAP lesion has been advocated, study of its effect on joint stability remains unknown. Recent studies compared translations of the glenohumeral joint with a simulated type II SLAP lesion to translations after its repair and to translations of the vented shoulder (107). A robotic/universal force testing system was used to simulate "load and shift tests" by applying anterior, posterior, and inferior loads. Glenohumeral translation was increased, regardless of severity, after simulation of type II SLAP lesions (105). Repair of the type II SLAP lesion only partially restored translation to that of the vented shoulder. In surgically treating a type II SLAP lesion, one should also consider repairing the passive stabilizers that may be injured with this lesion.

REFERENCES

1. Cook FF, Tibone JE. The Mumford procedure in athletes. An objective analysis of function. *Am J Sports Med* 1988;16: 97–100.
2. Bigliani LU, Kurzweil PR, Schwartzbach CC, et al. Inferior capsular shift procedure for anterior-inferior shoulder instability in athletes. *Am J Sports Med* 1994;22:578–584.

3. Montgomery WH 3rd, Jobe FW. Functional outcomes in athletes after modified anterior capsulolabral reconstruction. *Am J Sports Med* 1994;22:352–358.

4. Howell SM, Galinat BJ, Renzi AJ, et al. Normal and abnormal mechanics of the glenohumeral joint in the horizontal plane. *J Bone Joint Surg (Am)* 1988;70:227–232.

5. Poppen NK, Walker PS. Normal and abnormal motion of the shoulder. *J Bone Joint Surg (Am)* 1976;58:195–201.

6. Bey MJ, Song HK, Wehrli FW, et al. Intratendinous strain fields of the intact supraspinatus tendon: the effect of glenohumeral joint position and tendon region. *J Orthop Res* 2002; 20:869–874.

7. Colachis S, Strohm B, Brechner V. Effects of axillary nerve block on muscle force in the upper extremity. *Arch Phys Med Rehabil* 1969;50:647–654.

8. Halder AM, O'Driscoll SW, Heers G, et al. Biomechanical comparison of effects of supraspinatus tendon detachments, tendon defects, and muscle retractions. *J Bone Joint Surg (Am)* 2002;84:780–785.

9. Soslowsky LJ, Thomopoulos S, Tun S. Overuse activity injures the supraspinatus tendon in an animal model: a histologic and biomechanical study. *J Shoulder Elbow Surg* 2000;9:79–84.

10. Clark JM, Harryman DT. Tendons, ligaments, and capsule of the rotator cuff: gross and microscopic anatomy. *J Bone Joint Surg (Am)* 1992;74:713–725.

11. Testut L. Traite d'Anatomie Humaine. In: Tome Is, ed. *Osteologie, Arthrologie, Myologie.* Paris: Doin, 1921:504.

12. Walch G, Liotard JP, Boileau P. Fifth International Conference on Surgery of the Shoulder, Paris, France, 1992.

13. Eberly VC, Yang BY, McMahon PJ, et al. Effects of shoulder muscle forces on the glenohumeral joint force and translation. *Orthop Res Soc,* Anaheim, CA, 1999.

14. Lippett S, Vanderhooft J, Harris S, et al. Glenohumeral stability from concavity-compression: a quantitative analysis. *J Shoulder Elbow Surg* 1993;2:27–34.

15. Lee S-B, Kim K-J, O'Driscoll SW, et al. Dynamic glenohumeral stability provided by the rotator cuff muscles in the mid-range and end-range of motion: a study in cadavera. *J Bone Joint Surg (Am)* 2000;82:849–858.

16. Blasier R, Guldberg R, Rothman E. Anterior shoulder stability: contributions of rotator cuff forces and the capsular ligaments in a cadaver model. *J Shoulder Elbow Surg* 1992;1:140–150.

17. Warner JP, Bowen MK, Deng X, et al. Effect of joint compression on inferior stability of the glenohumeral joint. *J Shoulder Elbow Surg* 1999;8:31–36.

18. Eisenhart-Rothe RMV, Jäger A, Englmeier KH, et al. Relevance of arm position and muscle activity on three-dimensional glenohumeral translation in patients with traumatic and atraumatic shoulder instability. *Am J Sports Med* 2002;30(4):514–522.

19. Lee SB, An KN. Dynamic glenohumeral stability provided by three heads of the deltoid muscle. *Clin Orthop* 2002;400:40–47.

20. Turkel SJ, Panio MW, Marshall JL, et al. Stabilizing mechanisms preventing anterior dislocation of the glenohumeral joint. *J Bone Joint Surg (Am)* 1981;63:1208–1217.

21. Clarke I, Gruen T, Hoy A, et al. Problems in glenohumeral surface replacements—real or imagined? *Engineering in Medicine* 1979;8:161–175.

22. Cyprien JM, Vasey HM, Burdet A, et al. Humeral retrotorsion and glenohumeral relationship in the normal shoulder and in recurrent anterior dislocation (scapulometry). *Clin Orthop Rel Res* 1983:8–17.

23. Iannotti JP, Gabriel JP, Schneck SL, et al. The normal glenohumeral relationships. An anatomical study of one hundred and forty shoulders. *J Bone Joint Surg (Am)* 1992;74:491—500.

24. Jobe C, Iannotti JP. Limits imposed on glenohumeral motion by joint geometry. *J Shoulder Elbow Surg* 1995;4:281–285.

25. Freedman L, Munro RR. Abduction of the arm in the scapular plane: scapular and glenohumeral movements. A roentgenographic study. *J Bone Joint Surg (Am)* 1966;48:1503–1510.

26. Inman V, Saunders M, Abbott L. Observations on the function of the shoulder joint. *J Bone Joint Surg* 1944;27:1–30.

27. Schulz CU, Pfahler M, Anetzberger HM, et al. The mineralization patterns at the subchondral bone plate of the glenoid cavity in healthy shoulders. *J Shoulder Elbow Surg* 2002;11:174–181.

28. Reagan KM, Meister K, Horodyski MB, et al. Humeral retroversion and its relationship to glenohumeral rotation in the shoulder of college baseball players. *Am J Sports Med* 2002;30: 354–360.

29. Warner JJ, McMahon PJ. The role of the long head of the biceps brachii in superior stability of the glenohumeral joint. *J Bone Joint Surgery (Am)* 1995;77:366–372.

30. Kim SH, Ha KI, Kim HS, et al. Electromyographic activity of the biceps brachii muscle in shoulders with anterior instability. *Arthroscopy* 2001;17:864–868.

31. Soslowsky LJ, Flatow EL, Bigliani LU, et al. Articular geometry of the glenohumeral joint. *Clin Orthop Rel Res* 1992:181–190.

32. Bowen MK, Deng XH, Hannafin JA, et al. An analysis of the patterns of glenohumeral joint contact and their relationship to the glenoid "bare area." *Trans Orthop Res Soc* 1992;17:496.

33. Morrey B, An K-N. Biomechanics of the shoulder. In: Rockwood CJ, Matsen FS, eds. *The shoulder.* Philadelphia: WB Saunders, 1990:216.

34. Beltran J, Bencardino J, Padron M, et al. The middle glenohumeral ligament: normal anatomy, variants and pathology. *Skeletal Radiol* 2002;31:253–262.

35. DePalma AF, Callery G, Bennett GA. Variational anatomy and degenerative lesions of the shoulder joint. *Instr Course Lect* 1949;6:225–281.

36. Park YH, Lee JY, Moon SH, et al. MR arthrography of the labral capsular ligamentous complex in the shoulder: imaging variations and pitfalls. *Am J Roentgenol* 2000;175:667–672.

37. O'Brien SJ, Allen AA, Fealy S, et al. Developmental anatomy of the shoulder and anatomy of the glenohumeral joint. In: Matsen F, Rockwood CS, eds. *The shoulder,* vol 1. Philadelphia: WB Saunders, 1998:1–33.

38. Eberly VC, McMahon PJ, Lee TQ. Variation in the glenoid origin of the IGHL anterior band: implications for repair of the Bankart lesion. *Clin Orthop Rel Res* 2002;400:26–31.

39. Kuhn JE, Bey MJ, Huston LJ, et al. Ligamentous restraints to external rotation of the humerus in the late-cocking phase of throwing. A cadaveric biomechanical investigation. *Am J Sports Med* 2000;28:200–205.

40. McMahon PJ, Dettling JD, Sandusky MD, et al. Deformation and strain characteristics along the length of the anterior band of the inferior glenohumeral ligament. *J Shoulder Elbow Surg* 2001;10:482–488.

41. Pollock RG, Wang VM, Bucchieri JS, et al. Effects of repetitive subfailure strains on the mechanical behavior of the inferior glenohumeral ligament. *J Shoulder Elbow Surg* 2000;9:427–435.

42. Huber HP, Putz RV. Periarticular fiber system of the shoulder joint. *J Arthroscopy* 1997;13:680–691.

43. Moseley H, Overgaard B. The anterior capsular mechanism in recurrent anterior dislocation of the shoulder: morphological and clinical studies with special reference to the glenoid labrum and glenohumeral ligaments. *J Bone Joint Surg (Br)* 1962;44: 913–927.

44. Cooper DE, Arnoczky SP, O'Brien SJ, et al. Anatomy, histology, and vascularity of the glenoid labrum. An anatomical study. *J Bone Joint Surg (Am)* 1992;74:46–52.

45. Howell SM, Galinat BJ. The glenoid-labral socket. A constrained articular surface. *Clin Orthop Rel Res* 1989:122–125.

46. Halder AM, Kuhl SG, Zobitz ME, et al. Effects of the glenoid

labrum and glenohumeral abduction on stability of the shoulder joint through concavity-compression. *J Bone Joint Surg (Am)* 83:1062–1069.

47. Doody SG, Freedman L, Waterland JC. Shoulder movements during abduction in the scapular plane. *Arch Phys Med Rehabil* 1970;51:595–604.
48. Sugamoto K, Harada T, Machida V, et al. Scapulohumeral rhythm: relationship between motion velocity and rhythm. *Clin Orthop* 2002;401:119–124.
49. McClure PW, Michener LA, Sennett BJ, et al. Direct 3-dimensional measurement of scapular kinematics during dynamic movements *in vivo*. *J Shoulder Elbow Surg* 2001;10:269–277.
50. Laumann U. Kinesiology of the shoulder. In: Kobel RS, ed. *Shoulder replacement*. Berlin: Springer-Verlag, 1985:23.
51. Cleland FRS. Notes on raising the arm. *J Anat Physiol* 1884;18:275.
52. Rockwood C, Green D. *Fractures in adults*. Philadelphia: JB Lippincott, 1984.
53. Spencer EE, Kuhn JE, Huston LJ, et al. Ligamentous restraints to anterior and posterior translation of the sternoclavicular joint. *J Shoulder Elbow Surg* 2002;11:43–47.
54. Hong DA, Cheung TK. EMR. A three-dimensional, six-segment chain analysis of forceful overarm throwing. J Electromyogr Kinesiol 2001;11:95–112.
55. Bradley JP, Perry J, Jobe FW. The biomechanics of the throwing shoulder. *Perspect Orthop Surg* 1990;1:49–59.
56. Gainor BJ, Piotrowski G, Puhl J, et al. The throw: biomechanics and acute injury. *Am J Sports Med* 1980;8:114–118.
57. Glousman R, Jobe F, Tibone J, et al. Dynamic electromyographic analysis of the throwing shoulder with glenohumeral instability. *J Bone Joint Surg (Am)* 1988;70:220–226.
58. Gowan ID, Jobe FW, Tibone JE, et al. A comparative electromyographic analysis of the shoulder during pitching. Professional versus amateur pitchers. *Am J Sports Med* 1987;15:586–590.
59. Jobe FW, Bradley JP. Rotator cuff injuries in baseball. Prevention and rehabilitation. *Sports Med* 1988;6:378–387.
60. Jobe FW, Moynes DR, Tibone JE, et al. An EMG analysis of the shoulder in pitching. A second report. *Am J Sports Med* 1984;12:218–220.
61. Jobe FW, Tibone JE, Perry J, et al. An EMG analysis of the shoulder in throwing and pitching. A preliminary report. *Am J Sports Med* 1983;11:3–5.
62. Pappas AM, Zawacki RM, Sullivan TJ. Biomechanics of baseball pitching. A preliminary report. *Am J Sports Med* 1985;13:216–222.
63. DiGiovine NM, Jobe FW, Pink M, et al. An electromyographic analysis of the upper extremity in pitching. *J Shoulder Elbow Surg* 1992;1:15–25.
64. Weiser WM, Lee TQ, McMaster WC, et al. Effects of simulated scapular protraction on anterior glenohumeral stability. *Am J Sports Med* 1999;27:801–805.
65. Saha A. Dynamic stability of the glenohumeral joint. *Acta Orthop Scand* 1971;42:491–505.
66. Feltner M, Dapena J. Dynamics of the shoulder and elbow joints of the throwing arm during the baseball pitch. *Int J Sports Biomech* 1986;2:235–259.
67. Janda DH, Wojtys EM, Hankin FM, et al. Softball sliding injuries. A prospective study comparing standard and modified bases. *JAMA* 1988;259:1848–1850.
68. Bassett RW, Browne AO, Morrey BF, et al. Glenohumeral muscle force and moment mechanics in a position of shoulder instability. *J Biomechanics* 1990;23:405–415.
69. Bartlett LR, Storey MD, Simons BD. Measurement of upper extremity torque production and its relationship to throwing speed in the competitive athlete. *Am J Sports Med* 1989;17:89–91.

70. Pink M, Jobe FW, Perry J, et al. The normal shoulder during the backstroke: an EMG and cinematographic analysis of twelve muscles. *Clin J Sports Med* 1992;2:6–12.
71. Meister K. Injuries to the shoulder in the throwing athlete. Part I: biomechanics/ pathophysiology/ classification of injury. *Am J Sports Med* 2000;28:265–275.
72. Escamilla RF, Fleisig GS, Barrentine SW, et al. Kinematic comparisons of throwing different types of baseball pitches. *J Appl Biomech* 1998;14:1–23.
73. Murray TA, Cook TD, Werner SL, et al. The effects of extended play on professional baseball pitchers. *Am J Sports Med* 2001;29:137–142.
74. Lyman S, Fleisig GS, Andrews JR, et al. Effect of pitch type, pitch count, and pitching mechanics on risk of elbow and shoulder pain in youth baseball pitchers. *Am J Sports Med* 2002;30:463–468.
75. Barnes DA, Tullos HS. An analysis of 100 symptomatic baseball players. *Am J Sports Med* 1978;6:62–67.
76. McMahon P, Jobe F, Pink M, et al. Comparative electromyographic analysis of shoulder muscles during planar motions: anterior glenohumeral instability versus normal. *J Shoulder Elbow Surg* 1996;5:118–123.
77. Nobuhara K, Ikeda H. Rotator interval lesion. *Clin Orthop Rel Res* 1987:44–50.
78. Counsilman JE. Swimming power. *Swimming World and Junior Swimmer* 1977;18.
79. Douglas S. *Physical evaluation of the swimmer*. First Annual Vail Sports Medicine Symposium, Vail, CO, 1980.
80. Johnson D. Swimming, shoulder the burden. *Sportcare Fitness* 1988;May-June:24–30.
81. Tibone JE, Lee TQ, Csintalan RP, et al. Quantitative assessment of glenohumeral translation. *Clin Orthop* 2002;400:93–97.
82. Richardson AB, Jobe FW, Collins HR. The shoulder in competitive swimming. *Am J Sports Med* 1980;8:159–163.
83. Pink M, Perry J, Jobe FW, et al. The normal shoulder during freestyle swimming: an EMG and cinematographic analysis of twelve muscles. *Am J Sports Med* 1991;19:569–575.
84. Hawkins RJ, Hobeika PE. Impingement syndrome in the athletic shoulder. *Clin Sports Med* 1983;2:391–405.
85. Snyder SJ, Karzel RP, Del Pizzo W, et al. SLAP lesions of the shoulder. *Arthroscopy* 1990;6:274–279.
86. Pink M, Jobe FW, Perry J, et al. The painful shoulder during the butterfly stroke. An electromyographic and cinematographic analysis of twelve muscles. *Clin Orthop Rel Res* 1993:60–72.
87. Bahamonde RE. Changes in angular momentum during the tennis serve. *J Sports Sci* 2000;18:579–592.
88. Bankart ASB. Recurrent or habitual dislocation of the shoulder joint. *Br Med J* 1923;2:1132–1133.
89. Perthes G. Operationen bei habitueller schulterluxation. *Deutsch Ztschr Chir* 1906;85:199–227.
90. Speer KP, Deng X, Borrero S, et al. Biomechanical evaluation of a simulated Bankart lesion. *J Bone Joint Surg (Am)* 1994;76:1819–1826.
91. Black KP, Schneider DJ, Yu JR, et al. Biomechanics of the Bankart repair: the relationship between glenohumeral translation and labral fixation site. *Am J Sports Med* 1999;27:339–344.
92. O'Brien SJ, Schwartz RS, Warren RF, et al. Capsular restraints to anterior-posterior motion of the abducted shoulder: a biomechanical study. *J Shoulder Elbow Surg* 1995;4:298–308.
93. Aston JW, Gregory CF. Dislocation of the shoulder with significant fracture of the glenoid. *J Bone Joint Surg (Am)* 1973;55:1531–1533.
94. Itoi E, Lee S-B, Berglund LJ, et al. The effect of a glenoid defect on anteroinferior stability of the shoulder after Bankart repair: a cadaveric study. *J Bone Joint Surg (Am)* 2000;82:35–46.
95. Reeves B. Experiments on the tensile strength of the anterior

capsular structures of the shoulder in a man. *J Bone Joint Surg (Br)* 1968;50:858–865.

96. Stefko JM, Tibone JE, Cawley PW, et al. Strain of the anterior band of the inferior glenohumeral ligament during capsule failure. *J Shoulder Elbow Surg* 1997;6:473–479.

97. Bigliani LU, Pollock RG, Soslowsky LJ, et al. Tensile properties of the inferior glenohumeral ligament. *J Orthop Res* 1992;10: 187–197.

98. Mow VC, Bigliani LU, Flatow EL, et al. Material properties of the inferior glenohumeral ligament and the glenohumeral articular cartilage. In: Matsen FA, Fu FH, Hawkins RJ, eds. *The shoulder: a balance of mobility and stability.* Rosemont, IL: AAOS, 1993:29–68.

99. McMahon PJ, Dettling JR, Sandusky MD, et al. The anterior band of the inferior glenohumeral ligament: assessment of its permanent deformation and the anatomy of its glenoid attachment. *J Bone Joint Surg (Br)* 1999;81:406–413.

100. Andrews JR, Carson WG Jr, McLeod WD. Glenoid labrum tears related to the long head of the biceps. *Am J Sports Med* 1985;13:337–341.

101. Tibone JE, Grossman MG, McGarry M, et al. *A cadaveric model of the throwing shoulder: a possible etiology of SLAP lesions.* 19th Annual Meeting of ASES. Pebble Beach, CA, 2002.

102. Maffet Mw, Gartsman GM, Moseley B. Superior labrum-biceps tendon complex lesions of the shoulder. *Am J Sports Med* 1995; 23:93–98.

103. Parentis MA, Mohr KJ, ElAttrache NS. SLAP Lesions in the new millennium: review and treatment guidelines. *Clin Orthop Rel Res* 2002;400:77–87.

104. Pagnani MJ, Deng XH, Warren RF, et al. Effect of lesions of the superior portion of the glenoid labrum on glenohumeral translation. *J Bone Joint Surg* 1995;77:1003–1010.

105. McMahon PJ, Burkart A, Musahl V, et al. Glenohumeral translations are increased after a type II SLAP lesion: a cadaveric study of severity of passive stabilizer injury. *J Shoulder Elbow Surg* 2002.

106. Rodosky MW, Harner CH, Fu FH. The role of the long head of the biceps muscle and superior glenoid labrum in anterior stability of the shoulder. *Am J Sports Med* 1994;22:121–130.

107. Burkart A, Debski RE, Musahl V, et al. Glenohumeral instability is only partially restored after repair of the type II SLAP lesion. *Am J Sport Med* 2002.

3

CLINICAL EXAMINATION OF THE OVERHEAD ATHLETE: THE "DIFFERENTIAL-DIRECTED" APPROACH

JOHN M. TOKISH
SUMANT G. KRISHNAN
RICHARD J. HAWKINS

INTRODUCTION

The organization of this chapter on the clinical evaluation of the shoulder in overhead athletes is different than more traditional textbook approaches. Although we remain committed to a comprehensive, organized approach to the shoulder, the direction here is driven by chief complaint, such that a differential diagnosis is deduced at the beginning of the interview, rather than at the end. This "differential-directed" approach allows the examiner to test the premise of the initial diagnosis throughout the history and physical examination, and allows for a more focused approach to the shoulder as it pertains to the overhead athlete. Although this differs in style from established texts that describe the history and physical examination followed by formation of the differential diagnosis, we intend for this approach to lead to the same destination: an accurate diagnosis for an overhead athlete with shoulder dysfunction. For an organized, comprehensive, traditional approach to examination of the shoulder, refer to *Musculoskeletal Examination: An Organized Approach to Musculoskeletal Examination and History Taking* (1) and "Clinical Evaluation of Shoulder Problems" in "The Shoulder" (2).

Physical examination of the overhead shoulder for some has become somewhat of a lost art because of the difficulty of the examination itself, the subtleties of the normal athletic shoulder that often make comparison to the opposite side unreliable, and the ever-increasing reliance on magnetic resonance imaging (MRI) for definitive diagnosis. As helpful a tool as MRI is, it is of concern that completely asymptomatic shoulders demonstrate pathology that might be erroneously attributed to an athlete with symptoms. Sher and co-workers demonstrated a 34% rate of tears of the rotator cuff in painless volunteers (3). Miniaci and colleagues showed that 79% of asymptomatic professional baseball pitchers had abnormalities of the glenoid labrum

(4). Furthermore, partial thickness rotator cuff tears, a diagnosis common to the throwing and overhead shoulder, may be missed by MRI up to 44% of the time (5). Hence, even with the technologic advances available, we remain convinced that the diagnosis of a shoulder problem in the overhead athlete is made by a proper history and physical examination, not by the scanner.

Although a classic tenet of physical examination is to compare the symptomatic side with the opposite normal side, this is not always reliable in the overhead athlete. There are a number of physiologic adaptations that occur in throwers and other overhead athletes, which, although asymmetric, are not pathologic. These include hypertrophy of the dominant arm, elbow flexion contracture, increased external rotation, and decreased internal rotation (6). Striving to create symmetry in these athletes may "correct" physiologic adaptations that protect the overhead arm and might lead to further problems and dysfunction.

One theme that is emphasized in this chapter is the importance of communication with the athlete to a correct understanding of the athlete's problem. Many athletes present with shoulders that contain multiple pathologies such as labral tears, impingement, and instability. Communication with the athlete is critical to understanding which of these may be the most important in their disability. Communication is also critical in differentiating between objective signs on physical examination and clinical symptoms. For example, laxity (a physical examination *sign*) is present in many overhead athletes. It can often be demonstrated on physical examination as a positive sulcus sign or increased translation of the humeral head on the glenoid. Although often more pronounced than in the average person, this finding may be totally asymptomatic, and attempts to "correct" this may do more harm than good. In contrast, symptomatic laxity is instability (a clinical *symptom*). The key difference is symptomatology. An athlete who can be shifted over the glenoid rim with a posterior translation maneuver demonstrates laxity. This patient must demonstrate reproduction of symptoms with such a maneuver to raise the level of suspicion to diagnose instability (2). It is only with communication during such maneuvers that these subtle differences can be reliably interpreted.

Another important area of communication exists between physicians and the athlete's team trainers or physical therapists. A treating physician might be unimpressed with a pitcher's signs or symptoms in the office only to find out that, once the player throws at more than half speed, he becomes ineffective. Trainers and therapists can often provide key feedback on the mechanism of injury, the degree of disability, and the athlete's progression with conservative treatment. They are helpful with decisions concerning return to play or when to say rehabilitation is not working and other options should be considered. Such benefits only happen with open lines of communication.

This chapter first describes a throwing athlete who cannot throw well. From this initial presentation, we describe an organized yet focused differential-directed approach to understanding the cause for the dysfunction, which forms the basis for how to resolve the problem. Although much of this chapter is focused on the throwing shoulder, it is important to keep in mind that these principles apply both to the examination of shoulders involved in any repetitive overhead activity (e.g., tennis, volleyball, handball, swimming) and to athletes of all ages and levels of participation.

RATIONALE FOR THE DIFFERENTIAL-DIRECTED APPROACH

One of the early skills taught to medical students is how to perform a history and physical examination. It forms the structure and base of the clinical encounter, wherein a diagnosis is formulated and treatment subsequently planned. Students are taught to be organized and thorough, and although much of the necessary knowledge base comes later, the structure must be stressed early and often to have a framework from which to fill in new knowledge. Traditionally, this framework follows a fairly strict order of history, physical examination, review of imaging, and creation of a differential diagnosis. This differential diagnosis is the end result of the sum total of information gained throughout the encounter. One common directive in teaching students is to not let them see any of the past notes or diagnostic conclusions during their evaluation, because such information might "tip them off" as to what to look for during the encounter, leading the student to focus on the expected findings of the examination and be too quickly directed toward the diagnosis. This teaches the young clinician completeness and avoids the pitfall of jumping to conclusions or making assumptions that the diagnosis purported by another clinician is correct. Even though this

process is valuable to the development of any promising diagnostician, once the framework is ingrained, the clinician learns which findings in each specific clinical encounter are pertinent and which are superfluous. To perform every aspect of the physical examination on every patient is unrealistic and often results in a great amount of data with no comprehension of what those data mean. It is far easier "to find what you are looking for when you know what you seek." This premise is the basis for the differential-directed approach. If one can be taught to develop a suspicion of what may be problematic in the overhead shoulder at the beginning of the clinical encounter, one stays directed, efficient, and accurate. We *do not* sacrifice thoroughness and completeness, because often other pathologic diagnoses may not have been suspected at the beginning of the examination and may only be elucidated with appropriate physical examination maneuvers. However, we use this differential-directed approach to allow for patient-appropriate specific versus "screening" examination techniques, and we believe that the development of these initial suspicions is not only possible but is the natural history of becoming more "focused" as a diagnostician. This focus comes with experience but can be accelerated by modifying the approach to both the history and physical examination. It becomes obvious that the success of the evaluation is directly related to the initial differential diagnosis. The quality of the differential diagnosis is dependent upon the clinician's understanding of shoulder pathologies and the various tests that are available for each. The better one's understanding of the pathologies presented in this book, the higher the quality of the initial differential diagnosis and the better the clinician becomes. This creates a dynamic relationship between knowledge and skill that can continue to improve throughout one's career. The experienced clinician learns to "go for the money" and yet not miss more subtle diagnoses.

The differential for pathology in the overhead shoulder is initially formed from two important pieces of information: (a) the athlete's chief complaint and (b) the athlete's age. For example, in a 60-year-old male tennis player with shoulder pain, even though a diagnosis is not guaranteed with such limited information, the astute clinician has a working differential diagnosis from the beginning of the examination. Throughout the examination, certain findings are expected to be positive. In this example, impingement signs with associated weakness with supraspinatus testing would strongly suggest a rotator cuff tear. At the same time, features of the examination that focus on subtle glenohumeral instability might be less emphasized. This format emphasizes attention on a set of expected findings and makes the diagnosis that much more specific.

The first step in the differential-directed approach is to understand how pathologies present as chief complaints, so that the initial differential is complete but focused. This is rarely as easy as in the aforementioned simple example. If a

20-year-old baseball pitcher with pain is the example, rather than suspecting just a rotator cuff tear, the initial differential might include instability, labral pathology, impingement, internal impingement, or a combination of these. Thus, a deeper understanding of the chief complaint and how it relates to the history is necessary to come to an accurate differential. Even in difficult presentations, we still formulate an initial differential that may "tip us off" to what we are looking for while keeping us directed toward the appropriate diagnosis.

Once this differential is formulated, the remainder of the history proceeds in an organized fashion with expectations already in mind. If the differential is correct, answers to queries within the history validate the initial diagnosis. If, however, the answers given by the athlete are not as expected, the clinician is alerted early to suspect another diagnosis and thus take the examination in a different direction. By the completion of the history, the clinician should have clear expectations of what to look for and emphasize in the physical examination.

It would be ideal if we could exactly reproduce an athlete's symptoms during the physical examination, but this is only occasionally possible. Many tests for pain are not specific enough to be reliable, and patients with instability are often too guarded to allow provocative testing. In the throwing and overhead athletic population, many pathologies coexist and make presentations confusing. It is therefore important for the physical examination to remain organized and systematic. One of the dangers of having a short list of differential diagnoses in mind is that the clinician's attempts to be focused could result in an incomplete examination. Although we recommend reorganizing the examination according to the differential, the essential tenets of "inspect, palpate, and move" the shoulder remain (1,2).

Diagnostic injections can be helpful in determining the source of symptoms. The goal is to eliminate the athlete's clinical signs and physical symptoms with the use of a short-acting local anesthetic placed in the specific anatomic area that seems to be responsible for the symptoms. This maneuver is the equivalent of the Neer subacromial "impingement test" (Fig. 3-1) and can be applied to a variety of other conditions in the differential diagnosis. There are limitations, in that differential injections are time consuming and often are not applicable for diagnoses such as instability. When pain is the presenting complaint, a diagnostic injection in a specific location that quickly (within 5 to 10 minutes) takes away nearly 100% of the athlete's pain often leads to the area of pathology and the correct diagnosis.

The organization of this chapter is according to chief complaint, followed by the specific historical questions and physical examination maneuvers that are applicable to each entity. This is an alternative approach from traditional texts wherein it is more common to separate the history from the physical examination and from diagnostic injections. Nevertheless, we believe that this organization more closely

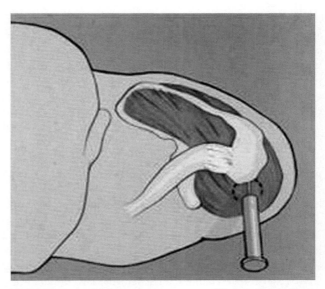

FIGURE 3-1. Neer impingement test. Instillation of local anesthetic into the subacromial space alleviates the previous pain that was demonstrated with Neer's impingement sign, indicating the pathology of subacromial impingement.

resembles how we approach the evaluation of the throwing and overhead shoulder.

PRINCIPLES OF THE HISTORY

Regardless of how one approaches the history, it is crucial that this approach is organized and systematic so that the clinician is thorough yet efficient. The general categories of chief complaint, history of present illness, past medical history, and review of systems (followed by the physical examination) remain the backbone of the clinical evaluation. We organize this evaluation according to the chief complaint for several reasons. First, it is the impetus behind the athlete's request for help, so organization by chief complaint keeps the interview patient-directed. Second, organization by chief complaint keeps the clinician focused and efficient. Third, knowing the age and the chief complaint provides a high index of suspicion for the diagnostic probabilities (1–3,5). Such an understanding provides an immediate differential diagnosis that can be tested throughout the history and physical to arrive at the correct diagnosis. It allows each step in the examination to help confirm or refute the diagnosis, providing dynamic confirmation when the initial diagnosis is right, and a series of red flags throughout the examination when the initial diagnosis is erroneous.

The Chief Complaint

A complete understanding of the chief complaint is critical to arriving at the correct diagnosis. This cannot be overemphasized due to the multiple pathologies in the shoulder of the throwing and overhead athlete. An operative "shotgun" approach to the wrong problems can end such an athlete's career, because more surgery undertaken in these patients may lessen the chances of their returning to high levels of participation. These overlapping pathologies present the so-called athlete's dilemma, emphasizing why the athlete's shoulder is so challenging. It is therefore critical to sort out which pathologies are dominant and might be corrected surgically and which should be left for rehabilitation.

These are difficult decisions that can be successfully made only with a thorough understanding of the athlete's chief complaint and how it relates to the rest of the athlete's history. For example, a chief complaint of pain in the shoulder may intimidate a novice examiner because there are so many possibilities. This assumption would be compounded if the examiner went from the chief complaint of pain directly to an MRI study, which showed acromioclavicular (AC) degenerative changes, a partial thickness undersurface tear of the rotator cuff, and a patulous capsule. However, if that same examiner seeks to gain a thorough understanding of the chief complaint, he or she might ask about where exactly is the pain, when does it hurt, and how is the pain produced. These simple questions might reveal an athlete who has pain on the top of the shoulder with bench press and is tender to palpation of the AC joint, leading to an initial suspicion of AC pathology. In contrast, the patient might say the shoulder hurts at the back when he or she starts to come forward with a fastball pitch, in which case the initial suspicion might be one of internal impingement. Thus, understanding the chief complaint should give the examiner a reliable early differential of the problem.

Once this is established, this differential can guide the examiner through the physical examination, providing clues to what findings should be positive on provocative testing and which should be negative. In the first example, symptoms of AC joint pathology were suggested. The examiner notes this by the chief complaint of pain on top of the AC joint and reproduction with the bench press. He or she then expects that during the physical examination the patient is likely to have tenderness to palpation of the AC joint and reproduction with crossed-arm adduction and an "augmented" AC joint maneuver. It does not mean that the clinician neglects to examine for symptoms of instability or impingement; it just highlights and sharpens the focus for the upcoming remainder of the history and physical. If the examiner notes that these findings on examination are indeed positive, especially in the absence of other findings, his or her suspicion is strengthened and he or she is closer to arriving at a correct diagnosis. If, however, the physical examination does not show the "expected" findings, the clinician must reconsider the diagnosis and perhaps consider one of the other diagnoses in the differential. Perhaps the chief complaint was not fully understood, and the clinician should revisit this first step before proceeding with the workup.

History of Present Illness and Injury

After establishing the chief complaint, the next step of the history-taking should include history of present illness. History of present illness reconstructs the story of the chief complaint (from onset to present) so that the examiner has a clear understanding of how things started, what has been previously done, and the current state of the problem. The athlete may be unclear as to how or why symptoms started and may describe an insidious onset. When a single traumatic event is responsible for the injury, appropriate time spent on the mechanism, degree, and events surrounding the event provide reliable information. For example, in the patient whose chief complaint is that his shoulder "came out," appropriate questions might include:

- Did the shoulder come out because of a significant injury?
- What position was the arm in when it came out?
- Could you move the shoulder after the injury?
- Did the shoulder "slide out of joint" or did it "pop?"
- Did the shoulder feel like it came all the way out of joint?
- Did you feel any numbness or tingling in the arm or hand?
- Did you have to go to the hospital or have something else done to have it "put back in?"
- Did you have x-rays?
- Has this ever happened to your shoulder before?

The answers to these questions not only may establish the diagnosis but also may determine different courses of treatment. For example, an athlete who presents with a shoulder that came "partly" out of joint 1 week ago in a posterior direction that spontaneously reduced would be approached differently than an athlete who complains of the shoulder coming "all the way" out of joint on the field. This short illustration demonstrates how similar chief complaints could result in entirely different management plans based on an appropriate history of present illness.

Clinical Course and Progression of the Problem

Once the circumstances surrounding the onset are established, the clinical course of the complaint is determined from its inception to the present. During this period, the effects and timing of various treatments are carefully considered. Any response to treatment, even if temporary, is important. For example, if a lidocaine and steroid injection was administered to the subacromial space for shoulder pain, it is important to note whether this was effective, even if only temporarily, because this yields diagnostic as well as therapeutic information. One should evaluate other interventions such as the effect of antiinflammatories, modalities, and physical therapy. This information should lead the examiner to an understanding of what has already been done and the progression of the treatment instituted. A patient who is improving after 6 weeks of physical therapy prescribed for impingement is a much different case than a patient who is getting worse with 6 months of the same therapy. It is important to realize that, although some athletes have the luxury of having highly trained therapists and athletic trainers who supervise their rehabilitation on a daily basis, others are often left to do an independent, poorly guided therapy regimen that is often incomplete or even misdirected. It is not enough to ask if "physical therapy" has been done. One must delve into the specifics of that therapy to make an accurate assessment of whether it was an adequate regimen that was correctly followed.

Current Status of the Problem and Degree of Disability

It is important also to note the current status of the complaint. This current status should be understood in light of the athlete's current level of activity, where the athlete is in relation to the sport season, and how long he or she has until the shoulder has to be in "playing condition." A college football quarterback who dislocates his shoulder for the first time early in his senior year might pursue a different treatment course than the same player who dislocates his shoulder in the first week of the off-season after his junior year. Such an understanding requires thorough communication with the athlete and an understanding of his or her goals, and will guide the patient and the physician to the best choice for their desired outcome.

The final aspect to the current status of the problem is the *degree of disability* incurred by the athlete from their injury. Athletes, and patients in general, present with complaints on the spectrum from minimal annoyance with high-level sports to complete disability with activities of daily living. Understanding where the patient is on this spectrum greatly aids in guiding how aggressive the diagnostic workup is and how invasive the treatment plan should be. It is important to note that an accurate assessment of the degree of disability may require communication with the athletic trainer or physical therapist, because some athletes may attempt to "play through" injuries that render them ineffective and put themselves in danger of further injury. These are sometimes difficult decisions for an athlete to make, and often a trainer's input is valuable in defining the degree of disability.

Past Medical History and Review of Systems

Although we should be confident with a solid differential diagnosis at this point and although athletes are among the healthiest patients in our population, questions about past medical history should not be neglected. These include questions about medications, allergies, and congenital or other medical problems. Finding out that a swimmer with shoulder pain has Ehlers-Danlos syndrome might not only point to multidirectional instability (MDI) as a diagnosis but might also influence the treatment of such a shoulder. Although often negative, a review of systems and queries regarding past medical history can avoid missing key aspects affecting the diagnosis and eventual treatment of the overhead athlete.

PRINCIPLES OF THE PHYSICAL EXAMINATION

Once the examiner completes an organized history, there should be a clear idea of the differential, which should direct which aspects of the physical examination should be emphasized. Just as in the history, there will be certain expected responses (both positive and negative) for the differential-directed physical. During the examination, one should note whether the physical examination expectations are met (in which case the suspicion of the correct diagnosis is strengthened) or whether the expectations are not met (in which case one must reconsider the appropriate diagnosis). Although we organize our approach based on complaint, there are certain aspects to the physical examination that should be ingrained in any competent examiner. Depending on the differential, some of these areas are more emphasized than others. Nevertheless, especially in the overhead athlete in whom multiple pathologies often exist and there is considerable overlap for many chief complaints, we repeatedly emphasize that the following tenets should be remembered:

1. *Introduction to the patient and cursory assessment of general aspects.* This allows the examiner to "see the big picture," to remember the whole patient, and to avoid making the mistake of focusing too narrowly on the shoulder.
2. *Features of inspection such as muscle wasting, deformity, and previous surgical scars.* This is especially important when the chief complaint is weakness related, which can lead to a number of other chief complaints, such as pain and instability.
3. *Palpation of known anatomic sites.* This is crucial in the patient who complains of pain, but also can be used for other pathologies (e.g., to diagnose rotator cuff tears in patients complaining of weakness).
4. *Range of motion (active and passive) with careful documentation.* This is an often overlooked area of the examination, but is often the key finding in overhead athletes with tight posterior capsules leading to pain and other complaints.
5. *Strength testing and neurologic examination.* This should be a part of every shoulder examination in the athlete.
6. *Stability assessment and laxity measurements.* Because laxity and "microinstability" are the "great imitators" in the athlete's shoulder, this is critical to every examination.

Instability can underlie many chief complaints in the overhead athlete.

7. *Special tests.* These tests may be the decisive blow in ruling in or out a diagnosis; familiarity with the special tests for each diagnosis separates the beginner from the advanced diagnostician.

8. *Lower extremities and trunk.* Although outside the scope of this chapter, it is emphasized that the kinetic chain begins in the legs and proceeds through the trunk before it ever gets to the shoulder. The examiner is reminded that problems in the shoulder may only be a manifestation of more proximal pathology in the chain that must be corrected to allow the athlete to return to proper overhead performance.

The patient should be prepared by removing the outer garment for a view of the bare shoulders. For women, a sports bra or designed halter top type gown preserves modesty while allowing the examiner to pick up on often subtle aspects of the examination such as atrophy or winging (Fig. 3-2). Attention to the asymptomatic side remains important, but the examiner must remember those physiologic adaptations that often are present in overhead athletes. With this in mind, the examiner should attempt to reproduce the conditions that bring on the chief complaint. This may involve more emphasis on range of motion when instability is suspected, or palpation and special tests when pain is the chief complaint.

This does not mean that we ignore range of motion in the patient with pain or palpation in the patient with instability—it is just that a different set of red flags and expectations arise for each patient with this approach.

In this section, we define the various chief complaints common to the overhead athlete and discuss what initial differential corresponds to each chief complaint. Next, we describe the specific historical questions that should narrow the focus and sharpen the differential. Finally, we demonstrate the various physical examination techniques that may rule in or rule out a specific diagnosis in the overhead athlete. This differential-directed approach is intended to provide an organized template for the correct diagnosis right from the initial history, to tip off the examiner on what to expect and what not to expect throughout the physical examination, to reinforce each step of the workup, and to create solid evidence for the diagnosis by the completion of the encounter.

CHIEF COMPLAINT: PAIN

Perhaps no chief complaint is as common as pain in the shoulder and none has a broader list of possible causes. Many of these causes overlap or play a role in the pathology of other processes. In addition, there is often more than one source of pain in the throwing athlete, making the approach not nearly as clear as one would like (4). The following dis-

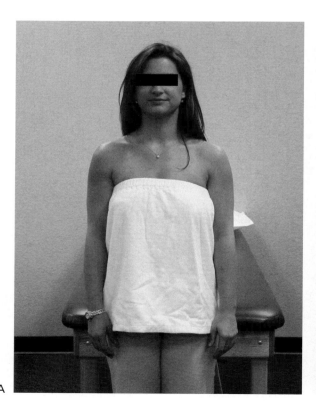
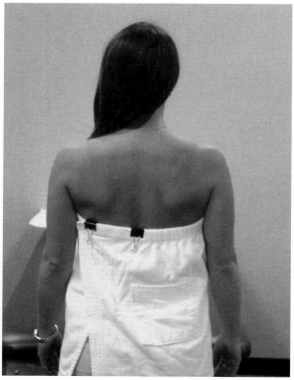

FIGURE 3-2. A,B: Direct inspection of shoulder.

TABLE 3–1. COMMON CAUSES FOR PAIN AS CHIEF COMPLAINT

Impingement
Classic outlet impingement
Internal impingement
Subcoracoid impingement
Rotator cuff
Tendinosis
Partial thickness tearing
Full thickness tearing
Instability
Anterior
Posterior
Multidirectional instability (MDI)
Acromioclavicular (AC) joint pathology
Biceps and labral pathology
Chondral defects
Neurologic
Cervical spine root compression
Brachial neuritis
Thoracic outlet syndrome
Suprascapular nerve entrapment

cussion describes the differential for pain and how to narrow down the list to a few diagnoses to test on physical examination. See Table 3-1 for a list of common causes for pain as chief complaint. Such a list can be daunting unless the examiner stays organized. With a few early questions, the differential can be established and narrowed down. One question to begin with is simply, "Where is the pain?" Although this is a seemingly basic question, it is often difficult to get the patient to be specific about this. We often ask patients to point with one finger to the area. Most patients respond in one of the following ways listed in Table 3-2.

TABLE 3–2. COMMON DESCRIPTIONS OF PAIN ABOUT THE SHOULDER

Patient Description	Likely Source of Pain
Whole hand over deltoid in rubbing motion	Impingement/rotator cuff
Greater tuberosity	Impingement/rotator cuff
One finger on top of distal clavicle	AC joint
In the back when the arm is in the throwing position (points to posterior capsule with arm in abduction/external rotation)	Internal impingement/ SLAP tear
Down the neck and scapula medial border	Neck pathology
In front within deltopectoral groove	Biceps tendon, subscapularis pathology
"Deep inside"	Labral or articular cartilage pathology
Vague and diffuse down arm	Brachial neuritis/thoracic outlet Syndrome (neurologic)

AC, acromioclavicular; SLAP, superior labrum anterior to posterior.

Palpation to Reproduce Pain

Once the patient has identified the area of the pain, the next step may be to find the point of maximal tenderness by palpating each of the following areas. Some areas of the shoulder are naturally tender, so comparison with the asymptomatic side might be helpful (Table 3-3) (Fig. 3-3).

The patient may say that the pain is "deep" and not really palpable (think intraarticular superior labrum anterior-to-posterior [SLAP], labral tear, articular cartilage injury). In addition to finding (or not finding) the point of maximal tenderness, there are a number of additional maneuvers that should be performed to further narrow the differential.

Provocative Tests to Reproduce Pain

Subacromial Impingement-Producing Maneuvers

When an athlete presents with tenderness over the greater tuberosity (especially with vague complaints involving the whole deltoid with overhead activity), one should already strongly suspect impingement. The following are provocative maneuvers that should lead one toward the diagnosis of subacromial impingement.

Neer's Sign (Fig. 3-4). This test is performed by placing the symptomatic arm in maximum passive forward flexion. A positive test is signified by production of pain. Neer's sign

TABLE 3–3. COMMON SITES OF TENDERNESS AND LOCATIONS/PEARLS

Point of Maximal Tenderness	Location/Pearl
Greater tuberosity (Codman's point) (Fig. 3-3)	Just anterior to anterolateral corner of acromion with dorsum of hand on buttock
Lesser tuberosity	Subscapularis pathology, biceps
AC joint	Follow posterior part of clavicle to acromion. AC joint just anterior to this. Push the clavicle down hard enough to move it.
Acromion	Do not forget about symptomatic os acromiale
Posterior capsule	Internal impingement lesions are tender posteriorly; SLAP tears may also be tender here
Biceps tendon	Directly anterior when arm internally rotated 10°
Coracoid	Subcoracoid impingement
Erb's point	Medial to coracoid, inferior to clavicle

AC, acromioclavicular; SLAP, superior labrum anterior to posterior.

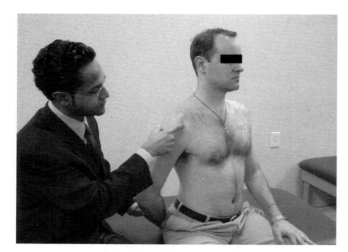

FIGURE 3-3. Codman's point.

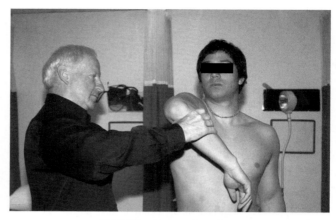

FIGURE 3-5. Hawkins sign.

has been shown to be 88.7% sensitive for subacromial impingement and 85% sensitive for rotator cuff tearing, but it has poor specificity (7,8).

Hawkins Sign (Fig. 3-5). This test is performed by placing the arm in 90 degrees of forward flexion, with the elbow flexed 90 degrees. The examiner then internally rotates the arm maximally. A positive test is signified by production of pain. This test has been shown to reflect contact between rotator cuff and the coracoacromial ligament (2). It has been shown to have a sensitivity of 92% for subacromial impingement and 88% for rotator cuff tearing (8). Like the Neer sign, however, this test is not very specific for these conditions.

Painful Abduction Arc Sign (Fig. 3-6). This test is performed by having the patient perform resisted abduction in or just posterior to the coronal plane. Reproduction of the

patient's symptoms of pain constitutes a positive sign (2,9). Unlike the Neer and Hawkins signs, this test is more specific than it is sensitive (7).

If these signs are positive, subacromial impingement may be strongly suspected and can be strengthened further with a Neer impingement test (Fig. 3-1), especially if the tests become negative after injection.

One should be mindful that subacromial impingement syndrome may be associated with a tear of the rotator cuff. Because rotator cuffs are often painful, any workup for impingement should include testing for a tear of the cuff. Although these tests are usually looking for weakness, any impingement examination should include an evaluation of the cuff.

Tests for Weakness

Jobe's Test (Fig. 3-7). This test is performed by placing the patient in 90 degrees of elevation in the scapular plane, classically with the thumbs pointed down. This position is

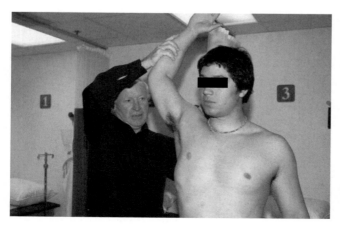

FIGURE 3-4. Neer's sign.

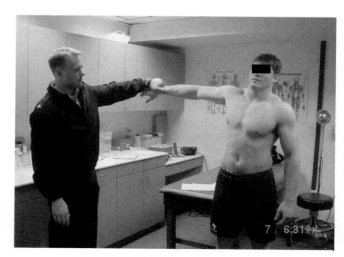

FIGURE 3-6. Painful abduction arc sign.

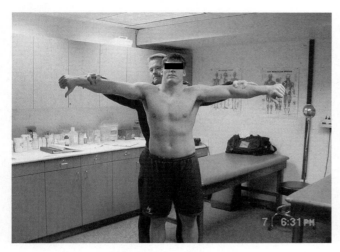

FIGURE 3-7. Jobe's test.

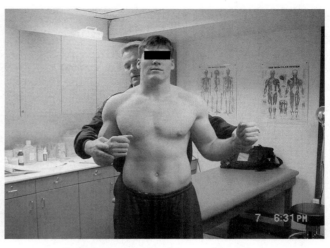

FIGURE 3-9. Resisted External Rotation.

held against downward resistance. This test isolates the supraspinatus (10) and is positive when there is asymmetric weakness. Caution should be used in the patient with pain, because pain can simulate weakness in patients with painful subacromial impingement.

Full Can Test (Fig. 3-8). Because Jobe's test can be painful in patients with impingement, the full can test has been proposed as an alternative. This test is performed like the Jobe's test, except the thumbs are pointed up. This test has been shown to isolate the supraspinatus as well as Jobe's test, but it produces less pain (11).

Resisted External Rotation (Fig. 3-9). This test is performed with the patient's elbows at his or her side and flexed 90 degrees. A positive test is signified by asymmetric weakness.

Lift-off Test (Fig. 3-10). This test is performed by having the patient place his or her arm behind the back, resting on the small of the lumbar spine. The patient's hand is lifted off the back, without extending the elbow, and the patient attempts to hold the arm off of the back once the examiner lets go. Gerber and colleagues (12) found that this test reliably diagnosed or ruled out clinically significant subscapularis ruptures. This test is of limited value in patients with painful internal rotation or with stiffness that does not allow the patient to achieve the starting position. Careful attention should be paid to the technique, because it is possible to "lift off" the hand by extending the elbow, which can be misleading.

Belly-Press Test. (Fig. 3-11). This test has been proposed as an alternative to the lift-off test in patients with either too much pain or stiffness to attempt the lift-off maneuver. It is performed by having the patient place both hands on the

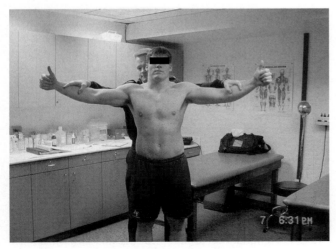

FIGURE 3-8. Full can test.

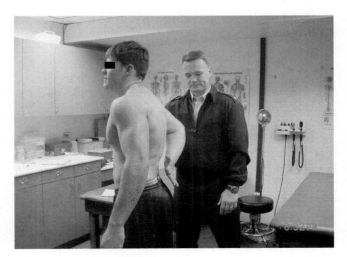

FIGURE 3-10. Lift-off test.

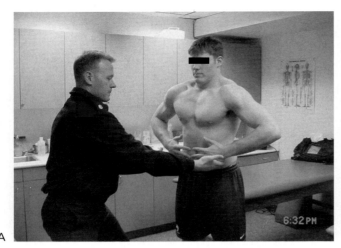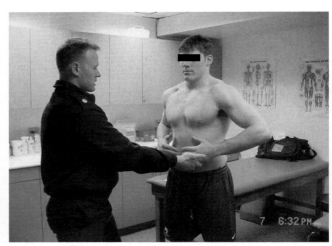

FIGURE 3-11. Belly-press test. Normal **(A)** and abnormal **(B)**, right side.

belly with flat wrists. The elbows should remain anterior to the trunk while the patient pushes posterior against the belly. Patients with subscapularis weakness demonstrate a dropped elbow, because they use shoulder extension to compensate for weak internal rotation.

The lift-off test and the belly-press test have both been validated as tests for the subscapularis. The lift-off test is more specific for the lower subscapularis, whereas the belly-press test is superior for the upper subscapularis (13).

Lag Signs. These are three signs that have been shown as reliable and efficient alternatives to more traditional rotator cuff testing (14). The external rotation lag sign (ERLS) is performed by placing a patient in 20 degrees of elevation, 90 degrees of elbow flexion, and near maximal external rotation. A patient who cannot maintain this position (even with a 5-degree lag) has a positive test suggesting a supraspinatus or infraspinatus tear (14). The "drop sign" is evaluated much the same way, except that the patient holds the affected arm in 90 degrees of elevation, 90 degrees of elbow flexion, and near full external rotation. If a drop occurs when the examiner releases the wrist, the sign is considered positive for infraspinatus weakness. Finally, the internal rotation lag sign (IRLS) is similar to the previous description of the lift-off test, noting a 5-degree drop toward the back. Hertel (14) noted that the ERLS and drop signs had a positive predictive value of 100% for both, and a negative predictive value of 56% and 32%, respectively. He also noted that the IRLS had a positive predictive value of 97% and a negative predictive value of 69%.

Rent Test. This test described by Codman (2,15) attempts to palpate a "rent" through the deltoid in a patient with a supraspinatus tear. Palpation is accomplished in a relaxed patient at the anterolateral border of the acromion. Wolf and colleagues (16) have reported on the diagnostic accuracy of

this test, noting a sensitivity of 95.7%, a specificity of 96.8%, and a diagnostic accuracy of 96.3% for rotator cuff tear.

Patients may demonstrate "pseudoweakness" on examination because many of these tests are subacromial impingement-producing. It can be difficult to distinguish true weakness due to a rotator cuff tear from pseudoweakness due to impingement-type pain. In those cases, use of the Neer impingement test, as described later, can be helpful, because it may eliminate the pain, differentiating true weakness from that which is produced by pain.

Acromioclavicular Joint Testing

If the patient has complaints of pain on the top of the shoulder, which is reproduced with pressing down on the clavicle, one should consider AC joint pathology. Palpation tenderness is a reliable sign for this condition, because a clinically significant AC joint problem is rarely nontender (17). Three additional tests are good stressors of the AC joint:

AC Compression Test (Fig. 3-12). This is a cross body adduction maneuver that compresses the AC joint. A positive test produces pain on top of the shoulder. An "augmented" AC compression test can be performed with palpation of the AC joint during forced cross body adduction.

AC Distraction Test ("bad cop" test). This is accomplished by placing the arm in maximal internal rotation and applying slight pressure upward. Again a positive test is signified by pain on top of the shoulder.

Active Compression Test (O'Brien's test) (Fig. 3-13). This test is performed by having the athlete place his or her arm forward flexed to 90 degrees with 10 degrees of horizontal adduction and internal rotation (thumb down) (18). A positive test is signified by pain on top of the shoulder when the

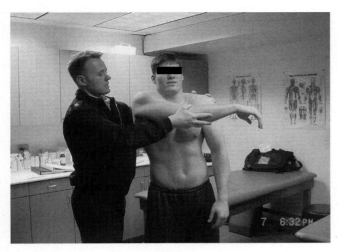

FIGURE 3-12.

arm is pushed in a downward direction, which is lessened when the test is repeated with the arm in external rotation (thumb up). This test has been shown to be positive in 89% of patients successfully treated for AC joint pathology (18).

When performing the aforementioned tests, it is important for the examiner to specifically look for pain at the top of the shoulder at the AC joint, because the first two tests often produce pain in the shoulder with impingement whereas O'Brien's test often produces "deep" pain in the presence of a superior labrum anterior to posterior (SLAP) tear (see SLAP tests). When the tests are positive, strong consideration should be given to injecting the AC joint with 1 to 3 mL of lidocaine to help confirm the diagnosis as described later.

Biceps Tendon Pathology (Non-Anchor Related)

If the presenting complaint is pain at the front of the shoulder, especially if the point of maximal tenderness is repro-

duced with palpation in the area of the biceps tendon as described earlier, then a biceps tendon problem should be considered. Although the biceps tendon is normally difficult to palpate, a number of provocative maneuvers can be considered to help confirm or rule out biceps tendon pathology. Many of these signs coexist with subacromial impingement.

Speed's Test (Fig. 3-14). This is accomplished by having the patient hold the supinated arm in 90 degrees of forward flexion. A positive test is marked by reproduction of pain with resisted forward flexion. This test has been shown to be 90% sensitive but only 14% specific for biceps tendon pathology (19).

Yergason's Test (Fig. 3-15). This test is performed by grasping the patient's hand as if to shake hands. The patient is asked to supinate while the examiner resists. A positive test is reproduction of the pain at the front of the shoulder.

Ludington's Test. This is an observational test to look for a ruptured long head of the biceps. The patient is asked to place both palms of the hands on his or her head and flex the biceps. A positive test is marked by the asymmetric biceps contour.

If the aforementioned tests are positive, strong consideration should be given to an injection of the biceps tendon sheath as described later. If such an injection provides near complete relief in the office, especially with the subsequent normalization of the aforementioned tests, one can be confident that the diagnosis of biceps tendon pathology is correct. This does not always address intraarticular biceps pathology (see SLAP tears), and this differentiation can be confusing.

It is difficult to exactly palpate the biceps tendon in its groove and, thus, an injection can be difficult to place in the right anatomic location. Matsen and colleagues have shown that the location of the biceps tendon and bicipital groove is commonly found with direct anterior palpation approxi-

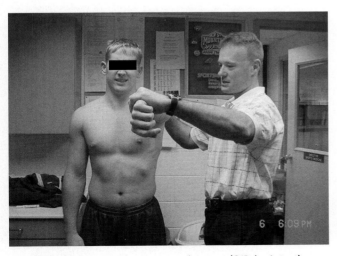

FIGURE 3-13. Active compression test (O'Brien's test).

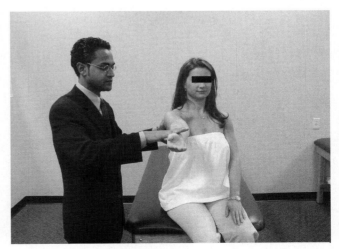

FIGURE 3-14. Speed's test.

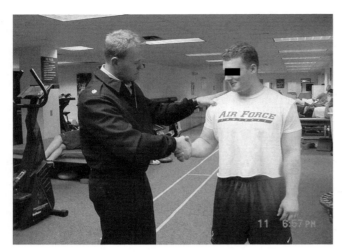

FIGURE 3-15. Yergason's test.

mately 2 cm distal to the anterolateral corner of the acromion when the arm is in 10 degrees of internal rotation (2,20) (Fig. 3-16). Because this is very close to the insertions of the subscapularis and pectoralis major, care must be taken to rule out strains of these two muscles before assuming a diagnosis of biceps tendinitis.

Superior Labral Pathology (SLAP Tears)

When a patient presents with a complaint of "deep" pain in the shoulder, especially in the absence of impingement signs or specific palpable points of tenderness, consideration should be given to the possibility of a SLAP tear. Since its description in 1990 (21), there has been an aggressive search by authors to find an accurate physical examination technique for superior labral tears. Some of the more commonly used techniques are described herein.

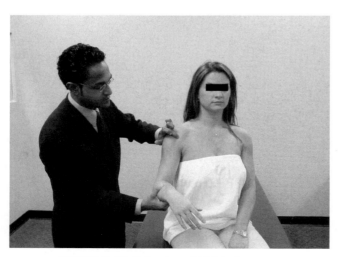

FIGURE 3-16. Palpation of bicipital groove.

In the presence of these tests being strongly positive, especially in the relative absence of impingement signs, consideration should be given to performing an intraarticular injection as described later. Complete relief suggests an intraarticular source and points strongly to a diagnosis of a SLAP tear or internal impingement.

Active Compression test (O'Brien's test). (Fig. 3-13). Described earlier as an AC joint provocative test, this test often produces dramatic pain "deep inside" in the presence of a SLAP tear. This test has been shown to be positive in 95% of patients who demonstrate superior labral pathology at arthroscopy (18). We find this test to be sensitive for labral tears, but not very specific, because it is often positive in patients with impingement.

"SLAP"prehension Test. This test is similar to the active compression test, but the arm is placed in 45 degrees of adduction and 90 degrees of shoulder flexion, with the elbow extended and forearm pronated, and a downward force on the arm is resisted by the patient (2,22). A positive test produces either apprehension, pain referable to the bicipital groove, or an audible or palpable click. The test is repeated with the forearm supinated, which must cause diminution of the pain. The authors of this test found this test to be 87.5% sensitive for unstable SLAP lesions.

Biceps Load Test. This test is performed by placing the supine patient's arm in 120 degrees of elevation and maximal external rotation with the elbow flexed 90 degrees and the forearm supinated (2,23). The patient is asked to flex the elbow against resistance and is considered positive if this reproduces or accentuates the patient's pain. In one prospective study, this test was shown to be 90% sensitive and 97% specific for a type II SLAP lesion. We have not been able to reproduce the accuracy of this test for SLAP lesions in our practice.

Anterior Slide Test. This test is performed by having the patient place both hands on the hips with the thumbs facing forward. The examiner directs an axial force at the elbow in an anterior and superior direction. A positive test is marked by pain with this maneuver. The anterior slide test has been shown to be 78% sensitive and 92% specific (24) for lesions of the superior labrum in throwing athletes.

O'Driscoll's SLAP Test. This test is similar to the test for valgus instability of the elbow. The patient is supine or upright and the shoulder is placed in the extreme abducted, externally rotated position. From this position, a moving valgus stress is applied, and a positive response is signified by pain in the shoulder. We have found this test to be quite sensitive, but not very specific for SLAP lesions (2).

Pain at Coracoid (Subcoracoid Impingement)

Although a rare cause of pathology, subcoracoid impingement has been recognized as a source of anterior shoulder pain (25). One test for this is the "coracoid impingement sign," which is performed with the patient standing with the shoulder abducted 90 degrees with horizontal adduction in the coronal plane and maximally internally rotated (tennis "follow-through" position, similar to the Hawkins sign with less horizontal adduction). A positive test is marked by pain around the coracoid process.

Pain Secondary to Instability

As previously stated, we believe that the best approach to problems with the evaluation of the shoulder is to begin with the patient's chief complaint, allowing it to immediately focus the clinical examination. It may seem odd, then, to describe a few tests for instability in a section on pain, but because pain is often the chief complaint in the athlete with instability, we remain consistent in our approach. Instability can coexist with conditions such as internal impingement or SLAP tears, which often present as posterior pain when the patient is in maximum abduction and external rotation. In addition, athletes are not immune from the diagnosis of multidirectional instability, which can present with pain. Thus, although we recommend tests that traditionally produce instability, pain in these positions may have instability as the underlying cause.

Relocation Test for Pain (Fig. 3-17). This test is performed by placing the patient supine in maximum abduction and external rotation. If this position produces posterior pain that is relieved by a posteriorly directed force on the humerus and again is recreated by removing the pres-

sure and allowing the humerus to slide forward, then a diagnosis of internal impingement may be considered. Paley and co-workers (26) demonstrated contact of the undersurface of the rotator cuff and the posterosuperior glenoid in the relocation position in 100% of patients undergoing arthroscopy for internal impingement.

This test is differentiated from a standard apprehension test, which is a measure of instability described later.

Inferior Sulcus Test for Pain. This test is performed by applying downward pressure on the humerus at both 0 and 90 degrees of abduction. Patients with MDI usually have reproduction of their symptoms with this maneuver with a positive sulcus sign (Fig. 3-18). It is critical to keep in mind that a positive sulcus sign, or visible dimpling between the inferior acromion and superior humeral head, itself is not enough to establish the diagnosis of MDI. Patients with a combined SLAP and Bankart lesion often show an increase in the sulcus sign, as do some asymptomatic patients. It is therefore important to differentiate between shoulder laxity, which is a sign, and instability, which is a symptom. Because MDI requires inferior instability plus at least one other direction of instability, the reproduction of the patient's pain with a sulcus test suggests the diagnosis.

The inferior sulcus test can also be used to diagnose pain secondary to rotator interval laxity and pathology. A sulcus sign (with the shoulder in the standard position of adduction and neutral rotation) that does not disappear when the sulcus is again tested in adduction and 25 to 30 degrees of external rotation indicates a deficient or lax rotator interval.

Pain Secondary to Cervical Spine Pathology

One potentially confusing cause of pain in the shoulder is that which is referred from the cervical spine. Herniated

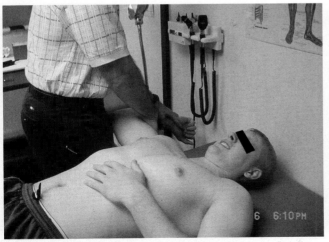
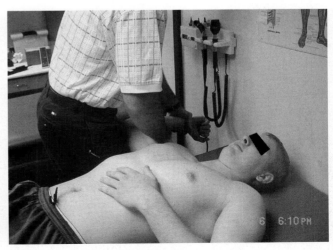

A   B

FIGURE 3-17. Relocation test for pain: with anterior translation **(A)** and with posterior stabilization **(B)**.

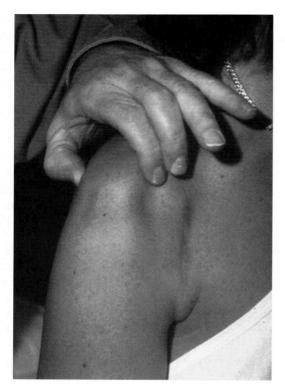

FIGURE 3-18 Sulcus sign.

discs can cause pressure on the C5- T1 nerve roots, which can cause vague symptoms in the anterior and posterior shoulder girdle. Patients may interpret this as shoulder pain, and thus it is incumbent upon the examiner to determine exactly where the pain comes from. In such cases, the patient often does not localize the pain. There are various tests that are good indicators of cervical pathology.

Provocative Tests

When the examiner suspects cervical pathology, testing should begin with gently stressing the limits of range of motion, especially in extension, because patients with cervical pathology often have pain. In addition, posterior cervical tenderness is often present in these patients. Finally, specific maneuvers can help define cervical pathology as the source of the pain.

The "Neer Relief" Test. In patients with cervical spine pathology, symptoms are often relieved when the patient places his or her arm above the head. This maneuver may relieve tension on an inflamed nerve, but in the shoulder with impingement, it would be expected to exacerbate pain. This test may help differentiate between pain from a cervical spine source and pain from shoulder pathology, and it can be elicited by history as well as by physical examination.

Spurling's Test (Fig. 3-19). This test is performed by stressing the neck in lateral flexion, rotation to the side tested, and compression. A positive test is heralded by reproduction of the patient's specific symptoms with special attention to radiation of pain or numbness into the dermatome of a specific nerve root or into the shoulder. In one evaluation of Spurling's test (27), it was shown to have a sensitivity of only 30%, but showed a specificity of 93%. The authors concluded that the test is not useful as a screening test, but it may be helpful in confirming the diagnosis of cervical radiculopathy. We find this test, when positive, to be the most helpful to us in determining the presence of cervical spine disease.

Valsalva Maneuver. This maneuver is performed by asking the patient to bear down, thereby increasing intrathecal pressure. Such an increase would be more likely to exacerbate pain from a cervical spine source than a shoulder cause.

Compression and Distraction tests. In the patient with cervical pain, compression of the top of the spine in extension would be expected to exacerbate the patient's symptoms, whereas distraction in flexion might provide relief.

Pain Secondary to Other Neurologic Conditions

The organization of this chapter by chief complaint requires some redundancy, in that some underlying conditions may lead to several chief complaints. One such area is neurologic pathology of the shoulder. Some neurologic conditions present primarily as pain, although they may also present as weakness and paresthesias (28).

In addition to nerve compression at the level of the cervical spine, athletes can present with neurologic pain that is from a more distal source. The initial differential diagnosis

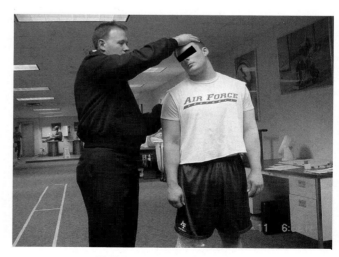

FIGURE 3-19. Spurling's test.

might include compression of the suprascapular nerve, "burners" or "stingers," thoracic outlet syndrome, and brachial neuritis.

Compression of the Suprascapular Nerve

This condition more commonly presents as weakness and atrophy in the supraspinatus, infraspinatus, or both, and is therefore covered more extensively in the section on weakness. However, when an athlete presents with posterior shoulder pain, especially in the presence of weakness of the spinati, consideration of compression of this nerve should be considered (29–31). There are no provocative maneuvers that exacerbate the specific pain associated with compression of the suprascapular nerve, but with a high index of suspicion, an injection of lidocaine into the area of the suprascapular notch may alleviate shoulder pain and be diagnostic. There are two common sites of compression for this nerve. The proximal site, at the suprascapular notch, both the nerve to the supraspinatus and infraspinatus can be compressed, leading to pain and weakness of both muscles. More distal compression can occur at the spinoglenoid notch, most commonly from a spinoglenoid notch cyst (usually associated with a posterosuperior labral tear), and can lead to isolated infraspinatus weakness.

Burners (Stingers)

Burners or stingers are common causes of pain and burning dysesthesias in the upper extremity. These injuries are most commonly the result of a violent stretch (31) of the brachial plexus. These injuries are usually transient, lasting only a few seconds. Because these often occur in game situations, especially in football, the athlete should be kept out of competition until symptoms resolve. The diagnosis of this condition is made almost on history alone, although a player might run off the field with a characteristic "dead arm" at his side. Symptoms usually are unilateral, extremely painful with burning and paresthesias down the extremity, and transient. They may also be accompanied by weakness in of the deltoid, biceps, spinati, and brachioradialis. It is important to distinguish a burner from cervical radiculopathy caused by compression of a nerve root. The former is usually self-limiting, but the latter is of more concern. Most patients with findings attributable to cervical radiculopathy such as tenderness in the cervical spine, pain with motion, a positive Spurling's test, or pain with compression, should be considered for early workup with cervical spine radiographs, MRI, and electromyography (EMG).

Thoracic Outlet Syndrome

This condition should be suspected in a patient who complains of diffuse shoulder pain, especially accompanied by radiating paresthesias in the ulnar nerve distribution below the elbow. Because paresthesias are more frequently the chief complaint in this condition, thoracic outlet syndrome is covered in detail under that discussion.

Brachial Neuritis

Occasionally, athletes present with an acute onset of severe pain with no apparent traumatic history. This pain can be severe and follows a variable distribution throughout the brachial plexus. In such a patient, a brachial neuritis can be the source. It has no known etiology and usually resolves over several weeks. In addition, it can often present with weakness, especially of the proximal musculature. This is generally a diagnosis of exclusion, and the examiner often makes this diagnosis only after obtaining imaging studies of the neck and EMG studies to rule out a specific source of compression.

Pain in the Presence of Scapular Dyskinesia

Most overhead athletes with shoulder problems have some degree of scapular dysfunction. Given this, it is important to examine all athletes, as well as any patient with shoulder pain, for scapular winging. Winging, which is discussed more thoroughly in the section on weakness, can be either the cause or the effect of shoulder pain. Thus, it is incumbent on the examiner to determine whether scapular winging, when present, contributes to a patient's symptoms. This is done by examining the patient from the back and asking the patient to elevate the arms at about half speed. Winging can be maximally demonstrated with resisted forward flexion at approximately 30 degrees of forward flexion (Fig. 3-20). It can also be

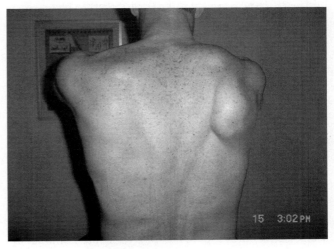

FIGURE 3-20. Scapular winging.

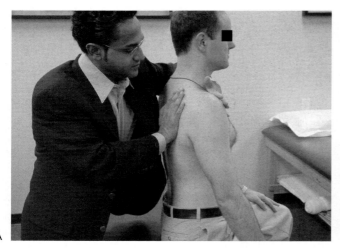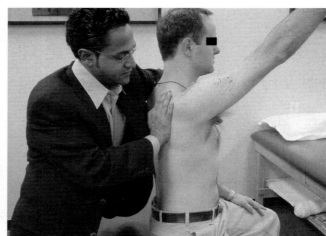

FIGURE 3-21. A,B: Scapular stabilization test.

observed with a push-up or wall push, or when patients use their arms to rise from a seated position.

Scapular Stabilization Test (Fig. 3-21). This test is performed by asking the patient to elevate the painful shoulder both before and after the examiner stabilizes the scapula against the thorax. If the patient's pain is relieved by this maneuver, then it is likely that the source of the pain is from the dysfunctional scapular platform.

Pain of Uncertain Origin

Some pain evaluations remain difficult even when armed with all of the techniques described. Some patients simply cannot specifically describe their pain and in others the shoulder is so inflamed that everything seems to produce positive signs. It is in these patients that the injection tests may have their greatest utility. Before discussing these, however, there is an additional test that is reported to accurately delineate between intraarticular and extraarticular sources of pain. This test is called the *internal rotation resisted strength test (IRRST)* (32), in which the patient places his or her shoulder in a position of 90 degrees abduction and 80 to 85 degrees of external rotation, with the elbow at 90 degrees of flexion. A manual isometric muscle test is performed for external rotation and then compared with one for internal rotation in the same position. Apparent weakness in internal rotation compared with external rotation notes a positive IRRST, and intraarticular pathology is then suspected. This test has been reported to be 88% sensitive, 96% specific, and 94.5% accurate in differentiating between intraarticular and subacromial sources for shoulder pain (32). We occasionally use this test in the presence of a difficult examination often to help direct which injection to begin with,

although we rely more heavily on the subsequent injection test to delineate the source of pain.

Injection Tests

The injection of a short-acting local anesthetic provides an excellent litmus test of one's clinical examination. The presumption is that if a local anesthetic is specifically placed into an area causing pain, that pain will be temporarily and nearly completely relieved. As importantly, the converse is true, making injection tests sensitive and specific. Performing a successful injection test has several important factors, including the accurate placement of the anesthetic, time for the anesthetic to take effect, reexamination for the elimination of the various provocative maneuvers, and subjective assessment of the patient's relief.

Accurate placement of the anesthetic takes time and experience to achieve consistency. One study has shown that attempts at subacromial injection can be unsuccessful in 17% of shoulders, and attempts at acromioclavicular injections can be unsuccessful 33% of the time (33). Therefore, meticulous attention must be paid to technique. A second pitfall to the successful employment of the injection test is a failure to give the anesthetic time to take effect. With today's emphasis on the 10-minute office visit, the importance of providing this time is often put aside, and the outcome of the injection test is postponed for a future visit. Asking the patient to recall the immediate response to the injection several weeks after the fact may be inaccurate and misleading. Finally, accuracy of interpretation of the injection test demands that the patient be reexamined during the same office visit. A repeat of the particular diagnostic maneuvers that were specific to the patient's symptoms are repeated. The patient is asked what percentage of their symptoms were

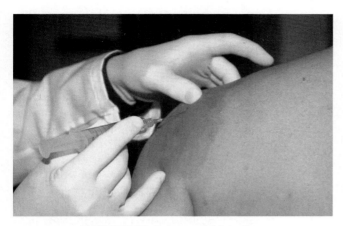

FIGURE 3-22. Subacromial injection.

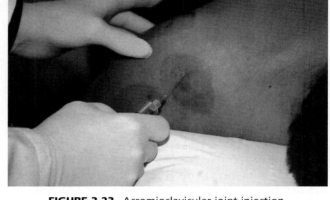

FIGURE 3-23. Acromioclavicular joint injection.

relieved by the injection, and that agreed upon level is recorded in the note. In our experience, 80% to 100% relief should be obtained by the injection test. If significantly less relief is gained, the examiner should reconsider the diagnosis and consider an additional injection.

Subacromial Injection (Fig. 3-22). We normally perform this injection from the back using the posterior lateral angle of the acromion as a landmark, although an anterior approach was originally described by Neer. The area is prepped sterilely, and 5 mL of 1% lidocaine and 5 mL of 0.25% Marcaine are placed into the subacromial space by advancing the needle directly under the acromion anteriorly and slightly medially. In exceptionally large individuals, the needle must be long enough to reach the anterior one third of the subacromial area because the pathology exists anteriorly. Alternatively, lateral and anterior injections can be placed into the subacromial space. Once an adequate time interval has passed (usually 5 minutes), reexamination of the patient is performed. We inquire about any resting relief that the patient experiences with the injection. Next, we ask the patient to move the arm into positions that caused pain before the injection, to see whether they obtain relief. This generally includes reassessment of Neer's, Hawkins, and painful abduction arc tests, as well as palpation over the greater tuberosity (Codman's point). The patients are asked to grade their relief as less than 25%, 25% to 75%, or greater than 75% relief. Rotator cuff strength testing is also repeated. Weakness in these tests when there is no pain is highly suggestive of rotator cuff tear and is often met with a more aggressive treatment plan.

AC Joint Injection (Fig. 3-23). Injection of the AC joint is performed by palpating the end of the clavicle, prepping the area sterilely, and attempting to inject 3 mL of lidocaine into the joint. This can be a difficult joint to inject, because there may be considerable degenerative spurring or an abnormal angle of entry. Plain x-ray films of the area help

direct the angle of injection. In addition, if in the joint, one should be able to perform a "refill test." This is done by allowing the increased intraarticular pressure created by the injection to refill the syringe when pressure is taken away from the piston. This test is positive whenever a closed space is entered and distended, and is a routine part of any closed space injection we perform. The AC joint is variable in its volume, and enough local anesthetic should be used to meet firm resistance with a 20-gauge needle. This injection test is among the most dramatic in the office when positive, and when steroid is added, often provides dramatic lasting relief.

Biceps Tendon Sheath Injection (Fig. 3-24). As previously mentioned, the biceps tendon is difficult to feel in all but the most thin individuals. However, the position of the tendon and its groove have been shown to be reproducibly located directly anterior on the shoulder, 2 cm distal to the anterolateral corner of the acromion, when the arm is held in 10 degrees of internal rotation (20). Injection is accomplished by sterilely prepping the area, and placing a 20g

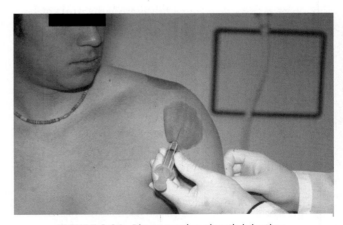

FIGURE 3-24. Biceps tendon sheath injection.

needle down to bone, then drawing back until resistance is released. This step is important because it is not desirable to inject directly into the tendon, and the release of tension during injection should signify the needle moving out of the tendon and into the surrounding area. We have seen several tendons rupture after this injection, and although this is of concern if the patient is not properly consented, it often provides lasting relief.

Suprascapular Nerve Injection. This is a rarely used injection, in that it serves to diagnose a rare condition, that is suprascapular nerve compression that presents as pain. Although primarily a motor supplier, the suprascapular nerve does contain sensory and pain fibers, which go to the subacromial bursa. Thus, in a patient who presents with posterior shoulder pain or what seems like subacromial pain that does not respond to subacromial injection, and when one has ruled out other causes, consideration may be given to compression of the suprascapular nerve as the source of the pain (29). The diagnostic injection to confirm this is performed by palpation of the AC joint and injection of 5 mL of 1% lidocaine beginning at a point just posterior to this joint with the needle directed 2 cm medial and 2 cm inferiorly. Weakness of the spinati confirms infiltration of the nerve, and temporary resolution of symptoms confirms the diagnosis of entrapment.

Intraarticular Glenohumeral Joint Injection. This injection can be very effective in isolating the source of pain to an intraarticular location. Internal impingement, SLAPs and other labral tears, and chondral lesions all are relieved with an intraarticular injection. This injection can be difficult for the inexperienced clinician, because the joint is deep and the injection is uncomfortable for the patient. We stress the importance of intraarticular placement of the local anesthetic by injecting 20 mL of fluid into the joint and allowing the refill test to confirm this placement.

We approach this injection posteriorly. The posterolateral corner of the acromion is identified and sterilely prepped. Next, a point 2 cm inferior and 1 cm medial to this point is identified and infiltrated with 5 mL of lidocaine in the skin and along the path of the needle. An 18-gauge spinal needle is then introduced and directed anteriorly, aiming for the coracoid process. Often, the needle hits a bony stop, and it must be determined whether this is the humerus or the glenoid. This can be determined by rotating the arm slightly internally and externally. If the needle moves with this rotation, the path must be redirected more medially to avoid the humerus. If it does not, it signifies that the needle is in the glenoid and must be directed more laterally. This is the same technique as we use in establishing a posterior portal for shoulder arthroscopy.

Our choice of an 18-gauge needle is important for several reasons. First, a smaller gauge needle may not be stout enough to maintain its shape as it traverses through the pos-

terior muscle mass and can be bent along its course. Second, an 18-gauge needle is large enough that once in the joint, intraarticular distention provides enough pressure to refill the syringe, whereas a smaller gauge needle often provides too much resistance to do this. Because the intraarticular placement of the needle is so critical, its position must be confirmed by this maneuver. Again it is critical to allow time for the local anesthetic to set up in the shoulder and then to reexamine the patient, especially those maneuvers that reproduced the patient's symptoms before the injection. If those provocative tests have been eliminated by the injection, one can be quite confident that the source of the pain is intraarticular. Given the high incidence of so-called pathologic findings on MRI studies of asymptomatic individuals, such injections can differentiate between variations of anatomy and symptomatic pathology. Such differentiation is the key to the clinical evaluation.

If an abnormal connection exists between two distinct anatomic spaces, an injection in one may relieve pain in another, leading to confusion in the interpretation of the injection test. An example of this is in the patient with the full thickness rotator cuff tear who receives a subacromial injection. The tear allows infiltration not only in the subacromial space but also in the shoulder joint proper. Thus, it is incumbent on the examiner to interpret the result of an injection in light of these possibilities.

Subscapular Injection. In patients who present with posterior scapular pain with or without an associated "snapping scapula" (see section on "Noise" as chief complaint), subscapular bursitis may be considered. This condition may produce impressive popping and may have associated pain. Five milliliters of 1% lidocaine can be directed into the more common superomedial or less common inferior angle bursa. This is done by palpating the medial border of the scapula and inserting the needle 1 cm medial to this. The goal is to hit the most anterior portion of the scapula and slide just anterior to this for medication infiltration. Care should be taken not to direct the needle too far anteriorly, because penetration of the thoracic cavity is an undesired consequence. The patient should wait several minutes and attempt to reproduce the pain and noise from the shoulder. Relief of pain helps confirm a subscapular source.

CHIEF COMPLAINT: "SLIPPING," "LOOSENESS," AND "COMING OUT OF JOINT"—INSTABILITY

One of the most challenging culprits in the athletic overhead shoulder is instability. Note that instability is a diagnosis and not generally a chief complaint. Because it is the goal of this chapter to begin always with the chief complaint, one must understand the multitude of ways that the athlete can communicate underlying instability.

Although the athlete may complain that his or her shoulder "comes out of joint," most often a presentation of instability is far subtler and often is not understood by the patient as instability. The classic patterns of "TUBS" and "AMBRI" (2,34) often do not apply to the athletic overhead shoulder. Instability in the overhead athlete is usually subtler than complete dislocation and may present as pain, slipping, sliding, or even as numbness or loss of control or velocity. Conditions such as the "dead arm syndrome" are also indicative of instability. With such a varied complaint set, the astute examiner must remain adherent to the principles of understanding the chief complaint and attempting to reproduce symptoms on physical examination. Instability may be the "great imitator" of the athletic shoulder, in that it can lead to so many different chief complaints. Because it underlies so many pathologies, it is important to look for it in most situations. For example, a patient with internal impingement complains of pain, but his or her pain may be associated with underlying instability. Some surgeons address this assumption surgically by doing thermal capsulorrhaphy or capsular plication to stabilize all patients with internal impingement, whereas others do so only in the presence of internal impingement and increased laxity compared to the opposite side. Although it is not yet clear how aggressive one should be with subtle instability that underlies other pathologies, it is important for the examiner to be aware of its many forms and become skilled in laxity testing and the findings of instability on examination.

Finally, when an athlete complains that the shoulder "comes out," one should also consider a large labral tear or chondral defect, because these pathologies can sometimes masquerade as feelings of instability.

Pertinent Questions: Instability

When the chief complaint leads to the suspicion of instability, the examiner often does not have the luxury of being able to palpate for symptom reproduction, as is the case with other causes of pain. Because instability is a dynamic process, our approach begins with asking the patient to reproduce the sensation. Particular attention is paid to the position that the patient assumes when attempting to reproduce the symptoms, and in throwers, the phase of throwing where problems arise. Often the patient knows that his or her shoulder slides, and he or she is usually right. Determining which direction the shoulder slides can be more difficult to discern.

In most cases in which anterior instability is the underlying problem, symptoms are maximally reproduced in the abducted and externally rotated position, that is, the apprehension position. Patients may place their arm in the cocking position of throwing or state that symptoms occur when they move into the acceleration of the throw. Follow-up questions should include whether the symptoms happen at the beginning of activity in this position or whether the

symptoms get worse as activity continues. The former is consistent with static sources and more severe instability, whereas the latter may represent instability that is masked by dynamic stabilizers such as the rotator cuff until they become fatigued.

Although anterior instability is far more common than in other directions, posterior and multidirectional instability may occur in the athlete. Throwers with posterior instability may describe their sensation to occur during the follow-through phase of a throwing motion, and other athletes may describe their symptoms as taking place during punching maneuvers or when the arm is forward flexed, adducted, and internally rotated. An additional curious complaint is of sliding or of "a hitch" in the lead arm at the top of an aggressive golf swing (35). Although atypical, these patients can be greatly helped if a correct diagnosis is made. Patients with MDI often have problems in all extremes of range of motion and can be some of the more difficult patients to evaluate and treat.

Examination of the Shoulder for Laxity and Instability

With laxity testing, it is important for the patient to be as relaxed as possible. We use a consistent grading system (described later) and ask the patient whether he or she can appreciate the translation (2). We then ask whether the translation reproduces symptoms. Although we use these tests primarily for laxity, grinding, or clicking pain may represent labral tears or chondral defects.

ANTERIOR TESTS

Apprehension Test (Fig. 3-25). This test is performed with the patient either supine (fulcrum) or sitting (crank) by stressing the symptomatic shoulder in maximum abduction and external rotation. The patient may exhibit guarding or other actions that may make the patient or the examiner apprehensive, resulting in a positive test. We believe that this is the best clinical test for anterior instability because it is easy to perform and is very sensitive for producing symptoms in the anteriorly unstable patient. We believe that it is also quite specific, except that the apprehension position is a possible impingement position and thus one must be specific in asking the patient the nature of his symptoms. Pain in this position is different than a feeling that the shoulder is going to come out of joint.

Relocation Test for Instability. (Fig. 3-25). This test is performed just as was described above for pain, except that a positive sign is signified by apprehension or a feeling that the shoulder will come out if further external rotation is applied. Such apprehension should disappear with a posteriorly directed force while holding the arm in the same

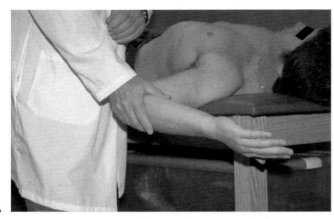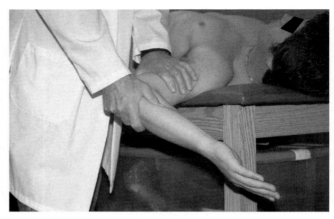

A   B

FIGURE 3-25. Apprehension test **(A)** and relocation test **(B)** for instability.

degree of external rotation; with this posteriorly directed force, the arm can be moved into further external rotation without discomfort. We often increase the external rotation slightly while holding the humerus back, then release this posterior pressure. This often reproduces the patient's symptoms exactly. We have found this test to be highly sug-

gestive of anterior instability, and we place a great deal of emphasis on it during our examination.

Load and Shift Test (Fig. 3-26). The load and shift test is a test for laxity or translation of the shoulder. It is performed with the patient in the supine and seated positions

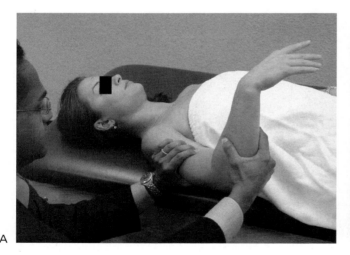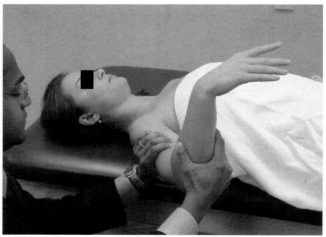

A   B

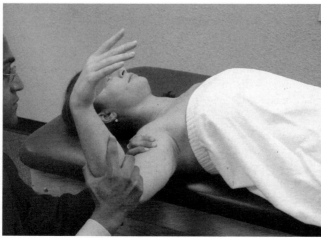

C

FIGURE 3-26. Load and shift test. Adduction supine **(A)**; 45 degrees supine **(B)**; 90 degrees supine **(C)**.

at various levels of glenohumeral abduction. In the seated position, the examiner stands behind the affected shoulder. One hand is used to stabilize the scapula by grasping the anterior and posterior acromion between the fingers. The other hand grasps the humeral head and by applying compression along with anterior and posterior force, the translational movement of the humerus on the glenoid can be appreciated. Grading of this passive translation includes motion up the face (normal or grade 0), up the face to the glenoid rim (grade 1), over the rim but spontaneously reducible (grade 2), and over the rim into a position of fixed dislocation that will not spontaneously reduce (grade 3) (2). This test can be repeated posteriorly with a similar grading system. It is important to compare the translational grades to the asymptomatic side, because gross differences may suggest abnormal laxity.

The load and shift may be repeated with the patient supine (our preference). In this position, the examiner holds the patient's wrist with one hand while the other hand grasps the humerus, and again provides some load with translational force. The test is done with the arm at the side at 45 degrees and at 90 degrees. We occasionally "dial in" the laxity by progressively abducting and rotating the arm while performing the load and shift test. Patients who continue to translate at increased glenohumeral abduction angles compared to the opposite side may indicate laxity of the inferior glenohumeral ligament. We always ask patients whether they can appreciate the translation, and if they respond "yes," we ask if this sensation reproduces their symptoms.

There are several aspects to this test that may limit its clinical utility. First, any patient who is guarded can make the test unreliable. Second, because anterior instability is normally a problem with the inferior glenohumeral ligament, it makes sense that the most useful portion of the test would be done at 90 degrees of abduction. However, achieving this position requires that one of the examiner's hands holds the patient's arm, which then prevents it from being used to stabilize the scapula. Thus, the mobility of the scapula on the thorax decreases the sensitivity of the test. Finally, although the load and shift test can be learned to detect subtle differences in side-to-side laxity, we do not treat laxity. As stated earlier, laxity is a clinical *sign*, whereas instability is a *symptom*.

POSTERIOR TESTS

The workhorse test for posterior instability is the *push-pull test* (Fig. 3-27). This is performed in the supine patient by holding the patient's arm at the wrist at 90 degrees abduction and neutral rotation (2,9). The examiner places the other hand on the proximal humerus and while pulling with the arm holding the patient's wrist, the examiner pushes with the arm on the proximal humerus. This is often enough to maximally translate the patient's

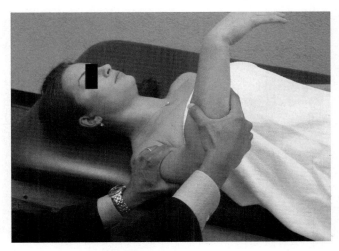

FIGURE 3-27. Push-pull test.

humeral head posteriorly. Again, the test is positive only when the maneuver reproduces the patient's symptoms, and in our experience, the patient's response to this test is not subtle. The only caution here is to be sure to differentiate between pain and instability, in that we have found the former to be consistently present with posterior and superior labral tears.

Jahnke or "Jerk" Test (Fig. 3-28). This test is performed in the seated or supine patient by placing the affected arm in maximal horizontal adduction with internal rotation (2,9). A posterior force is then applied. In the patient with posterior instability, this starting position subluxes or dislocates the shoulder posteriorly, and care is taken to ask the patient whether this maneuver reproduces specific symptoms. Next, the shoulder is brought back from horizontal adduction while maintaining the posterior force on the humerus at the elbow. As the shoulder approaches normal, a clunk may herald the reduction of the subluxed shoulder, which is a positive test. In our experience, this test has few false-positive results and therefore has a good positive predictive value.

TESTS FOR MULTIDIRECTIONAL INSTABILITY

Because patients with MDI often present with a chief complaint of pain, we believe that such tests are more appropriate in the section on pain. However, there are complementary data that should be included in the evaluation of the patient with MDI. The classic finding associated with MDI is a positive sulcus sign (Fig. 3-18). This is a visible dimpling between the bottom of the acromion and the top of the humeral head when an inferior traction force is placed on the arm. This is quantified by measur-

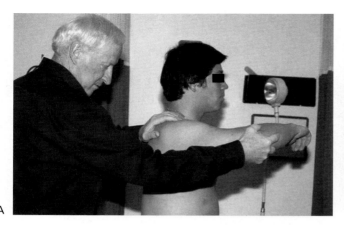
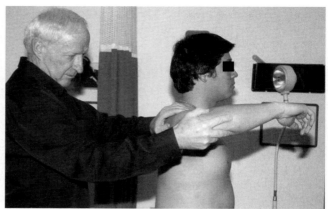

A   B

FIGURE 3-28. A,B: Jahnke (jerk) test.

ing this acromiohumeral distance in millimeters. The normal shoulder sits approximately 7 to 8 mm below the acromion, so that an acromiohumeral distance of 1.5 cm is really only 7 to 8 mm of excursion. It is again emphasized that instability implies symptoms and that a positive sulcus sign is not enough to grant the diagnosis. Nevertheless, it is an important adjunctive clue for the diagnosis, and when positive, attempts should be made to correlate it with symptoms. When instability is the underlying diagnosis in MDI, patients often complain that their shoulder comes "out the bottom," and we therefore ask patients about this specifically if we are concerned that MDI is the underlying diagnosis.

There are other clues and complexes to note when entertaining the diagnosis of MDI. Many of these patients have generalized ligamentous laxity, which can be measured with such tests as an ability to touch the thumb to the forearm (2,9,23) and hyperextension of the elbow or knee. These patients often have reproduction of their symptoms in all directions of translational testing, and they can be difficult to manage conservatively or operatively. Often patients with MDI demonstrate a sulcus sign, in which downward traction on the humerus produces a noticeable dimpling between the top of the humerus and bottom of the acromion, and demonstrates laxity in the anterior and posterior directions.

CHIEF COMPLAINT: "WEAKNESS," "HEAVINESS," OR "TIREDNESS"

These chief complaints can have several sources. With such complaints, we formulate an initial differential diagnosis of a muscle problem such as scapular dyskinesia, a neurologic problem such as suprascapular nerve palsy, or, in rare cases (especially with tiredness), a vascular problem, and our workup proceeds from here.

Muscle Sources

We recommend that the examiner begin by asking the patient during which activities and in what position he or she is weak. Because so many athletes are involved in year-round strength training, they are often sensitive to changes in their lifting abilities, and they often present early and with subtle findings. The examiner must use enough force to overcome the tested muscle. We use a standard approach to the muscular examination (36) including those listed in Table 3-4 (as well as the rotator cuff tests discussed earlier).

Scapular Dyskinesia

The function of the upper extremity is dependent on a number of factors. One of the most important of these is a stable and strong scapular platform to support the motions of the shoulder joint. Abnormalities of this platform may be as subtle as early activation of the scapular rotators to assist in glenohumeral elevation or as pronounced as severe and fixed scapular winging. Such dyskinesia can lead to a variety of chief complaints including pain, weakness, loss of control, and crepitance, among others. Given such a wide variety of chief complaints that can be attributed to this

TABLE 3–4. MUSCLE TESTS ABOUT THE SHOULDER

Muscle	Test
Trapezius	Shoulder shrug
Deltoid	Resisted abduction
Biceps	Resisted forearm supination
Triceps	Resisted elbow flexion
Brachialis	Resisted elbow extension
Wrist flexors	Resisted wrist flexion
Wrist extensors	Resisted wrist extension
Interossei	Resisted finger abduction

problem, it is rare for any patient *not* to warrant a careful look at the scapular platform.

Scapular dyskinesia is best tested by examining the disrobed patient from behind. The patient is asked to repetitively elevate and lower his or her arms at a moderate pace while the examiner notes the scapula for signs of dyskinesia or winging. Static winging often signifies either a long thoracic or spinal accessory nerve palsy, whereas dynamic winging or early substitution often points to compensation for a glenohumeral joint abnormality. Winging can be maximized by performing resisted shoulder flexion at about 30 degrees of elevation (Fig. 3-20), by asking the patient to perform a wall push-up, or by having the patient use his or her arms to elevate out of a chair.

When winging is noted on examination, it is helpful to guess whether it is primary, as in a nerve palsy, or secondary, as in compensating for a diseased glenohumeral joint. Findings associated with a primary cause include a static or fixed scapular wing that is often painless, whereas a compensatory dyskinesia is often more subtle, presenting as early substitution during elevation with associated glenohumeral abnormalities. In either case, it is important for the examiner to note these findings and to suggest correction of both the dyskinesia and the underlying shoulder abnormality.

Neurologic Sources of Weakness

Any athlete who presents with weakness about the shoulder should also be suspected of having a neurologic cause of the weakness. The most common sources in the athlete are compression at the level of the cervical spine and neuropathy of the suprascapular nerve (6,37).

A thorough understanding of the cervical spine neurologic examination is a baseline requirement for any shoulder surgeon. Because cervical spine pathology can present as pain, paresthesias, or weakness about the shoulder, it is consequently a part of the shoulder workup. Although provocative maneuvers for reproduction of radiculopathy are presented in the section on pain, the specific neuroanatomy pertinent to the sensory and motor examination of the cervical spine is listed below in Table 3-5.

It is uncommon for a radiculopathy to result in weakness without pain, and the examiner is referred to the cervical spine sources for shoulder pain in the section previously outlined. Any findings of weakness should be cross-checked for pain with the various cervical spine provocative tests to strengthen or discredit the suspicion of a cervical source for the shoulder symptoms.

Suprascapular Nerve

This is a common cause of weakness in the athlete and should be considered high on the list when an athlete presents with a complaint of weakness in external rotation or elevation, especially with an intact rotator cuff. The examiner should be mindful of the anatomy of the nerve, and know that it has two chief sites of entrapment. The first is at the suprascapular notch, where such compression would result in weakness of both supraspinatus and infraspinatus weakness and possibly atrophy; the second site of entrapment, the spinoglenoid notch, usually spares the supraspinatus. Thus, if one notes weakness in Jobe's position and in external rotation, the differential might include either a large tear of the rotator cuff or a suprascapular nerve entrapment. Such a large tear would normally require a history of significant trauma in the young athlete, and therefore the two diagnoses are often easily differentiated. Compression of this nerve has been reported in volleyball players (38), baseball players (39), and gymnasts (40). Sometimes a patient presents with isolated infraspinatus atrophy and weakness. In such patients, consideration should be given to an isolated compression of the suprascapular nerve at the spinoglenoid notch. A common cause of this in athletes is a ganglion cyst in conjunction with a posterior or posterosuperior labral tear (38). These tears usually cause pain, and often can demonstrate tenderness, atrophy, and weakness on examination (41).

Brachial Neuritis

Although not a true compressive neuropathy, the acute onset of brachial neuritis has been documented in athletes (42) and may manifest as weakness in a patchy distribution of C5 to T1 neurologic levels. A more complete discussion of this condition is presented in the section on pain, because that is the far more common presentation of this condition.

Finally, chief complaints of weakness, heaviness, or tiredness should lead the examiner to think of a vascular source.

TABLE 3–5. NEUROLOGIC LEVELS IN THE UPPER EXTREMITY (KRISHNAN, HAWKINS, BOKOR)

Nerve Root	Sensory	Motor	Reflex
C5	Lateral deltoid	Deltoid abduction	Biceps
C6	Thumb	Biceps/wrist extension	Brachioradialis/biceps
C7	Middle finger	Triceps/wrist flexors/ finger extension	Triceps
C8	Ulnar border of middle finger	Finger flexors	
T1	Medial side proximal arm	Finger abduction	

One such source is "effort thrombosis" (43), which is venous thrombosis of the axillary or subclavian veins in close proximity to the intersection of the clavicle and first rib. Specific findings in this diagnosis include venous engorgement of the arm, upper extremity swelling of several centimeters, discoloration, and palpable cords.

CHIEF COMPLAINT: "NUMBNESS OR TINGLING"—PARESTHESIAS

A number of conditions may lead the athlete to seek treatment for numbness or tingling. If one rules out the possible cervical pathologies discussed earlier, then the initial differential should concentrate on sources of peripheral nerve compression. The pertinent sources include thoracic outlet syndrome, burners, and brachial neuritis. If distal in the arm, compression of the median and ulnar nerves may also be considered.

Thoracic outlet syndrome is an uncommon but important source of paresthesias in the athlete. It is associated with neurologic symptoms in more than 90% of patients, and presents with primary vascular symptoms in only 3% to 5% of cases (43). This syndrome often presents in throwers and racquet sports athletes, is often insidious, and can present as pain, or heaviness. Neurologic findings can vary, but usually involve the lower brachial plexus and affect the forearm and hand (44). However, thoracic outlet syndrome has also been reported to manifest as a high radial nerve palsy with triceps weakness in tennis players (45,46).

Provocative Maneuvers for Thoracic Outlet Syndrome

Perhaps the best test for thoracic outlet syndrome is with overhead exercises consisting of slow repetitive opening and closing of the hand in the elevated position looking for reproduction of symptoms (9). In addition, several maneuvers have been described to detect the neurovascular symptoms that result from compression of the thoracic outlet.

Adson's Maneuver (Fig. 3-29). This is accomplished by palpating the patient's radial pulse in a seated position with the arm at the side. The patient is instructed to hold his or her breath while the arm is extended and the head rotated toward the side being examined. The examiner documents a diminution in the radial pulse, which is recorded as a positive finding for vascular compression (fielding). We modify this test by turning the patient's head away from the side being examined (2,9), and deem a positive test not only by a decrease in pulse but also by reproduction of symptoms.

Hyperabduction Syndrome Test. In this test, the radial pulses are again monitored for change with the arms brought from resting to a hyperabducted position. It should

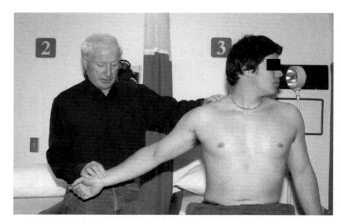

FIGURE 3-29. Modified Adson's maneuver.

be noted that 20% of individuals demonstrate a diminution of the radial pulse in this position, so attention should be paid to asymmetry (2).

Wright's Test. This test is performed by abducting, extending, and externally rotating the arm (47). It is traditionally a test to monitor decrease in radial pulse, but we again modify this for reproduction of the patient's specific symptoms to call the test positive.

In addition to these findings, thoracic outlet syndrome can rarely present with vascular symptoms such as engorgement and increased arm circumference, raising suspicion of thrombosis as described earlier.

Although burners and brachial neuritis more commonly present as pain and dysesthesias, some patients have a difficult time describing their symptoms, so that such complaints should illicit some suspicion of these diagnoses.

CHIEF COMPLAINT: "CATCHING" OR "CLUNKING"

When a patient presents with catching or clunking, the differential should include a SLAP tear or other labral lesions, a loose body, an osteochondral defect, or instability. Note that these mechanical symptoms are different from "popping" or "crackling," which is a common finding with subacromial crepitance. It is usually not difficult to differentiate between the two, because the noise from the subacromial space is usually not accompanied by much disability, whereas true mechanical symptoms generally are immediately, although often temporarily, disabling. The patient should be asked to attempt to reproduce the symptoms. This is an important step, in that the active shoulder motions that can get the shoulder to catch are often not demonstrated on passive movement of the joint. If the symptoms can be reproduced by the patient, we attempt to temporarily provide relief with an injection. Because most causes of mechanical symptoms of the shoulder are intraarticular, we generally begin with an intraarticular injection. The injection should relieve any painful or disabling symptoms with the provocative maneuvers, and it may temporarily relieve the mechanical symptom itself because the increase in intraarticular fluid often cushions the inside of the joint. If the injection is effective, an imaging modality sometimes provides the specific cause of the mechanical symptom.

CHIEF COMPLAINT: "NOISE"

One common chief complaint, or at least a common concern for athletes, is "popping," "crunching," or "grinding" in the shoulder. These can run the spectrum from being completely asymptomatic, inaudible noise to being painful cracks that concern both the patient and the examiner. Crepitus in the shoulder girdle should suggest an initial differential of subacromial (impingement), glenohumeral (degenerate joint disease, chondral defect, loose body), or scapulothoracic (subscapular bursitis) sources. The goal of the examiner in these cases is to find out whether the noise is associated with an additional chief complaint such as pain. By having the patient or examiner reproduce the noise, it can usually be localized to its origin. The examiner should ask the patient whether the popping is associated with the pain, or whether it simply occurs but is not painful. One might ask, if the popping is taken away, would the shoulder be perfect? Is the patient there regarding the noise, or for some other reason, like pain? The most common source of crepitus in the shoulder is subacromial associated with impingement. Although the patient may associate the noise with symptoms, the patient with impingement often demonstrates the crepitus for the examiner to hear, and the demonstration of crepitus is not nearly as painful as it is during maneuvers like the Neer's test. This patient is contrasted with the one who is reluctant to demonstrate his or her crepitus, because such a demonstration hurts. This noise is often less like grinding and more like a series of larger "cracks," which are obviously painful with each iteration. This second type may be associated with an intraarticular source, and one should think of loose body or a cartilage defect. It is rare to treat such noise in the absence of pain or disability.

Once the examiner has a good sense of the degree of disability of the popping as an isolated entity, he should move on to trying to reproduce the popping. This may be done by placing a hand on the top of the shoulder and asking the patient to reproduce the noise. A patient who moves his or her glenohumeral joint through a range of motion to demonstrate the noise is likely to have a subacromial source. This is a softer crepitus than in the patient who has the painful bone-on-bone grind of arthritis. The examiner should pay particular note to a patient who, when asked to reproduce the noise, moves only slightly from the glenohumeral joint, but reproduces the crepitus by moving the scapula or shrugging the shoulders. This is a classic finding in a patient with subscapular crepitus.

Once demonstrated, the patient should be specifically asked whether the crepitus is the chief complaint. Patients with subacromial symptoms are often able to differentiate the two, but patients with intraarticular sources often are not. If pain is the true chief complaint, with the crepitus being coexistent, the examiner should attempt to use the aforementioned techniques to narrow the source of the pain and to use various injection tests to eliminate the pain and arrive at a diagnosis. Crepitus may or may not be silenced by the injection, and attention should again be directed to alleviation of the patient's symptoms, not the associated noise.

CHIEF COMPLAINT: LOSS OF CONTROL OR LOSS OF VELOCITY

When a patient presents with this complaint, the initial differential should include dynamic instability often associated with SLAP tears and internal impingement, as well as muscle weakness and scapular dyskinesia. Throwing is an extremely complex athletic maneuver, relying on the specific coordination of the entire kinetic chain. This chief complaint is often among the most difficult to discern, because, by its nature, it implies that the athlete is able to throw and thus the impediment is usually a subtle one. In addition, because this often is a dynamic complaint (i.e., only demonstrated when the patient is throwing), reproducing the patient's symptoms may not be possible in the office. It is sometimes necessary to go to the field or the weight room to elicit signs or reproduce the patient's symptoms. Despite the difficulty of symptom reproduction, there are some techniques that help in the approach to this chief complaint.

Does the loss of control or decreased speed happen in initial or in later innings? In the thrower who complains of decreased velocity or loss of control that is present at the outset of throwing, the initial differential should point more toward a static condition affecting the kinetic chain. The chain starts in the core with the legs and trunk, and although herein we emphasize the shoulder, it is important to appreciate that such problems often originate lower in the chain. The astute examiner will do well to inquire and examine the lower extremities and trunk for causes of shoulder pathology. If the core is functioning properly, then the shoulder differential should include causes of weakness, subtle instability, SLAP tears, and cuff problems. Refer to those sections for the focused examinations for those pathologies.

If a pitcher starts out normally but loses command later, the problem is more likely dynamic. This makes the evaluation more challenging, in that findings may be minimal in an office evaluation. The importance of "revving up" the shoulder is emphasized. The initial differential includes dynamic fatigue or instability. As a pitcher continues to throw, he may become fatigued in any segment of his kinetic chain, leading to compensatory maneuvers such as "dropping the elbow," using a straighter lead leg, or using less external rotation at the shoulder (48). These compensations, which have been noted by pitching coaches for years, lead to increasing strains in the shoulder when the athlete continues to pitch. This may lead to new shoulder problems that are difficult to completely eliminate until the more proximal elements of the chain are evaluated and rehabilitated.

CHIEF COMPLAINT: "STIFFNESS"

True stiffness, defined as a mechanical block to passive motion, can present with or without pain, and can be global or in selected motions. In most athletes, stiffness occurs in the presence of a painful shoulder. When stiffness does coincide with pain, refer to the pain as chief complaint section, because diagnosis and treatment of the pain source often leads to resolution of the stiffness. Occasionally, stiffness can contribute to pain, especially in the throwing athlete. For example, posterior capsular tightness in pitchers is likely an adaptive change from the powerful forces created in repetitive pitching. This stiffness can be measured as the distance between the coracoid and the antecubital fossa when the athlete is in a position of maximal horizontal adduction with a straight elbow (Fig. 3-30). Other causes of stiffness in the shoulder include adhesive capsulitis, osteoarthritis, and synovitis. In addition, patients who have had previous anterior stabilizations should be closely examined for overtightening, especially limiting external rotation, because these patients can present with such selective stiffness.

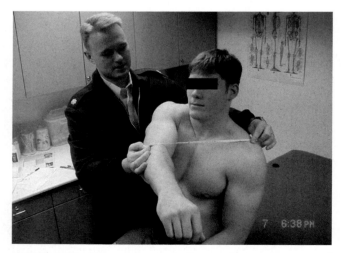

FIGURE 3-30. Coracoantecubital distance for measurement of posterior capsular tightness.

CONCLUSION

This chapter presents a focused approach to the evaluation of the athlete's shoulder that begins with an understanding of the patient's chief complaint and, based on this, the immediate formation of a differential diagnosis. The accuracy of this differential is enhanced by asking the right questions in the history such as onset, character, duration, clinical course, degree of disability, and response to clinical intervention. This differential-directed approach then guides the remainder of the encounter.

The physical examination of the throwing athlete remains a challenging art. However, with a knowledge of various tests and techniques, the examiner can often narrow its focus. The examination should be organized and comprehensive, but with expectations for findings directed by the differential (i.e., "going for the money"). Finally, when possible, and especially when pain is a chief complaint, we are liberal in our use of local anesthetic to temporarily and completely relieve the patient's chief complaint as an aid to narrowing the diagnosis.

The advantage of the differential approach is that it establishes a suspected diagnosis at the beginning of the encounter and leads the examiner regarding what to look for during the examination. When one elicits positive findings that are expected, one's suspicions of the diagnosis are strengthened. However, even when the examiner is surprised by unexpected findings, it will redirect him or her toward another diagnosis that is also in the differential.

Formulating a differential at the beginning of the encounter, however, does have its risks. One must be careful not to be convinced too quickly, because overconfidence leads to a biased interpretation of the physical examination findings and can result in a misdiagnosis. In addition, the quality of the differential and the skill of validating it depend largely on the examiner's knowledge of shoulder pathology and the various forms in which it presents. In describing this process of a focused approach, we intend for the examiner to become better able to formulate a short list of diagnoses early in the encounter, so that the examiner will be more directed, efficient, and accurate in the approach to the athlete's shoulder.

REFERENCES

1. Hawkins RJ. *Musculoskeletal examination: an organized approach to musculoskeletal examination and history taking.* Boston: Mosby–Year Book, 1995.
2. Krishnan SG, Hawkins RJ, Bokor DJ. Clinical evaluation of shoulder problems. In: Rockwood CA, Matsen FA, eds. *The shoulder*, 3rd ed. Philadelphia: WB Saunders, 2004.
3. Sher JS, Uribe JW, Posada A, et al. Abnormal findings on magnetic resonance images of asymptomatic shoulders. *J Bone Joint Surg (Am)* 1995;77(1):10–15.
4. Miniaci A, Mascia AT, Salonen DC, et al. Magnetic resonance

imaging of the shoulder in asymptomatic professional baseball pitchers. *Am J Sports Med* 2002;30:66–73.

5. Traughber PD, Goodwin TE. Shoulder MRI: arthroscopic correlation with emphasis on partial tears. *J Comput Assist Tomogr* 1992;16:129–133.

6. King JW, Brelsford HJ, Tullos HS. Analysis of the pitching arm of the professional baseball pitcher. *Clin Orthop* 1969;67:116–123.

7. Calis M, Akgun K, Birtane M, et al. Diagnostic values of clinical diagnostic tests in subacromial impingement syndrome. *Ann Rheum Dis* 2000;59:44–47.

8. MacDonald PB, Clark P, Sutherland K. An analysis of the diagnostic accuracy of the Hawkins and Neer subacromial impingement signs. *J Shoulder Elbow Surg* 2000;9:299–301.

9. Boublik M, Silliman JF. History and physical examination. In: Hawkins RJ, Misamore GW, eds. *Shoulder injuries in the athlete.* New York: Churchill Livingstone, 1996:9–22.

10. Yocum LA. Assessing the shoulder. History, physical examination, differential diagnosis, and special tests used. *Clin Sports Med* 1983;2:281–289.

11. Itoi E, Kido T, Sano A, et al. Which is more useful, the "full can test" or the "empty can test," in detecting the torn supraspinatus tendon? *Am J Sports Med* 1999;27:65–68.

12. Gerber C, Krushell RJ. Isolated rupture of the tendon of the subscapularis muscle. Clinical features in 16 cases. *J Bone Joint Surg* 1991;73:389–394.

13. Tokish JM, Decker M, Ellis H, et al. The belly press test for the physical examination of the subscapularis muscle: electromyographic validation and comparison to the lift-off test. Presented at the American Shoulder and Elbow Surgeons 3rd Biennial Open Meeting, Orlando, FL, 2002.

14. Hertel R, Ballmer FT, Lombert SM, et al. Lag signs in the diagnosis of rotator cuff rupture. *J Shoulder Elbow Surg* 1996;5:307–313.

15. Codman EA. *The shoulder: rupture of the supraspinatus tendon and other lesions in or about the subacromial bursa.* Chapter V. Original edition, Boston: Thomas Todd, 1934:123–177. Reprint edition, Melbourne, FL: Krieger, 1984.

16. Wolf EM, Agrawal V. Transdeltoid palpation (the rent test) in the diagnosis of rotator cuff tears. *J Shoulder Elbow Surg* 2001;10:470–473.

17. Petersson CJ. The acromioclavicular joint in rheumatoid arthritis. *Clin Orthop* 1987;223:86–93.

18. O'Brien SJ, Pagnani MJ, Fealy S, et al. The active compression test: a new and effective test for diagnosing labral tears and acromioclavicular joint abnormality. *Am J Sports Med* 1998;26:610–613.

19. Bennett WF. Specificity of the Speed's test: arthroscopic technique for evaluation the biceps tendon at the level of the bicipital groove. *Arthroscopy* 1998;14:789–796.

20. Matsen FA, Kirby R. Office evaluation and management of shoulder pain. *Orthop Clin North Am* 1982;13:45.

21. Snyder SJ, Karzel RP, Del Pizzo W, et al. SLAP lesions of the shoulder. *Arthroscopy* 1990;6:274–279.

22. Berg EE, Ciullo JV. A clinical test for superior glenoid labral or "SLAP" lesions. *Clin J Sport Med* 1998;8:121–123.

23. Kim SH, Ha KI, Ahn JH, et al. Biceps load test II: a clinical test for SLAP lesions of the shoulder. *Arthroscopy* 2001;17:160–164.

24. Kibler WB. Specificity and sensitivity of the anterior slide test in throwing athletes with superior glenoid labral tears. *Arthroscopy* 1995;11:296–300.

25. Dines DM, Warren RF, Inglis AE, et al. The coracoid impingement syndrome. *J Bone Joint Surg (Br)* 1990;72:314–316.

26. Paley KJ, Jobe FW, Pink MM, et al. Arthroscopic findings in the overhand throwing athlete: evidence for posterior internal impingement of the rotator cuff. *Arthroscopy* 2000;16:35–40.

27. Tong HC, Haig AJ, Yamakawa K. The Spurling test and cervical radiculopathy. *Spine* 2002;15:156–159.

28. Porter P, Fernandez GN. Stretch-induced spinal accessory nerve palsy: a case report. *J Shoulder Elbow Surg* 2001;10:92–93.

29. Post M, Mayer J. Suprascapular nerve entrapment: diagnosis and treatment. *Clin Orthop* 1987;223:125–136.

30. Ringel SP, Treihaft M, Carry M, et al. Suprascapular neuropathy in pitchers. *Am J Sports Med* 1990;18:80–86.

31. Rowe CR, ed. *The shoulder.* New York: Churchill Livingstone, 1988:419.

32. Zaslav KR. Internal rotation resistance strength test: a new diagnostic test to differentiate intra-articular pathology from outlet (Neer) impingement syndrome in the shoulder. *J Shoulder Elbow Surg* 2001;10:23–27.

33. Partington PF, Broome GH. Diagnostic injection around the shoulder: hit and miss? A cadaveric study of injection accuracy. *J Shoulder Elbow Surg* 1998;7:147–150.

34. Matsen FA, Thomas SC, Rockwood CA, et al. Glenohumeral instability. In: Rockwood CA, Matsen FA, eds. *The shoulder*, 2nd ed. Philadelphia: WB Saunders, 1998:611–754.

35. Hovis WD, Dean MT, Mallon WJ, et al. Posterior instability of the shoulder with secondary impingement in elite golfers. *Am J Sports Med* 2002;30:886–890.

36. Netter FH. The CIBA collection of medical illustrations: musculoskeletal system part I: anatomy, physiology and metabolic disorders. Ciba-Geigy Corporation, 1991:29.

37. Fielding JW, Francis WR, Hensinger RN. The cervical and thoracic spine. In: Cruess RJ, Rennie WRJ, eds. *Adult orthopaedics*, vol 2. New York: Churchill Livingstone, 1984:747–841.

38. Feretti A, Cerullo G, Russo G. Suprascapular neuropathy in volleyball players. *J Bone Joint Surg (Am)* 1987;69:260.

39. Bryan WJ, Wild JJ. Isolated infraspinatus atrophy: a common cause of posterior shoulder pain and weakness in the throwing athlete. *Am J Sports Med* 1989;17:130.

40. Lauland T, Fedders O, Sgaard I, et al. Suprascapular nerve compression syndrome. *Surg Neurol* 1984;22:308.

41. Piatt BE, Hawkins RJ, Fritz RC, et al. Clinical evaluation and treatment of spinoglenoid notch ganglion cysts. *J Shoulder Elbow Surg* 2002;11:600-604.

42. Hershman EB, Wilbourn AJ, Bergfeld JA. Acute brachial neuropathy in athletes. *Am J Sports Med* 1989;17:655–659.

43. DiFelice GS, Paletta GA, Phillips BB, et al. Effort thrombosis in the elite throwing athlete. *Am J Sports Med* 2002;30:708–712.

44. Duralde XA, Bigliani LU. Neurologic disorders. In: Hawkins RJ, Misamore GW, eds. *Shoulder injuries in the athlete.* New York: Churchill Livingstone, 1996:243–265.

45. Mitsunga MM, Nakano K. High radial nerve palsy following strenuous muscular activity. *Clin Orthop* 1982;98:39.

46. Priest JD. The shoulder of the tennis player. *Clin Sports Med* 1988;7:387.

47. Wright IS. The neurovascular syndrome produced by hyperabduction of the arm. *Am Heart J* 1945;29:1.

48. Murray TA, Cook TD, Werner SL, et al. The effects of extended play on professional pitchers. *Am J Sports Med* 2001;29:137–142.

4

IMAGING OF THE OVERHEAD ATHLETE

CHARLES P. HO
ERIC D. SMITH

INTRODUCTION

The shoulder has the most complex and greatest range of motion of any joint in the body. This range and versatility is possible because of the articulation of the relatively large humeral head and smaller and shallow glenoid fossa. The inherently unequal osseous articulation must rely on the glenoid labrum to deepen and enlarge the glenoid socket and on the capsular–labral complex, glenohumeral ligaments, and rotator cuff to provide additional stability as well as power for shoulder function. This complex anatomy and function are vital to the overhead athlete as well as overhead use in occupational endeavors and activities of daily living. Overhead function produces extensive demands on the soft tissues and osseous structures of the shoulder, often leading to pain and dysfunction. The clinical evaluation of these symptoms is complex and at times inconclusive. Imaging evaluation, both with conventional radiographs and magnetic resonance imaging (MRI), has proven an invaluable aid for both diagnosis and reassessment after treatment.

The approach to imaging of the overhead athlete applies to swimmers, gymnasts, climbers, throwing athletes, paddlers, players of racquet sports, and athletes who engage in weight training either as the primary sport or as supplemental training. Repetitive overhead activity in the workplace as performed by painters, carpenters, or laborers subjects the shoulder to similar stresses and leads to similar patterns of injury as in the sports participants. This large cohort of patients is subject to the same injuries as occur in nonoverhead athletes as well as more activity-specific injuries.

RADIOGRAPHIC EVALUATION

The goals of any radiographic examination are to provide the treating physician with the necessary supporting diagnostic information to facilitate treatment with as little expense, complexity, time delay, and patient discomfort as possible. It is equally important for both the imaging specialist and treating specialist to be confident in the validity and repro-ducibility of the techniques used. Patients must be able to tolerate the length and positioning of the examination.

Conventional radiographs are the starting point for the imaging evaluation of nearly all musculoskeletal complaints. In the evaluation of the shoulder, they are rarely the final imaging step. They do demonstrate osseous anatomy, but their projectional rather than tomographic nature limits the evaluation of three-dimensional relationships. They provide the most limited evaluation of soft tissue. Most pathologic processes affecting the overhead athlete only demonstrate radiographic changes at the late stages, long after the optimal period for intervention.

Radiographs are most helpful in initial screening for fractures or advanced osseous degenerative change. They are also helpful in the demonstration of dystrophic or heterotopic calcification and in the evaluation and characterization of primary osseous or chondral neoplasms.

Computed tomography (CT) has optimal spatial resolution and is the most sensitive technique for showing cortical bone, complex fracture anatomy, and small amounts of calcification or ossification. Without the introduction of intraarticular contrast (gas or iodinated contrast), CT is well suited to detection of intraarticular osseous or calcific bodies, whereas intraarticular contrast may assist in evaluation of soft tissue internal bodies or debris. However, the limited soft tissue characterization of CT makes it primarily a specialty, problem-solving tool in shoulder evaluation.

In recent years, high-resolution ultrasound of the musculoskeletal system has gained in popularity and use. One of the first areas of clinical utility was in the evaluation of the rotator cuff. In experienced hands, ultrasound is highly accurate in the diagnosis of rotator cuff tears. It has high patient satisfaction, low cost, and comparatively fewer equipment requirements. However, it is less well suited for evaluating osseous anatomy, articular cartilage, and labral abnormalities that affect overhead athletes. It also has a much higher level of operator dependence. The images obtained are often more difficult for clinical colleagues to appreciate because they bear less resemblance to surgical anatomy.

MRI has become the most widely accepted technique for evaluation of the shoulder. No other technique combines its soft tissue resolution and multiplanar capability. It is the imaging gold standard for evaluation of internal derangements and shows the highest correlation with surgical results.

GENERAL SHOULDER MRI

MRI of the shoulder poses greater technical difficulty and is more often the focus of debate and controversy than imaging of other areas of the musculoskeletal system. The highly complex and variable nature of the labral and capsular structures also makes interpretation complex. There is a growing diversity of both hardware and software alternatives that make generalization about technique and establishment of standard imaging protocols difficult.

The demand for lower cost MRI combined with technical advances has led to the development of a great diversity of magnets. These include whole-body magnets as well as extremity-only scanners. Whole-body scanners are available in two basic configurations: open and closed. Closed magnets are more common and have been the predominant design for high field strength imaging. Open systems are designed to reduce the risk of claustrophobia. They are often permanent magnets that operate at room temperature and generally cost less than closed, superconducting magnets. However, the trade-off for lower field strength in the open systems is longer imaging time to achieve equal signal-to-noise and spatial resolution (1). The longer imaging time may in turn contribute to patient discomfort and motion with resulting image degradation. Lower field strength systems also restrict the ability to perform spectral fat suppression.

Coil selection is an important part of MR image quality. As with scanners, multiple different designs are available. Phased-array coils offer the highest signal-to-noise ratio. Flex coils are versatile and well suited to a range of shoulder configurations and positions. In most all situations, a single surface coil is used.

SPECIFIC SHOULDER MRI CONSIDERATIONS

The bore size of closed whole body MR systems only allows for the shoulder to be imaged with the arm at the patient's side or overhead. Open systems allow for more flexibility in patient positioning. The shoulder is most commonly imaged with the patient supine and the arm at the patient's side. Positioning of the hand determines the degree of external rotation. The extent of rotation is controversial. External rotation with the thumb away from the patient can be uncomfortable, tightens the anterior capsule, and can cause gas to form in the joint via vacuum phenomenon. Internal rotation with the thumb directed toward the patient causes the infraspinatus tendon to overlap the supraspinatus tendon and causes the subscapularis tendon to be redundant, folding on itself. Neu-

tral positioning with the thumb directed up is usually best tolerated by the patient and minimizes motion artifacts.

Routine shoulder MRI is usually performed in three planes. A plane axial to the glenohumeral joint serves as a localizer for obtaining the oblique sagittal and coronal planes. The oblique coronal plane follows the orientation of the supraspinatus and infraspinatus muscle bellies. It is usually obtained by aligning with the scapular spine and orthogonal to the glenoid fossa plane on a mid glenoid slice of the axial localizer. The oblique sagittal plane is also obtained from an axial localizer, but is parallel to the articular surface of the glenoid and perpendicular to the scapular spine. Even though an attempt is made to evaluate all structures in all planes, certain anatomic features are best demonstrated in one projection. The axial plane is best suited for evaluation of the acromion base, anterior and posterior labrum, glenohumeral articular surface, intertubercular biceps tendon, and subscapularis tendon. The oblique coronal plane optimizes evaluation of the superior and inferior labrum, labral-biceps anchor, acromioclavicular (AC) joint, and supraspinatus and infraspinatus muscles. The oblique sagittal plane is best for evaluation of the coracoacromial arch, intraarticular long biceps tendon, and rotator interval.

The overhead position (also referred to as *ABER* for abduction and external rotation) is achieved in a supine patient by positioning the patient's hand over or behind his head (2). Oblique axial images are obtained by aligning sections with the long axis of the humerus and orthogonal to the glenoid fossa plane using a coronal localizer. The plane is particularly helpful for demonstrating the undersurface of supraspinatus and infraspinatus tendons. It also shows the inferior glenohumeral ligament as well as the anterioinferior labrum under tension. It is also helpful to appreciate the cuff undersurface to posterior-superior glenoid and labral relationships in the overhead position that may contribute to clinical posterior-superior (internal) impingement. However, the position is often poorly tolerated by the patient with a painful shoulder and adds additional time to the imaging examination.

Sequence options for shoulder imaging include spin-echo, fast spin-echo, gradient echo, and short tau inversion recovery (STIR). Each of these techniques has strengths and weaknesses.

Conventional T1-, proton density (PD)-, and T2-weighted spin-echo sequences have been the primary imaging sequences for the shoulder. T1-weighted spin-echo is relatively rapid, can be used on both high and low field strength systems, and offers high fat water contrast. However, T1-weighted images suffer from relatively poor soft tissue contrast. T1-weighted spin-echo is also used to show areas of enhancement after intravenous or intraarticular administration of gadolinium (Gd)-based contrast. Frequency selective fat suppression is often used to provide contrast between fat and Gd-enhanced tissues. Fat suppression also enhances contrast between articular cartilage and joint fluid. T2-weighted spin-echo generates contrast on the basis of differences in free and bound water. It is more sensitive for inflammation, infection, and trauma. T2-weighted images are relatively unaffected by magic angle phenomenon. The disadvantages are long imaging time and limited signal-to-noise ratio.

The development of fast spin-echo allowed development of T2-weighted images in a fraction of the time of conventional spin-echo with greater spatial resolution. Fast spin-echo is the least vulnerable to magnetic susceptibility effects amongst available pulse sequences. Fat also remains high in signal intensity on fast spin-echo T2-weighted images. This lowers the contrast between fat and fluid. Use of frequency selective fat suppression can be added, but magnetic field heterogeneity can produce uneven fat suppression.

STIR imaging provides fat suppression that is less susceptible to magnetic field inhomogeneities. The technique is extremely sensitive to free water. It can be obtained on both low and high field scanners. However, signal-to-noise ratio is relatively low and excessive signal loss in soft tissues can reduce overall diagnostic utility of the images.

Gradient echo images are another alternative to conventional T2-weighted spin-echo images. They are considerably faster, thus permitting thinner image sections. They also accentuate edges, which may be helpful in labral evaluation. However, they are vulnerable to magic angle effects, have a low sensitivity for evaluation of articular cartilage, and have high sensitivity to magnetic susceptibility effects.

MR ARTHROGRAPHY AND CONTRAST IMAGING

In addition to standard MRI of the shoulder, MR arthrography can be performed either by direct or indirect approach. Direct arthrography uses intraarticular injection of contrast material whereas indirect arthrography uses intravenous injection of Gd-based contrast agents. Direct MR arthrography has been the most widely used technique and is analogous to other forms of arthrography. Typically 15 to 20 mL of a Gd-saline solution (diluted to about 1/200) is injected into the joint under fluoroscopic visualization. Saline only may also be used for MR arthrography. T1-weighted images are then obtained in two to three planes, typically with frequency selective fat saturation. After injection, PD- or T2-weighted images with fat suppression are acquired in two to three planes. This technique distends the joint to provide better definition of labrocapsular structures and may improve sensitivity of some rotator cuff tears. The disadvantages of direct arthrography include the need for fluoroscopic guidance, which adds to procedure time and may be unavailable at some outpatient imaging centers. Direct arthrography converts a noninvasive standard MRI examination to a somewhat invasive procedure. The beneficial effects of direct arthrography are also limited to the space or compartment injected. There is also potential discomfort and apprehension on behalf of the patient. Some patients may experience a symptomatic synovitis after the intraarticular injection, particularly when an initial test injection of iodinated radiographic contrast is done to confirm intraarticular position before infusing the saline or Gd-saline solution.

An alternative to direct arthrography is indirect arthrography in which a standard dose of Gd contrast is injected intravenously and allowed to diffuse into the joint fluid through the synovial lining. The diffusion process typically takes 20 to 30 minutes. Active mobilization speeds the diffusion process. Indirect arthrography is less invasive and less time consuming, and may have greater patient acceptance. However, indirect arthrography does not produce joint distention to separate adjacent labral structures.

Yet another alternative may be direct contrast enhancement imaging immediately after intravenous injection of standard dose Gd contrast. The patient is imaged immediately after the Gd contrast is given intravenously, rather than after a period of waiting or exercise. This technique anticipates and uses direct enhancement of well-vascularized or hyperemic tissues by intravenous Gd contrast, and actively highlights areas of inflammation, granulation tissue, and developing scarring. Examples include the synovial tissue overgrowth associated with labral and capsular tears as well as disruptions of the bursal and articular margins of the rotator cuff (Fig. 4-1). The immediate, direct enhancement imaging is "active" contrast enhancement pointing to the area of derangement, as opposed to the "passive" contrast enhancement distending the joint indiscriminately in arthrography,

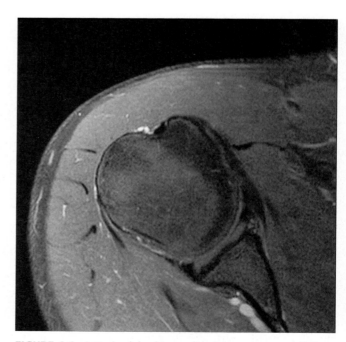

FIGURE 4-1. Anterior labral tear after intravenous gadolinium. Axial fat-suppressed T2-weighted image after intravenous gadolinium administration highlights anterior labral tearing.

either direct or indirect. The active enhancement is not confined to the joint space or compartment injected, but encompasses the entire imaged field of view. The longer the delay between intravenous contrast administration and image acquisition, the more the direct enhancement diffuses away from the area of maximal inflammation. After the standard delay of 20 to 30 minutes, the direct technique has transformed into the passive contrast of indirect arthrography.

In most patients, none of the above invasive or minimally invasive contrast-enhanced procedures are necessary. The noncontrast shoulder MRI examination is generally comprehensive and diagnostic. The additional procedures are best used as specialty problem-solving tools to increase conspicuity in the patient whose case is a diagnostic dilemma. As always, cost, risk, benefit, and patient satisfaction must be considered.

Given the variety of hardware and software alternatives available, there are many possibilities for efficient and thorough shoulder imaging. The senior author uses the following protocol on high field scanners: PD-weighted and frequency selective fat-suppressed PD-weighted oblique sagittal images, PD-weighted and second echo T2-weighted oblique coronal images, and PD-weighted and gradient echo axial images.

OSSEOUS ACROMIAL OUTLET

MRI provides the optimal imaging evaluation of the osseous acromial outlet as well as soft tissues of the cora-coacromial arch that may be associated with rotator cuff impingement (3). Osseous changes that can lead to extrinsic impingement and are well evaluated by MRI include anteriorly hooked acromion, lateral downsloping acromion, low-lying acromion, subacromial enthesophytes, and an os acromiale. Capsular and osseous hypertrophy of the AC joint as well as an enlarged coracoid process may also contribute to rotator cuff impingement.

The shape of the acromion and subacromial enthesophyte formation are best determined on oblique sagittal images located lateral to the AC joint. Any lateral downsloping or subacromial enthesophyte formation is best seen on oblique coronal images. Osteophytes or callus under the AC joint can predispose to impingement. However, AC arthrosis is not specific for impingement and is common in asymptomatic individuals. An inferolaterally sloping acromion has been associated with lateral supraspinatus injury near the greater tuberosity in overhead athletes who perform forceful abduction.

The os acromiale is an accessory ossification center along the outer edge of the acromion that has failed to fuse by age 25 years. Its prevalence ranges from 1% to 15% (4). It is uncertain what percentage of these are symptomatic. The synchondrosis may be fibrous or cartilaginous. The variant is bilateral 60% of the time. An association between os acromiale and impingement and rotator cuff pathology has been found, but identifying the os does not implicate it as the source of shoulder pain. The os is best seen on the axial and sagittal planes (Fig. 4-2).

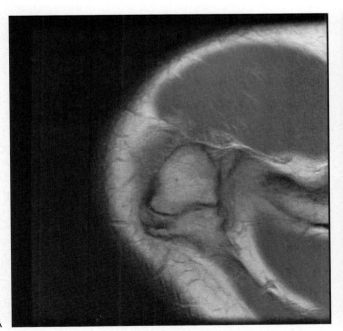
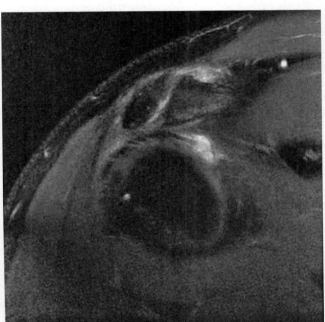

A   B

FIGURE 4-2. Os acromiale. **A:** Axial proton density–weighted image shows unfused distal acromial synchondrosis as well as acromioclavicular joint. **B:** Coronal fat-suppressed T2-weighted image through the os acromiale.

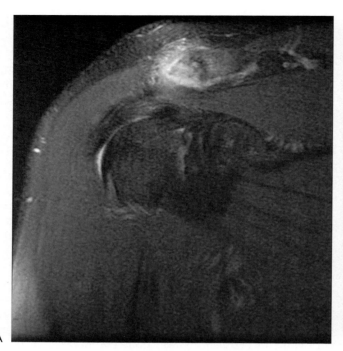
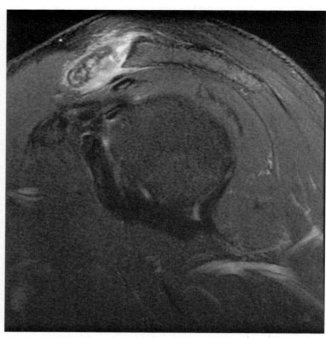

A   B

FIGURE 4-3. A,B: Acromioclavicular joint synovitis. Coronal and sagittal fat-suppressed T2-weighted images show articular cartilage loss, bone trabecular edema, and surrounding synovial edema at the acromioclavicular joint.

A thickened coracoacromial ligament has been associated with impingement. However, objective criteria for thickening have been elusive. Others suggest that the thickening is a secondary result of impingement. The ligament and coracoacromial arch are best seen on oblique sagittal images.

The AC joint itself may be symptomatic and is well evaluated on coronal and axial images. Arthrosis manifests as prominent osteophyte formation with capsular and synovial hypertrophy and scarring. Cystic change of the acromion and distal clavicle about the joint may be seen, with reactive bone edema. Synovitis may manifest as joint effusion and debris, as well as surrounding bone edema (Fig. 4-3).

Stress-related or posttraumatic synovitis with bone edema and hyperemia may suggest developing resorption and osteolysis in overhead athletes (Fig. 4-4).

ROTATOR CUFF

Impingement Syndromes

Clinical extrinsic impingement is a syndrome that results from compression of the supraspinatus tendon, as well as the biceps tendon and subacromial bursa, between the humeral head and subacromial arch. It is common in overhead athletes and in those whose occupations require overhead motion. There are multiple types of impingement. Primary extrinsic impingement is caused by entrapment of the supraspinatus tendon by the coracoacromial arch. This is exacerbated by subacromial enthesophyte, downsloping acromion, anteriorly hooked acromion, AC joint osteophytes, os acromiale, or thickened coracoacromial ligament. The final common pathway is mechanical narrowing, friction, and impaction on the bursal surface of the supraspinatus with increased wear, degeneration, and tearing.

Secondary extrinsic impingement can be caused by narrowing of the coracoacromial outlet from glenohumeral or scapulothoracic instability. It is most common in young patients and those who perform repetitive overhead movements. It is commonly associated with anterior or multidirectional instability (5). Chronic instability is associated with capsular laxity and weakening, which forces the rotator cuff to play a greater role in stabilization. This leads to wear on the tendons with excessive humeral head translation, which results in undersurface degeneration and tearing.

Internal or posterior superior impingement can also lead to undersurface rotator cuff tears. This also is most common in overhead athletes. The process involves compression of the articular side of the rotator cuff and greater tuberosity against the posterosuperior glenoid labrum in the overhead throwing position. The associated pathology includes articular sided tears of the posterior supraspinatus, infraspinatus, degenerative tearing of posterosuperior labrum, and osteochondral cystic changes and remodeling in the posterolateral humeral head to greater tuberosity (6) (Fig. 4-5).

A final form of impingement may be supraspinatus muscle hypertrophy. This is most common in weightlifters and

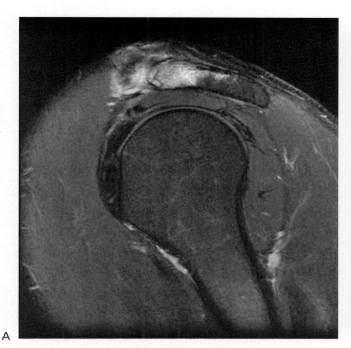
A

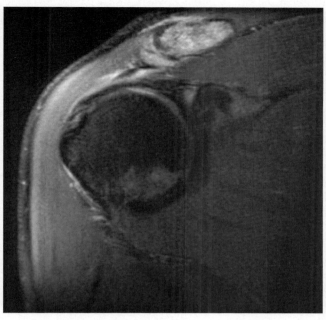
B

FIGURE 4-4. A,B: Distal clavicular edema. Sagittal and coronal fat-suppressed T2-weighted images through the acromioclavicular joint show bone trabecular edema in the distal clavicle. This can be seen in acute injuries and in chronic stress from weightlifting or repetitive overhead activity.

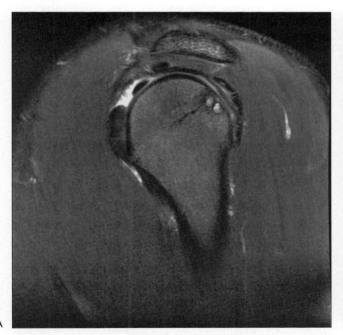
A

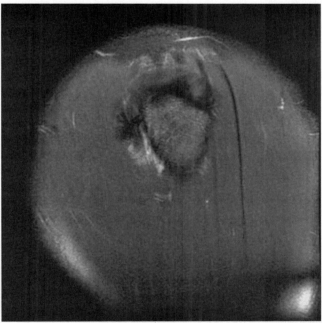
B

FIGURE 4-5. Posterior superior glenoid (internal) impingement. Sagittal T2-weighted **(A)** and fat-suppressed **(B)** images shows subcortical cystic change in the posterior and superior humeral head. This is a finding of posterior superior impingement. A non–fat-suppressed proton density–weighted sagittal image through the greater tuberosity shows tendinosis of the supraspinatus and infraspinatus tendons.

swimmers as well as other athletes who perform forceful overhead movements. This can occur with a normal cora-coacromial arch. The supraspinatus can be seen to be deformed at the myotendinous junction beneath the AC joint on oblique coronal images.

Tendinosis

All forms of impingement may lead to cuff derangement and characteristic imaging findings. When a tendon has abnormal increased signal intensity without focal defect to suggest partial tear, tendinosis (or chronic degeneration and scarring, likely from repetitive stress) or tendinopathy is described (7). The signal intensity is intermediate between fluid and healthy tendon on T2-weighted images (Fig. 4-6). There is most commonly thickening of the tendon, although more advanced cases show attrition. The word *tendinitis* has fallen out of favor except in those specific cases when tendon inflammation can be inferred from high signal on T2-weighted images (Fig. 4-7).

Partial Thickness Tears

Partial thickness tears can be articular sided, bursal sided, or interstitial. Articular sided tears are most common in overhead athletes. Findings suggestive of a partial thickness tear include focal increased signal intensity with morphologic disruption extending through a portion of nonretracted tendon, irregularity, or thinning or thickening of the tendon. Fat saturation improves detection of partial thickness tears with the potential pitfall of overestimating degree of tearing. Increased fluid in the glenohumeral joint or subacromial-subdeltoid bursa is common but not specific for both full and partial thickness tears (Fig. 4-8).

Full Thickness Tears

A full-thickness tear involves complete tendon thickness disruption to both bursal and articular margins. MR findings include tendon discontinuity and replacement with a fluid-filled gap to tendon retraction, fatty atrophy, and absence of tendon in chronic large tears. Some partial and full thickness tears do not demonstrate fluid signal intensity because of tendon debris or granulation tissue. Fat saturation has been shown to increase sensitivity for detection of (but may overestimate) full thickness tears. Tendon retraction, fatty infiltration, and muscle atrophy are specific signs of chronic tendon tears. They are also important determinants for therapeutic planning.

Isolated infraspinatus tendon tears are rare. When seen they are most common in young overhead athletes. The infraspinatus may also be affected by posterosuperior impingement. These tears are best demonstrated in the oblique sagittal and coronal planes (Fig. 4-9).

Subscapularis tears are uncommon. They are usually seen in association with large tears of the other rotator cuff

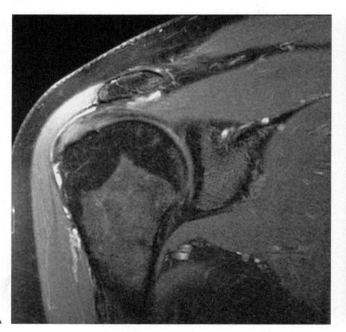
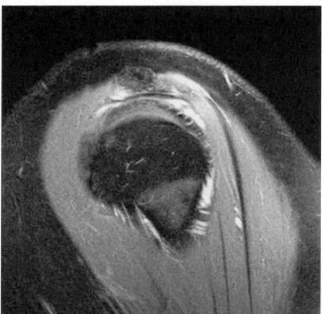

A

B

FIGURE 4-6. Tendinosis of the posterolateral rotator cuff. **A:** Fat-suppressed T2-weighted coronal and sagittal images through the posterior supraspinatus tendon and infraspinatus tendon show thickening and intermediate signal characteristic of tendinosis. **B:** There is associated subacromial bursitis.

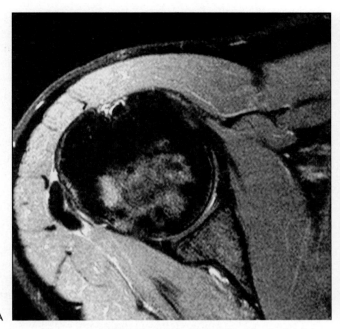
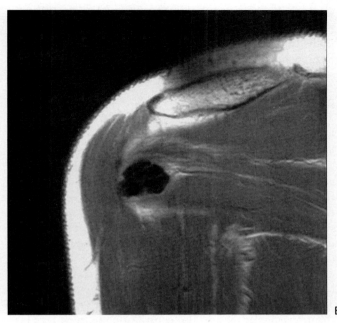

A B

FIGURE 4-7. Calcific tendonitis. **A:** Axial fat-suppressed T2-weighted and coronal proton density–weighted images through the infraspinatus tendon show a globular focus of low signal consistent with calcification. **B:** There is adjacent inflammation and edema.

tendons or as a result of recurrent shoulder dislocation (8). However, the overhead throwing athlete may also more commonly be subject to anterosuperior subscapularis tears and anterior supraspinatus tears about the rotator interval. These tears may be full or partial thickness. Small partial thickness tears of the anterosuperior portion of the deep portion of the subscapularis at the lesser tuberosity adjacent

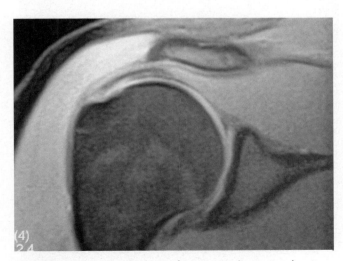

FIGURE 4-8. Partial articular surface supraspinatus tendon tear. Coronal fat-suppressed T2-weighted image through anterior supraspinatus demonstrates partial (less than 50%) thickness articular surface tear.

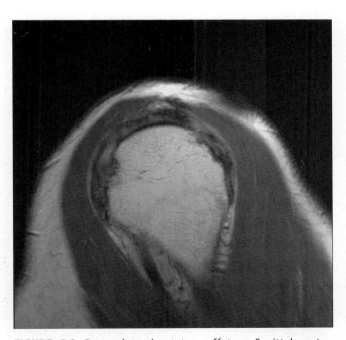

FIGURE 4-9. Posterolateral rotator cuff tear. Sagittal proton density–weighted image shows discontinuity in the infraspinatus tendon near the greater tuberosity attachment site. This is a full thickness infraspinatus tendon tear.

to the far lateral rotator interval have been described. These tears may be difficult to appreciate clinically or arthroscopically, and may be evaluated and documented by MRI. Sagittal and axial images are most helpful.

ROTATOR INTERVAL

Shoulder function relies on the soft tissues for stabilization. The muscles and tendons of the rotator cuff provide power and contribute to stability. The rotator cuff tendons fuse along their distal attachments at the greater and lesser tuberosities to provide a continuous cuff. Before their fusion, the anatomic space between the supraspinatus and subscapularis along the anterosuperior aspect of the shoulder is the rotator interval. The long head of the biceps tendon enters the shoulder through the rotator interval to extend to the labral-biceps anchor. The interval is bridged by the rotator interval capsule, which fuses with the coracohumeral ligament and which together serve as a roof over the intraarticular biceps. Also contributing to the interval is the superior glenohumeral ligament, which forms the floor of the biceps pulley.

Injuries to the Rotator Interval

The many structures that define and course through the rotator interval may be injured together. The athlete who uses repetitive or forceful overhead motion stresses the rota-

tor interval and long head of biceps. Occupational injuries or, occasionally, a fall on an outstretched hand may sprain or tear the interval capsule, coracohumeral ligament, and superior glenohumeral ligament with resulting deficiency of the long biceps pulley mechanism (Fig. 4-10). Biceps tendon dislocation with disruption of the transverse humeral ligament, biceps tendon tears and superior labrum anterior-to -posterior (SLAP) tears may be seen (9).

The normal coracohumeral ligament and interval capsule should be thin, smooth, and low in signal on sagittal images. In acute injuries such as anteroinferior dislocation, the interval capsule and coracohumeral ligament become thickened, irregular, and increased in signal intensity. Complete disruption with surrounding edema and hemorrhage is also possible.

With chronic injury, irregular thickening and scarring of both capsule and ligament may be seen. Prominent low to intermediate signal thickening of synovial hypertrophy or debris may be seen in the medial to far lateral portions of the interval.

The normal long biceps tendon is a smooth, oval, low signal structure in cross section. In sequential sagittal images it may be followed within the interval from medial to lateral to the bicipital groove, after which axial images are best for following the tendon along the humeral shaft. Acute long biceps strain or tearing may be outlined by high signal joint fluid and synovitis within the interval or within the biceps tendon sheath. Absence of the biceps tendon in cross section with an empty rotator interval or biceps tendon sheath may

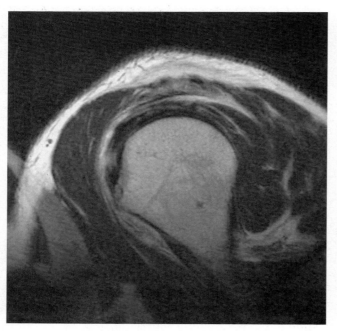
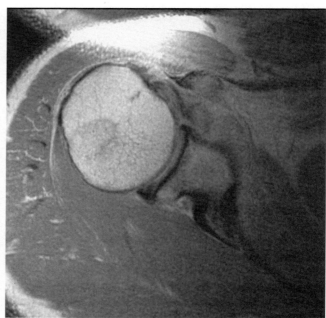

A   B

FIGURE 4-10. Rotator interval lesion. **A:** Coronal fat-suppressed T2-weighted image shows tearing of the distal subscapularis tendon and medial dislocation of the biceps tendon into the joint. **B:** Axial proton density–weighted images reveal medial dislocation of the biceps tendon.

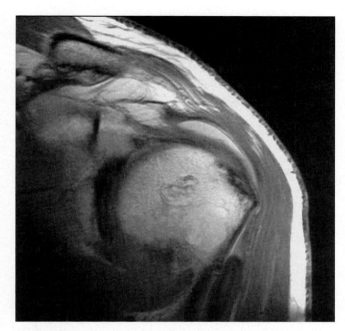

FIGURE 4-11. Long biceps tendon tear. Coronal proton density–weighted weighted image shows the torn, retracted long head of the biceps tendon lying within the superior portion of the bicipital groove. The proximal tendon is thickened both from tendinosis and loss of tension ("hourglass biceps").

indicate complete tear with distal retraction. Often a small proximal remnant is left at the labral-biceps anchor. A severely degenerated long biceps tendon with thinning and longitudinal tearing may also be seen as an apparently empty interval to biceps tendon sheath. When a complete tear is detected, the location of the distal tendon end should be located for surgical planning (Fig. 4-11).

With more chronic derangement, tendinosis may appear as thickening with intermediate signal of the long biceps tendon sheath. Synovitis usually accompanies chronic degeneration while longitudinal splitting is seen as well (9).

Traumatic injuries may disrupt or strip the far lateral interval capsule, coracohumeral ligament, and superior glenohumeral ligament. The biceps tendon is then susceptible to anteromedial luxation out of the proximal bicipital groove, often accompanied by strain or tearing of the biceps tendon. This is best evaluated on high proximal axial images and far lateral sagittal images. The far lateral superior margins of the subscapularis tendon also may be torn from the lesser tuberosity insertion ("hidden lesion" of the subscapularis). More severe injury may avulse the entire subscapularis tendon from the lesser tuberosity. The long biceps tendon may dislocate into the substance of the subscapularis tendon tear (10) (Fig. 4-12).

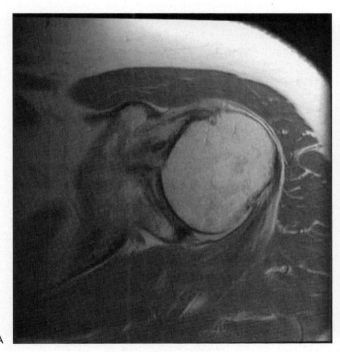

A

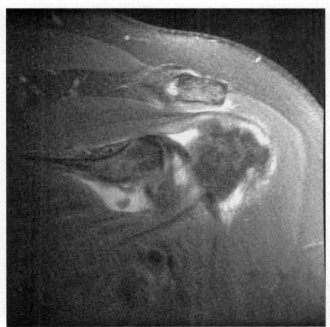

B

FIGURE 4-12. Subscapularis tendon tear and biceps tendon dislocation. **A:** Axial proton density–weighted image shows partial tearing of the subscapularis and medial dislocation of the intraarticular long biceps tendon. **B:** Coronal fat-suppressed T2-weighted images show the medial course of the dislocated biceps tendon after failure of biceps pulley mechanism.

With more chronic repetitive stress or overhead usage, degeneration and tearing with insufficiency of the biceps ligamentous pulley may develop. The transverse humeral ligament and superficial fibers of the subscapularis may tear off the lesser tuberosity. The biceps tendon may develop intermittent luxation out of the bicipital groove under either a deficient or lax transverse humeral ligament. Degenerative partial tears of the subscapularis may develop, with the long biceps residing in or coursing obliquely through the delaminated tendon. Intermittent luxation may be difficult to demonstrate on standard MR images. Stress positioning with external shoulder rotation, abduction, and simulated throwing may be helpful.

With rotator interval dysfunction or disruption, tearing of the distal anterior supraspinatus tendon at the greater tuberosity may be seen. Partial thickness or small full thickness tears may be difficult to detect on coronal images, and the far lateral sagittal images are most helpful (11).

The long biceps merges with the superior labrum at the labral biceps anchor after coursing through the rotator interval. The incidence of SLAP lesions is increased when long biceps or rotator interval pathology is detected. Discrete tears of superior labrum and biceps anchor may result from acute trauma, whereas repetitive overuse results in chronic degeneration and tearing, characterized by heterogeneous intermediate signal and fraying (see SLAP Lesions).

GLENOHUMERAL INSTABILITY

Instability can be classified in a number of ways. It may be classified with respect to direction: unidirectional (anteroinferior or posterior) or multidirectional. It may be classified in broad clinical categories—traumatic, unidirectional, associated Bankart lesion and often improve with surgical treatment (TUBS) or atraumatic, multidirectional, bilateral, recurrent instability (AMBRI) (12). The most important reason to image instability is to define the anatomic lesion leading to the problem. A proliferation of lesions resulting from dislocation and contributing to recurrent instability have been defined.

Anatomy

The glenohumeral ligaments represent a condensation of the shoulder capsule and are variable in appearance on imaging. The inferior glenohumeral ligament complex (IGHLC) courses from the anatomic neck of the humerus and inserts on the inferior portion of the glenoid and labrum. The anteroinferior and posteroinferior labrum are a fibrous thickening of the IGHLC at the attachment to the glenoid. The IGHLC is further divided into anterior and posterior bands. Visualization of the insertion of the anterior band is important in the evaluation of instability in that this site is often damaged during dislocation.

The middle glenohumeral ligament is variable and may be absent in as many as 30% of people (13). It may also take on a cordlike or sheetlike appearance. It runs deep to the subscapularis tendon and inserts on the tip of the anterosuperior glenoid or medially on the scapular neck. It is best evaluated on the axial images.

The superior glenohumeral ligament blends with the superior labrum and biceps anchor medially. It courses laterally along the rotator interval and fuses with the interval capsule to attach at the greater and lesser tuberosities, contributing to the long biceps ligamentous pulley. It serves as a constraint on the biceps tendon and limits external rotation when the shoulder is adducted. It is best seen on oblique sagittal images running obliquely near the coracoid process.

The labrum is an important structure for joint stability. It is the attachment site of the IGHLC. It deepens the shallow glenoid fossa and may act as a pressure seal. It is usually triangular in shape. However, many variations have been described. The area of greatest variability is in the anterosuperior quadrant. The anterosuperior labrum may be smaller than the rest of the labrum. It may be firmly attached or there may be a recess of variable depth. The labrum may be completely detached from the glenoid as a normal variant. This is referred to as a *sublabral hole or foramen*. Isolated injury of the anterosuperior labrum is thought to be uncommon, but when present it is often seen in high level throwing athletes. Importantly, the sublabral hole is not associated with biceps anchor abnormality, mid or inferior labral abnormality, or residual labral tissue on the glenoid rim (14).

The Buford complex is described as a cordlike middle glenohumeral ligament with a diminutive or absent anterosuperior labrum. This is best seen on sequential axial images. It is important not to misinterpret this as a torn labrum.

Anatomic Lesions of Instability

Bankart Lesions

Instability can result from a disruption of rotator cuff muscles, labral ligamentous structures, or bony glenoid. The most common lesion resulting from an anterior dislocation is the Bankart lesion (15). This refers to an avulsion of the labral ligamentous complex from its attachment to the anteroinferior glenoid. This may be accompanied by a fracture of the anteroinferior glenoid. Acutely, the MRI appearance often shows a hemorrhagic effusion and elevation of the labrum and capsule from the glenoid. There may be a discrete labral tear, but labral fragmentation and inhomogeneity are also common. In chronic cases, the Bankart lesion may be partially healed and scarred to the glenoid, making detection more difficult (Fig. 4-13).

In the classic Bankart lesion, the scapular periosteum is ruptured; in the variant lesions, the periosteum remains intact. If the labral ligamentous complex is displaced medially and shifted inferiorly, the lesion is called an *ALPSA* for anterior labroligamentous periosteal sleeve avulsion (16). In

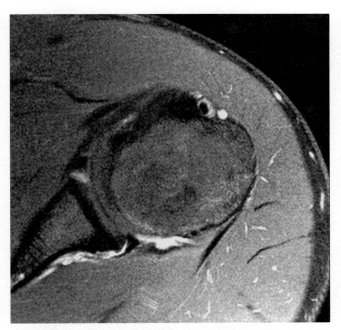

FIGURE 4-13. Intravenous gadolinium (Gd) showing acute and chronic labral tears. Axial fat-suppressed T2-weighted image immediately after intravenous Gd administration shows linear tearing of both the anterior and posterior glenoid labrum. There is intermediate signal in the anterior labral tear consistent with resynovialization or scar formation. This is a subacute to chronic tear. Contrast this with the fluid signal seen in the acute posterior labral tear and capsular stripping.

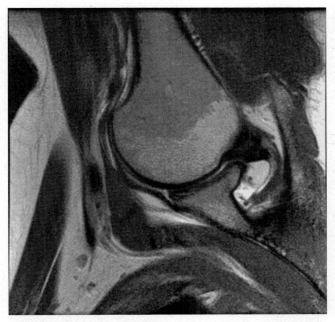

FIGURE 4-14. Perthes lesion in the overhead (ABER) position. Proton density–weighted image with the arm overhead shows a tear of the anterior inferior labrum with an intact scapular periosteum. There is a glenohumeral effusion with synovial debris posteriorly.

chronic ALPSA, fibrous tissue is deposited on the medially displaced labral ligamentous complex and the entire articular surface is resynovialized. This can complicate both imaging and arthroscopic diagnosis.

Perthes Lesions

The Perthes lesion is another Bankart variant with an intact scapular periosteum. The periosteum is stripped medially and becomes redundant. The lesion may scar down with the periosteum displaced medially and the labrum either in a normal position on the glenoid or displaced with the creation of a pseudojoint into which the humeral head can repeatedly sublux (Fig. 4-14).

HAGL Lesions

Humeral avulsion of the inferior glenohumeral ligament (HAGL) is less common than the classic Bankart lesion. It may occur with or without an associated anterior labral tear. The identification of the anterior band of the IGHL complex is best seen on oblique coronal and oblique sagittal images; it is facilitated by fluid within the joint. The injured IGHL may be seen as redundant or retracted, or as a poorly defined mass of intermediate signal tissue.

Hill-Sachs Lesions

With anteroinferior dislocation, the posterolateral superior humeral head impacts against the anteroinferior glenoid. This leads to a Hill-Sachs impaction fracture of the humeral head in 80% of cases (17). This lesion is seen as a focal concavity or defect with subjacent bone edema along the posterolateral superior humeral head. It is best demonstrated on axial images. If the humeral defect has its long axis parallel to the anterior glenoid rim within the athletic range of motion, it can be defined as *engaging*, which can contribute to recurrent instability.

GLAD lesions

Labral tears may be associated with glenoid articular chondral injury. When the humeral head impacts against the glenoid in abduction and external rotation, a nondisplaced anteroinferior labral tear and chondral defect can result. This is termed a *GLAD* lesion for glenolabral articular disruption. The labrum remains attached to the anterior scapular periosteum, distinguishing it from a Bankart lesion.

Posterior Lesions

Posterior instability is a risk when the shoulder is in a position of adduction and internal rotation. An anterior impacting force can overwhelm the already taut posterior

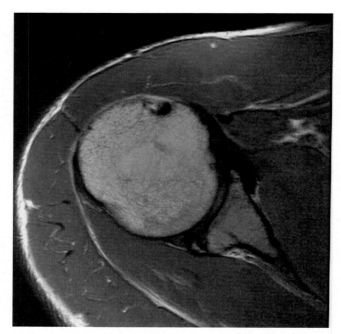

FIGURE 4-15. Posterior labral tear. Axial proton density–weighted image shows linear high signal in the posterior labrum consistent with a posterior labral tear.

capsule and labrum. The labral capsular disruption is called a *reverse Bankart*, and the impaction injury to the anterior humeral head is a *reverse Hill-Sachs* (Fig. 4-15). The subscapularis may also be torn, either as a full thickness or a partial thickness articular sided tear. Less commonly the posterior portion of the inferior glenohumeral ligament may be torn from the humerus. This is a *reverse HAGL* (18).

SLAP LESIONS

The long head of the biceps tendon originates through and is continuous with the superior labrum. The superior labrum is best seen on coronal images and should be a smooth, low-signal, triangular structure. The attachment of the superior labrum is variable with a spectrum from superior labrum adherent to superior glenoid (creating a potential space between free edge of labrum and biceps tendon) to a meniscoid superior labrum bound tightly to biceps tendon. A superior labral tear that involves both anterior and posterior labral quadrants is termed a *SLAP* lesion, for superior labrum from anterior to posterior (relative to the biceps tendon). There may be associated pathology in the biceps tendon and rotator cuff. Snyder originally described four types of SLAP lesions (19). Type I consists of degenerative fraying of the superior labrum. These lesions show free edge fraying and blunting or intermediate signal on MRI. Type II lesions have detachment of the superior labrum and biceps tendon from the superior glenoid (Fig. 4-16), which

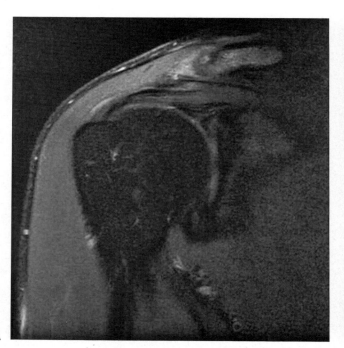

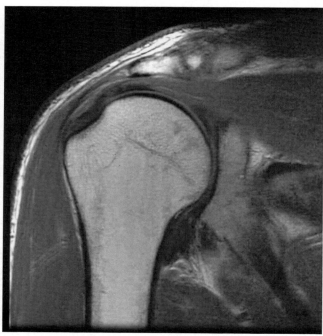

A   B

FIGURE 4-16. SLAP (superior labrum anterior-to-posterior) lesion. Coronal proton density–weighted images both with **(A)** and without **(B)** fat saturation show irregular increased signal within the superior labrum consistent with a type II SLAP lesion.

may result in instability. Fluid signal can be seen tracking between the labral-bicipital complex and the osseous glenoid. Type III lesions have a bucket-handle tear of the superior labrum with a normal biceps tendon. A type IV lesion is a type III tear with extension into the biceps tendon. Five additional SLAP lesions have been characterized. It is often difficult to completely characterize the lesions according to subtype on MRI. The goal of imaging is to evaluate both the labrum and biceps tendon and to characterize the anatomic abnormality as completely as possible. The superior labrum is best evaluated on coronal images, with extension of tears more inferiorly along the anterior or posterior labrum best seen on axial images.

Paralabral Cysts

Labral tears including SLAP lesions may be associated with paralabral cysts. They are most common in the posterosuperior labrum, but may occur anywhere. The cysts form when joint fluid extravasates through a labral tear and is trapped by a ball-valve mechanism. Water is reabsorbed and the remaining fluid increases in protein content. The cyst can remodel adjacent bone or cause impingement on the suprascapular nerve in either the suprascapular or spinoglenoid notches. The labral tear that gave rise to the cyst may have scarred at the time of cyst diagnosis and may be difficult to appreciate on imaging or at arthroscopy (Fig. 4-17).

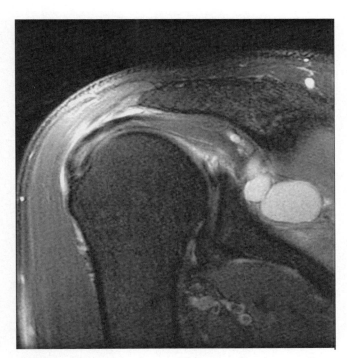

FIGURE 4-17. Paralabral cyst with denervation changes. Coronal fat-suppressed T2-weighted image shows a superior labral tear with an associated multiloculated paralabral cyst. The cyst has dissected to the spinoglenoid notch where it is impinging on the suprascapular nerve. The increased signal within the infraspinatus muscle belly is due to subacute denervation change.

MICROINSTABILITY

Microinstabilities are a spectrum of disorders that occur in the anterosuperior aspect of the shoulder joint and overlaps with the spectrum of previously discussed rotator interval lesions. This includes the biceps anchor, superior labrum, rotator interval, and rotator cuff. Pathologic lesions associated with microinstability include the classic SLAP lesion, posterior labrum peel-back (a posterior SLAP), anterosuperior labral detachments and cuff tears (see SLAC Lesions), superior glenohumeral ligament laxity or tear, middle glenohumeral detachment, and articular partial thickness cuff tears (20).

Peel-Back SLAP lesions

The posterior peel-back SLAP lesion usually occurs as a result of repetitive overhand throwing. It may overlap with previously discussed internal impingement syndrome findings. A posterosuperior labral detachment allows for laxity in the posterosuperior direction and pseudolaxity anteroinferiorly. A partial articular-sided posterior rotator cuff tear develops subsequently.

SLAC Lesions

The association between superior labral tears and anterior cuff lesions was also noted in overhead athletes. The initial lesion is thought to be an injury to the anterior superior labrum that involves the insertion of the superior glenohumeral ligament and the anterior portion of the biceps tendon. The resultant laxity of the superior glenohumeral ligament and interval structures leads to abnormal translation and chafing on the glenoid rim. This results in the partial thickness anterior cuff tears. This complex has been termed the *SLAC* lesion for superior labrum anterior cuff. This complex of findings is well evaluated on MRI with integration of all three (sagittal, axial, and coronal) imaging planes.

LATISSIMUS DORSI AND OTHER MUSCLE INJURIES

Strain injuries of the latissimus dorsi, teres major, and subscapularis are an uncommon cause of pain in the thrower's shoulder. The latissimus dorsi and teres major function similarly to the subscapularis in the throwing motion. Both show high levels of activity during acceleration and deceleration with reduced activity during wind-up and follow-through. Acute injuries show intramuscular edema and may show localized hemorrhage. Discrete muscle or muscle tendon junction tears may also be seen, although less commonly. The most common site of latissimus injury is at the myotendinous junction, just proximal to its attachment on the humeral shaft (21). This is best demonstrated on axial and oblique sagittal images.

REFERENCES

1. Hoult DI, Chen CN, Sank VJ. The field dependency of NMR imaging. *Magn Res Med* 1986;3:742–746.
2. Tirman PFJ, Bost FW, Garvin GJ, et al. Posterosuperior glenoid impingement: MRI and MR arthrographic findings with arthroscopic correlation. *Radiology* 1994;193:431–436.
3. .Banas MP, Miller RJ, Totterman S. Relationship between the lateral acromial angle and rotator cuff disease. *J Shoulder Elbow Surg* 1995:4:454–461.
4. Edelson JG, Zuckerman J, Hershkovitz I. Os acromiale: anatomy and surgical implications. *J Bone Joint Surg (Br)* 1993;75:551–555.
5. Jobe FW, Kvitne RS, Giangarra CE. Shoulder pain in the overhand or throwing athlete: the relationship of anterior instability and rotator cuff impingement. *Orthop Rev* 1989;18:963–975.
6. Walch G, Boileau P, Noel E, et al. Impingement of the deep surface of the supraspinatus tendon on the posterosuperior glenoid rim: an arthroscopic study. *J Shoulder Elbow Surg* 1992;1:238–245.
7. Kannus P, Jozsa L. Histopathological changes preceding spontaneous rupture of a tendon: a controlled study of 891 patients. *J Bone Joint Surg (Am)* 1991;73:1507–1525.
8. Deutsch A, Altchek DW, Veltri DM, et al. Traumatic tears of the subscapularis tendon: clinical diagnosis, magnetic resonance imaging findings, and operative treatment. *Am J Sports Med* 1997;25:13–22.
9. Ho C. MR imaging of the thrower's shoulder. *MRI Clin North Am* 1999;7:39–47.
10. Walch G, Nove-Josserand L, Levigne C, et al. Tears of the supraspinatus tendon with "hidden" lesions of the rotator interval. *J Shoulder Elbow Surg* 1994;3:353.
11. Patten RM. Tears of the anterior portion of the rotator cuff (the subscapularis tendon): MR imaging findings. *AJR* 1994;162:351.
12. Silliman J, Hawkins R. Classification and physical diagnosis of instability of the shoulder. *Clin Sports Med* 1991;10:693–705.
13. Crues JV, Ryu RK. The shoulder. In: Stark D, Bradley WG, eds. Magnetic resonance imaging. St. Louis: Mosby, 1991:2424–2458.
14. Tirman P, Feller J, Palmer W, et al. The Buford complex-a variation of normal shoulder anatomy: MR arthrographic imaging features. *AJR* 1996;166:869—873.
15. Bankart ASB. Recurrent of habitual dislocation of the shoulder joint. *Br Med J* 1923;2:1132.
16. Neviaser TJ. The anterior labroligamentous periosteal sleeve avulsion lesion: a cause of anterior instability of the shoulder. *Arthroscopy* 1993;9:17–21.
17. Neviaser RJ, Neviaser TJ, Neviaser JS. Anterior dislocation of the shoulder and rotator cuff rupture. *Clin Orthop Rel Res* 1993;291:103–106.
18. Tirman P. Glenohumeral instability. In: Steinbach L, Tirman P, Peterfy C, et al, eds. *Shoulder magnetic resonance imaging.* Lippincott Williams & Wilkins? 1998:135–167.
19. Snyder SJ, Karzel RP, Del Pizzo W, et al. SLAP lesions of the shoulder. *Arthroscopy* 1990;6:274–279.
20. Nottage WM. Controversial topics in shoulder arthroscopy—microinstability. *Arthroscopy* 2002;18:65–67.
21. Schickendantz MS, Ho CP, Keppler L, et al. MR imaging of the thrower's shoulder. *MRI Clin North Am* 1999;7:39–47

5

THE ASSESSMENT OF OUTCOMES FOR THE TREATMENT OF THE OVERHEAD ATHLETE

JOHN E. KUHN

INTRODUCTION

In recent years, a great deal of attention has been paid to the concept of outcomes research. The emphasis on outcomes research has stemmed from the impression that health care expenditures in the United States are excessive. Research conducted in the 1970s and 1980s demonstrated that there is significant regional variation in the use of certain medical services. This implies that, in high-use areas, inefficient or unnecessary services are being provided and that, in low-use areas, patients may not be receiving adequate medical care.

The mission of outcomes research has many fronts: (a) developing standardized methods of reported data, using validated and reliable assessment tools so that different studies can be combined or compared, (b) restructuring measures of outcome so that more emphasis is placed on the *athlete's* perception of the outcome, and (c) developing methods to allow for an analysis of the varying rates of application of medical services and costs. In essence, we need to report accurate data following accepted standards. We need to know whether the procedures being done are beneficial to the athlete from the athlete's perspective. And, we need to be cost effective.

The concept of outcomes research is not new. One of the foremost early shoulder surgeons, Dr. Ernest Anthony Codman, was also a pioneer in the field of outcomes research. In 1913, he delivered his landmark address, "The Product of a Hospital," to the Philadelphia County Medical Society (1). In this address, Codman called for the "standardization of reporting data" so that the work done at different hospitals could be compared. He recognized "regional variation of medical services" and discussed "fiscal and clinical efficiency" while offering insight into the cause of such variation. Finally, he recognized that the "result to the patient" is the critical result when assessing the outcomes of medical and surgical treatments. Interestingly, Codman's ideas were not well accepted in his time. In fact, Codman's career suffered after-

ward; in his frustration, he presented a cartoon of an ostrich with its head buried in the sand to his colleagues who undoubtedly were threatened by this brash young surgeon who demanded accountability (2). For many years, Codman's efforts went underappreciated, yet these pivotal issues raised in 1913 are the same issues being examined today.

GENERAL CONCEPTS REGARDING OUTCOMES ASSESSMENTS
Validity, Reliability, and Responsiveness

When assessing outcomes of treatment, researchers typically use questionnaires or scoring systems (also known as *assessment tools*) to allow for the presentation and publication of data. Ideally, these assessment tools would be standardized and generally accepted for specific populations, so that the outcomes from different studies could be compared. Of equal importance, although rarely done in the past, all assessments should be tested for *reliability, validity*, and *responsiveness* before clinical use (3).

Reliability assures that repeated administration of an assessment will give the same results. An assessment has *Test-retest reliability* if it produces the same results when given different times under the same conditions. *Internal reliability* occurs when an assessment evaluating similar conditions produces similar results.

Validity assures that the assessments measure outcomes accurately— that is, does the test measure what it was designed to measure? The three approaches used to measure validity include *content validity*, which determines whether all of the important aspects of a condition are covered by the assessment, *criterion validity*, which assures that the scores produced by the assessment correlate with accepted standards, and *construct validity*, which demonstrates that the assessment produces results consistent with the existing understanding of the field or with other assessments.

Responsiveness refers to the ability of an assessment tool to measure changes over time. The *responsiveness index* is one method of evaluating the responsiveness of an assessment tool and is determined by the mean change score divided by the variability in scores among stable subjects (4,5). Other methods include the *standard response mean*, which is the mean change in the score divided by the standard deviation of the change scores (6), the *relative efficiency*, which is the squared ratio of the *t* statistic (7), and the *effect size*, which is determined by the mean change score divided by the standard deviation of baseline scores (8). An assessment tool that is highly responsive detects even small changes in outcome over time, increasing the statistical power of the study and allowing researchers to perform studies with fewer subjects.

Of the many available assessment tools developed for evaluating the shoulder, only those developed recently have been assessed for reliability, validity, and responsiveness. Examples include the Self-Administered Questionnaire for Assessment of Symptoms and Function of the Shoulder (9), the Western Ontario Shoulder Instability Index (10), the American Shoulder and Elbow Surgeons Standardized Shoulder Assessment Form (11), the Simple Shoulder Test (12–14), and the Constant-Murley evaluation (15,16). Clearly, the use of a valid and reliable assessment tool is of great value in the assessment of outcomes for the treatment of the athlete's shoulder, but the question remains: which of the many assessments should be used?

The Hierarchy of Assessment Tools

Assessment tools used in orthopaedic surgery generally tend to fall into a hierarchy of three different levels of sensitivity:

1. General health assessments
2. Joint-specific assessments
3. Disease- or population-specific assessments (Table 5-1)

Like the different powered lenses on a microscope, each of these levels of assessment provides a different perspective on the patient's outcome (17–19). General health assessments are best suited to discriminate the outcomes of differing treatments for systemic diseases or conditions, such as rheumatoid arthritis. Other conditions (e.g., shoulder pain when throwing) may not affect general health, but rather would be better assessed by disease-specific or population-specific assessment tools. Joint- or extremity-specific assessments are common in orthopedic surgery, and try to provide a method of assessing all potential disorders for a particular joint or extremity. There are a number of global shoulder assessments in the orthopedic literature (Table 5-1). Disease- or population-specific assessment tools are likely the most sensitive because they are designed to apply to a very specific population of patients.

TABLE 5–1. HIERARCHY OF ASSESSMENT TOOLS USED TO EVALUATE THE SHOULDER

Each level of assessment provides different information, and improved sensitivity, particularly for the athlete's shoulder, not that the validity and reliability has not been evaluated for many of these assessments.

General health measures
SF-36
Arthritis Impact Measurement Scale
Nottingham Health Profile
Sickness Impact Profile

Joint specific shoulder assessments
Without scoring systems
   American Shoulder and Elbow Surgeons Assessment
   Simple Shoulder Test
With scoring systems
   Imatani Scoring System
   Severity Index for Chronically Painful Shoulders
   Swanson Score
   HSS Shoulder-Rating Score
   UCLA End-Result Score
   Constant Score
   American Shoulder and Elbow Surgeons Index
   Shoulder Pain and Disability Index
HSS Self-Administered Questionnaire for Assessment of Symptoms and Function of the Shoulder

Assessments for specific shoulder conditions/populations
Instability
   Rowe Bankart Repair Scoring System
   Walch-Duplay Rating Sheet
   Western Ontario Shoulder Instability Score
Impingement/Rotator Cuff Disease
   HSS Impingement Shoulder Rating Score
   Western Ontario Rotator Cuff Index
Glenohumeral Osteoarthritis
   Swanson Score
   Western Ontario Osteoarthritis of the Shoulder Index
The Athlete's Shoulder
   The Athletic Shoulder Outcome Rating Scale
   The Athlete's Shoulder Assessment Tool

Modified from Kuhn JE, Blasier RB. Measuring outcomes in shoulder arthroplasty. *Semin Arthroplasty* 1995;6:245–264, with permission.

General Health Assessments

General health assessments report a score for the general health of the patient. The best known example of a general health assessments is the standard form (SF) 36 questionnaire (20), which measures eight different aspects of health, scoring them on a 100-point scale (Appendix 5-1). These aspects of general health include assessment of the following: (a) limitations in physical activities due to health problems, (b) limitations in social activities due to physical or emotional problems, (c) limitations in usual role activities due to physical health problems, (d) limitations in usual role activities due to mental health problems, (e) general mental health and well-being, (f) bodily pain, (g) vitality, and (h) general health perceptions (20). Not unexpectedly,

This survey asks you your views about your health. Please answer every question by making the appropriate answer.

1. In general, would you say your health is:
   __Excellent   __Very Good   __Good   __Fair   __Poor

2. Compared to one year ago, how would you rate your health in general now?
   __Much better now than one year ago
   __Somewhat better now than one year ago
   __About the same as one year ago
   __Somewhat worse than one year ago
   __Much worse than one year ago

The following items are about activities you might do during a typical day. Does your health now limit you in these activities? If so, how much?

	Yes limited a lot	Yes limited a little	No, not limited at all
3. Vigorous activities, such as running, lifting heavy objects, participating in strenuous sports	____	____	____
4. Moderate activities, such as moving a table, pushing a vacuum cleaner, bowling or playing golf	____	____	____
5. Lifting or carrying groceries	____	____	____
6. Climbing several flights of stairs	____	____	____
7. Climbing one flight of stairs	____	____	____
8. Bending, kneeling or stooping	____	____	____
9. Walking more than a mile	____	____	____
10. Walking several blocks	____	____	____
11. Walking one block	____	____	____
12. Bathing or dressing yourself	____	____	____

During the past 4 weeks, have you had any of the following problems with your work or other regular daily activities as a result of your physical health?

	Yes	No
13. Cut down on the amount of time you spent on work or other activities	___	___
14. Accomplished less than you would like	___	___
15. Were limited in the kinds of work or other activities	___	___
16. Had difficulty performing the work or other activities (for example, it took extra effort)	___	___

APPENDIX 5-1. Standard Form (SF) 36 General Health Assessment. This assessment consists of 36 questions that investigate the patient's general health and well-being. (From Ware JE, Shervourne CD. The MOS 36-item short-form health survey [SF-36]: I. Conceptual framework and item selection. *Med Care* 1992;30:473–483, with permission.)

During the past 4 weeks, have you had any of the following problems with your work or other regular daily activities as a result of any emotional problems (such as feeling depressed or anxious)?

	Yes	No
17. Cut down the amount of time you spent on work or other activities	___	___
18. Accomplished less than you would like	___	___
19. Didn't do work or other activities as carefully as usual	___	___

20. During the past 4 weeks, to what extent has your physical health or emotional problems interfered with your normal social activities with family, friends, neighbors, or groups?
    ___Not at all   ___Slightly   ___Moderately   ___Quite a bit   ___Extremely

21. How much bodily pain have you had during the past 4 weeks?
    ___None   ___Very Mild   ___Mild   ___Moderate   ___Severe   ___Very Severe

22. During the past 4 weeks, how much did pain interfere with your normal work (including both work outside the home and housework)?
    ___Not at all   ___Slightly   ___Moderately   ___Quite a bit   ___Extremely

These questions are about how you feel and how things have been with you during the past 4 weeks. For each question please give the one answer that comes closest to the way you have been feeling.

How much of the time during the past 4 weeks	All of the time	Most of the time	A good bit of the time	Some of the time	A little of the time	None of the time
23. Did you feel full of pep?	___	___	___	___	___	___
24. Have you been a very nervous person?	___	___	___	___	___	___
25. Have you felt so down in the dumps that nothing could cheer you up?	___	___	___	___	___	___
26. Have you felt calm and peaceful?	___	___	___	___	___	___
27. Did you have a lot of energy?	___	___	___	___	___	___
28. Have you felt downhearted and blue?	___	___	___	___	___	___
29. Did you feel worn out?	___	___	___	___	___	___
30. Have you been a happy person?	___	___	___	___	___	___
31. Did you feel tired?	___	___	___	___	___	___

During the past 4 weeks, how much of the time has your physical health or emotional problems interfered with your social activities (like visiting with friends, relatives, etc.)?

___All of the time ___Most of the time ___Some of the time ___A little of the time ___None of the time

APPENDIX 5-1. *(continued)*

How TRUE or FALSE is each of the following statements for you?	Definitely true	Mostly true	Don't know	Mostly false	Definitely false
33. I seem to get sick a little easier than other people	____	____	____	____	____
34. I am as healthy as anybody I know	____	____	____	____	____
35. I expect my health to get worse	____	____	____	____	____
36. My health is excellent	____	____	____	____	____

APPENDIX 5-1. *(continued)*

the ability to perform overhead sports is not weighted heavily on this assessment; general health assessments are much more sensitive when assessing the effects of a systemic disease (e.g., arthritis). Other examples of general health assessments include the Arthritis Impact Measurement Scale (21), the Nottingham Health Profile (22), and the Sickness Impact Profile (23)—all of which may be more relevant to orthopedic treatments than the SF-36 assessment (24,25). However, because the SF-36 assessment has been well validated and successfully used to evaluate a number of medical conditions, its use is increasing for the general health evaluation of patients with orthopedic conditions. With regard to the shoulder however, the SF-36 form does not seem to correlate well with other measures of shoulder disability (26,27).

Global Shoulder Assessment Tools

The next level of assessment in measuring outcomes in orthopedic surgery focuses on a particular joint or extremity. Assessments at this level may be more sensitive for evaluating the treatment of orthopedic conditions. A number of different global shoulder assessment methods have been used (Table 5-1). These assessments are designed for the evaluation of most disorders of the shoulder and as such may have some application to overhead athletes. Some

global shoulder assessments produce a final numeric grade, which allows statistical comparison of the overall preoperative and postoperative condition of the shoulder and allows for comparison of different methods of treatment (9,15, 16,28–30). Other assessments serve as guides to assure that none of the important elements in the evaluation of outcome are neglected and, although comprehensive, may be lengthy and cumbersome (29). Yet other assessments for the shoulder take a different approach and are designed to be as simple as possible (12–14).

One major concern with these different assessments is that they are inconsistent, emphasizing different components of shoulder well-being (17–19,31,32) (Table 5-2). Whereas some scoring assessments place most emphasis on the patient's pain, others place more emphasis on function or range of motion. This occurs because the investigator who has developed each measure has his or her own ideas on the best parameters to measure success. This bias determines the most important elements of the assessment. Because this bias exists, the scoring systems in use are not comparable and, worse, may not reflect the athlete's perspective of his or her outcome. For example, the assessments that place relatively high emphasis on pain may be ideal for assessing outcomes in athletes with rotator cuff pathology, but they may not be sensitive for assessing those with glenohumeral instability. In addition, some assessment

TABLE 5–2. POINT ALLOCATION FOR VARIOUS COMPONENTS OF GENERAL SHOULDER SCORING SYSTEMS USED IN EVALUATING THE ATHLETE'S SHOULDER

Assessment Tool	Pain	Range of Motion	Strength	Function	Patient Satisfaction	Other	Total Points
Rowe	10 (10%)	10 (10%)		50 (50%)		Stability 30 (30%)	100
ASES Index	50 (50%)			50 (50%)			100
UCLA	10 (28.6%)	5 (14.3%)	5 (14.3%)	10 (28.6%)	5 (14.3%)		35
Constant	15 (15%)	20 (20%)	25 (25%)	20 (20%)			100
HSS Self-Assessment	40 (40%)			45 (45%)		Global 15 (15%)	100

Percentages indicate the relative weight given to each component of the scoring systems.
Modified from Kuhn JE, Blasier RB. Measuring outcomes in shoulder arthroplasty. *Semin Arthroplasty* 1995;6:245–264, with permission.

tools may show bias related to age or gender (33). As a result, scores from one assessment tool cannot be equated to scores from another assessment tool (33).

This is particularly true in the case of the overhead athlete who may have a normal range of motion, normal strength, and ability to perform the simple tasks of daily living without pain but in whom pain develops only with overhead sports. In this case, a shoulder assessment that emphasizes pain or emphasizes function as determined by the ability to perform activities of daily living may not detect patient dissatisfaction that results from an inability to perform athletics. As a result, these evaluations, although applicable to most shoulder conditions, may not be sensitive enough to evaluate the problems in the athlete's shoulder. For these reasons, no published shoulder scoring system has been universally accepted (33,34).

To illustrate this point, a National Library of Medicine MEDLINE search of the literature conducted by the author using the key words *athlete* and *shoulder* identified 38 clinical studies over the past 10 years in which athletes were evaluated and treated for shoulder pathology (review articles were excluded). These manuscripts were reviewed to identify the following: (a) scoring systems used to grade the outcome, (b) whether patient satisfaction was reported, (c) whether return to play was reported and, if so, whether the level of play was identified, and (d) whether the recurrence of symptoms was reported. In most studies, the overhead athlete was a small subset of the entire population under study.

There is no consensus on which of the outcomes assessment tools should be used; 14 different outcomes assessment tools were used in these studies (Table 5-3). The most popular was the Rowe Score (35), an assessment tool for the population of patients with instability, which has not been tested for validity and reliability and which has significant flaws (10). The ability to return to play was reported in 89% of the studies, and these data were stratified according to intensity of play in 71%. Even though the ability to return to play and the intensity of play are important variables to report in assessing the outcomes of treating the ath-

lete's shoulder, patient satisfaction was reported in only 21% of the studies.

The most popular global shoulder assessment tool used to evaluate the shoulder in the athletes in this small study was the American Shoulder and Elbow Surgeons Standardized Shoulder Assessment Form (Appendix 5-2). This assessment tool was developed by the Research Committee of the American Shoulder and Elbow Surgeons as a standardized method for evaluating the shoulder (29). This effort was undertaken to create a universal method to measure the condition of the shoulder that would be easy to use, would assess activities of daily living, and would include a subjective component completed by the patient. This assessment is based primarily on the early work of Neer (36,37); however, many other scoring systems were reviewed during the development of this assessment (1,12,35,38,39).

The subjective (or patient-completed) assessment includes an inquiry about pain, symptoms of instability, and activities of daily living (Appendix 5-2). Both pain and instability are graded on a 10-point visual analog scale. The functional assessment includes 10 questions regarding activities of daily living. The patient grades his ability to perform each of these activities on a four-point scale. The objective or physician-completed part of the form reviews range of motion, specific physical findings, strength, and stability.

Range of motion is analyzed passively and actively using a goniometer in forward elevation, cross-body adduction, external rotation with the arm at the side, external rotation with the arm at 90 degrees of abduction, and also assesses internal rotation at the levels of the spinous processes. Strength is measured using the five-level Medical Research Council Grades in forward elevation, abduction, internal rotation, and external rotation. Instability is graded on a four-point scale in three planes: anterior, posterior, and inferior.

The Research Committee of the American Shoulder and Elbow Surgeons (ASES) has isolated components of this assessment to produce a score called the *Shoulder Score Index* (29). This scoring system uses the subjective visual

TABLE 5–3. RESULTS OF LITERATURE SURVEY IN ASSESSING OUTCOMES IN THE ATHLETE'S SHOULDER

Reported Outcome Data	Number of Studies Reporting Data	Number of Assessments Used	Number of Studies Used	Assessment Tool	Number of Times Used
Return to play	34/38 = 89%	0	6/38 = 16%	Rowe	24
Return to play— stratified by intensity	27/38 = 71%	1	16/38 = 42%	ASES	12
Recurrence of symptoms	33/38 = 87%	2	8/38 = 21%	UCLA	6
Patient satisfaction	8/38 = 21%	3	5/38 = 13%	Constant	5
		3	3/38 = 8%	SF-36	3
				8 Others	1–2

Name_____ Date_____
Age_____ Hand Dominance R__ L__ Ambi__ Sex M__ F__
Diagnosis_____ Initial Assess? Y__ N__
Procedure/Date_____ Follow-up M___ Y___

PATIENT SELF-EVALUATION

Are you having pain in your shoulder (circle correct answer) Yes   No
Mark where your pain is

Do you have pain in your shoulder at night? Yes   No
Do you take pain medication (aspirin, Advil, Tylenol etc.)? Yes   No
Do you take narcotic pain medication (codeine or stronger)? Yes   No
How many pills do you take each day (average)? _____pills
How bad is your pain today (mark line)?

I   I   I   I   I   I   I   I   I   I   I

No pain at all   Pain as bad as it can be

Does your shoulder feel unstable (as if it is going to dislocate)? Yes   No
How unstable is your shoulder (mark line)?

I   I   I   I   I   I   I   I   I   I   I

Very stable   Very Unstable

Circle the number that indicates your ability to do the following activities:
0= unable to do; 1= very difficult to do; 2= somewhat difficult; 3= not difficult

Activity	Right Arm	Left Arm
1.) Put on a coat	0 1 2 3	0 1 2 3
2.) Sleep on your painful or affected side	0 1 2 3	0 1 2 3
3.) Wash back/do up bra in back	0 1 2 3	0 1 2 3
4.) Manage toileting	0 1 2 3	0 1 2 3
5.) Comb hair	0 1 2 3	0 1 2 3
6.) Reach a high shelf	0 1 2 3	0 1 2 3
7.) Lift 10 lbs. above shoulder	0 1 2 3	0 1 2 3
8.) Throw a ball overhand	0 1 2 3	0 1 2 3
9.) Do usual work - List:_____	0 1 2 3	0 1 2 3
10.) Do usual sport - List:_____	0 1 2 3	0 1 2 3

PHYSICIAN ASSESSMENT

RANGE OF MOTION	RIGHT		LEFT	
	active	passive	active	passive
Total shoulder motion with goniometer				
Forward elevation (max. arm trunk angle)				
External rotation (arm at side)				
External rotation (arm at 90° abduction)				
Internal rotation (highest with thumb)				
Cross-body adduction				

APPENDIX 5-2. The American Shoulder and Elbow Surgeons Standardized Shoulder Assessment and Shoulder Score Index. (From Richards RR, An KN, Bigliani LU, et al. A standard method for the assessment of shoulder function. *J Shoulder Elbow Surg* 1994;3:347–352, with permission.)

SIGNS
0=none; 1=mild; 2=moderate; 3=severe

SIGN	RIGHT	LEFT
Supraspinatus/greater tuberosity tenderness	0 1 2 3	0 1 2 3
AC joint tenderness	0 1 2 3	0 1 2 3
biceps tendon tenderness (or rupture)	0 1 2 3	0 1 2 3
Other tenderness - List:_____	0 1 2 3	0 1 2 3
Impingement I (passive FE in slight internal rot)	Y	N
Impingement II (passive internal rotation, 90° FE)	Y	N
Impingement III(90° active abduction/painful arc)	Y	N
Subacromial crepitus	Y	N
Scars - location_____	Y	N
Atrophy - location_____	Y	N
Deformity - describe:_____	Y	N

STRENGTH
(record MRC grade)
0=no contraction; 1=flicker; 2=movement with gravity; 3=movement against gravity;
4= movement against some resistance; 5=normal power

	RIGHT	LEFT
Testing affected by pain?	Y	N
Forward elevation	0 1 2 3 4 5	0 1 2 3 4 5
Abduction	0 1 2 3 4 5	0 1 2 3 4 5
External rotation (arm at side)	0 1 2 3 4 5	0 1 2 3 4 5
Internal rotation (arm at side)	0 1 2 3 4 5	0 1 2 3 4 5

INSTABILITY

0=none; 1=mild (0 - 1 cm translation); 2=moderate (1 - 2 cm translation); 3=severe (>2 cm translation or over the rim of the glenoid)

SIGN	RIGHT	LEFT
Anterior translation	0 1 2 3	0 1 2 3
Posterior translation	0 1 2 3	0 1 2 3
Inferior translation (sulcus sign)	0 1 2 3	0 1 2 3
Anterior apprehension	0 1 2 3	0 1 2 3
Reproduces symptoms?	Y	N
Voluntary instability?	Y	N
Relocation test positive?	Y	N
Generalized ligamentous laxity?	Y	N

Other physical findings:

Examiner's name_____   Date_____

The Shoulder Score Index is derived by
   5 X (10 - Visual analog scale pain score)   +   (5/3 X Cumulative ADL Score)
And has a total maximum of 100 points.

APPENDIX 5-2. *(continued)*

analog scale for pain for 50% of the total score and scores the activities of daily living questionnaire for the other 50%, producing a 100-point total.

Some concerns have been raised about the ASES Standardized Shoulder assessment, however (40,41). Although motion is measured passively and actively, it is not clear whether this motion is measured in the sitting or supine position, which may affect the active range. Because motion is referenced to the thorax (to negate spine motion), the range of motion reported by this assessment may appear less than range of motion reported by other assessments. Internal rotation as measured by the vertebral levels on the back may not be accurate (42). Internal rotation measured with the arm at 90 degrees of abduction was part of Neer's original evaluation but was neglected from the ASES evaluation, presumably because this position is difficult for many patients (41). However, this information may be particularly important in assessing the overhead athlete because some researchers believe posterior capsular tightness is of paramount importance to the development of pathology. In addition, functional testing in the ASES Standardized Shoulder Assessment may be altered by elbow and wrist abnormalities and may not reflect abnormalities in shoulder function when such maladies exist.

The ASES Standardized Shoulder Assessment, unlike the Neer evaluation, does not include a subjective measure of improvement or patient satisfaction with treatment, which might be helpful in serial evaluations and is critically important in assessing the athlete's perception of the outcome of treatment. Finally, because the scoring index may not be sensitive enough to detect some specific disorders of the shoulder, such as pain when throwing, it is recommended that authors report the specific findings in the different components of the ASES Standardized Shoulder Assessment.

Realizing these limitations, the Research Committee of the ASES has recommended modifying or customizing this assessment to fit individual clinician's needs, so that any specific or unusual conditions can be addressed. For example, when using this assessment to evaluate the effect of a treatment in overhead athletes, the authors should add measurements of internal rotation for the abducted arm and include patient satisfaction when reporting outcomes.

The patient-completed subjective portion of this assessment was recently evaluated and was found to be reliable, valid, and responsive (11). Therefore, the ASES Standardized Shoulder Assessment will likely become the standard global shoulder assessment for evaluating outcomes in the treatment of shoulder disorders in the United States.

Population- or Disease-Specific Assessment Tools

The final and most focused method of assessing outcomes is to use assessment tools that specifically assess a particular population in question. Most commonly, this population is defined by the diagnosis. For example, there are evaluation systems for assessing the outcome after instability surgery (10,34,43,44), rotator cuff pathology (37,45,46), and osteoarthritis of the shoulder (47–49). These methods of assessing outcomes have been developed for use in disease-specific populations of patients and should not be used as global shoulder assessments or for other populations of patients.

The Rowe evaluation is an example of a shoulder evaluation designed for the assessment of outcomes following treatment for shoulder instability (34) (Appendix 5-3). This scoring system, albeit popular (Table 5-3), has not been validated, has not undergone testing for reliability or responsiveness, and has multiple flaws (30). One assessment tool developed to measure outcomes for shoulder instability that has undergone this testing is the Western Ontario Shoulder Instability Index (WOSI) (10) (Appendix 5-4). This assessment tool has excellent reliability and validity, and is more responsive than other outcome measures for instability. As such, the WOSI is preferred for the evaluation of patients with glenohumeral joint instability (30).

Whereas the diagnosis of glenohumeral joint instability can be used to define a specific population of patients, the overhead athlete likely represents a separate population. Even though some overhead athletes may have symptoms of instability and the two populations may overlap, the constellation of pathology in the thrower's shoulder is somewhat different than that of a patient with traumatic anterior glenohumeral joint instability. Therefore, it seems reasonable to have an assessment tool designed to evaluate the population of overhead athletes with shoulder problems. Overhead, noncollision athletes represent a specific and identifiable population, and specific assessment tools could be designed to be very sensitive for this population.

There have been two attempts at developing an assessment for the athlete's shoulder. The first was developed by Tibone and Bradley (50) and is presented in Appendix 5-5. This assessment tool was designed specifically for evaluating the athlete's shoulder.

In this assessment, a final score is determined that is heavily weighted toward subjective categories. Objective measures of range of motion account for 10% of the total score. This assessment was developed with equal weighting for the athlete's subjective perceptions of pain, strength and endurance, stability, and intensity. In addition, the patient's

Scoring System	Units	Excellent (100-90)	Good (89-75)	Fair (74-51)	Poor (50 or less)
Stability					
No recurrence, subluxation, or apprehension	50	No recurrences	No recurrences	No recurrences	Recurrence of dislocation
					or
Apprehension when placing arm in certain positions	30	No apprehension when placing arm in complete elevation and external rotation	Mild apprehension when placing arm in elevation and external rotation	Moderate apprehension during elevation and external rotation	Marked apprehension during elevation and external rotation
Subluxation (not requiring reduction)	10	No subluxation	No subluxation	No subluxation	
Recurrent dislocation	0				
Motion					
100% of normal external rotation, internal rotation, and elevation	20	100% of normal external rotation; complete elevation	75% of normal external rotation; complete elevation	50% of normal external rotation; complete elevation	No external rotation; 50% of elevation
75% of normal external rotation, and normal elevation, and internal rotation	15				
50% of normal external rotation, 75% of normal elevation, and internal rotation	5				
50% of normal elevation and internal rotation, no external rotation	0				
Function					
No limitation in work or sports; little or no discomfort	30	Performs all work and sports; no limitation in overhead activities shoulder strong in lifting, swimming, tennis, throwing; no discomfort	Mild limitation in work and sports, shoulder strong; minimum discomfort	Moderate limitation doing overhead work and heavy lifting; unable to throw, serve hard in tennis, or swim; moderate disabling pain	Marked limitation unable to perform overhead work and lifting; cannot throw, play tennis or swim; chronic discomfort
Mild limitation and minimum discomfort	25				
Moderate limitation and discomfort	10				
Marked limitation and pain	0				

Total (of 100 possible) _____ (Excellent = 90-100, Good = 75-89, Fair = 51-74, Poor = 50 or less)

APPENDIX 5-3. The Rowe Score for Evaluating the Bankart Operation. (From Rowe CR, Patel D, Southmayd WW. The Bankart procedure. *J Bone Joint Surg (Am)* 1978;60:1–16, with permission.)

Section A: Physical Symptoms

1. How much pain do you experience in your shoulder with overhead activities?

   No pain _____ Extreme pain

2. How much aching or throbbing do you experience in your shoulder?

   No aching/throbbing _____ Extreme aching/throbbing

3. How much weakness or lack of strength do you experience in your shoulder?

   No weakness _____ Extreme weakness

4. How much fatigue or lack of stamina do you experience in your shoulder?

   No fatigue _____ Extreme fatigue

5. How much clicking, cracking, or snapping do you experience in your shoulder?

   No clicking _____ Extreme clicking

6. How much stiffness do you experience in your shoulder?

   No stiffness _____ Extreme stiffness

7. How much discomfort do you experience in your neck muscles as a result of your shoulder?

   No discomfort _____ Extreme discomfort

8. How much feeling of instability or looseness do you experience in your shoulder?

   No instability _____ Extreme instability

9. How much do you compensate for your shoulder with other muscles?

   Not at all _____ Extreme

10. How much loss of range of motion do you have in your shoulder?

    No loss _____ Extreme loss

Section B: Sports/Recreation/Work

11. How much has your shoulder limited the amount you can participate in sports or recreational activities?

    Not limited _____ Extremely limited

12. How much has your shoulder affected your ability to perform the specific skills required for your sport or work? (If your shoulder affects both sports and work, consider the area that is most affected).

    Not affected _____ Extremely affected

13. How much do you feel the need to protect your arm during activities?

    Not at all _____ Extreme

APPENDIX 5-4. Western Ontario Shoulder Instability Index. Patients are instructed to place an X on the horizontal line. Each question is scored from 0 to 100 based on the placement of the X on the line. The best score possible is 0; the worst score possible is 2100. (From Kirkley A, Griffin S, McLintock H, et al. The development and evaluation of a disease-specific quality of life measurement tool for shoulder instability. *Am J Sports Med* 1998;26(6):764–772, with permission.)

14. How much difficulty do you experience lifting heavy objects below shoulder level?

_____

No difficulty   Extreme difficulty

Section C: Lifestyle
15. How much fear do you have of falling on your shoulder?

_____

No fear   Extreme fear

16. How much difficulty do you experience maintaining your desired level of fitness?

_____

No difficulty   Extreme difficulty

17. How much difficulty do you have "roughhousing or horsing around" with family or friends?

_____

No difficulty   Extreme difficulty

18. How much difficulty do you have sleeping because of your shoulder?

_____

No difficulty   Extreme difficulty

Section D: Emotions
19. How conscious are you of your shoulder?

_____

Not conscious   Extremely conscious

20. How concerned are you about your shoulder becoming worse?

_____

Not concerned   Extremely concerned

21. How much frustration do you feel because of your shoulder?

_____

No frustration   Extremely frustrated

APPENDIX 5-4. *(continued)*

subjective impression of his or her *performance* is weighted heavily (50% of the total score). This emphasis on function of the shoulder is important; Gill and colleagues showed high-level function to be the most important concern for patients with shoulder instability (43).

The second athlete's shoulder assessment tool, developed by Kuhn and Hawkins (51) (Appendix 5-6), is a modification of the assessment tool of Tibone and Bradley (50). The modification of the athlete's shoulder score was done to try to scale instability and function using the *ability to compete in the athlete's usual sport* as a reference. The intent was to try to improve the sensitivity of the instrument in this select population of athletes with shoulder pathology. This assessment tool is currently under investigation for validation, reliability, and responsiveness in a population of athletes who compete in shoulder intensive sports. Like the Tibone and Bradley assessment tool, the domain with the highest emphasis is the athlete's subjective impression of function (70% of the total score) with subdivisions of athletic performance (50% of the score), intensity (10%), and strength during sport (10%).

SUMMARY AND RECOMMENDATIONS

The goal of outcomes research is important. There is no question that we should be able to compare studies from different institutions using standardized and accurate

Name_____Age_____Sex_____

Dominant Hand (R)_____ (L)_____ (Ambidextrous)_____

Date of Examination_____ Surgeon_____

Type of Sport_____ Position Played_____

Years Played_____ Prior Injury_____

Activity Level
1.) Professional (Major League)
2.) Professional (Minor League)
3.) College
4.) High School
5.) Recreational (Full Time)
6.) Recreational (Occasionally)

Diagnosis
1.) Anterior Instability
2.) Posterior Instability
3.) Multidirectional Instability
4.) Recurrent Dislocations
5.) Impingement Syndrome
6.) Acromioclavicular Separation
7.) Acromioclavicular Arthritis
8.) Rotator Cuff Tear (Partial)
9.) Rotator Cuff Tear (Complete)
10.) Biceps Tendon Rupture
11.) Calcific Tendinitis
12.) Fracture

SUBJECTIVE (90 Points)

Pain (10 Points)

No pain with competition	10
Pain after competing only	8
Pain while competing	6
Pain preventing competing	4
Pain with ADLs	2
Pain at rest	0

Strength/Endurance (10 points)

No weakness, normal competition fatigue	10
Weakness after competition, early competition fatigue	8
Weakness during competition, abnormal competition fatigue	6
Weakness or fatigue preventing competition	4
Weakness or fatigue with ADLs	2
Weakness or fatigue at rest	0

Stability (10 points)

No looseness during competition	10
Recurrent subluxation while competing	8
Dead-arm syndrome while competing	6
Recurrent subluxation prevent competition	4
Recurrent subluxation during ADLs	2
Dislocation	0

Intensity (10 points)

Preinjury versus postinjury hours of competition (100%)	10
Preinjury versus postinjury hours of competition (<75%)	8
Preinjury versus postinjury hours of competition (<50%)	6
Preinjury versus postinjury hours of competition (<25%)	4
Preinjury and postinjury hours of ADL (100%)	2
Preinjury and postinjury hours of ADL (<50%)	0

Performance (50 points)

APPENDIX 5-5. The Athletic Shoulder Outcome Rating Scale. (From Tibone JE, Bradley JP. Evaluation of treatment outcomes for the athlete's shoulder. In: Matsen FA III, Fu FH, Hawkins RJ, eds. *The shoulder: a balance of mobility and stability.* Rosemont, IL: American Academy of Orthopaedic Surgeons, 1993:519–529, with permission.)

At the same level, same proficiency	50
At the same level, decreased proficiency	40
At the same level, decreases proficiency, not acceptable	30
Decreased level with acceptable proficiency at that level	20
Decreased level, unacceptable proficiency	10
Cannot compete, had to switch sport	0

OBJECTIVE (10 Points)

Range of Motion (10 Points)

Normal external rotation at 90°-90° position, normal elevation	10
Less than 5° loss of external rotation; normal elevation	8
Less than 10° loss of external rotation; normal elevation	6
Less than 15° loss of external rotation; normal elevation	4
Less than 20° loss of external rotation; normal elevation	2
More than 20° loss of external rotation; any loss of elev.	0

OVERALL RESULTS

Excellent	90-100
Good	70-89
Fair	50-69
Poor	Less than 50

APPENDIX 5-5. *(continued)*

outcomes measures that importantly reflect the athlete's perception of the result of treatment. As the field of outcomes research advances, a consensus may eventually be reached on the most appropriate method to assess the results and effectiveness of treatments for the athlete's shoulder. The most appropriate assessment must emphasize the patient's perception of the outcome. Scoring systems should place emphasis on the components of shoulder well-being according to the relative importance of these components as assigned by the patients (43). Once reasonable levels of importance are determined, all assessment tools must undergo reliability, validity, and responsiveness evaluations. Finally, when all of this is completed, a consensus must be produced by the experts in that field. Despite years of study, there is still no current consensus on the best method of assessing outcomes in the overhead athlete. Nevertheless, some guidelines can be offered.

When designing a study to review a treatment method in this special population of overhead athletes, it would be wise to collect outcomes data using validated, reliable, and responsive assessment tools for all levels of the hierarchy of sensitivity. Because the SF-36 form is the most widely accepted assessment tool for general health and well-being, it should be included in the data analysis. In addition, the ASES Standardized Shoulder Assessment, which has been found to be reliable, responsive, and valid, is rapidly becoming an accepted measure for the general assessment of the shoulder in the United States. However, it is important to add criteria relative to the overhead athlete's shoulder to this assessment, for example, by adding measures of internal rotation with the arm abducted to 90 degrees and a subjective patient satisfaction scale to the original assessment.

The final level of assessment is most important: the most sensitive instrument to measure the outcome of a treatment in the overhead athlete will be an assessment tool that is specifically designed to evaluate this population. At this time, however, the assessment tools that are specific for the overhead athlete's shoulder have not yet been validated. On the other hand, some disease-specific tools have been validated and should be considered. We expect to soon have a validated, reliable, and responsive outcomes assessment tool to use in the evaluation of treatments for shoulder pathology in the distinct population of the overhead athlete.

Name: _____ Date: _____

Involved Shoulder: __Right __Left Hand Dominance: __Right __Left

Sports Participation Information

Primary Sport Played: _____ Years Played: _____ Position Played:_____

What is the Level of Intensity of your Sport?
___Recreational/Part-time
___Recreational/Full-time
___High School
___College
___Professional Minor League
___Professional Major League

At what Regional Level do you compete?
___Local
___Regional
___National
___International

Pain Evaluation (10 points)

How does your pain affect your ability to compete in your sport?
___No pain with competition (10 points)
___Pain only after competition (8 points)
___Mild pain with competition (6 points)
___Moderate pain with competition (4 points)
___Severe pain with competition (2 points)
___Pain prevents competition (0 points)

Shoulder Instability Evaluation (10 points)

Do you feel looseness or instability in your shoulder, and if so, how does it affect your ability to compete in your sport?
___I do not have a feeling of looseness or instability and have no problems during competition (10 points)
___I have a feeling of looseness, but can continue to compete without stopping (8 points)
___I rarely have to stop competing (6 points)
___I occasionally have to stop competing (4 points)
___I frequently have to stop competing (2 points)
___I cannot compete due to the looseness or instability in my shoulder (0 points)

Functional Evaluation (70 points: Performance = 50; Strength/Endurance = 10, Intensity = 10)

At what level can you now participate in your sport?
___Equal to or above my pre-injury level (50 points)
___Slightly below my pre-injury level (40 points)
___Moderately below my pre-injury level (30 points)
___Significantly below my pre-injury level (20 points)
___I cannot compete in my usual sport (10 points)
___I cannot compete in any sport (0 points)

Describe your current strength or endurance of your shoulder when competing in your usual sport:
___I have no weakness or fatigue playing my usual sport (10 points)
___I have mild weakness or fatigue playing my usual sport (8 points)
___I have moderate weakness or fatigue playing my usual sport (6 points)
___I have severe weakness or fatigue playing my usual sport (4 points)
___Weakness or fatigue prevents me from competing in my usual sport (2 points)
___Weakness or fatigue prevents me from competing in any sport (0 points)

At what intensity level do you now compete in your usual sport compared to your pre-injury level?
___Same or better than my pre-injury level (10 points)
___75-100% of my pre-injury level (8 points)
___50-75% of my pre-injury level (6 points)
___25-50% of my pre-injury level (4 points)

APPENDIX 5-6. Athlete's Shoulder Assessment Tool. Of the total 100 points available, 90 are based on the patient's subjective assessment of the shoulder. In addition, 70 points are based on the function of the shoulder during the patient's usual sport. (From Hawkins RJ. Consideration of the athlete's shoulder: how it differs. In: Hawkins RJ, Misamore GW, eds. *Shoulder injuries in the athlete.* New York: Churchill Livingstone, 1996:1–8.)

___<25% of my pre-injury level (2 points)
___I can no longer compete at any intensity (0 points)

Range of Motion Evaluation (Completed by Examining Physician)
___No loss of external rotation at 90/90 position, no loss of elevation (10 points)
___Less than 5 degrees loss of external rotation at 90/90 position, no loss of elevation (8 points)
___5-10 degree loss of external rotation at 90/90 position, no loss of elevation (6 points)
___10-15 degree loss of external rotation at 90/90 position, no loss of elevation (4 points)
___15-20 degree loss of external rotation at 90/90 position, no loss of elevation (2 points)
___>20 degree loss of external rotation at 90/90 position, any loss of elevation (0 points)

OVERALL RESULTS

Excellent	90-100
Good	70-89
Fair	50-69
Poor	Less than 50

APPENDIX 5-6. *(continued)*

REFERENCES

1. Codman EA. The product of a hospital. *Surg Gynecol Obstet* 1914;18:491–496.
2. Mallon W. *Ernest Amory Codman*. Philadelphia: WB Saunders, 2000.
3. Fitzpatrick R. Patient satisfaction and quality of life measures. In: Pynsent P, Fairbank J, Carr A, eds. *Outcome measures in orthopaedics*. Oxford: Butterworth-Heinemann, 1993:45–58.
4. Guyatt GH, Mitchell A, Irvine EJ, et al. A new measure of health status for clinical trials in inflammatory bowel disease. *Gastroenterology* 1989;96:804–810.
5. Guyatt GH, Walter S, Norman G. Measuring change over time: assessing the usefulness of evaluative instruments. *J Chronic Dis* 1987;40:171–178.
6. Liang MH, Fossel AH, Larson MG. Comparisons of five health status instruments for orthopedic evaluation. *Med Care* 1990;28: 632–642.
7. Liang MH, Larson MG, Cullen KE, et al. Comparative measurement efficiency and sensitivity of five health status instruments for arthritis research. *Arthritis Rheum* 1985;28: 542–547.
8. Kazis LE, Anderson JJ, Meenan RF. Effect sizes for interpreting changes in health status. *Med Care* 1989;27:S178–S189.
9. L'Insalata JC, Warren RF, Cohen SB, et al. A self administered questionnaire for assessment of symptoms and function of the shoulder. *J Bone Joint Surg (Am)* 1997;79:738–748.
10. Kirkley A, Griffin S, McClintock JH, et al. Development of a disease-specific quality of life measurement tool for shoulder instability: the Western Ontario Shoulder Instability Index (WOSI). *Am J Sports Med* 1998;26:764–772.
11. Michener LA, McClure PW, Sennett BJ. American shoulder and elbow surgeons standardized shoulder assessment form, patient self-report section: reliability, validity, and responsiveness. *J Shoulder Elbow Surg* 2002;11:587–594.
12. Lippitt SB, Harryman DT II, Matsen FA III. A practical tool for evaluating function: the simple shoulder test. In: Matsen FA III, Fu FH, Hawkins RJ, eds. *The shoulder: a balance of mobility and stability*. Rosemont, IL: American Academy of Orthopaedic Surgeons, 1993:501–518.
13. Matsen FA, Lippitt SB, Sidles JA, et al. Evaluating the shoulder. In: Matsen FA, Lippitt SB, Sidles JA, et al, eds. *Practical evaluation and management of the shoulder*. Philadelphia: WB Saunders, 1994:1–17.
14. Matsen FA, Ziegler DW, BeBartolo SE. Patient self-assessment of health status and function in glenohumeral degenerative joint disease. *J Shoulder Elbow Surg* 1995;4(5):345–351.
15. Constant CR. *Age related recovery of shoulder function after injury*. Thesis. Cork, Ireland, University College, 1986.
16. Constant CR, Murley AHG. A clinical method of functional assessment of the shoulder. *Clin Ortho* 1987;214:160–164.
17. Kuhn JE, Blasier RB. Measuring outcomes of shoulder arthroplasty. *Semin Arthroplasty* 1995;6(4):245–264.
18. Kuhn JE, Blasier RB. Evaluating outcomes in the shoulder. In: Tom Norris, ed. *Orthopaedic knowledge update, the shoulder and elbow*. Rosemont, IL: American Academy of Orthopaedic Surgeons, 1997:47–59.
19. Kuhn JE, Blasier RB. Assessment of outcome in shoulder arthroplasty. *Orthop Clin North Am* 1998;29(3):549–563.
20. Ware JE, Shervourne CD. The MOS 36-item short-form health survey (SF-36): I. Conceptual framework and item selection. *Med Care* 1992;30:473–483.
21. Meenan RF, Gertman PM, Mason JH, et al. The arthritis impact measurement scales: further investigation of a health status measure. *Arthritis Rheum* 1982;25:1048–1053.
22. Hunt SM, McEwen J, McKenna SP. Measuring health status. A new tool for clinicians and epidemiologists. *J R Coll Gen Pract* 1985;35:185–188.
23. Bergner M, Bobbitt RA, Carter WB, et al. The sickness impact profile: development and final revisions of a health status measure. *Med Care* 1981;19:787–805.
24. Deyo RA, Inui TS, Leininger JD, et al. Measuring functional outcome in chronic disease: a comparison of traditional scales and a self administered health status questionnaire in patients with rheumatoid arthritis. *Med Care* 1983;21:180–192.
25. McDowell IW, Martini CJM, Waugh WA. A method for self-assessment of disability before and after hip replacement operations. *Br Med J* 1978;2:857–859.
26. Beaton DE, Richards RR. Measuring shoulder function: a cross-sectional comparison of five questionnaires. *J Bone Joint Surg (Am)* 1996;78:882–890.
27. Richards RR, Beaton DE. Measuring shoulder function: a cross-sectional comparison of five different questionnaires. *J Shoulder Elbow Surg* 1994;4(Part 2):561.

28. Patte D. Directions for the use of the index severity for painful and/or chronically disabled shoulders. Abstracts of the First Open Congress of the European Society of Surgery of the Shoulder and the Elbow, Paris, 1987:36–41.
29. Richards RR, An KN, Bigliani LU, et al. A standard method for the assessment of shoulder function. *J Shoulder Elbow Surg* 1994; 3:347–352.
30. Roach KE, Budiman-Mak E, Songsiridej N, et al. Development of a shoulder pain and disability index. *Arthritis Care Res* 1991; 4(4):143–149.
31. Kirkley A. Scoring systems for the functional assessment of the shoulder. *Techniques Shoulder Elbow Surg* 2002;3(4):220–233.
32. Uhorchak JM, Arciero RA, Huggard D, et al. Recurrent shoulder instability after open reconstruction in athletes involved in collision and contact sports. *Am J Sports Med* 2000;28(6):794–799.
33. Binker MR, Cuomo JS, Popham GJ, et al. An examination of bias in shoulder scoring instruments among healthy collegiate and recreational athletes. *J Shoulder Elbow Surg* 2002;11(5):463–469.
34. Romeo AA, Bach BR, O'Halloran KL. Scoring systems for shoulder conditions. *Am J Sports Med* 1996;24(4):472–476.
35. Rowe CR, Patel D, Southmayd WW. The Bankart procedure: a long-term end-result study. *J Bone Joint Surg (Am)* 1978;60:1–16.
36. Neer CS II. Anterior acromioplasty for the chronic impingement syndrome in the shoulder: a preliminary report. *J Bone Joint Surg (Am)* 1972;54:41–50.
37. Neer CS II, Watson KC, Stanton FJ. Recent experience in total shoulder replacement. *J Bone Joint Surg (Am)* 1982;64:319–337.
38. Altchek DW, Warren RF, Wickiewicz TL, et al. Arthroscopic acromioplasty. Technique and results. *J Bone Joint Surg (Am)* 1990;72:1198–1207.
39. Ellman H, Hanker G, Bayer M. Repair of the rotator cuff: end-result study of factors influencing reconstruction. *J Bone Joint Surg (Am)* 1986;68:1136–1144.
40. Gerber C. Integrated scoring systems for the functional assessment of the shoulder. In: Matsen FA III, Fu FH, Hawkins RJ, eds. *The shoulder: a balance of mobility and stability.* Rosemont, IL: American Academy of Orthopaedic Surgeons, 1993:531–550.
41. MacDonald DA. The shoulder and elbow. In: Pynsent P, Fairbank J, Carr A, eds. *Outcome measures in orthopaedics.* Oxford: Butterworth-Heinemann, 1993:144–173.
42. Mallon WJ, Herring CL, Sallay PI, et al. Use of vertebral levels to measure presumed internal rotation at the shoulder: a radiographic analysis. *J Shoulder Elbow Surg* 1996;5:299–306.
43. Gill TJ, Micheli LJ, Gebhard F, et al. Bankart repair for anterior instability of the shoulder. Long-term outcome. *J Bone Joint Surg* 1997;79(6):850–857.
44. Walch G. Directions for use of the quotation of anterior instabilities of the shoulder. First Open Congress of the European Society of Surgery of the Shoulder and Elbow, Paris, 1987: 51–55.
45. Kirkley A, Griffin S. Alvarez C. The development and evaluation of a disease-specific quality of life measurement tool for rotator cuff disease: The Western Ontario Rotator Cuff Index (WORC). In: *Annual meeting book of abstracts.* New Orleans: American Academy of Orthopaedic Surgeons, 1998.
46. Marechal E. Ruptures degeneratives de la coiffe des rotateurs l'epaule: Evaluation foncitionnelle: Resultats du traitement chirurgical. Universite Claude Bernard, Lyon I, France, Facultee de Medecine Grange, Blanche, These N. 5, 1990.
47. Amstutz HL, Sew Hoy AL, Clark IC. UCLA anatomic total shoulder arthroplasty. *Clin Orthop* 1981;155:7–20.
48. Lo IKY, Griffin S, Kirkley A. The development and evaluation of a disease specific quality of life measurement tool for osteoarthritis of the shoulder: the Western Ontario Osteoarthritis of the Shoulder Index (WOOS). *Arthritis Cartilage* 2001;9:771–778.
49. Swanson AB, DeGroot Swanson G, Sattel AB, et al. Bipolar implant shoulder arthroplasty. *Clin Orthop* 1989;249:227–247.
50. Tibone JE, Bradley JP. Evaluation of treatment outcomes for the athlete's shoulder. In: Matsen FA, Fu FH, Hawkins RJ, eds. *The shoulder: a balance of mobility and stability.* Rosemont, IL: American Academy of Orthopaedic Surgeons, 1994:519–529.
51. Hawkins RJ. Consideration of the athlete's shoulder: how it differs. In: Hawkins RJ, Misamore GW, eds. *Shoulder injuries in the athlete.* New York: Churchill Livingstone, 1996:1–8.

6

RESISTANCE TRAINING AND CORE STRENGTHENING

DONALD A. CHU
CHRISTINE BOYD
ANDREA HAMMER

INTRODUCTION

Resistance training programs for the overhead athlete should focus on developing strength, power, and outcome gains, which directly contribute to improved function and performance. It is a well-established fact that throwing and overhead activities follow an activation sequence known as the *kinetic chain*. The kinetic chain is a summation of all the forces developed within the body, applied in the proper sequence, which results in the outcome of throwing or overhead striking a ball or object. The overhead action really begins from the ground up.

The sequence of activation in the kinetic chain works from proximal to distal in overhead activities. The goal is to impart maximum force or velocity through each part of the proximal kinetic chain so that the distal segments (shoulder, arm, and hand) ultimately reach their maximum velocity. This process may be viewed as "cracking the whip."

Because the lower extremities are relatively large in terms of mass, they are responsible for most of the force developed in the kinetic chain. Hence, in activities such as baseball pitching, lower extremity force production (strength and power) is more highly correlated with ball velocity than is upper extremity force production. It follows that any program aimed at achieving an outcome of increased overhead velocity should first address the development of general, functional, and sport-specific strength in the lower extremities.

Kibler and colleagues describe the physiologic model for throwing and striking sports as a "motor" program (1). Motor programs activate muscles in a coordinated sequence of events that creates joint movements related to the movement task. The first event occurs at a single joint, which is stimulated by joint perturbations. These perturbations are resisted and force-couple activation among muscles occurs to stabilize the joint. Next, force-dependent patterns coordinate motions at several joints and use agonist–antagonist

activation to generate forces that are directly applied to throwing or striking an object. In combination, these two activities result in task orientation for the muscle contractions and include lower extremity and trunk muscle activation before and during arm motion.

The core is what transmits the forces generated from ground reaction and the lower extremities to the distal upper extremity segments or an object. The core must be strong and stable in order to effectively transmit forces that have as the outcome a functional task. In addition to generating and transferring force to distal segments, these motor programs create a stable base from which voluntary arm movements occur. This allows for maintenance of body equilibrium during the course of throwing or overhead striking an object. Sensory and proprioceptive information for positioning and feedback during the activity are also required for integration and activation of the complete throwing motion.

Resistance training and core strengthening must start as general training programs and advance to programs specific to position, motion, and function. These should include gravity resistance and joint integration to stimulate the appropriate functional patterns. Given the importance of trunk musculature as a conduit for ground reaction forces through the kinetic chain, there are many questions that must be addressed:

- Is the object of resistance training programs to develop maximal strength, strength-endurance, or actual power output?
- What modalities are the most effective at achieving these goals?
- What areas of the trunk should be addressed first and most frequently?
- How many exercises should be included in a core-strengthening program?
- What sorts of loads or intensities should be used with the exercises?

BACKGROUND

Historical

A significant portion of the functional outcome, strength, and power generated at the shoulder relies on contributions from more proximal body segments including the core. The term *core strength* traditionally encompasses the muscles of the torso that are involved in originating movement. These include the rectus abdominis, internal and external obliques, and erector spinae. Virtually all of the past and recent program developments in the area of core strengthening have been the result of attempting to reduce or mitigate low back pain. Even though the primary theme of this chapter is to address core-strengthening routines for overhead athletes who do *not* suffer from symptoms that limit range of motion or function, it would be a major oversight not to acknowledge those practitioners who helped define the field of core strengthening by treating low back pain. It is through their efforts that preventive programs have been developed and refined to avoid some of the long-term effects of degeneration while optimizing performance (2).

Among the first programs attempting to develop core strength were the "Williams Flexion Exercises" (3). These were among the primary modalities for the treatment of low back pain in the 1970s. The principal tenet of Paul Williams, MD, in 1937 was "Always sit, stand, walk, and lie in a way that reduces the lumbar lordosis to a minimum." He believed that lumbar lordosis placed unacceptable pressure on the posterior aspect of the intervertebral disc, which, in turn, accelerated the degenerative process. Williams' goal was to reduce lumbar lordosis as much as possible. Interestingly, he believed the same regarding the lordotic curve in the cervical spine.

The major thrust of his exercise routine consisted of a series of what Williams referred to as "first aid exercises." These exercises are as follows:

1. *Partial sit-up*—The athlete lies in a "hooklying" position (supine with knees bent and feet flat). With hands behind his or her head, the athlete elevates the upper torso until the scapulae clear the resting surface and stress is placed on the rectus abdominis. After returning to the start position, the sit-up is repeated for a prescribed number of repetitions (Fig. 6-1).
2. *Knee-to-chest*—From the hooklying position, the athlete places his or her hands over his or her knees and pulls them slowly toward the chest. This movement flattens the lumbar spine, stretching the low back, including the posterior hip, sacroiliac joints, and high hamstring area.
3. *Hamstring stretch*—Lying supine, the athlete places both hands around the back of one knee. The athlete straightens his or her knee and pulls the thigh toward his or her head so the hip goes into flexion. Williams believed that flexible hamstrings are necessary to accomplish full flexion of the lumbar spine. Although tight hamstrings limit

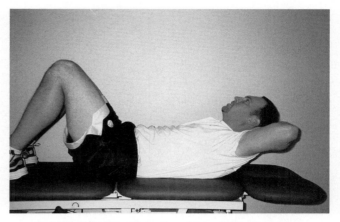

FIGURE 6-1. "Hooklying" position and partial sit-up.

lumbar flexion in standing with knees straight, we now know that tight hamstrings actually tilt the pelvis posteriorly and promote trunk flexion (Fig. 6-2).

4. *Seated flexion*—This exercise is performed by sitting in a chair and flexing forward in a slumped position. Maximum trunk flexion is obtained and direct stretching of the lumbosacral soft tissue structures occurs (Fig. 6-3).
5. *Squat*—Williams' squat position is with the feet placed shoulder width apart, the hips and knees are flexed to the maximum available range of motion, and the lumbar spine is rounded into flexion. Upon reaching maximum depth, the athlete "bounces the buttocks up and down" 15 to 20 times, with 2 to 3 inches of excursion on each bounce, then repeats three to four times. Williams believed that cultures that "hunkered down" in this position tended to have less back pain (Fig. 6-4).
6. *Lunges*—This exercise actually results in some extension of the lumbar spine when performed properly. Nonetheless, it is a good stretching exercise for the entire lower extremity, especially the iliopsoas, which may be a per-

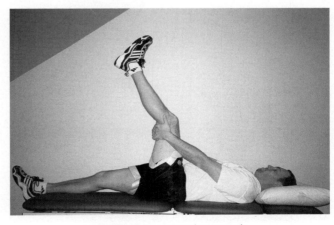

FIGURE 6-2. Hamstring stretch.

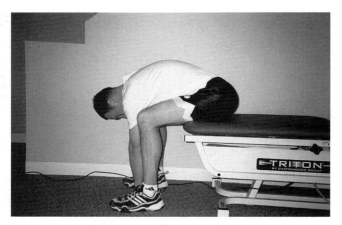

FIGURE 6-3. Williams' seated flexion.

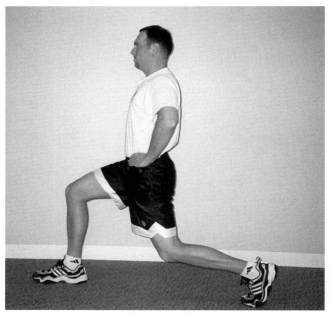

FIGURE 6-5. Williams' lunges.

petrator of low back pain if it is abnormally tight or in spasm (Fig. 6-5).

For years, the Williams Flexion Exercises were the mainstay of most low back pain prevention and care programs (4). They certainly accomplished the goal of flattening the lumbar spine and were advocated by physical therapists who worked with sports and industrial injuries. Although the success was limited, Williams' comprehensive program helped advance the idea that strong abdominal muscles are needed to prevent low back pain and improve core strength.

Robin McKenzie, MD, in 1981 followed Williams in the development of an exercise program for controlling back pain (4). Although at first it seems contradictory to Williams' program, they are similar in that both methods teach movement control techniques. Like Williams, McKenzie also claimed that the intervertebral disc is the major source of back pain.

However, he differed from Williams in that he claimed "flexion" to be the culprit in developing low back pain. According to McKenzie, prolonged sitting in a flexed position and frequency of flexion were the primary reasons for disc degeneration, and the lack of lumbar extension was a predisposition to low back pain. His discovery that some low back pain patients had reduced symptoms with extension movements was counter to Williams' line of thinking at that time.

The goal of McKenzie's exercises was to "centralize" pain. For example, in a patient with lower back pain that radiated to the left buttock, left posterior thigh, and left calf, the goal was to have the pain move proximally so that it only radiated from the lower back to the posterior thigh. Then, the goal was to centralize the pain so that it only radiated to the buttock, and then finally have the pain localized in the low back. This was accomplished through a system that emphasized extension movements of the lumbar, thoracic, and cervical spines. McKenzie postulated that extension of the spine corrects posteriorly displaced intradiscal mass, which was presumed to be the embryonic stage of disc herniation. This dynamic disc model provided an explanation for the commonly noted phenomenon of "centralization" in which disc pain is abolished and symptoms move more proximally, often in response to spinal extension exercises.

There is an entire McKenzie certification process and credential available for physicians and physical therapist to study and undergo with regard to the McKenzie system of assessment and evaluation. The exercises presented here are a sample of the myriad of movements proposed by Dr. McKenzie and are presented in the context of those relating to "core strength."

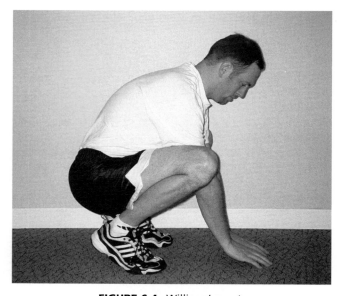

FIGURE 6-4. Williams' squat.

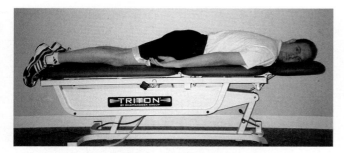

FIGURE 6-6. Prone lying.

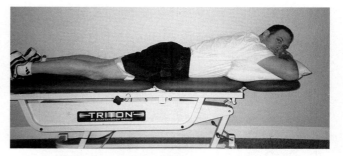

FIGURE 6-8. Progressive extension with pillows.

1. *Prone lying*—The athlete lies prone with arms along his or her sides and head turned to the most comfortable side. The athlete maintains this position for 5 to 10 minutes (Fig. 6-6).
2. *Prone lying on elbows*—The athlete lies prone with anterior hips touching the floor and his or her body weight on the elbows and forearms. With relaxation of the lower back muscles, the lumbar spine moves into extension. The athlete maintains this position for 5 to 10 minutes. If it causes pain, exercise 1 should be repeated and then this one tried again (Fig. 6-7).
3. *Progressive extension with pillows*—The athlete lies prone with a pillow under his or her chest. After 2 to 3 minutes, a second pillow is added. If this does not result in increased pain, a third pillow should be added. If possible, the athlete should stay in this position for up to 10 minutes. Pillows should be removed one at a time over several minutes (Fig. 6-8).
4. *Prone press-ups*—The athlete lies prone with palms near his or her shoulders, as if to do a standard push-up. While maintaining contact between hips and floor, the athlete slowly pushes up his or her shoulders and lets his or her back and stomach sag and move into extension. After reaching maximum extension range (before hips coming away from the resting surface), the athlete slowly

returns to the start position by lowering his or her shoulders (Fig. 6-9).
5. *Standing extension*—While standing, the athlete places his or her hands on the small of his or her back with fingers pointing toward the floor and resting over the buttocks. The athlete then leans backward over his or her hands and holds the position for 20 seconds. This exercise should be repeated 10 times and should be performed throughout the day after normal activities that place the athlete's back in a flexed position, that is, lifting, forward bending, sitting, and the like (Fig. 6-10).

Although both Williams' and McKenzie's systems may result in increases in trunk strength and range of motion, there is a fair share of controversy over their efficacy and effectiveness in treating low back pain (4). Looking at this issue from a historical perspective, they have both provided some benefits during the time of their peak popularity and both support the concept that "some movement is better than no movement."

Current Concepts

More recent work by Hodges and co-workers (4) has focused on differentiating the *local* stabilizing system of musculature for the intervertebral joints and sacroiliac region from the *global* stabilizing system of the spine (Table 6-1).

The efforts of Hodges and co-workers (4) are the most recent attempts to define mechanisms to stabilize the spinal

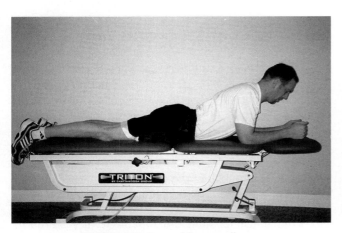

FIGURE 6-7. Prone lying on elbows.

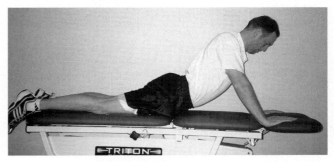

FIGURE 6-9. Prone press-ups.

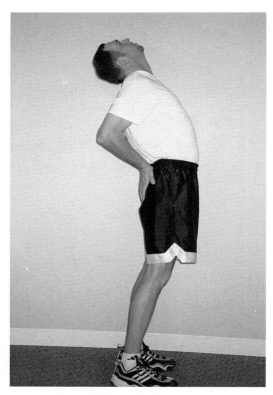

FIGURE 6-10. Standing extension.

segments for the purpose of reducing low back pain. They postulate that the global stabilizing system alone is unable to provide "core stability" and maintain an intersegmentally stable spine. Through their research, they have found that the transversus abdominis and multifidus are crucial in stabilizing the lumbar spine and lumbosacral regions, and poor function of these muscles has a direct effect on low back pain.

The transversus abdominis is the only abdominal muscle that directly attaches to the lumbar spine. It is a tonic muscle, and research has shown that, in individuals with healthy

backs, it should be the first muscle to fire before any other muscle in the abdominal area and before any movement in the body occurs. The transversus does not create movement, but rather, with its contraction, functions as a corset to stabilize the abdominal cavity. Hodges found that, in individuals with low back pain, the transversus either does not fire at all or fires too late in the sequence (e.g., the global muscles fire, then the transversus turns on).

The multifidus is the only muscle that can intersegmentally stabilize the lumbar spine. It is also a tonic muscle and is facilitated by and works with the transversus to locally stabilize the spine. Hodges' research found that, with a single incident of low back pain, atrophic changes might occur within the multifidus within 24 hours. Even long after symptoms have resolved, the multifidus may be inhibited and still cease to fire.

The sequence of the muscle recruitment is also crucial. The transversus should contract first, which should then facilitate the multifidus, and from that point the other core stabilizers begin to contract as needed.

These findings are significant because, given the use of many advanced dynamic exercises with the recent emphasis on "core strengthening," they indicate that an overhead athlete could perform very high-level core exercises without the transversus and multifidus firing. Assessment and treatment of the ability of these muscles to function requires specific training that is beyond the scope of this chapter. Knowledge of the existence of this information is important, however, especially for those overhead athletes with shoulder pain as well as persistent low back pain.

The work of Hodges and co-workers (4) exemplifies how far lumbar and "core" stability has come. Physical therapists such as Paul Hodges, Diane Lee, and Mark Commerford are all experts in manual therapy and have developed concepts on teaching and training musculature that most physicians and therapists were unaware of just 5 years ago. Core strengthening is an area of expertise that has grown, and the body of knowledge continues to expand as long as individuals suffer from low back pain.

TABLE 6–1. DIFFERENTIAL MUSCULAR STABILIZING SYSTEMS

Local Stabilizing System (Intervertebral Joints/ Sacroiliac Region)	Global Stabilizing System (Spine)
Transversus abdominis	Rectus abdominis
Internal oblique (posterior)	External oblique abdominis
Multifidus	Internal oblique abdominis
Intertraversaii, interspinales	Longissimus thoracis
Longissimus thoracis	Iliocostalis lumborum
Iliocostalis lumborum	Quadratus lumborum (lateral fibers)
Quadratus lumborum (medial fibers)	

OBJECT OF CORE STRENGTHENING

Strength is defined as the maximal force that a muscle or muscle group can generate at a specific velocity. *Power* refers to the amount of force that can be generated in a given time period (5). A one repetition maximum squat is a measure of absolute strength, whereas the force of a racquet on a ball at a given velocity determines the amount of power that is imparted to the ball. The crucial question is how core strength relates to each of these situations.

Muscles such as those classified by Hodges as *local stabilizers* are at work at all times, even while sitting, standing, and walking. Under these circumstances, they are under "low loads." Global stabilizers are under "high loads" in strength and power situations, such as lifting weights or performing movements under resistance.

According to Hodges, in order to develop an exercise program that focuses on lumbar stability, the following principles should be followed (4):

1. Use phasic *not* tonic contractions of the muscle.
2. Do not use ballistic movements.
3. Co-contraction, *not* unidirectional exercises, is the key to successfully training these muscles.
4. The focus should be on joint position.
5. Add proprioceptive cues to enhance training of these muscles.
6. Focus on low load exercises.
7. Gradually include more unstable positions to the exercise regimen.
8. Include proximal to distal segment movements (closed chain exercises).
9. Retrain general joint position control with everyday activities.

Assessing and Facilitating the Transversus Abdominis

Hodges and co-workers (4) and other researchers have spent years learning how the local stabilizing system functions and how to optimally facilitate it; they teach courses on the assessment and manual skills necessary to incorporate their techniques into treatment. The following is a brief description of what is involved in assessing and treating the local stabilizers and is by no means meant as instructions to the reader to competently perform what is described. One-on-one instruction is required as is a certain level of knowledge and manual skills.

The transversus can be palpated with the athlete in a hooklying position (Fig. 6-1) with the clinician's fingertips just medial to the anterosuperior iliac spine (ASIS). When the transversus fires, no movement should occur in the lumbar spine or pelvis. If movement is observed, other muscles have kicked in instead.

The athlete is asked to first breathe in, then exhale, and then (for a brief moment) stop breathing. This prevents the diaphragm from attempting to help brace the abdominal cavity. The athlete then gently pulls his navel toward the table as if he or she was putting on a tight pair of pants without sucking in his or her stomach. When the transversus contraction is palpated, it should be subtle and turn on very slowly. If a fast contraction is palpated, most likely the internal oblique attempted to compensate.

Because this is a difficult move to feel and perform, the athlete may be educated on how to contract his or her pelvic floor. When the muscles of the pelvic floor contract, they facilitate the transversus to turn on. A pelvic floor contraction, also known as a *Kegel*, can be described as contracting the muscles as if trying to stop the flow of urine (3).

After performing the breathing sequence described earlier, the athlete may be asked to only contract the pelvic floor. A gentle transversus contraction can then be palpated. Although using the pelvic floor is a good cue to learn how to first facilitate the transversus, the athlete should eventually be able to differentiate between a pelvic floor contraction and a transversus contraction.

Another, more objective method of retraining the transversus is to use a blood pressure cuff. There is a commercially produced model that is made specifically for these types of activities. The athlete lies prone and the blood pressure cuff is placed under his or her lower abdominals. The cuff is pumped up to 70 mm Hg of pressure. As the athlete performs a transversus contraction, the pressure should decrease 2 to 4 mm Hg. If it decreases more than that, other muscles are contributing. If the pressure increases, the athlete is most likely either contracting his or her rectus or using his or her diaphragm to increase abdominal pressure.

Assessing and Facilitating the Multifidus

There are a number of methods of assessing the multifidus. One method is by observation and palpation. An atrophied multifidus appears smaller and feels soft on palpation. It is possible, and often common, for the multifidus to be atrophied unilaterally and at only one or two levels (i.e., L4 and L5).

To see how the multifidus contracts, the athlete lies prone. Placing a hand under one ASIS, the clinician gently rotates the ileum posteriorly. The athlete is asked to maintain this position; with one hand the clinician maintains palpation to the ASIS to assess movement with the next step and, with the other hand, palpates the multifidus on the same side. The athlete, while maintaining the slight posterior pelvic rotation, extends his or her hip so that the excursion of his or her thigh is approximately 1 to 2 inches off the table surface (Fig. 6-11). If the multifidus is not firing appropriately, the clinician does not feel a contraction upon palpation of the muscle belly and feels the athlete's ASIS drop due to the inability of the multi-

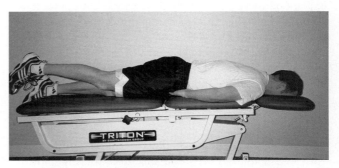

FIGURE 6-11. Assessment and exercise of multifidus.

fidus to maintain the position of the sacrum and the posteriorly rotated pelvis.

Although there are a number of methods for facilitating the multifidus, the easiest and most effective is using FES (functional electrical stimulation). It is done with the athlete in side-lying position and the electrodes placed unilaterally on the side farthest from the table. The athlete should be instructed to perform a transversus contraction simultaneously with the muscle is being contracted. This is because, just as the pelvic floor facilitates the transversus, a contraction of the transversus facilitates the multifidus. Once the muscle is facilitated, it is important for it to be trained and strengthened.

In the case of an injured athlete, an evaluation by a physical therapist knowledgeable in this area is recommended. When lumbar instability is present, "local stabilizers" usually lack muscular endurance and control rather than absolute strength deficits. This lack of muscular control places excessive and abnormal forces on ligaments, joint capsules, and intervertebral discs, along with other supportive soft tissue structures of the spine. Hypermobility is often apparent and the spine may appear "sloppy" due to poor motor control.

CORE STRENGTH MODALITIES

The overhead athlete is typically participating in a sport that demands repeated motion of the arm. Supporting this demand requires not only absolute strength of the core, but also a significant amount of strength-endurance to allow for maximal transfer of power from the ground to the distal segment on a repetitive basis. This strength-endurance also allows the athlete to maintain proper technique and stabilization to prevent injury, which often occurs as a result of fatigue. Just as the muscular component of an aerobic endurance-training program involves submaximal contractions extended over a large number of repetitions, core strength programs should begin the same way (5).

Body weight is sufficient to generate an adequate stimulus for initial core strengthening exercises. It is also necessary for the therapist, trainer or coach to recognize deficits, which must be addressed if the athlete is to successfully embark on this form of training. Strength-endurance is best accomplished when using a system of two to three sets of 15 to 18 repetitions for each exercise.

Given the cylindrical shape of the core musculature, the core cannot be worked in a one-dimensional plane. A comprehensive program should be multidirectional and cover all areas of the core. Weaknesses must be recognized and addressed with exercises specifically aimed at alleviating the problem.

An overriding theme of the current literature dealing with core stabilization is that machines for strengthening the low back and abdominals have little to no place in the development of functional core strength. Machines address the "global stabilizers" and may have minimal effect on the performance of the "local stabilizers." Machine-based exercises are generally performed non–weight bearing, have limited movement patterns and trunk excursion, and do not lend themselves to development of functional movement patterns (5). In reality, during functional movements, core muscles work eccentrically to decelerate and control movement. Machine-based exercises are unable to replicate this, and there is little transfer of stability gains obtained from machines to a weight-bearing, high-velocity, multiplane motion such as throwing a baseball or spiking a volleyball.

Common tools of the trade for lumbar stabilization programs include stabilization (physio) balls, foam rollers, and medicine balls. Because these modalities require dynamic stability and mimic the firing sequence of core musculature as it occurs in functional activity, they are considered better ways to train the core. However, it is important for an athlete to be taught the basic mechanics of how to recruit the local stabilizers, such as the transversus abdominis and the multifidus, to stabilize the spine before executing a movement or exercise. Free weights, pulley devices, and movement simulators such as elliptical trainers, StairMaster, and stationary bikes are all tools that may be included in core strength routines.

Currently, the trendiest tool in the war on weak cores is the exercise system developed by Joseph Pilates in the 1940s. Pilates was born in Germany in 1880, immigrated to New York, and developed a fitness regimen that bears his name. Simply know as *Pilates*, it is considered the exercise system of the Hollywood stars, and it is a sterling example of how things go full circle in the exercise world. The program was developed in his quest to overcome his own disabilities as a sick and frail child. The regimen puts emphasis on developing torso strength and flexibility (known as *centering*) to develop proper posture. This system caught the fancy of dancers because it does not use high numbers of repetitive exercises and focused on postural alignment as well as motor control of the abdominal and trunk musculature. Although recently commercialized, disciples of Josef Pilates have maintained his original precepts and the equipment used is basically the same as Pilates' original design. Although others have suggested that the methods of pelvic alignment and postural management might not be optimal in traditional Pilates classes, probably the most valuable contribution to the everyday user of this system of exercise is the bounty of stabilization and postural enhancement movements that come from the Pilates Mat Exercise Programs (5).

DESIGNING A CORE STRENGTHENING PROGRAM

A good rule to follow is to start small and perform well. Core strengthening is based on the quality of movements rather than the quantity. A three-stage approach to core strengthening appears to work best.

Stage One: Local Stabilizers

The athlete should first have an understanding of how the spine is stabilized and why it is important to learn how to perform such a specific and fine-tuned low-level contraction. The athlete should learn the basics of how to contract the local stabilizers of the spine, specifically the transversus abdominis and the multifidus. The contraction of these muscles is the foundation from which all movement patterns and exercises are performed. Once this has been learned, the principles should be applied to a program of four to six basic, fundamental abdominal and trunk strengthening exercises. Three to five repetitions are all that are needed to facilitate the learning component of each exercise. If deficits such as an inhibited multifidus have been identified, this stage should be used to work on overcoming them.

Exercises for Stage One

These exercises are basic, minimal, and small enough in number that they can easily be remembered. The key to success in stage one is to limit the complexity of the program and to reinforce basic fundamentals that will carry through to other programs:

1. Once the athlete knows how to correctly contract the transversus, he or she should be practicing a number of times a day. The athlete should work up to being able to hold an isometric contraction for 10 seconds. Initially however, the athlete may only be able to maintain an isolated contraction for a few seconds and may even fatigue after only a few repetitions. Fatigue occurs as soon as other muscles attempt to compensate.
2. Once the athlete knows how to correctly contract the multifidus, he or she can use the previously discussed assessment technique as an exercise. The athlete lies prone and rotates one side of the ileum slightly posteriorly. After performing a transversus contraction, the athlete extends his or her hip so that his or her thigh is approximately 1 inch off the table. The multifidus should contract in order to prevent the ASIS from lowering toward the table (Fig. 6-11).
3. It is important for the athlete to understand how to dissociate between hip mobility and pelvic mobility. Local core stability is needed to do this. In a hooklying position, the athlete contracts the transversus, and without the pelvis rotating or rocking, he or she slowly and under control brings one hip into abduction and external rotation. The thigh should only move as far as the athlete is able to control it while keeping the pelvis stable (Fig. 6-12).
4. Similarly, exercise 3 can be done in the prone position. With both knees flexed, the athlete contracts the trans-

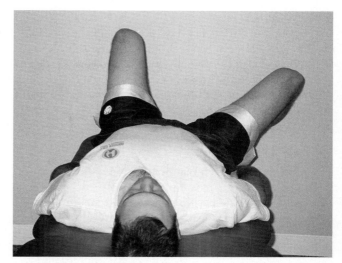

FIGURE 6-12. Transversus contraction with pelvis stabilized with hip abduction and external rotation.

versus and slowly and under control brings one foot toward the table so that the hip goes into internal rotation (foot moves out). Again, the pelvis and lumbar spine should not move (Fig. 6-13).

Stage Two: Global Stabilizers

Once the athlete can recruit the local stabilizers, he or she can be taught how to use the global stabilizers to maintain a stable base, or "core," from which to create and control movement in the lumbar spine and pelvis. The athlete should begin with low-level exercises in which the local stabilizers are fired first and then the global stabilizers neces-

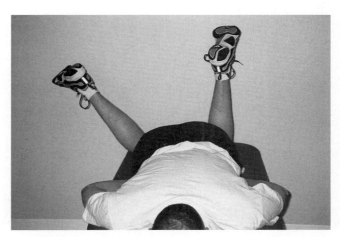

FIGURE 6-13. Transversus contraction with pelvis stabilized with prone hip internal and external rotation.

sary to perform a given exercise are fired. The athlete should not be progressed to higher-level stability exercises until the easier ones have been mastered. There should be 6 to 10 exercises in this stage that are done with 10 to 12 repetitions. The body is thought of as a cylinder and exercises are concentrated on the global stabilizers within the context of this program.

Exercises for Stage Two

5. *Partial sit-up*—Given that many athletes are focused on "doing crunches," it is important for them to be educated about spine positioning and core stability so that the crunches can be performed correctly and the athlete can achieve optimal gain. In a hooklying position with hands behind head, the athlete performs a transversus contraction and then a posterior pelvic tilt. The athlete then brings his or her head and arms up so that the chest is raised to clear the shoulder blades from the table. The athlete should maintain the same spine position through the entire range of the exercise and should *not* pull on his or her neck by bringing the elbows in and attempting to curl the body (Fig. 6-1).

6. *Bridging with knee extension*—In a hooklying position, the athlete performs a transversus contraction and pelvic tilt. While maintaining this position, the athlete lifts his or her pelvis, hips, and low back off the table into a bridge position. In the bridge position, the athlete then straightens one knee, ensuring that the pelvis stays stable and does not drop. If the pelvis (ASIS) on the moving limb side drops, it may also be indicative of contralateral glut weakness. This exercise can be progressed by increasing the amount of time the knee is extended or by increasing the number of consecutive repetitions the athlete can perform without lowering out of the bridge position (Fig. 6-14).

7. *"Dead bug" progression*—In a hooklying position with a transversus contraction and a posterior pelvic tilt, the athlete maintains the position of his or her spine while slowly extending one knee and sliding that heel along the table. The further the extremities get away from the core, the longer the lever arm and the stronger the abdominal contraction must be in order to maintain the same position of the spine. When moving, the lower extremities is mastered, the athlete can then combine opposite shoulder flexion. Hence, when the left knee is extended, the right shoulder is flexed. This provides two different lever arms in opposite direction, making the exercise even more difficult. It is important for lumbar spine stability to be maintained or else the purpose of the exercise is defeated. Quality of the movement pattern is more important than the number of repetitions (Fig. 6-15).

8. *Side-lying bridge*—The athlete lies on his or her left side with hips, knees, and shoulders in a single line. The left elbow is placed so that it is in line with the axilla of the left arm and the upper body weight is resting on it. After contracting the transversus and bracing the core, the athlete then places his or her right hand on the right hip and points the elbow upward toward the ceiling. Focusing on using the muscle on the underside of the body to draw the left side up, the athlete lifts his or her torso up off the table. The athlete should then slowly lower his or her body to the ground (Fig. 6-16).

9. *Standing lat pull-down*—The athlete stands facing a wall or standalone pulley mechanism. Arms are placed at 90 degrees of flexion, with hands facing toward the floor. The athlete is asked to stabilize the transversus abdominis by "hollowing" out the stomach. Maintain this position and pull the hands down with straight arms until the hands reach the thighs. The athlete should feel a stronger contraction from the core muscles as they go through the movement (Fig. 6-17).

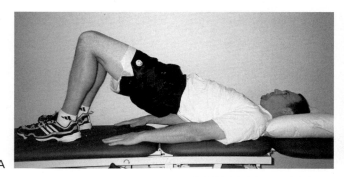
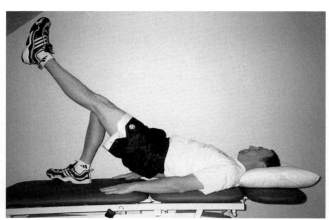

A   B

FIGURE 6-14. A: Bridging. **B:** Bridging with knee extension.

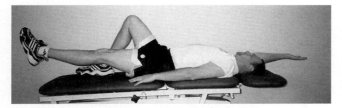

FIGURE 6-15. "Dead bug" progression.

Stage Three: Core Strengthening

This stage assumes a certain level of neuromuscular control and basic core stability and focuses on developing true core strength. Only those individuals who do not have symptoms associated with low back pain and who have mastered stages one and two should use this. This stage should progress toward power development by including speed of movement. In the next section, assessment and functional exercises are represented as part of the total core strengthening program.

SPORT-SPECIFIC CORE STRENGTHENING PROGRAM

When attempting to develop a core strengthening program for the elite overhead athlete, volume, intensity, and frequency of overhead activities become important variables that must be considered. Increasing the amount of load or weight against which muscles must work can increase intensity in any strengthening program. For example, using a medicine ball as an exercise modality increases the resistance and can even make the exercise "plyometric" in nature (6).

For an exercise to classify as plyometric, there must be an elongation of the muscle spindles to stimulate a stretch reflex (6). This can be done with lighter weights such as those provided by the catching of a medicine ball when it is thrown. After catching the ball, it must be returned to the thrower rapidly. This allows the athlete to take advantage of the stretch reflex to add power to the return. Table 6-2 lists

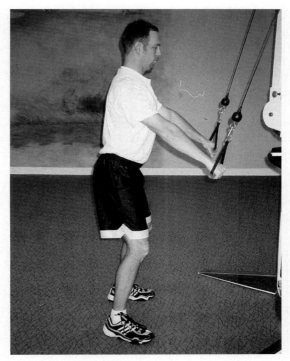

FIGURE 6-17. Standing lat pull-down.

recommended medicine ball weights based on the age of the athlete.

The medicine ball is an excellent tool for assessing a player's upper body and core strength through the use of "field tests." Field tests directly reflect the athlete's ability to use his or her entire body. The results of these tests are an indication of how effective the athlete is at using his or her core to transmit forces to the medicine ball. In comparison to laboratory testing, field testing may have a number of variables that are not taken into account. However, field tests are generally simple and relatively easy to administer, and the results can offer valuable information. In many cases, testing tools consist only of chalk to mark starting and finishing points, and a tape measure and stop watch to record distances and times. For example, testing of many

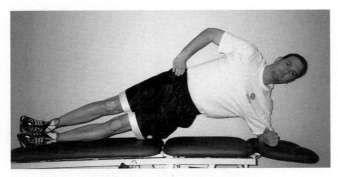

FIGURE 6-16. Side-lying bridge.

TABLE 6–2. RECOMMENDED MEDICINE BALL WEIGHTS BASED ON AGE

Age (yr)	Ball Weight
8–10	4 lb
10–12	4–6 lb
12–14	6 lb
14–16	6–8 lb
16–18	8–10 lb
18+	10–12 lb

tennis players over the years has convinced the senior author that the strength of a player's ground strokes is closely correlated with the best distance achieved by throwing the medicine ball in a similar way: an athlete who has a dominant forehand excels in throwing the medicine ball for distance from that side.

The purpose of self-testing is to give the athlete an idea of his or her strengths with each particular sport-specific shoulder motion. This may help in deciding where the athlete needs to spend time developing strength and power in a specific motion. If one throw is considerably less in distance than another, it is an indication that the athlete will benefit by emphasizing core work and strength development for that motion.

Sample Procedure for Testing Overhead Athletes (e.g., Tennis Player)

1. *Overhead throw for distance*—This is a measure of serving force from the ground reaction forces up the kinetic chain to the point of release. The athlete holds the medicine ball overhead with both hands. Placing one foot on the baseline as if setting up to serve, the athlete rocks back and takes one step forward while bringing the medicine ball from behind the head to an overhead release position. The athlete throws the ball into the court as far as possible. The distance the ball travels from the baseline is measured. It is immaterial if the athlete steps into the court on the follow-through because he or she does the same thing on the court while serving.
2. *Forehand throw for distance*—The athlete stands in an open or closed forehand stance with a foot on the baseline. Using a forehand motion, the athlete throws the medicine ball into the court as far as possible. The distance from the baseline to where the ball lands is measured.
3. *Backhand throw for distance*—The athlete stands in a backhand stance with the heel of a foot on the baseline. While keeping the back fairly straight and bending the knees, the athlete uses a backward, over-the-head

motion to throw the medicine ball into the court as far as possible. The distance from the baseline to where the ball lands is measured.

The aforementioned three tests are exercises in and of themselves. Each throw should be part of the athlete's workouts for 2 to 3 weeks and should be performed for 10 to 15 repetitions. After 2 to 3 weeks, another set of 10 to 15 throws should be added. Performing these exercises twice a week or as part of the athlete's strength workouts add to his or her ability to generate speed in rotational activities such as ground strokes.

Medicine Ball Exercises for Core Strengthening

The following drills represent those which can be grouped easily into a complete workout that should take no more than 15 to 20 minutes to complete. The athlete starts with 12 to 15 repetitions of each exercise and may increase to 25 throws or tosses per exercise. As the athlete matures, he or she may get to the point where two to three sets of each exercise can be performed in a circuit training model (i.e., performing one set of each exercise in the program and then repeating the same order two to three more times).

1. *Chest pass toss*—Coach or partner stands 10 to 15 feet away from the athlete with a medicine ball. The athlete sits on the ground with the knees bent and feet flat on the ground, leaning back on a 45-degree angle. The coach tosses the ball to the athlete who catches it and returns it without moving from the "lean-back" position. The pair continues to rapidly toss the ball back and forth (Fig. 6-18).
2. *Sit-up toss*—The athlete starts in the same position as in exercise 1, but when catching the ball, the athlete lets the momentum push him or her to the floor. The athlete then rapidly sits up and simultaneously returns the chest pass.
3. *Pullover tosses*—The athlete starts in the same position as in exercise 1, but has his or her hands above the head.

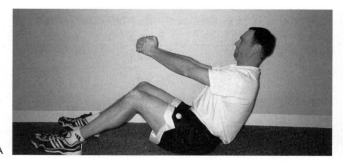
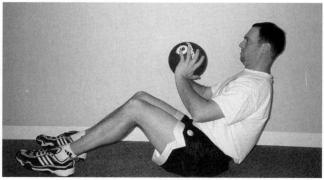

A   B

FIGURE 6-18. Chest pass toss.

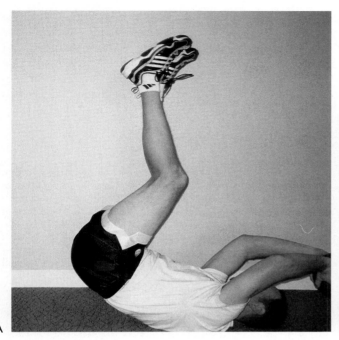
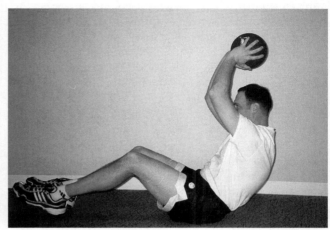

A   B

FIGURE 6-19. Pullover tosses.

While catching the ball, the athlete lets the momentum rock him or her backwards. The athlete's feet should come up and his or her body rolls back with the ball. The athlete uses full body momentum to then rock forward and releases the ball in an overhead throw position (Fig. 6-19).

4. *Side tosses*—The athlete sits on the ground with his or her legs straight out. The coach stands 10 to 15 feet away at a 90-degree angle from the athlete. The coach tosses a medicine ball at the athlete's knees, so that when the athlete catches the ball he or she lets momentum cause his or her trunk to rotate so that the ball is completely opposite the coach. The athlete then rotates back and quickly releases the ball back to the coach (Fig. 6-20).

5. *Double pump*—This exercise incorporates the same action as in exercise 4. However, the athlete rotates back and then rotates all the way over in the opposite direction before returning to the start and throwing the ball back. This guarantees a rotation in each direction before releasing the ball.

6. *Power drops*—The coach stands on a box 12 to 36 inches high and holds a medicine ball out over where the athlete is lying in a supine position with his or her head close to the box and arms outstretched vertically. The coach releases the ball and the athlete catches it as soon as possible and then releases it as quickly as possible by slightly flexing his or her arms and pushing the ball back up to the coach.

7. *Superman tosses*—While the coach stands about 3 to 4 feet in front of the athlete, the athlete lies prone on the floor.

The athlete arches back and up with his or her hands slightly elevated and in front of his or her face. The coach then tosses the ball into the athlete's hands, and the athlete must return it without losing the arched position.

8. *Backward throws*—The athlete stands with his or her back to the coach who is approximately 20 to 25 feet away. Using a squatting motion, the athlete lowers the ball between his or her knees and then rapidly extends his or her legs and torso to throw the ball backward over his or her head to the coach. The coach can roll the ball back to the athlete to repeat the exercises. The ball should be lowered between the knees quickly in order to achieve the stretching action.

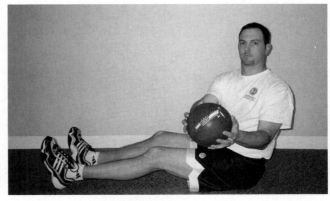

FIGURE 6-20. Side tosses.

SUMMARY

Core strengthening programs have a long history. With most exercise programs developing as a result of attempts to reduce or eliminate low back pain, current programs are centered on stabilization of spinal segments as they move during functional activities. General training programs for core strength tend to move toward more specific programs with regard to position, motion, and function.

Overhead athletes can all benefit from learning how to contract local stabilizing musculature of the lumbar spine and then advance to more global musculature as it relates to the sport activity.

The concept that the core musculature helps to form the walls of a cylinder that is commonly called *the trunk* allows one to incorporate exercises aimed at developing specific functions of the body. Outside resistance or loads are best kept to a minimum while performing these exercises so as not to limit range, function, and speed of activity. Global (as opposed to local) stabilizing exercises have the greatest emphasis in those individuals with no history of low back pain. Local stabilizing exercises are most effective when the athlete is a novice or has had a history of low back pain.

The core is certainly the "link" between the upper and lower extremities, and even though the development of ground reaction forces may be the most important biomechanical factor in effective overhead activities, the chain is only as strong as its weakest link.

REFERENCES

1. Kibler WB, McMullen J, Uhl T. Shoulder rehabilitation strategies, guidelines and practice. *Orthop Clin North Am* 2001;32(3):527–538.
2. Karayannis N, Anderson K, Carter S. Effectiveness of trunk stabilization and aerobic endurance exercises for the treatment of chronic low back pain. *Phys Ther Case Rep* 2001;4(2):77–89.
3. Lee D. *The pelvic girdle.* Edinburgh: Churchill Livingstone, 2000.
4. Richardson, C, Jull G, Hodges P, et al. Therapeutic exercise for spinal segmental stabilization in low back pain. London: Churchill Livingstone, 1999.
5. Siff MC. Functional training revisited. *Strength Conditioning J* 2002;24(5):42–46.
6. Chu DA. *Plyometric exercises with the medicine ball,* 2nd ed. Livermore, CA: 2003.

7

SPECIFIC EXERCISES FOR THE THROWING SHOULDER

KEVIN E. WILK
MICHAEL M. REINOLD

INTRODUCTION

Specific strengthening and flexibility exercises play a vital role in the ultimate function and injury prevention in the overhead throwing athlete. The most significant challenge facing the clinician (physical therapist, athletic trainer, strength and conditioning coach) is the achievement of a delicate balance between mobility and stability. The overhead throwing athlete must exhibit considerable glenohumeral joint mobility and laxity to allow the extreme motions necessary to throw effectively and without pain or injury.

The exercise program should include exercise drills to enhance flexibility, improve dynamic stabilization, increase muscular strength, enhance explosive power, and optimize muscular endurance. The clinician must carefully supervise so that the overhead athlete enhances flexibility, but not to the extent where excessive motion occurs; this may lead to glenohumeral joint instability. The strengthening exercises are designed to enhance muscular strength but not to create tightness and inflexibility. Other exercises such as plyometrics are designed to enrich explosive power and enhance the overhead thrower's ball velocity. Thus, the exercise program is a delicate balance of all these elements, which should produce the ultimate goal of pain-free, injury-free unrestricted throwing. Furthermore, the program should enhance the athlete's performance.

The repetitive microtraumatic stresses placed on the athlete's shoulder joint complex during the throwing motion challenges the physiologic limits of the surrounding tissues. During the overhead throwing motion, the athlete places excessive stresses at end ranges with tremendous angular velocities (Fig. 7-1). Fleisig and colleagues (1) reported the angular velocity of the overhead throw to reach 7,265 degrees per seconds, which is the fastest human movement. Furthermore, these forces are generated when the shoulder joint is in excessive external rota-tion, often at 145 to 165 degrees of external rotation. This results in high forces generated at the joint and placed on the supporting structure (i.e., capsule or musculature) (2). Fleisig and colleagues (1) reported anterior forces up to 1 times body weight during external rotation (late cocking) and up to 1½ times body weight distracting the joint during the follow-through phase. Frequently, injury may occur as a result of muscle fatigue, muscle weakness and imbalances, alterations in throwing mechanics, and excessive capsular laxity. A well-designed and properly implemented program may prevent some of these injuries.

OVERVIEW

Most overhead athletes exhibit significant laxity of the glenohumeral joint. This allows them to accomplish the necessary motions required to perform their sport. However, this appears to be potentially problematic. Because of the excessive mobility, the surrounding stabilizing structures must play a significant role. We believe the surrounding musculature functions to dynamically stabilize the glenohumeral joint, provide movements, and dissipate the large forces generated during the throw. Thus, the exercise program must include exercise drills to enhance dynamic stabilization, improve acceleration power, and upgrade eccentric muscular efficiency. Furthermore, the exercise drills must not solely be confined to the glenohumeral joint, but must include the scapular region, core stability, and lower extremities. These components contribute to increased force generation as well as proper mechanics and efficiency.

This chapter discusses our approach to the rehabilitation and preventive program for the overhead throwing athlete. The rehabilitation principles and guidelines, and the specific programs for selected injuries are also reviewed.

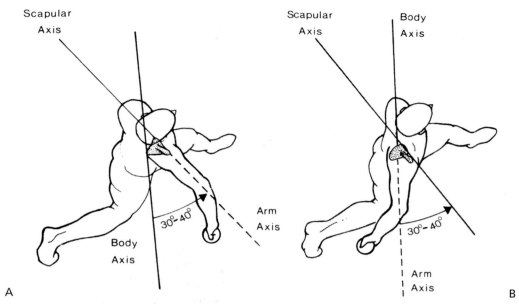

FIGURE 7-1. Hyperangulation during the overhead throwing motion. During the late cocking phase of the overhead throw, as the thrower's humerus excessively abducts horizontally, posterosuperior impingement of the shoulder joint may occur. To prevent this, the thrower must stay in the plane of the scapula. **A:** Normal angular relationship. **B:** Hyperangulation. (From Davidson PA, et al. Rotator cuff and posterior-superior glenoid injury associated with increased glenohumeral motion: a new site of impingement. *J Shoulder Elbow Surg* 1995:4:384–390, with permission.)

PHYSICAL CHARACTERISTICS OF THE OVERHEAD ATHLETE

The overhead throwing athlete exhibits several differences in physical characteristics than the nonoverhead athlete, specifically in shoulder range of motion, laxity, strength, and proprioception. These characteristics must be completely understood before an individualized rehabilitation program is developed. Briefly discussed are the typical characteristics of overhead athletes so that pathology may be appreciated on clinical examination and addressed through a structured rehabilitation program.

Range of Motion

One of the most characteristic differences between overhead athletes and nonoverhead athletes is shoulder range of motion. Most overhead athletes exhibit excessive external rotation and decreased internal rotation at 90 degrees of abduction in the throwing shoulder (3–6). Brown and colleagues (4) reported that the mean range of motion in 41 professional baseball pitchers was 141 degrees ± 15 degrees of shoulder external rotation at 90 degrees of abduction and 83 degrees ± 14 degrees of internal rotation. External rotation was 9 degrees greater in the throwing shoulder than in the nonthrowing shoulder, and internal rotation was 15 degrees less than in the nonthrowing shoulder. Furthermore, external rotation of the throwing shoulder was 9

degrees greater in pitchers than in positional players. Similarly, Bigliani and colleagues (3) evaluated the range of motion characteristics in 148 professional baseball players. The authors reported a mean of 118 degrees of external rotation at 90 degrees of abduction (range 95 to 145 degrees) in the throwing shoulder of pitchers and a mean of 108 degrees external rotation in positional players. A statistically significant increase in external rotation and decrease in internal rotation was observed between the dominant and nondominant shoulder.

Wilk and colleagues (7) reported the shoulder range of motion characteristics in 372 professional baseball players. The authors reported a mean of 129 degrees ± 10 degrees of external rotation and 61 degrees ± 9 degrees of internal rotation in the throwing shoulder at 90 degrees of abduction. The authors noted that external rotation was 7 degrees greater and internal rotation was 7 degrees less in the dominant arm when compared with the nondominant arm. The concept of "total motion" was introduced in this article. *Total motion* is the motion value of external and internal rotation (at 90 degrees of abduction) added together. The authors noted that total motion is equal bilaterally in most throwers, usually within 7 degrees.

Reinold and colleagues (8) recently noted that range of motion is affected by overhead throwing. The authors evaluated shoulder range of motion in 31 professional baseball pitchers before and immediately after baseball pitching. External rotation before throwing (133 degrees ± 11 degrees) did not significantly change after throwing (131 degrees ± 10 degrees). However, there was a statistically significant decrease in internal rotation range of motion after pitching (73 degrees ± 16 degrees before; 65 degrees ± 11 degrees after) and a subsequent decrease of 9 degrees of total motion. The authors hypothesized that this decrease in internal rotation range of motion is due to the large eccentric forces observed in the external rotators during the follow-through phase of throwing. Furthermore, the overall decrease in total motion observed after throwing may make the athlete more susceptible to injury.

Laxity

The excessive motion observed in overhead athletes is commonly attributed to an increase in glenohumeral laxity. Numerous theories regarding this increased laxity have been reported. Some authors have reported that the excessive external rotation and limited internal rotation are due to anterior capsular laxity and posterior capsule tightness (9). Others have reported that the excessive laxity in throwers is the result of repetitive throwing and have referred to this as *acquired laxity* (J. R. Andrews, *unpublished data*, 1996), whereas others have documented that overhead throwers exhibit congenital laxity (3).

Bigliani and colleagues (3) subjectively examined laxity in 72 professional baseball pitchers and 76 positional players. The authors reported 61% of pitchers and 47% of positional players exhibited a positive sulcus sign, indicating inferior glenohumeral joint laxity. This laxity was present bilaterally, indicating a certain degree of congenital laxity.

Crockett and colleagues (10) examined the amount of humeral version in the dominant and nondominant shoulders of professional baseball players and nonthrowers. Results indicated a retroversion of the humeral head that was present in the dominant shoulder of throwers and not in the nondominant shoulder or shoulders of nonthrowers. Posterior capsular translation was consistently greater than anterior translation in all of the shoulders. Thus, the authors reported that the excessive external rotation and limited internal rotation may not be attributed to anterior capsular laxity and posterior capsular tightness, but rather to osseous adaptations to the throwing arm.

Borsa and colleagues (*unpublished data*, 2002) recently assessed the amount of anterior and posterior capsular laxity in professional baseball pitchers using an objective mechanical translation device (Telos device). The authors reported that posterior capsular laxity was significantly greater than anterior capsular laxity. This was true despite gross limitation of internal rotation. Furthermore, the investigators reported total translation (anterior and posterior) was equal bilaterally, thus the throwing shoulder was not more lax than the nonthrowing shoulder.

Thus, it appears that the unique range-of-motion characteristics in overhead athletes cannot be explained as a result of capsular laxity entirely. Rather, it appears that the increased external rotation and decreased internal rotation observed is due in part to a combination of osseous adaptations, soft tissue adaptations (e.g., posterior rotator cuff), congenital laxity, and superimposed acquired laxity as a result of adaptive changes from throwing.

Muscle Strength

Several investigators have examined muscle strength parameters in the overhead throwing athlete with varying results and conclusions (4,11–17). Wilk and colleagues (16,17) have performed isokinetic testing on professional baseball players as part of their physical examinations during spring training. The investigators demonstrated that the external rotation strength of the pitcher's throwing shoulder is significantly weaker ($p < 0.05$) than the nonthrowing shoulder, by 6%. Conversely, internal rotation strength of the throwing shoulder was significantly stronger ($p < 0.05$), by 3%, compared with the nonthrowing shoulder. In addition, adduction strength of the throwing shoulder is also significantly stronger than in the nonthrowing shoulder, by approximately 10%. The authors reported the optimal antagonist-agonist ration between external and internal rotation strength should be 66% to 76%. Table 7-1 illustrates the expected muscle strength values of professional baseball players.

Magnusson and colleagues (18) used a handheld dynamometer to study the isometric muscle strength of professional baseball pitchers and compared results with those of a control group of nonthrowers. The authors noted a significant decrease in supraspinatus strength of the dominant shoulder when compared with the nondominant shoulder. Additionally, pitchers exhibited strength deficits for shoulder abductors, external rotators, internal rotators, and supraspinatus (empty can maneuvers) when compared with nonthrowers.

Reinold and colleagues (19) evaluated external and internal rotation strength at 0 degrees and 90 degrees of abduction in 23 professional baseball pitchers using a handheld dynamometer. The mean peak force output for external rotation at 0 degrees of abduction was approximately 37 Nm bilaterally. Similarly, internal rotation at 0 degrees for the bilateral shoulders was approximately 44 Nm. The authors noted a statistically significant decrease of approximately 7 Nm of external and internal rotation strength when measured at 90 degrees of abduction. The 90-degree abducted position may be better suited to perform manual strength testing in professional baseball pitchers when determining subtle strength deficits or imbalances of the shoulder rotators.

The scapular muscles also play a vital role during overhead throwing (20). Wilk and colleagues (21) documented the isometric scapular strength values of professional baseball players. The results indicated that pitchers and catchers exhibited significantly greater strength of the scapular pro-

TABLE 7-1. ISOKINETIC SHOULDER STRENGTH CRITERIA FOR OVERHEAD ATHLETES

Velocity (deg/sec)	Bilateral Comparisons (Dominant Arm/Nondominant Arm)			
	External Rotation (ER)	Internal Rotation (IR)	Abduction (Abd)	Adduction (Add)
180	98%–105%	110%–120%	98%–105%	110%–128%
300	85%–95%	105%–115%	96%–102%	111%–129%

Velocity (deg/sec)	Unilateral Muscle Ratios		
	ER/IR	Abd/Add	ER/Abd
180	66%–76%	78%–84%	67%–75%
300	61%–71%	88%–94%	60%–70%

Velocity (deg/sec)	Peak Torque to Body Weight Ratios			
	ER	IR	Abd	Add
180	18%–23%	28%–33%	26%–33%	32%–38%
300	12%–20%	25%–30%	20%–25%	28%–34%

tractors and elevators than positional players. Antagonist-agonist muscles values are also of importance in the scapular muscles. Table 7-2 illustrates the scapular muscle strength values of the overhead throwing athlete.

Proprioception

The overhead thrower relies on enhanced proprioception to influence the neuromuscular system to dynamically stabilize the glenohumeral joint in the presence of capsular laxity and excessive range of motion. Blasier and colleagues (22) reported that persons with generalized joint laxity are significantly less sensitive to proprioceptive testing.

Allegrucci and colleagues (23) examined shoulder proprioception in 20 healthy overhead athletes. Testing of joint repositioning was performed on a motorized system with the subject attempting to actively reproduce a specific joint angle. The investigators noted that the dominant shoulder exhibited diminished proprioception compared with the nondominant shoulder. The investigators also noted improved proprioception toward end range of motion compared with early and mid range.

Wilk and colleagues (*unpublished data*, 2000) studied the proprioceptive capability of 120 professional baseball players using active reproduction of passive joint positioning. The researchers noted no significant difference bilaterally, although greater proprioception was achieved at end range of motion compared with mid range. In addition, Wilk and colleagues (*unpublished data*, 2000) compared the proprioceptive ability of 60 professional baseball players with that of 60 nonthrowing athletes. The authors noted no significant difference between groups. However, the overhead athletes exhibited a trend toward greater proprioception at end range when compared towards non-throwing athletes, although not statistically significant.

REHABILITATION PRINCIPLES AND GUIDELINES

The rehabilitation program for the thrower's shoulder follows several principles and guidelines to maximize the athlete's return to competition. The following section briefly explains several principles and guidelines followed by an

TABLE 7-2. SCAPULAR MUSCLE STRENGTH VALUES AND THEIR UNILATERAL RATIOS[a]

	Scapular Muscle Values (ft-lb)								Unilateral Muscle Ratios (%)			
	Protraction		Retraction		Elevation		Depression		Protraction/Retraction		Elevation/Depression	
	D	ND	D	ND	D	ND	D	ND	D	ND	D	ND
Pitchers	71 ± 10	74 ± 13	62 ± 8	60 ± 7	83 ± 14	84 ± 5	22 ± 6	18 ± 5	87	81	27	21
Catchers	68 ± 10	73 ± 10	63 ± 5	59 ± 7	88 ± 15	85 ± 8	21 ± 4	16 ± 5	93	81	24	19
Positional players	58 ± 10	58 ± 11	57 ± 6	56 ± 6	65 ± 12	66 ± 11	19 ± 5	18 ± 5	98	94	29	27

[a]D, dominant extremity; ND, nondominant extremity.

overview of the thrower's rehabilitation program incorporating these principles.

Thrower's Ten Program

Strengthening exercises of the entire upper extremity, including shoulder, scapula, elbow, and wrist exercises, are essential for the overhead thrower. We have developed the Thrower's Ten Program (see Appendix 7-1 at end of book) based on numerous electromyographic (EMG) analysis studies to strengthen the muscles involved in the throwing motion (24–29). The exercise program involves several exercises with emphasis on the scapulothoracic and rotator cuff muscles, particularly the external rotators (30). This program serves as a foundation to the strengthening program, around which skilled and advanced techniques may be superimposed.

Dynamic Stabilization

The excessive mobility and compromised static stability observed within the glenohumeral joint often result in numerous injuries to the capsulolabral and musculotendinous structures of the throwing shoulder. Efficient dynamic stabilization and neuromuscular control of the glenohumeral joint is necessary for overhead athletes to avoid injuries during competition (25). Dynamic stability refers to the ability of the shoulder to stabilize during the throwing motion to avoid injuries. This involves neuromuscular control and the efferent (motor) output to afferent (sensory) stimulation from the shoulder.

Dynamic stabilization exercises for the thrower's shoulder begin with baseline proprioception and kinesthesia drills to maximize the athlete's awareness of joint position and movement in space. Rhythmic stabilizations are incorporated to facilitate cocontraction of the rotator cuff and dynamic stability of the glenohumeral joint. These dynamic stabilization techniques may be applied as the athlete progresses to provide advance challenge to the neuromuscular control system.

Neuromuscular control of the shoulder involves stability of not only the glenohumeral joint but also the scapulothoracic joint. The scapula provides a stable base of support for muscular attachment and dynamically positions the glenohumeral joint during upper extremity movement. Scapular strength and stability are essential to proper function of the glenohumeral joint. Therefore, isotonic strengthening and dynamic stabilization of the scapular musculature should also be included into rehabilitation programs for the thrower's shoulder to assure proximal stability.

Core Stabilization

Core stabilization drills are used to further enhance proximal stability with distal mobility of the upper extremity.

Core stabilization is used based on the kinetic chain concept in which imbalance within any point of the kinetic chain may result in pathology throughout. Movement patterns, such as throwing, require a precise interaction of the entire body kinetic chain to perform efficiently. An imbalance of strength, flexibility, endurance, or stability may result in fatigue, abnormal arthrokinematics, and subsequent compensation.

Core stabilization is progressed using a multiphase approach, progressing from baseline core and trunk strengthening, to intermediate core strengthening with distal mobility, to advanced stabilization in sport-specific movement patterns.

Closed Kinetic Chain Exercises

The integration of closed kinetic chain (CKC) exercises, or axial compression exercises, is another important principle in the rehabilitation of the overhead athlete (31). CKC exercises are used to stress the joint in a weight-bearing position, resulting in joint approximation. The goal of this is to stimulate articular receptors and facilitate cocontraction of the shoulder force couples, thus incorporating a combination of eccentric and concentric contractions to provide joint stability.

CKC exercises are progressed to gradually increase the amount of challenge to the shoulder. Static stabilization exercises on a stable surface are progressed to dynamic stabilization exercises on an unstable surface. Single plane movements with a wide base of support are progressed to multiplane movements with a narrow base of support, and bilateral support is advanced to unilateral support. Furthermore, manual resistance, rhythmic stabilizations, and perturbation training may also be included to provide a constant increase in challenge to the neuromuscular control system.

Plyometric Exercises

Plyometric exercises provide a quick, powerful movement involving a prestretch of the muscle, thereby activating the stretch shortening cycle of the muscle (32–34). Plyometrics replicates several functional movement patterns, such as throwing, that involve stretch-shortening cycles of the muscle tissue. The goal is to train the upper extremity to efficiently develop and withstand force.

Stretch-shortening muscle contractions use a prestretching of the muscle spindles and Golgi tendon organs to produce a recoil action of the elastic tissues, which results in improved muscle performance by the combined effects of the stored elastic energy and the myotactic reflex activation of the muscle.

There are three phases of stretch-shortening exercises. The first phase, the eccentric stretch phase, increases the activity of the muscle spindle. The second phase, the amortization phase, is the time between the eccentric and con-

TABLE 7–3. INTERVAL THROWING PROGRAM FOR BASEBALL PLAYERS: PHASE I

45 ft Phase
Step 1: A. Warm-up throwing
B. 45 ft (25 throws)
C. Rest 5–10 min
D. Warm-up throwing
E. 45 ft (25 throws)
Step 2: A. Warm-up throwing
B. 45 ft (25 throws)
C. Rest 5–10 min
D. Warm-up throwing
E. 45 ft (25 throws)
F. Rest 5–10 min
G. Warm-up throwing
H. 45 ft (25 throws)
60 ft Phase
Step 3: A. Warm-up throwing
B. 60 ft (25 throws)
C. Rest 5–10 min
D. Warm-up throwing
E. 60 ft (25 throws)
Step 4: A. Warm-up throwing
B. 60 ft (25 throws)
C. Rest 5–10 min
D. Warm-up throwing
E. 60 ft (25 throws)
F. Rest 5–10 min
G. Warm-up throwing
H. 60 ft (25 throws)
90 ft Phase
Step 5: A. Warm-up throwing
B. 90 ft (25 throws)
C. Rest 5–10 min
D. Warm-up throwing
E. 90 ft (25 throws)
Step 6: A. Warm-up throwing
B. 90 ft (25 throws)
C. Rest 5–10 min
D. Warm-up throwing
E. 90 ft (25 throws)
F. Rest 5–10 min
G. Warm-up throwing
H. 90 ft (25 throws)
120 ft Phase
Step 7: A. Warm-up throwing
B. 120 ft (25 throws)
C. Rest 5–10 min
D. Warm-up throwing
E. 120 ft (25 throws)

Step 8: A. Warm-up throwing
B. 120 ft (25 throws)
C. Rest 5–10 min
D. Warm-up throwing
E. 120 ft (25 throws)
F. Rest 5–10 min
G. Warm-up throwing
H. 120 ft (25 throws)
150 ft Phase
Step 9: A. Warm-up throwing
B. 150 ft (25 throws)
C. Rest 5–10 min
D. Warm-up throwing
E. 150 ft (25 throws)
Step 10: A. Warm-up throwing
B. 150 ft (25 throws)
C. Rest 5–10 min
D. Warm-up throwing
E. 150 ft (25 throws)
F. Rest 5–10 min
G. Warm-up throwing
H. 150 ft (25 throws)
180 ft Phase
Step 11: A. Warm-up throwing
B. 180 ft (25 throws)
C. Rest 5–10 min
D. Warm-up throwing
E. 180 ft (25 throws)
Step 12: A. Warm-up throwing
B. 180 ft (25 throws)
C. Rest 5–10 min
D. Warm-up throwing
E. 180 ft (25 throws)
F. Rest 5–10 min
G. Warm-up throwing
H. 180 ft (25 throws)
Step 13: A. Warm-up throwing
B. 180 ft (25 throws)
C. Rest 5–10 min
D. Warm-up throwing
E. 180 ft (25 throws)
F. Rest 5–10 min
G. Warm-up throwing
H. 180 ft (20 throws)
I. Rest 5–10 min
J. Warm-up throwing
K. 15 Throws progressing from 120 ft → 90 ft
Step 14: Return to respective position or progress to step 14.

All throws should be on an arc with a crow-hop
Warm-up throws consist of 10–20 throws at approximately 30 ft
Throwing program should be performed every other day, 3 times per week unless otherwise specified by a physician or rehabilitation specialist.
Perform each step _____ times before progressing to next step.
Flat Ground Throwing for Baseball Pitchers
Step 14:
A. Warm-up throwing
B. Throw 60 ft (10–15 throws)
C. Throw 90 ft (10 throws)
D. Throw 120 ft (10 throws)

E. Throw 60 ft (flat ground) using pitching mechanics (20–30 throws)
Step 15:
A. Warm-up throwing
B. Throw 60 ft (10–15 throws)
C. Throw 90 ft (10 throws)
D. Throw 120 ft (10 throws)
E. Throw 60 ft (flat ground) using pitching mechanics (20–30 throws)
F. Throw 60–90 ft (10–15 throws)
G. Throw 60 ft (flat ground) using pitching mechanics (20 throws)

Progress to Phase II—Throwing Off the Mound
45 ft = 13.7 m; 60 ft = 18.3 m; 90 ft = 27.4 m; 120 ft = 36.6 m; 150 ft = 45.7 m; 180 ft = 54.8 m.

centric contractions. This phase relies on the rate of stretch rather than the length of stretch. Excessive amortization time may result in the dissipation of energy as heat and a deactivation of the stretch reflex. The last phase, the concentric response phase, is the summation of the previous phases producing a facilitated shortening contraction.

Plyometric exercises may serve several benefits to the overhead athlete including increasing the speed of the myotactic stretch-reflex, desensitizing the Golgi tendon organ, and increasing neuromuscular coordination. Furthermore, plyometrics serve as an excellent transitional exercise from slow isotonic movement to high-speed functional movements in throwing. Thus, the athlete exhibits improved neural efficiency and coordination of muscle groups.

Plyometric activities are advanced exercises requiring full range of motion, strength, and dynamic stability. Exercises for the thrower's shoulder are initiated with two-hand, short-axis drills before progressing to more advanced one-hand, long-axis drills.

REHABILITATION PROGRAM FOR OVERHEAD ATHLETES

The rehabilitation process for overhead athletes must include the restoration of range of motion, muscular strength, and muscular endurance, as well as a gradual restoration of proprioception, dynamic stability, and neuromuscular control. As the athlete advances, sport-specific drills are emphasized to prepare for a gradual return to competition through an interval sport program. Neuromuscular control drills are performed throughout and advanced as the athlete progresses to provide continuous challenge to the neuromuscular control system. The following section provides an overview of a functional rehabilitation progression for overhead athletes following injury or postoperatively incorporating the previously discussed principles and guidelines. The program is divided into four separate phases with specific goals and criteria for advancement for each phase. The use of a criteria-based rehabilitation program allows for individualization to each patient and specific pathology. It is imperative to modify each program based on each patient's pathology or surgical procedure. Alterations in exercise activities, positioning, and rate of progression are based on the type of injury, surgical procedure performed, healing constraints involved, and tissues being stressed during rehabilitation.

Acute Phase

The acute phase of rehabilitation begins immediately after injury or surgery. The duration of the acute phase depends on the healing constraints of the involved pathologic tissues. Rehabilitation precautions vary based on the exact pathology and postoperative limitations. The initial goals of the acute phase are (a) to diminish pain and inflammation and progress to include the normalization of motion and muscular balance and (b) to restore baseline proprioceptive and kinesthetic awareness.

Range-of-motion exercises are performed immediately in a restricted range of motion based on the theory that motion assists in the enhancement and organization of collagen tissue and the stimulation of joint mechanoreceptors, and that such exercises may assist in the neuromodulation of pain. The rehabilitation program should allow for progressive applied loads, beginning with gentle passive range of motion. Active-assisted range-of-motion exercises are taught to the patient, including cane or L-Bar (Breg Corporation, Vista, California) range of motion for flexion, external rotation, and internal rotation. As the athlete advances, flexion progresses as tolerated and shoulder rotation range of motion is progressed from 0 degrees of abduction to 30 degrees and 45 degrees of abduction. Also, pendulum and rope and pulley exercises are used as needed.

Flexibility exercises for the posterior shoulder musculature are also performed. As previously mentioned, the soft tissue of the posterior shoulder is subjected to extreme repetitive eccentric contractions during throwing, which may result in soft tissue adaptations and loss of internal rotation range of motion (8). Common stretches performed include horizontal adduction stretching across the body and light internal rotation stretching at 90 degrees of shoulder abduction. The cross-body horizontal adduction stretch may be performed in a straight plane adduction motion as well as being integrated with a component of internal rotation at the shoulder as well (Fig. 7-2).

Self-capsular stretches may be performed for the anterior, posterior, and inferior glenohumeral joint complex as appropriate. Also, gentle joint mobilization and contract-relax or hold-relax stretching techniques may be performed during the early stages of rehabilitation for pain modulation and to maintain symmetric capsular mobility.

Strengthening begins with submaximal, pain-free isometrics for shoulder flexion, extension, abduction, external rotation, internal rotation, and elbow flexion. Isometrics are used to retard muscular atrophy and restore voluntary muscular control, while avoiding detrimental shoulder forces. Isometrics should be performed at multiple angles throughout the available range of motion, with particular emphasis on contraction at the end of the currently available range of motion.

Manual rhythmic stabilization drills are performed for the shoulder internal and external rotators with the arm in the scapular plane at 30 degrees of abduction. Alternating isometric contractions are performed to facilitate cocontraction of the anterior and posterior rotator cuff musculature. Rhythmic stabilization drills may also be performed with the patient supine and arm elevated to approximately 90 to 100 degrees and 10 degrees of horizontal abduction.

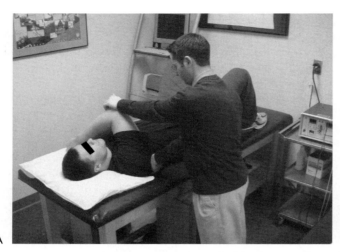
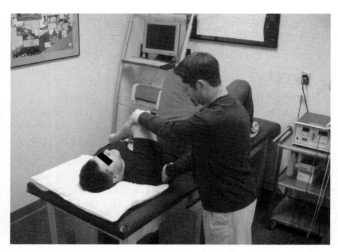

A

B

FIGURE 7-2. Horizontal adduction stretch. **A:** The clinician stabilizes the scapula while bringing the shoulder into horizontal adduction. **B:** The stretch may also be performed in an across body and slightly downward motion with shoulder internal rotation.

This position is chosen for the initiation of these drills because the combined centralized line of pull of both the rotator cuff and deltoid musculature at this angle causes a humeral head compressive force during muscle contraction. The rehabilitation specialist employs alternating isometric contractions in the flexion, extension, horizontal abduction, and horizontal adduction planes of motion. As the patient progresses, the drills can be performed at variable degrees of elevation such as 45 degrees and 120 degrees.

Active range-of-motion activities are permitted when adequate muscular strength and balance have been achieved. Active motion is initiated in the acute phase with joint reproduction exercises. With the athlete's eyes closed, the rehabilitation specialist passively moves the upper extremity in the planes of flexion, external rotation, and internal rotation, pauses, and then returns the extremity to the starting position. The patient is then instructed to actively reposition the upper extremity to the previous location. The rehabilitation specialist may perform these joint repositioning activities in variable degrees throughout the available range of motion and notes the accuracy of the patient.

Also performed during the acute phase are CKC exercises. Initial exercises are performed below shoulder level, such as weight bearing on a table while standing. The athlete may perform weight shifts in the anteroposterior and mediolateral directions. Rhythmic stabilizations may also be performed during weight shifting. As the athlete progresses, a medium-sized ball may be placed on the table and weight shifts may be performed on the ball. Weight-bearing exercises are progressed from the table to the quadruped position.

Ice, high-voltage stimulation, iontophoresis, ultrasound, and nonsteroidal antiinflammatory medications may also be employed to control pain and inflammation.

Intermediate Phase

The intermediate phase begins once the athlete has regained near-normal passive motion and sufficient balance of strength of the shoulder musculature. Baseline proprioception, kinesthesia, and dynamic stabilization are also needed before progressing, because emphasis will be placed on regaining these sensory modalities throughout the athlete's full range of motion, particularly at end range. The goals of the intermediate phase are to enhance functional dynamic stability, reestablish neuromuscular control, restore muscular strength and balance, and regain and maintain full range of motion.

Range-of-motion exercises are continued and the athlete is encouraged to perform active-assisted range of motion with a cane or L-bar to maintain motion. External and internal range of motion may be performed at 90 degrees of abduction. Joint mobilizations and self-capsular stretches continue to be performed to prevent asymmetric glenohumeral joint capsular tightness.

Strengthening exercises are advanced to include external and internal rotation with exercise tubing at 0 degrees of abduction and active range of motion exercises against gravity. These exercises initially include standing scaption in external rotation (full can), standing abduction, side-lying external rotation, and prone rowing. As strength returns, the program may be advanced to a program that includes full upper extremity strengthening with emphasis on posterior rotator cuff and scapular strengthening, such as the Thrower's Ten Program (Appendix 7-1).

Rhythmic stabilization exercises are performed during the early part of the intermediate phase. Drills performed in the acute phase may be progressed to include stabilization at end ranges of motion and with the patient's eyes closed. Proprioceptive neuromuscular facilitation (PNF) D2 patterns are performed in the athlete's available range of motion and progressed to include full arcs of motion. Rhythmic stabilizations may be incorporated in various degrees of elevation during the PNF patterns to promote dynamic stabilization.

Also performed during the intermediate phase is manual resistance external rotation. By applying manual resistance to specific exercises, the rehabilitation specialist can vary the amount of resistance throughout the range of motion and incorporate concentric and eccentric contractions, as well as rhythmic stabilizations at end range (Fig. 7-3). The application of manual resistance assists in the reinforcement of proper resistance, form, and cadence based on the symptoms of each athlete. As the athlete regains strength and neuromuscular control, external and internal rotation with tubing may be performed at 90 degrees of abduction. All stabilization drills may be advanced by removing the patient's visual stimulus.

Scapular strengthening and neuromuscular control are also critical to regaining full dynamic stability of the glenohumeral joint. Isotonic exercises for the scapulothoracic joint are performed as well as manual resistance prone rowing. Also, neuromuscular control drills and PNF patterns may be applied to the scapula.

Closed kinetic chain exercises are also advanced. Weight shifting on a ball is progressed to a push-up on a ball or unstable surface on a table top. Rhythmic stabilizations are performed by the rehabilitation specialist at the upper extremity as well as the uninvolved shoulder and trunk to incorporate a combination of upper extremity and trunk stabilization. Wall stabilization drills are performed with the athlete's hand on a small ball (Fig. 7-4). Further axial compression exercises include table and quadruped exercises using a towel around the hand, slide board, or unstable surface.

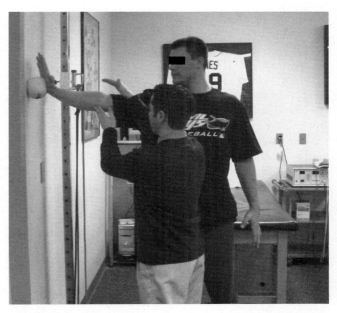

FIGURE 7-4. Wall stabilization drills. The patient stabilizes the shoulder while holding a small ball against the wall in the scapular plane. The clinician imparts perturbations to the upper extremity.

Lower extremity, core, and trunk strength and stability are critical to efficiently perform overhead activities by transferring and dissipating forces in a coordinated fashion. Therefore, full lower extremity strengthening and core stabilization activities are also performed during the intermediate phase. Basic exercises such as abdominal crunches and pelvic tilts are initiated during the late acute to early intermediate phase and progressed to include crunches with an altered center of gravity and with medicine ball throws.

Double and single leg balance on unstable surfaces such as foam or a balance beam is also performed. As core stability progresses, upper extremity movement and medicine ball throws may be included to alter the athlete's center of gravity and train the athlete to control unexpected forces.

Advanced Phase

The third phase of a functional rehabilitation program, the advanced phase, is designed to advance the athlete through a series of progressive strengthening and neuromuscular control activities, while preparing the athlete to begin a gradual return to athletic activity. Criteria to enter this phase include minimal pain and tenderness, full range of motion, symmetrical capsular mobility, good (4/5 on manual muscle testing) strength and endurance of the upper extremity and scapulothoracic musculature, and sufficient dynamic stabilization.

Full motion and capsular mobility are maintained through range-of-motion and self-stretching techniques. These include manual stretching and L-bar exercises. Spe-

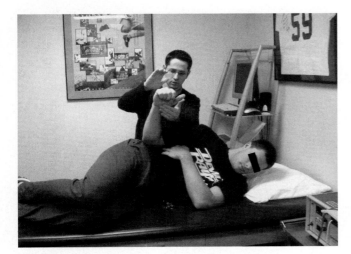

FIGURE 7-3. Manual resistance side-lying external rotation with rhythmic stabilizations.

cific emphasis on soft tissue mobility of the posterior musculotendinous structures should be made through exercises such as horizontal adduction stretching while stabilizing the scapula (Fig. 7-2).

Strengthening exercises include the Thrower's Ten Program (Appendix 7-1) as well as exercises for the lower extremities and trunk, which are continued with a gradual increase in resistance. Exercises such as internal and external rotation with exercise tubing at 90 degrees of abduction may be progressed to also incorporate eccentric and high-speed contractions.

Aggressive strengthening of the upper body may also be initiated depending on the needs of the individual patient. Common exercises include isotonic weight machine exercises such as bench press, seated row, and latissimus dorsi pull-downs within a restricted range of motion. During bench press and seated row, the athlete is instructed to not extend the upper extremities beyond the plane of the body to minimize stress on the shoulder capsule. Latissimus pull-downs are performed in front of the head, and the athlete is instructed to avoid full extension of the arms to minimize the amount of traction force applied to the upper extremities.

Plyometric activities for the upper extremity may be initiated during this phase to train the upper extremity to produce and dissipate forces. Plyometric exercises are initially performed with two hands. Specific exercises include a chest pass, overhead throw, and alternating side-to-side throw with a 3- to 5-pound medicine ball. Two-hand drills are progressed to one-hand drills as tolerated by the athlete, usually between 10 and 14 days after the initiation of two-hand drills. Specific one-hand plyometrics include baseball style throws in the 90/90 position with a 2-pound ball (Fig. 7-5) and stationary and semicircle wall dribbles. Wall dribbles are also beneficial to increase upper extremity

endurance while overhead and may be progressed to include dribbles in the 90/90 position.

Axial compression exercises are progressed to include the quadruped and triped positions. Rhythmic stabilizations of the involved extremity as well as at the core and trunk may be applied. Unstable surfaces, such as tilt boards, foam, large exercise balls, or the Biodex stability system (Biodex Corp., Shirley, New York), may be incorporated to further challenge the athlete's stability system while in the closed chain position.

Dynamic stabilization and neuromuscular control drills are progressed to include reactive neuromuscular control drills and functional, sport-specific positions. Concentric and eccentric manual resistance may be applied as the athlete performs external rotation with exercise tubing with the arm at 0-degree abduction. Rhythmic stabilizations may be included at end range to challenge the athlete to stabilize against the force of the tubing as well as the therapist. This exercise may be progressed to the 90/90 position to require the athlete to stabilize the shoulder at end range in a more sport-specific position (Fig. 7-6). Also, rhythmic stabilizations may be applied at end range during the 90/90 wall dribble exercise. The athlete performs a predetermined number of repetitions before the therapist applies a series of rhythmic stabilizations at external rotation end range. These drills are designed to impart a sudden perturbation to the throwing shoulder at near end range to develop the athlete's ability to dynamically stabilize the shoulder to prevent the shoulder from translating into excessive ranges of motion.

Lower extremity and core strengthening and stability are continued. Exercises are progressed to provide further challenge and to include sport-specific positions. An unstable surface or balance beam may be used while performing upper extremity isotonic, manual resistance, and plyomet-

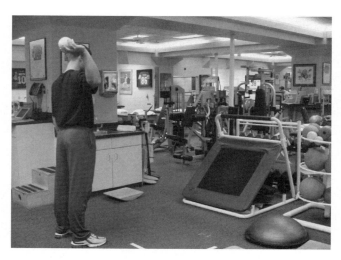

FIGURE 7-5. One-hand plyometric ball throws in the 90-degree abducted shoulder position using a 2-pound ball.

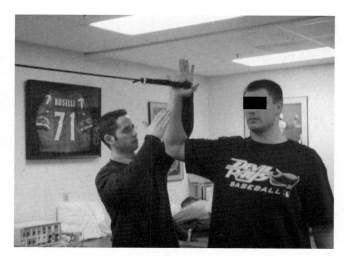

FIGURE 7-6 External rotation against exercise tubing in the 90-degree abducted shoulder position while the clinician applies manual resistance and rhythmic stabilizations at end range.

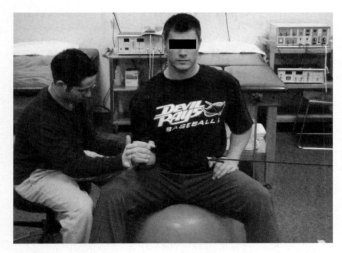

FIGURE 7-7. External rotation against exercise tubing while the clinician applies manual resistance and rhythmic stabilizations at end range while stabilizing the core on an exercise ball.

ric exercises to challenge core stability while performing upper extremity movements (Figs. 7-7 and 7-8).

Near the end of the advanced phase, the athlete may begin basic sport-specific drills. Various activities such as underweight and overweight ball throwing or implement swinging for baseball, golf, and tennis players may be performed.

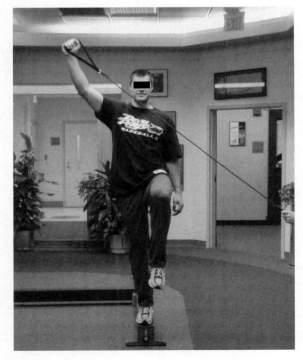

FIGURE 7-8. Proprioceptive neuromuscular facilitation patterns with exercise tubing while stabilizing the core and balancing on a beam.

Return to Activity Phase

Upon completion of the previously outlined rehabilitation program and the successful evaluation of the injured shoulder, the athlete may begin the final phase of the rehabilitation program—the return to activity phase. Specific criteria during the clinical examination that need to be fulfilled to begin an interval sport program include minimal complaints of pain or tenderness, full range of motion, balanced capsular mobility, adequate proprioception, dynamic stabilization, neuromuscular control, and full muscular strength and endurance based on an isokinetic examination. We routinely perform a combination of isokinetic testing for our overhead athletes, which we refer to as the *Thrower's Series* (16,17). Criteria to begin an interval sport program includes an external rotation/internal rotation strength ratio of 66% to 76% or greater at 180 degrees per second, an external rotation to abduction ratio of 67% to 75% or greater at 180 degrees per second (16,17).

Interval sport programs (ISPs) are designed to gradually return motion, function, and confidence in the upper extremity after injury or surgery by slowly progressing through graduated sport-specific activities (35). These programs are intended to gradually return the overhead athletes to full athletic competition as quickly and safely as possible. An athlete is allowed to begin an ISP following a satisfactory clinical examination.

A gradual return to throwing is performed using an interval throwing program as described by Reinold and colleagues (35). The athlete begins with a long toss program (Table 7-3) designed to gradually increase the distance and number of throws. Athletes typically begin at 45 feet and gradually progress to 60, 90, and 120 feet. At this time, pitchers may begin a mound throwing program (Table 7-4) and positional players progress to greater distances of long toss and positional drills. Throwing off the mound includes a gradual progression in the number of pitches, intensity of effort, and, finally, type of pitch. Each player progresses at an individualized pace depending on the type and extent of injury. Typically, a player throws three times a week with a day off in between, performing each step two to three times before progressing to the next step.

The athlete should supplement the interval throwing program with a high-repetition, low-resistance maintenance exercise program including the Thrower's Ten Program. The rehabilitation program should follow a sequential order of alternating days. All strengthening, plyometric, and neuromuscular control drills should be performed three times per week (with a day off in between) on the same day as the ISP. The athlete should warm up, stretch, and perform one set of each exercise before the ISP, followed by two sets of each exercise after the ISP. This provides an adequate warm-up and ensures maintenance of necessary range of motion and flexibility of the upper extremity. Cryotherapy may be used following the completion of the rehabilitation program to minimize pain and inflammation.

TABLE 7–4. INTERVAL THROWING PROGRAM: PHASE II—THROWING OFF THE MOUND

STAGE ONE: FASTBALLS ONLY:
Step 1: Interval throwing
  15 Throws off mound 50%[a]
Step 2: Interval throwing
  30 Throws off mound 50%
Step 3: Interval throwing
  45 Throws off mound 50%
Step 4: Interval throwing
  60 Throws off mound 50%
Step 5: Interval throwing
  70 Throws off mound 50%
Step 6: 45 Throws off mound 50%
  30 Throws off mound 75%
Step 7: 30 Throws off mound 50%
  45 Throws off mound 75%
Step 8: 10 Throws off mound 50%
  65 Throws off mound 75%
STAGE TWO: FASTBALLS ONLY
Step 9: 60 Throws off mound 75%
  15 Throws in batting practice

Use Interval Throwing 120 ft (36.6 m) phase as warm-up.

Step 10: 50–60 Throws off mound 75%
  30 Throws in batting practice
Step 11: 45–50 Throws off mound 75%
  45 Throws in batting practice
STAGE THREE
Step 12: 30 Throws off mound 75% warm-up
  15 Throws off mound 50% BEGIN BREAKING BALLS
  45–60 Throws in batting practice (fastball only)
Step 13: 30 Throws off mound 75%
  30 Breaking balls 75%
  30 Throws in batting practice
Step 14: 30 Throws off mound 75%
  60–90 Throws in batting practice (gradually increase breaking balls)
Step 15: Simulated game: progressing by 15 throws per workout (pitch count)
All throwing off the mound should be done in the presence of the pitching coach or sport biomechanist to stress proper throwing mechanics
(Use speed gun to aid in effort control.)

[a]Percentage effort.

TABLE 7–5. REHABILITATION PROGRAM COMMONLY USED FOR OVERHEAD ATHLETES

Monday	Tuesday	Wednesday	Thursday	Friday	Saturday	Sunday
Throwers 10* Plyometrics Neuromuscular control drills Stretching ISP	LE strengthening Cardiovascular Core stability Stretching Posterior RTC/scapula strengthening[b]	Throwers 10 Plyometrics Neuromuscular control drills Stretching ISP	LE strengthening Cardiovascular Core stability Stretching Posterior RTC/scapula strengthening[a]	Throwers 10 Plyometrics Neuromuscular control drills Stretching ISP	LE strengthening Cardiovascular Core stability Stretching Posterior RTC/scapula strengthening[a]	Light ROM Stretching

[a]Consists of a set of specific exercises designed to increase strength and flexibility of the upper extremity.[7,10,11]
[b]Strengthening of the posterior rotator cuff and scapular muscles are incorporated on alternating days during the early phases of rehabilitation. As the overhead athlete progresses to more of a maintenance program, these exercises are discontinued on these days.
ISP, Interval sport program; LE, lower extremity; ROM, range of motion; RTC, rotator cuff.

TABLE 7–6. SIX CRITERIA TO INITIATE AN INTERVAL THROWING PROGRAM

1. Appropriate healing time
2. No pain or tenderness
3. Sufficient range of motion and flexibility
4. Satisfactory clinical examination
5. Adequate muscular strength (isokinetic)
6. Appropriate rehabilitation progression

The following day is used for lower extremity, cardiovascular, and core stability training. In addition, the athlete performs range of motion and light strengthening exercises emphasizing the posterior rotator cuff and scapular muscles. The cycle is repeated throughout the week with the seventh day designated for rest, light range of motion, and stretching exercises (Table 7-5).

CRITERIA TO INITIATE A THROWING PROGRAM

One of the concerns of clinicians is knowing when to allow an overhead athlete to initiate his or her interval throwing program. At our center, we address this concern through several clinical tests and parameters. Specific criteria are listed in Table 7-6 and Table 7-7.

The first criterion is based on healing constraints. Based on extensive clinical experience, we believe specific time is necessary to allow tissue healing before initiating an aggressive activity such as throwing. For example, it takes at least 12 weeks for tissue stiffness properties to return after thermal capsular shrinkage (36), so no throwing is allowed for 16 weeks (37,38). Repair of a full thickness rotator cuff tear may require 5 to 6 months before throwing is allowed depending on the size of the tear, tissue quality, and concomitant lesions. The treatment for nonoperative lesions, such as internal impingement, varies significantly depending on the severity of the injury. Minor tendinitis may necessitate that the thrower refrain from throwing for 7 to 14 days, whereas other injuries may require 8 to 12 weeks.

The second criterion to consider is the presence of pain or tenderness. We prefer our throwing athletes to exhibit no pain or tenderness on clinical examination or during their exercise program before they start a throwing program. Common locations of tenderness of the thrower's shoulder are proximal biceps tendon, greater tuberosity, and infraspinatus at the joint line. These locations should be nontender or only slightly painful before a throwing program is allowed.

Third, the athlete should exhibit sufficient range of motion and flexibility. If a thrower begins throwing activities when feeling "tight," then the thrower exhibits abnormal mechanics, risks injury, and probably will become sore. The range-of-motion criteria that we have used for several years include the following: external rotation at 90 degrees abduction to at least 115 degrees, internal rotation at 90

TABLE 7–7. CRITERIA TO INITIATE INTERVAL THROWING PROGRAMS

1. Full, Non-painful range of motion
2. Satisfactory Isokinetic test
3. Satisfactory clinical examination
4. Appropriate rehabilitation progression

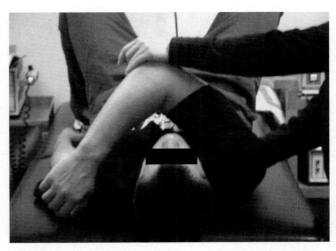

FIGURE 7-9. The clinical assessment of horizontal shoulder adduction. The overhead athlete should exhibit approximately 135 degrees of shoulder horizontal adduction.

degrees abduction to at least 50 degrees, horizontal adduction at 90 degrees to at least 135 degrees (Fig. 7-9). Additionally, we prefer full overhead flexion and external rotation at 45 degrees of abduction to at least 95 degrees. If the athlete does not exhibit these range-of-motion measurements, a rigorous stretching and range-of-motion program is initiated.

The fourth criterion is a satisfactory clinical examination. This includes stability assessment, labrum testing, neurovascular testing, strength assessment, and palpation. The clinician should examine the shoulder complex, scapular region, and trunk carefully before allowing an athlete to begin functional training.

The fifth criterion is an objective muscular strength assessment. We use isokinetic testing to objectively quantify the athlete's muscular strength. We perform the "thrower's series isokinetic test"(39), which consists of shoulder abduction, adduction, and external rotation and internal rotation at 90 degrees of abduction. We use test speeds of 180 degrees per second and 300 degrees per second. The isokinetic report generates numerous values based on previous studies (16,17,21). We have determined five parameters necessary to evaluate: torque-to-body weight ratios, unilateral muscular ratios, bilateral comparisons, acceleration rates for internal rotation and adduction, and deceleration rates for external rotation. Specific values are listed in Table 7-1.

The sixth and final criterion that we use is an empirical assessment of the athlete's rehabilitation or exercise progression, making sure that the athlete has been performing the proper exercises, has been applying adequate resistance, and has gradually increased the resistance. Another important progression is that the athlete has been performing plyometric drills for at least 2 to 4 weeks before initiating an interval-throwing program. We believe the plyometric drills prepare the athlete's tissue for the quick, ballistic, and repetitive forces that occur during throwing. Thus, plyometric exercises serve as a precursor activity to throwing.

SPECIFIC REHABILITATION GUIDELINES

In this section, we elaborate on the specific rehabilitation programs we use for common shoulder injuries seen in the thrower. To successfully rehabilitate the overhead thrower, an accurate differential diagnosis is imperative. Furthermore, the rehabilitation specialist must establish a list of abnormalities and positive clinical findings determined on the examination, which may be contributing to the problem. Once this has been established, an appropriate rehabilitation program can be formulated. Often, the programs must be modified based on the specific disorder exhibited by the thrower.

Posterosuperior Glenoid Impingement

Posterosuperior glenoid impingement, often referred to as *internal impingement,* is one of the most frequently observed injuries to the overhead throwing athlete (40–47). We believe that one of the underlying causes of symptomatic internal impingement is excessive anterior shoulder laxity. One of the primary goals of the rehabilitation program is to enhance the athlete's dynamic stabilization abilities, thus controlling anterior humeral head translation. In addition, another essential goal is to restore flexibility to the posterior rotator cuff muscles of the glenohumeral joint. The stretch we think is most beneficial is the horizontal adduction stretch and the horizontal adduction with internal rotation. This stretch probably stretches the posterior rotator cuff and posterior capsular structures. We strongly suggest caution against aggressive stretching of the anterior and inferior glenohumeral structures, which may result in increased anterior translation. Additionally, the program emphasizes muscular strengthening of the posterior rotator cuff to reestablish muscular balance and improve joint compression abilities. The scapular muscles must be an area of increased focus as well. In particular, the scapular retractors and depressors are targeted to reposition the scapular in retraction and with a posterior tilt. Restoring dynamic stabilization is an essential goal to minimize the anterior translation of the humeral head during the late cocking and early acceleration phases of throwing. Exercise drills such as PNF patterns with rhythmic stabilization are incorporated (48–50). Also, stabilization drills performed at end range external rotation are beneficial in enhancing dynamic stabilization (Fig. 7-6). Perturbation training to the shoulder joint is performed to enhance proprioception, dynamic stabilization, and neuromuscular control. It is the senior author's (K.E.W.) opinion that this form of training has been extremely effective in treating the thrower with pos-

terosuperior impingement. Plyometric throwing drills are incorporated into the program before the initiation of an interval throwing program. The plyometrics are designed to normalize throwing mechanics and prepare the tissue for the repetitive stresses of throwing (32).

Once we have restored posterior flexibility, normalized glenohumeral strength ratios, enhanced scapular muscular strength, and diminished the patient's symptoms, an interval throwing program may be initiated (30,35). Jobe (43) suggested abstaining from throwing for 2 to 12 weeks depending on the thrower's symptoms. Once the thrower begins the interval throwing program, the clinician or pitching coach should observe the athlete's throwing mechanics frequently. Occasionally, throwers who exhibit internal impingement allow their arm to lag behind the scapula, thus throwing with excessive horizontal abduction and not throwing with the humerus in the plane of the scapula (Fig. 7-1). Jobe (43,50–52) referred to this phenomenon as *hyperangulation* of the arm. This type of fault leads to excessive strain on the anterior capsule and internal impingement of the posterior rotator cuff (43,51,52). Correction of throwing pathomechanics is critical to returning the athlete to asymptomatic and effective throwing.

Subacromial Impingement

Primary subacromial impingement in the young overhead throwing athlete is unusual but may occur (46,53). Subacromial impingement complaints in this group of athletes usually represent primary hyperlaxity, which leads to secondary impingement (53). Neer (55) and Bigliani and colleagues (56) reported that abnormal acromial architecture may lead to rotator cuff disease. In cases of abnormal acromial architecture, the athlete may require surgical treatment. Also, Hawkins and Kennedy (57) as well as Penny and Welsh (58) stated the coracoacromial ligament can be a primary source of pathology in the athlete.

The nonoperative treatment for subacromial impingement should focus on a five-step program:

1. Abstain from irritating activities, such as throwing or other overhead motions, for 7 to 10 days until inflammation is diminished.
2. Normalize glenohumeral motion and capsular mobility. Harryman and colleagues (59) reported that posterior capsular tightness results in anterosuperior migration of the humeral head leading to subacromial impingement. The senior author (K.E.W.) has noted patients with inferior capsular tightness frequently complain of subacromial pain. Thus, the rehabilitation program must focus on restoring normal capsular and soft tissue mobility posteriorly and inferiorly (60).
3. Enhance dynamic stability of the glenohumeral and scapulothoracic joints. Jobe and colleagues (54) noted subacromial impingement may be secondary to hypere-

lasticity of the capsular ligaments. Hence, the rehabilitation program must focus on rotator cuff strength to adequately compress and stabilize the humeral head within the glenoid fossa (60,61). Furthermore, scapular strengthening should also be an area of focus. During arm elevation, the scapula upwardly rotates, retracts, and posteriorly tilts. Lukasiewicz and colleagues (63) reported that patients with subacromial impingement exhibit less posterior tilting than subjects without impingement. We have also clinically noted this phenomenon for some time. Thus, the rehabilitation program should include pectoralis minor stretching and inferior trapezius strengthening to ensure posterior scapular tilting. We believe the exercises that target the lower trapezius the best are the prone horizontal abduction movement with external rotation, the standing table lift (Fig. 7-10), and side-lying neuromuscular control drills with manual resistance. This is especially true in the recreational baseball player who performs a sedentary job.

4. Emphasize the scapular retractors and correct any forward head posture. Solem-Bentoft and colleagues (64) using magnetic resonance imaging have demonstrated that excessive scapular protraction produces anterior tilt of the scapula and diminishes the acromial-humeral space, whereas scapular retraction increases the subacromial space. Consequently, we use scapular retraction strengthening exercises. The exercises we use for this muscle group are prone horizontal adduction, seated rowing, posterior deltoid flies, and side-lying manual resistance for scapular muscles.

5. The last step is a gradual return to throwing activities once pain has significantly diminished.

Overuse Syndrome Tendinitis

Occasionally, throwers describe the symptoms and exhibit the signs of overuse tendinitis of the shoulder muscles. The tendinitis signs and symptoms can be of the rotator cuff or long head of the biceps brachii muscles (65). Frequently this occurs early in the season when the athlete's arm may not be in the best condition. This can also occur at the end of the competitive season when the athlete begins to fatigue. Additionally, this condition develops when the athlete does not perform his or her in-season strengthening program while throwing. Mere participation in throwing activities does not ensure the maintenance of proper shoulder muscular strength and flexibility. Frequently, specific muscles (external rotators, scapular muscles) become weak and painful as a result of the stresses involved with throwing.

The rehabilitation program for overuse rotator cuff tendinitis should concentrate on treating the causes of the tendinitis and not merely the symptoms. Often, the athlete is instructed to discontinue throwing for a short period of time (2 to 4 weeks) to reduce inflammation and restore strength and flexibility. Other times, the athlete is instructed to reduce the number of throws during competition or practice. Thus, a strict pitch count is enforced. The rehabilitation program is successful if the cause is identified, throwing activities are modified, and proper strength and flexibility are restored.

Often, the thrower complains of bicipital pain, occasionally referred to as "groove pain." The biceps brachii appear to be moderately active during the overhead throwing motion. DiGiovine and colleagues (20) reported peak EMG activity of 44% ± 32% maximum voluntary isometric contraction (MVIC) during the deceleration phase of throwing. In the senior author's opinion, bicipital tendinitis present in the overhead thrower usually represents a secondary condition. The primary disorder may be instability or a SLAP (superior labrum anterior-to-posterior) lesion. The rehabilitation of this condition focuses on improving dynamic stabilization of the glenohumeral joint through muscular training drills. Knatt and colleagues (66) described a glenohumeral joint capsule and biceps reflex in the feline. The authors reported that stimulation of the anterior capsule caused a reflexive biceps contraction. Furthermore, Guanche and colleagues (67) studied the synergistic action of the capsule and shoulder muscles in the feline. The investigators demonstrated that the biceps brachii were the first muscled to reflexively respond to stimulation of the capsule, occurring in 2.7 msec. Therefore, it is the belief of those authors that the biceps brachii are activated to a greater extent when the thrower exhibits hyper-

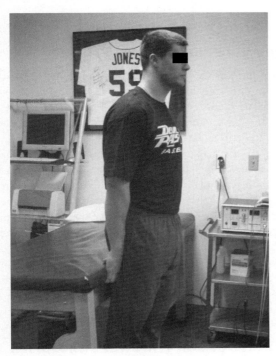

FIGURE 7-10. Standing table lift exercise. The patient may rotate head away from involved shoulder to assist lower trapezius activity.

laxity or inflammation of the capsule. Glousman and colleagues (68) reported that throwers with instability exhibited a higher level of biceps EMG activity than throwers without instability. Additionally, Gowan and colleagues (69) noted higher EMG activity in amateur throwers than in skilled throwers. Nonoperative rehabilitation for this condition usually consists of a reduction in throwing activities, reestablishing dynamic stability, and modalities such as ice, ultrasound, and electrical stimulation to reduce bicipital inflammation.

Posterior Rotator Cuff Musculature Tendinitis

The successful treatment of posterior rotator cuff tendinitis depends on its differential diagnosis from internal impingement. Frequently, the athlete complains of pain in the same location for both lesions. However, subjectively the athlete notes posterior shoulder pain during ball release or the deceleration phase of throwing. Conversely, in athletes who exhibit internal impingement, the pain complaint is during late cocking and early acceleration. During the deceleration phase of the overhead pitch, the distractive forces at the glenohumeral joint approach 1 to 1½ times body weight (1). These are excessive forces that must be dissipated and opposed by the posterior rotator cuff muscles. Pitchers occasionally exhibit this condition. Upon examination, the most common findings are significant posterior rotator cuff weakness, weakness of the lower trapezius and scapular retractors, and tightness of the posterior rotator cuff muscles.

The rehabilitation program focuses on several key areas. First, throwing activities are discontinued until the athlete exhibits proper muscular strength ratios between the external and internal rotator muscles. This ratio should be at least 64% (optimal goal 66% to 75%) (17).

Second, the athlete is placed on an aggressive strengthening program for the posterior rotator cuff muscles, the scapular retractors, and the scapular depressors. We emphasize side-lying external rotation, prone rowing into external rotation, prone horizontal abduction with external rotation, scapular retraction, and prone horizontal abduction. Fleisig and colleagues (26) have shown that teres minor EMG activity can be enhanced with the use of a towel roll placed between the humerus and side of the body. Once strength levels have improved, the exercise program should emphasize eccentric muscular training. In particular, the external rotators and lower trapezius are the focus of the eccentric program (Fig. 7-11). DiGiovine and colleagues (20) determined that the EMG activity of the teres minor is 84% and lower trapezius 78% of a maximum voluntary contraction during the deceleration phase of the throw. These two muscles are the most active during this phase and hence must be the focus of the strengthening program.

Third, flexibility and stretching exercises for the posterior rotator cuff muscles are performed. We also use heat

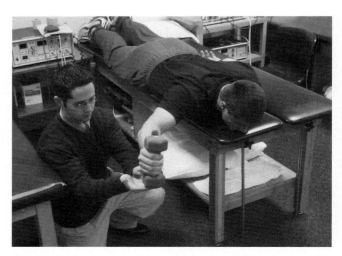

FIGURE 7-11. Eccentric prone horizontal abduction at 100 degrees with external rotation. The clinician assists the patient lifting an overloaded weight followed by the patient slowly returning to the starting position.

and ultrasound before stretching to enhance tissue extensibility while increasing circulation to the area. Once flexibility and muscular strength are improved and the athlete's pain and inflammation have abated, an interval throwing program can be initiated. The interval throwing program should be progressed slowly so that the stresses of throwing are gradually increased. The athlete is instructed to be sure to follow through properly and not to terminate the deceleration phase abruptly because this may lead to increased stresses on the posterior rotator cuff muscles.

Primary Instability

Most skillful throwers exhibit significant hyperelasticity of their anterior glenohumeral joint capsule. This laxity is more than likely congenital laxity. This allows excessive external rotation and proper throwing mechanics. Because of the repetitive microtraumatic forces of throwing, the hyperelasticity may progress to primary instability and associated lesions (e.g., labral tears, internal impingement, tendinitis) and complaints. This is a very common occurrence in the overhead thrower. The nonoperative treatment for this condition is discussed in the rehabilitation program in this paper. The key aspects remain the same: reduce throwing activity to diminish inflammation, normalize motion, restore proper strength of glenohumeral and scapular muscles, enhance proprioception, and gradually return to throwing. In most cases, this treatment is effective and surgery is avoided.

Bennett's Lesion (Thrower's Exostosis)

The successful nonoperative treatment of throwing athletes with ossification of the posterior capsule is often difficult. It has been our clinical experience that the thrower with symptomatic thrower's exostosis can be conservatively managed for some time; however, long-term success is limited and often surgical debridement of the ossification becomes necessary (70). Nonoperative treatment includes abstaining from throwing until pain subsides, restoring posterior capsular and muscular flexibility, improving posterior rotator cuff and scapular strength, and gradually returning to throwing activities. The acute management of pain may be accomplished through modalities such as iontophoresis, ultrasound, and muscle stimulation.

SLAP Lesions

The nonoperative treatment of SLAP lesions depends on the type of lesion present. Using the classification system developed by Snyder and colleagues (71), type I SLAP lesions present as fraying of the labrum and often respond favorably to a nonsurgical treatment regimen. Throwers who exhibit this type of lesion receive treatment similar to the posterosuperior glenoid impingement protocol (previously discussed). Conversely, players with a type II or type IV SLAP lesion are probably best served with surgical intervention. If rehabilitation is indicated before surgery, the program should emphasize restoration of range of motion through stretching exercises within the patient's tolerance. Due to potential "joint snapping" and pain, avoidance of overhead motions with excessive internal and external rotation is enforced. A strengthening program should be performed to prevent muscular atrophy. The strengthening exercises should be performed by the patient below shoulder level to prevent further damage to the glenoid labrum. Strengthening exercises such as external and internal rotation with the arm at the side or scapular plane, scapular strengthening, and deltoid exercises to 90 degrees of abduction can be safely performed. Exercises such as shoulder press, bench press, and latissimus dorsi pull-downs (behind the neck) are avoided because of increased stress applied to the superior labrum and anterior glenohumeral joint capsule. Furthermore, the clinician should be cautious with CKC exercises that result in excessively high joint compressive loads, which could result in further compromise of the superior glenoid labrum.

Improper Mechanics

Throwing with improper or faulty mechanics can lead to shoulder pain or injury as a result of abnormal stresses applied across various tissues. To determine whether the thrower exhibits improper throwing mechanics, the clinician should carefully observe the athlete throw. Obvious flaws can be seen occasionally. The clinician may require assistance from an experienced and knowledgeable baseball coach or athletic trainer with extensive baseball experience. Frequently, the skilled eye of an experienced coach or ath-

letic trainer can determine subtle abnormalities in the throwing mechanics. Perhaps the most objective analysis is a high-speed video biomechanical evaluation. This can be done at a biomechanics laboratory using specialized high-speed video cameras and computer analysis of the data.

When evaluating an athlete's throwing mechanics, we commonly look at several different aspects of the movement. The clinician can use a video recorder to film the thrower and analyze the biomechanics during slow motion playback to pinpoint improper mechanics. Filming should be performed from multiple views to accurately assess the athlete, including a lateral (facing the athlete), posterior, and anterior view. We normally analyze several aspects of the throwing motion in sequential order to detect subtle pathomechanical deviations throughout the phases of throwing.

Biomechanical analysis of the throwing motion begins with the lateral view; there are several critical moments to observe from this view. During the wind-up phase, the pitcher should be in a balanced position when the lead leg reaches the highest point. Forward movement should not begin until the lead leg is fully raised. Rushing the delivery by falling toward home plate during the wind-up phase may decrease the amount of energy generated by the lower body and result in a loss of velocity. As the athlete begins the early cocking phase, the path of motion as the thrower removes the ball from the glove should be smooth with the elbow flexed and fingers on top of the ball. As the lead leg comes in contact with the ground, the knee should be slightly flexed and the elbow should be level with the shoulder. A right-handed pitcher shows the ball to the shortstop and a left-handed thrower shows the ball to the second baseman. The stride should be long enough (approximately equal to the height of the thrower) to allow sufficient rotation and force generation from the hips and trunk. At maximal external rotation during the late cocking phase, the arm should be abducted approximately 90 to 100 degrees. Fleisig (1) reported that throwing with reduced external rotation at the time of foot contact causes an increase in strain on the shoulder during acceleration and ball release. Furthermore, the thrower should begin straightening the elbow before shoulder internal rotation during the acceleration phase. At this time, the lead leg extends, or straightens, to stabilize the body and provide a fulcrum for body rotation.

During the deceleration and follow-through phases, the throwing shoulder should internally rotate and horizontally adduct across the body. The upper extremity should cross the front of the body and end outside of the lead leg. Abbreviating the follow-through and ending with the hand toward the target may increase the stresses applied to the shoulder.

Observing the thrower from a posterior view allows the clinician to observe two instants during the throwing motion. As the thrower removes the ball from the glove during early cocking, the arm path should move smoothly in a down, back, and upward motion as the athlete strides toward the target. A thrower whose arm moves behind the body may result in excessive anterior capsular straining and possible internal impingement. Also of interest from the posterior view is the hand position during late cocking. As previously stated, the ball should be facing toward the shortstop for right-handed and toward the second baseman for left-handed throwers.

An anterior view of the throwing motion is helpful to the clinician to determine the position of the stride leg as the foot comes into contact with the ground. At this time, the lead foot should be pointed toward the target. Often, young and inexperienced throwers overrotate and place the lead foot on the first base side of the mound. This results in the pitcher's "opening up too soon" and causes the hips to rotate early, resulting in loss of velocity and increased strain to the anterior shoulder. Fleisig (1) has shown that, as the lead foot angle becomes more open, the thrower tends to throw across the body and increases the loads applied to the shoulder. Furthermore, "leading with the elbow" (increased horizontal adduction and elbow flexion) during the acceleration phase correlated with decreased loads at the shoulder but increased loads on the medial aspect of the elbow (1).

Also, during the anterior view of the throwing motion, the orientation of the shoulder can be assessed at the moment of ball release. The throwing elbow should be in line with the shoulder with minimal flexion of the elbow. The nonthrowing elbow should be tucked at the side. As the athlete progresses into the deceleration and follow-through phases, the throwing arm should follow a long arc of deceleration—allowing proper dissipation of forces from the arm to the trunk and lower extremities.

SUMMARY

Overhead throwing athletes typically present with a unique musculoskeletal profile. The overhead thrower frequently experiences shoulder pain as a result of anterior capsular laxity and increased demands placed on the dynamic stabilizers. This may be the result of repetitive high stresses imparted to the shoulder joint and may lead to the development of injuries. Most commonly, these injuries are overuse injuries and can be successfully managed with a well-structured rehabilitation program. The rehabilitation program should focus on the correction of adaptive changes seen in the overhead thrower, such as loss of internal rotation and muscular weakness of the external rotators and scapular muscles. The athlete may then initiate a gradual throwing program to return back to competition. The athlete's overhead throwing motion should be examined to determine whether improper biomechanics are contributing to the injury. Lastly, education of the athlete in the area of year-round conditioning is imperative. The throwing athlete should be instructed when to begin conditioning and throwing to prepare for the next competitive season and prevent subsequent injury.

REFERENCES

1. Fleisig GS, Andrews JR, Dillman CJ, et al. Kinetics of baseball pitching with implications about injury mechanisms. *Am J Sports Med* 1995;23:233–239.
2. Wilk KE, Meister K, Fleisig GS, et al. Biomechanics of the overhead throwing motion. *Sports Med Arthroscopic Rev* 2000;8(2):124–134.
3. Bigliani LU, Codd TP, Connor PM, et al. Shoulder motion and laxity in the professional baseball player. *Am J Sports Med* 197;25:609–613.
4. Brown LP, Niehues SL, Harrah A, et al. Upper extremity range of motion and isokinetic strength of the internal and external shoulder rotators in major league baseball players. *Am J Sports Med* 1988;16:577–585.
5. Johnson L. Patterns of shoulder flexibility among college baseball players. *J Athl Train* 1992;27:44–49.
6. Wilk KE, Arrigo C. Current concepts in the rehabilitation of the athletic shoulder. *J Orthop Sports Phys Ther* 1993;18:365–378.
7. Wilk KE, Meister K, Andrews JR. Current concepts in the rehabilitation of the overhead throwing athlete. *Am J Sports Med* 2002;30:136–151.
8. Reinold MM, Wilk KE, Reed J, et al. Change in shoulder and elbow range of motion of professional baseball pitchers before and after pitching. *J Orthop Sports Phys Ther* 2003;33(2):A-50.
9. Tyler TF, Roy T, Nicholas SJ, et al. Reliability and validity of a new method of measuring posterior shoulder tightness. *J Orthop Sports Phys Ther* 1999;29(5):262–269.
10. Crockett HC, Gross LB, Wilk KE, et al. Osseous adaptation and range of motion at the glenohumeral joint in professional baseball pitchers. *Am J Sports Med* 2002;30:20–26.
11. Alderink GJ, Kuck DJ. Isokinetic shoulder strength of high school and college-aged pitchers. *J Orthop Sports Phys Ther* 1986;7:163–172.
12. Barlett LR, Storey MD, Simons DB. Measurement of upper extremity torque production and its relationship to throwing speed in the competitive athlete. *Am J Sports Med* 1989;17:89–91.
13. Cook EE, Gray UL, Savinar-Nogue E, et al. Shoulder antagonistic strength ratios: a comparison between college-level baseball pitchers and non-pitchers. *J Orthop Sports Phys Ther* 1987;8:451–461.
14. Davies CJ. *Compendium of isokinetics in clinical usage,* 4th ed. Onalaska, WI: S&S Publishing, 1992:445.
15. Hinton RY. Isokinetic evaluation of shoulder rotational strength in high school baseball pitchers. *Am J Sports Med* 1988;16:274–279.
16. Wilk KE, Andrews JR, Arrigo CA. The abductor and adductor strength characteristics of professional baseball pitchers. *Am J Sports Med* 1995;23:307–311.
17. Wilk KE, Andrews JR, Arrigo CA, et al. The strength characteristics of internal and external rotator muscles in professional baseball pitchers. *Am J Sports Med* 1993;21:61–66.
18. Magnusson SP, Gleim GW, Nicholas JA. Shoulder weakness in professional baseball pitchers. *Med Sci Sports Exerc* 1994;26:5–9.
19. Reinold MM, Wilk KE, Hooks TR, et al. Comparison of bilateral shoulder external and internal rotation strength at 0 degrees versus 90 degrees of shoulder abduction in professional baseball pitchers. *J Orthop Sports Phys Ther* 2003;33(2):A-51.

20. DiGiovine NM, Jobe FW, Pink M, et al. An electromyographic analysis of the upper extremity in pitching. *J Shoulder Elbow Surg* 1992;1:15–25.

21. Wilk KE, Suarez K, Reed J. Scapular muscular strength values in professional baseball players [abstract]. *Phys Ther* 1999;79[Suppl 5]:81–82(abst).

22. Blasier RB, Carpenter JE, Huston LJ. Shoulder proprioception: effect of joint laxity, joint position, and direction of motion. *Orthop Rev* 1994;23:45–50.

23. Allegrucci M, Whitney SL, Lephart SM, et al. Shoulder kinesthesia in healthy unilateral athletes participating in upper extremity sports. *J Orthop Sports Phys Ther* 1995;21:220–226.

24. Blackburn TA, McLeod WD, White B, et al. EMG analysis of posterior rotator cuff exercises. *Athl Training* 1990;25:40–45.

25. Davies GJ, Dickoff-Hoffman S. neuromuscular testing and rehabilitation of the shoulder complex. *J Orthop Sports Phys Ther* 1993;18:449–458.

26. Fleisig GS, Jameson GG, Cody KE, et al. Muscle activity during shoulder rehabilitation exercises. In: Proceedings of NACOB '98, The Third North American Congress on Biomechanics. Waterloo, Ontario, Canada, August 14, 1998, pp 223–234.

27. Malanga GA, Jenp YN, Growney ES, et al. EMG analysis of shoulder positioning in testing and strengthening the supraspinatus. *Med Sci Sports Exerc* 1996;28:661–664.

28. Townsend H, Jobe FW, Pink M, et al. Electromyographic analysis of the glenohumeral muscles during a baseball rehabilitation program. *Am J Sports Med* 1991;19:264–272.

29. Moseley JB, Jobe FW, Pink M, et al. EMG analysis of the scapular muscles during a shoulder rehabilitation program. *Am J Sports Med* 1992;20(2):128–134.

30. Wilk KE, Andrews JR, Arrigo CA, et al. *Preventive and rehabilitative exercises for the shoulder and elbow,* 6th ed. Birmingham, AL: American Sports Medicine Institute, 2001.

31. Wilk KE, Arrigo CA, Andrews JR. Closed and open kinetic chain exercises for the upper extremity. *J Sport Rehabil* 1996;5:88–102.

32. Wilk KE, Voight ML, Keirns MA, et al. Stretch-shortening drills for the upper extremities: theory and clinical application. *J Orthop Sports Phys Ther* 1993;17:225–239.

33. Wilk KE. Conditioning and training techniques. In: Hawkins RJ, Misamore GW, eds. *Shoulder injuries in athletes.* New York: Churchill Livingstone, 1996:333–364.

34. Wilk KE, Arrigo CA, Andrews JR. Functioning training for the overhead athlete. Sports Physical Therapy Home Study Course 1995, Chapter 5, Sports Section, American Physical Therapy Association, Indianapolis, IN.

35. Reinold MM, Wilk KE, Reed J, et al. Interval sport programs: guidelines for baseball, tennis, and golf. *J Orthop Sports Phys Ther* 2002;32:293–298.

36. Hecht P, Hayashi K, Lu Y. Monopolar radiofrequency energy effect on joint capsular tissue: potential treatment for joint instability: an *in vivo* mechanical morphological and biomechanical study using an ovine model. *Am J Sports Med* 1992;27:761–771.

37. Wilk KE, Reinold MM, Andrews JR. Postoperative treatment principles in the throwing athlete. *Sports Med Arthroscopic Rev* 2001;9(1):1–27.

38. Wilk KE, Reinold MM, Dugas JR, et al. Rehabilitation following thermal-assisted capsular shrinkage of the glenohumeral joint: current concepts. *J Orthop Sports Phys Ther* 2002;32(6):268–292.

39. Wilk KE, Arrigo CA. Standardized isokinetic testing protocol for the throwing shoulder: the thrower's series. *Isokin Ex Sci* 1991; I(2):63–71.

40. Andrews JR, Angelo RL. Shoulder arthroscopy for the throwing athlete. *Techn Orthop* 1988;3:75–79.

41. Andrews JR, Kupferman SP, Dillman CJ. Labral tears in throwing and racquet sports. *Clin Sports Med* 1991;10:901–911.

42. Baker CL, Liu SH, Blackburn TA. Neuromuscular compression syndrome of the shoulder. In: Andrews JR, Wilk KE, eds. *The athlete's shoulder.* New York: Churchill Livingstone, 1994: 261–273.

43. Jobe CM. Posterior superior glenoid impingement: expanded spectrum. *Arthroscopy* 1995;11:530–536.

44. Jobe FW, Bradley JP, Tibone JE. The diagnosis and nonoperative treatment of shoulder injuries in athletes. *Clin Sports Med* 1989; 8:419–438.

45. Jobe FW, Moynes DR. Delineation of diagnostic criteria and a rehabilitation program for rotator cuff injuries. *Am J Sports Med* 1982;10:336–339.

46. Meister K. Injuries to the shoulder in the throwing athlete. Part One. Biomechanics/pathophysiology/classification of injury. *Am J Sports Med* 2000;28:265–275.

47. Walch G, Boileau P, Noel E, et al. Impingement of the deep surface of the supraspinatus tendon on the posterosuperior glenoid rim: an arthroscopic study. *J Shoulder Elbow Surg* 1992;1: 238–245.

48. Wilk KE, Arrigo CA, Andrews JR. Closed and open kinetic chain exercises for the upper extremity. *J Sport Rehabil* 1996;5: 88–102.

49. Wilk KE. Restoration of functional motor patterns and functional testing in the throwing athlete. In: Lephart SM, Fu FH, eds: *Proprioception and neuromuscular control in joint stability.* Champaign, IL: Human Kinetics, 2000:415–438.

50. Wilk KE, Meister K, Andrews JR. Current concepts in the rehabilitation of the overhead athlete. *Am J Sports Med* 2002; 30(1).

51. Wilk KE. Rehabilitation of the shoulder. In: Andrews JR, Zarins B, Wilk KE, eds. *Injuries in baseball.* Philadelphia: Lippincott-Raven, 1998:451—468.

52. Jobe CM. Superior glenoid impingement. *Orthop Clin North Am* 1997;28:137–143.

53. Jobe CM. Superior glenoid impingement [Current concepts]. *Clin Orthop* 1996;330:98–107.

54. Jobe FW, Tibone JE, Jobe CM, et al. The shoulder in sports. In Rockwood CA Jr, Matsen FA III, eds. *The shoulder.* Philadelphia: WB Saunders, 1990:961–990.

55. Neer CS III, Welsh RP. The shoulder in sports. *Orthop Clin North Am* 1977;8:583–591.

56. Bigliani LU, Ticker JB, Flatow EL, et al. The relationship of acromial architecture to rotator cuff disease. *Clin Sports Med* 1991;10:823–838.

57. Hawkins RJ, Kennedy JC. Impingement syndrome in athletes. *Am J Sports Med* 1980;8:151–158.

58. Penny JN, Welsh RP. Shoulder impingement syndromes in athletes and their surgical management. *Am J Sports Med* 1981;9: 11–15.

59. Harryman DT II, Sidles JA, Clark JM, et al. Translation of the humeral head on the glenoid with passive glenohumeral motion. *J Bone Joint Surg (Am)* 1990;72:1334–1343.

60. Wilk KE Arrigo CA, Andrews JR. Current concepts: The stabilizing structures of the glenohumeral joint. *J Orthop Sports Phys Ther* 1997;25:364–379.

61. Kibler WB. The role of the scapula in athletic shoulder function. *Am J Sports Med* 1998;26:325–337.

62. Kibler WB. Role of the scapular in the overhead throwing motion. *Contemp Orthop* 1991;22:525–532.

63. Lukasiewicz AC, McClure P, Michener L, et al. Comparison of 3-dimensional scapular position and orientation between subjects with and without shoulder impingement. *J Orthop Sports Phys Ther* 1999;29:574–586.

64. Solem-Bertoft E, Thuomas KA, Westerberg CE. The influence of

scapular retraction and protraction on the width of the subacromial space: an MRI study. *Clin Orthop* 1993;296:99–103.

65. Wilk KE. Shoulder injuries in baseball. In: Andrews JR, Wilk KE, eds. *The athlete's shoulder.* New York: Churchill Livingstone, 1994:369–390.
66. Knatt T, Guanche C, Solomonow M, et al. The glenohumeral-biceps reflex in the feline. *Clin Orthop* 1995;314:247–252.
67. Guanche C, Knatt T, Solomonow M, et al. The synergistic action of the capsule and shoulder muscles. *Am J Sports Med* 1995;23 (3):301–306.
68. Glousman R, Jobe F, Tibone JE, et al. Dynamic electromyo-graphic analysis of the throwing shoulder with glenohumeral instability. *J Bone Joint Surg (Am)* 1988;70:220–226.
69. Gowan ID, Jobe FW, Tibone JE, et al. A comparative electromyographic analysis of the shoulder during pitching: professional versus amateur pitchers. *Am J Sports Med* 1987;15: 586–590.
70. Meister K, Andrews JR, Batts J, et al. Symptomatic thrower's exostosis arthroscopic evaluation and treatment. *Am J Sports Med* 1999;27(2):133–136.
71. Snyder SJ, Karzel RP, Del Pizzo W, et al. SLAP lesions of the shoulder. *Arthroscopy* 1990;6:274–279.

8

INTERVAL PROGRAM AND ITS IMPLICATION FOR THE THROWING ATHLETE

MICHAEL W. ALLEN
SUMANT G. KRISHNAN

The kinematics and kinetics of full effort pitching are well documented (1). Shoulder internal rotation velocity can exceed loads of 7,000 degrees per second, while ball velocity approaches 90 to 100 mph (2,3). Despite continued advancements in rehabilitation techniques, these forces are impossible to reproduce in a clinical or training room setting. Therefore, a gradual transition to sport-specific functional programs must be developed. Interval throwing programs (ITP) assist athletes in their physiologic and neuromuscular reconditioning. This process is based on "specific adaptation to imposed demand," or the SAID principle (4). It requires progressive adaptations by increasing loads to the skeletal, articular, neural, and soft tissue systems. Establishing a sufficient strength and endurance base with appropriate functional intervention is essential in returning an athlete to preinjury/surgery status expeditiously and with minimal complications (Fig. 8-1).

In developing an ITP, the chronologic and physiologic time of healing following a surgery or injury must be well understood. Table 8-1 depicts time frames established for initiation of ITP for throwing athletes. Clinicians must be patient during this often difficult and lengthy phase of rehabilitation. The time frame in returning the athlete to a "competitive" level wherein performance matches or exceeds preinjury/surgery status is often longer than anticipated. It is common for an athlete to endure several setbacks or regressions during the ITP. Creating a well-designed rehabilitation approach is an essential element in returning a throwing athlete to full, unrestricted participation. This chapter outlines a concise, methodical, reproducible model for returning to competition at a high level of performance.

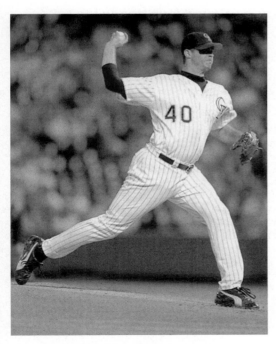

FIGURE 8-1. Game participation.

TABLE 8–1. EXAMPLE OF GENERAL TIME FRAMES FOR INITIATION OF INTERVAL THROWING AFTER COMMON SURGICAL PROCEDURES

Shoulder	
Subacromial decompression	6 weeks—as tolerated
Anterior heat capsulorrhaphy	4 months
Posterior heat capsulorrhaphy	4 months
Heat capsulorrhaphy with SLAP repair	4 months
Rotator cuff repair	4 months
Knee	
Knee meniscectomy	1–2 weeks
Meniscus repair	3 months
ACL reconstruction	3 months
Patella tendon fenestration	3 months
Microfracture condyle	3 months
Microfracture trochlear groove	3 months
Elbow	
Arthroscopic debridement	6 weeks—as tolerated
UCL reconstruction	3–4 months

ACL, anterior cruciate ligament; UCL, ulnar collateral ligament.

Nonsurgical versus Postsurgical Approach

In establishing an appropriate strategy for returning the throwing athlete to competition, we must first turn our attention to the basic science of healing. Nonsurgical progression through the ITP is more rapid and based on the athlete's symptoms. Postsurgical progression is generally slower and based on the physiologic healing process involved for that particular procedure. Nonsurgical athletes may bypass lower levels of the program whereas postsurgical athletes generally follow each level sequentially.

For both nonsurgical and surgical intervention, the clinician must first give strong attention to the global deconditioning process that occurs when an athlete is injured and unable to throw for an extended period of time. Arm strength and, in particular, endurance is lost rapidly. This is extremely important to understand because complications can arise when an athlete is progressed too rapidly through the program.

Criteria for Entry into the Interval Throwing Program

Before the initiation of the ITP, a well-designed strength and endurance program must be completed. Initiating the ITP for either the nonsurgical or postsurgical athlete requires the following six criteria:

1. No subjective complaints
2. Full pain-free range of motion (ROM)
3. Full strength
4. Negative clinical examination
5. Adequate endurance
6. Maintenance program in strength, flexibility, and conditioning

Allowing an athlete to return without meeting these six criteria assures certain failure and potential reinjury. Moreover, the athlete should have these variables reassessed frequently as they progress through the program. Close monitoring of these criteria enables the therapist or trainer to "back down" or modify the athlete's program appropriately. Table 8-2 lists modifications to programs when complications arise.

Controlling Exercise Variables

Before initiating the ITP, the primary focus for the throwing athlete is centered on restoring full ROM, strength, flexibility, and endurance. It is common for an athlete to be involved in some aspect of rehabilitation, strength, or conditioning 3 to 8 hours per day for 4 to 6 days per week. Without question, total training volume can reach high levels, which, if not controlled, can lead to fatigue and overuse. The end result is decreased performance, frustration, and possibly injury. The ITP must be considered an exercise modality in itself. Once initiated, it must have first priority in the athlete's rehabilitation program. Table 8-3 establishes appropriate sequencing. The ITP should follow a 10-minute cardiovascular warm-up and thorough upper and lower extremity stretch. Global weight room strength and conditioning are modified and likely reduced. The total volume of rotator cuff and scapular strengthening must also

TABLE 8–2. GUIDELINES FOR PROBLEM-BASED MODIFICATION OF A THROWING PROGRAM

Soreness at beginning of session but subsides after warm up:
Treatment intervention: continue session at that level
Soreness at beginning of session that does not resolve:
Treatment intervention: attempt to reduce sore level, if soreness persists, end session. Take appropriate measures to reduce inflammation. Reassess range of motion (ROM), strength, flexibility, and endurance. Resume throwing at one level lower once a negative clinical examination is present.
Soreness during a session associated with pain:
Treatment intervention: end session. Pain is often associated with a rapid decrease in performance. Throwing mechanics change: change in velocity, location, arm action, or body lean. Take appropriate measures to reduce inflammation.
Reassess ROM, strength, flexibility, and endurance. Resume throwing at one level lower once a negative clinical examination is present.
Soreness during a session associated with fatigue:
Treatment intervention: The athlete reports a gradual increase in fatigue in the latter portions of the throwing session. The fatigue is usually reported in the posterior shoulder region as a response to sports-specific reconditioning of the rotator cuff decelerators. The timing of this subjective report during a session is an excellent measure of the athlete's improvement in throwing endurance (i.e., a later onset of fatigue equates to improved endurance). The athlete should stay at the current level of throwing until he is able to complete the level without significant reports of fatigue.
No soreness during session, soreness and fatigue the next day, no pain
Treatment intervention: This is the expected post-throwing response. Continue at the current level of throwing. Soreness should resolve within 24 hours.
No soreness during session, soreness, fatigue and pain lasting greater than 2 days
Treatment intervention: Take one session off. If symptoms resolve, resume throwing at one level lower. If symptoms continue, discontinue throwing until a negative clinical examination is present. Initiate antiinflammatory measures and address strength, ROM, flexibility, and endurance deficits.

TABLE 8–3. APPROPRIATE SEQUENCING FOR A REHABILITATION PROGRAM

- 10-minute cardiovascular warm-up to increase core temperature
- Upper and lower extremity stretch
- 5–10 minutes of warm-up throwing 30–60 ft
- Interval throwing program
- Rotator cuff and scapular strengthening: weights, bands, manuals, or combination.
- Weight room and cardiovascular training

TABLE 8–4. INTERVAL THROWING PROGRAM

PHASE I: Long Toss
Level 1: 30–45 ft
5–8 minute warm-up throwing
3 sets × 15 progressing to 25 throws
3–5 minute rest interval between sets
Level 2: 60 ft
5–8 minute warm-up throwing
3 sets × 15 progressing to 25 throws
3–5 minute rest interval between sets
Level 3: 75–90 ft
5–8 minute warm-up throwing
3 sets × 15 progressing to 25 throws
3–5 minute rest interval between sets
Level 4: 100–110 ft
5–8 minute warm-up throwing
3 sets × 15 progressing to 25 throws
3–5 minute rest interval between sets
Level 5: 120 ft
5–8 minutes warm-up throwing
3 sets × 15 progressing to 25 throws
3–5 minute rest interval between sets
Level 6: Traditional long toss 150–180 ft/
PHASE II: Flat Ground Work
5–8 minutes warm-up throwing
10–12 minutes of progressive throwing to 150–180 ft
1 set progressing to 3 sets × 15 at 60 ft on flat ground
PHASE III: Mound Work
Level 1:
8–10 minutes warm-up throwing
3 sets × 15 progressing to 25 throws at 50%
Fast balls only
Level 2:
8–10 minutes warm-up throwing
3 sets × 15 progressing to 25 throws at 75%
Fast balls only
Level 3:
8–10 minutes warm-up throwing
3 sets × 15 progressing to 25 throws at 90%–100%
Fast balls and change-up
Level 4:
8–10 minutes warm-up throwing
3 sets × 15 progressing to 25 throws
75% fast balls; 25% breaking balls
Level 5:
8–10 minute warm-up throwing
3 sets × 15 progressing to 25 throws
60% fast balls; 40% breaking balls
Focus on velocity and location
Level 6:
8–10 minutes warm-up throwing
3 sets × 25 unrestricted throws
Focus on velocity and location
PHASE IV: Simulated Game Activity
PHASE V: Game Progression
PHASE VI: Return Maintenance

decrease. Plyometric exercises for the upper extremity are decreased or eliminated. Although these essential components are being deemphasized, it is essential that the throwing athlete not be allowed to regress in flexibility, strength, or overall conditioning. Undoubtedly, controlling and monitoring these variables is difficult but essential to successfully directing the program.

INTERVAL THROWING PROGRAM

The ITP is divided into surgical and nonsurgical groups and is broken into six phases within each group:

1. Long toss
2. Flat ground work
3. Progressive mound work
4. Simulated game activity
5. Game progression
6. Return maintenance

Phase I: Long Toss

The long toss component provides a low-intensity, high-endurance intervention to establish foundational arm strength (5). This is an extension of the concept that running longer distances improves a sprinter's performance and reduces injury. Axe and colleagues (5) studied young athletes and concluded that the faster the athlete throws, the further distance he can throw. It is our assumption that the inverse of this hypothesis is true. Our long toss program has been developed and modified from the work of Andrews and Wilk (6). There are six levels within the long toss phase (Table 8-4).

Postsurgical Long Toss

All postsurgical athletes begin at level 1 and progress systematically to level 6. However, surgical interventions not requiring ongoing physiologic protection (i.e., arthroscopic subacromial decompression, elbow debridement, or meniscectomy) may independently progress more rapidly. The athlete uses a "crow hop" technique with proper follow-through (Fig. 8-2). Strong effort is placed on "throwing on

a line" thus, minimizing trajectory on the ball to promote arm strength. Each phase consists of three sets of 15 to 25 throws, with a 3- to 5-minute rest between each set. The rest interval is based on full recovery, but is less than the 10 minutes currently recommended in the literature (6). This

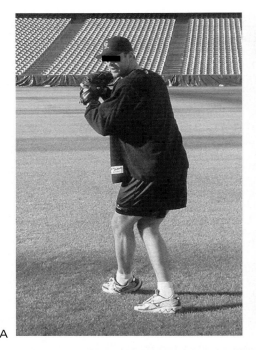

A

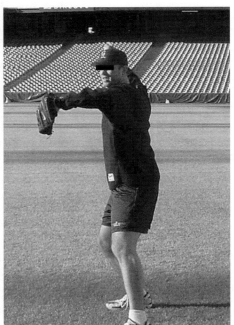

B

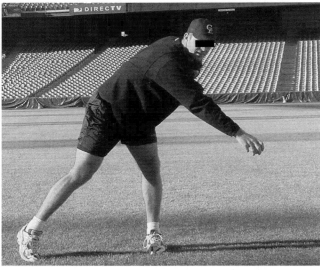

C

FIGURE 8-2. "Crow hop" technique with proper follow-through.

allows the athlete to complete the program in a reasonable timeframe without significantly "cooling off" within the session. The athlete throws three times per week with one rest day between each session and must be able to throw three sets of 25 throws at each distance before advancing to the next level. The athlete must remain symptom free and maintain adequate ROM, strength, and flexibility. Two to three sessions at each level are necessary for postsurgical athletes. Progression to the next level is based on symptoms, maintenance of arm strength, endurance, and mechanics. Close evaluation of the athlete's tolerance at each level is essential. Constant monitoring of appropriate throwing mechanics and fatigue provides information to avoid too

rapid of a progression, which can potentially result in injury. The trainer or therapist must develop functional evaluation skills to determine volume threshold for the athlete.

Four indicators of fatigue include the following:

1. Decreased velocity: the athlete puts more arc on the ball
2. Altered mechanics: change in arm angle, arm mechanics, or body lean
3. Increased time between throws
4. Poor location of each throw

Once the athlete completes level 5, he is transitioned into a traditional long toss program, which consists of a 10-

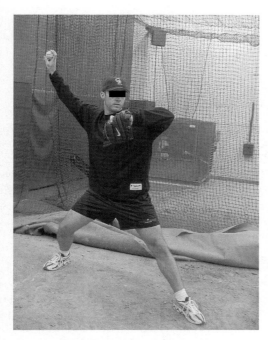

FIGURE 8-3. Flat ground work.

takes 7 days to 2 weeks to advance through this phase. This time is necessary to establish enough arm strength and endurance to endure mound work or positional throws for infielders or outfielders.

Phase II: Flat Ground Work

Flat ground work (Fig. 8-3) is incorporated into level 6 of both the postsurgical and nonsurgical long toss programs to gradually transition the throwing athlete into normal pitching mechanics. The work of Fleisig and colleagues (7) established that partial effort pitching in training, warm-up, and rehabilitation significantly reduces force and torque throughout the entire kinematic chain. This includes less shoulder external rotation at foot contact, more elbow varus torque during arm cocking, a more upright trunk at ball release, and less shoulder and elbow compressive forces during deceleration (7). Flat ground work requires a reduction in distance to 60 feet and intensity is established at 50%, with a progressive increase based on SAID principles.

Phase III: Progressive Mound Work

To initiate mound work, the athlete must successfully complete the long toss program and continue to demonstrate a negative clinical examination and maintain full ROM, strength, and flexibility. There are six levels within the mound work phase (Table 8-4). Intensity is gradually increased.

Postsurgical Mound Work

Pitchers are given instruction to begin throwing at 50% intensity. What constitutes 50%, 75%, and 100% is vague. Fleisig and colleagues conducted a kinematic and kinetic comparison of full effort and partial effort baseball pitching. At 75% effort, pitchers produced approximately 90% of the velocity and 85% of the force and torque as produced during full effort. At 50% effort, pitchers produced approximately 85% velocity and 75% force and torque. Reduced effort pitching also corresponded with reduced arm rotation during cocking, increased horizontal adduction, and a more upright trunk (less knee flexion and less trunk lean) at ball release.

There is a gradual increase in intensity and duration in each subsequent throwing session (Table 8-4). Sessions are conducted two to three times per week (Fig. 8-4). Frequency is individualized and based upon subjective reports of recovery and tolerance to the previous throwing session. There is a normal warm-up and a 10-minute progressive toss session, increasing to 120 feet before beginning mound work. The athlete's mound work is conducted before a traditional long toss throwing session of 12 to 15 minutes. Continuing to advance arm strength with the long toss program is essential during the mound work phase.

to 12-minute throwing session consisting of 50 to 60 throws, gradually backing up to 150 to 180 feet. The athlete throws 6 to 10 repetitions at the maximum distance. Level 6 is also conducted on an every other day basis. At this junction in the ITP, flat ground mound work is incorporated to assist in the transition to normal pitching mechanics (Fig. 8-3). One to three sets of 15 throws from the wind-up position at 60 feet with the catcher down is added to the end of the long toss session. Typically the postsurgical athlete needs 4 to 6 weeks in the long toss program before initiating mound work. Positional and outfield players need the same duration in the long toss program before beginning positional throws.

Nonsurgical Long Toss

The nonsurgical long toss program consists of the same six levels as the postsurgical program; the difference lies in the speed of progression and adjustments of the training variables. Once an athlete is cleared to begin throwing, he starts at a level 1 or level 2. Based on tolerance during that first session (30 to 60 feet), he quickly advances to level three (90 feet) at the next session as long as he or she remains symptom free. Subsequent progressions are based on symptoms. Nonsurgical throwing sessions may be conducted on successive days, 5 to 6 days per week. Typically a rest day is needed every two to three sessions. Once the athlete has established that he can throw with good strength, endurance, and location for three sets of 25 throws at 120 feet, he is advanced to level 6. Two to three sessions at level 6 are needed before initiating mound work. Typically, it

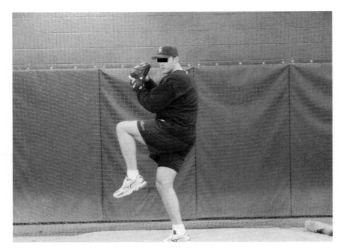

FIGURE 8-4. Progressive mound work.

Example of the ITP for a week is as follows:

Monday: Level (1 to 6) mound work
Tuesday: 12- to 15-minute long toss
Wednesday: Light recovery day, 10 minutes at 60 feet
Thursday: Level (1 to 6) mound work
Friday: 12- to 15-minute long toss
Saturday: Light recovery, 10 minutes at 60 feet
Sunday: Off

Once the throwing athlete has established good arm strength and control with fast balls, he can begin working on breaking balls. The athlete can begin more traditional side sessions, throwing 15% to 25% breaking balls. Following completion of levels 1 to 6 mound work and three to four unrestricted side sessions without symptoms, the athlete is ready to begin simulated game activity. Typically it takes 4 to 6 weeks of progressive mound work to begin simulated game activity.

Nonsurgical Mound Work

The nonsurgical pitcher advances through the identical postsurgical mound work phase, but progression is much more rapid. The athlete is allowed to throw to tolerance at each level, and advancement is based on symptom reproduction. The athlete is allowed to initiate breaking balls as soon as strength and endurance with the fastball pitch is established. Two to three side sessions are needed before facing live batting with simulated game activity. Rest intervals between mound sessions differ from those of the postsurgical program. Side sessions may be conducted every other day, with long toss or recovery throwing between sessions based on the athlete's fatigue. Consideration of the pitcher's role as a starter or reliever plays a factor in the amount of

rest as well as the total number of pitches within a side session. Close monitoring by the pitching coach is essential during this phase of throwing.

Postsurgical and Nonsurgical Positional Throws

Positional players continue with the same long toss program as pitchers. However, instead of initiating mound work, they begin a functional throwing program based on position. Infielders gradually work up to 30 to 50 throws in a session, and outfielders increase to 15 to 20 long throws from their respective position, in addition to long toss sessions.

Phase IV: Simulated Game Activity

Following successful completion of the mound work phase, the pitcher is ready to face live batting. The pitcher increases intensity—thus placing increased physiologic stress on the recovering area. Whereas reviewing videotapes on a player's previous throwing mechanics or tabulating isokinetic evaluation scores may provide objective information, these do not functionally relate to the athlete's sport-specific strength and endurance. An objectively formulated simulated game satisfies the requirements of a functional evaluation procedure (4). The simulated game requires a specific number of innings, a specific number of pitches per inning, a pitch selection ratio, and a rest interval between innings (4). The strength and power component is evaluated in the fastball velocity after injury versus before injury. Endurance is reflected in the miles-per-hour change from first to last innings pitched, and accuracy is determined by fastballs-to-strikes ratio. Coordination with the coaching staff during this phase and continual evaluation of the pitching mechanics is essential. The pitcher performs three to six simulated innings (15 throws each inning) with 8 to 10 minutes of rest between each inning (4). Starting pitchers throw four to six innings initially, whereas middle or late relief pitchers throw three to four innings. For nonsurgical athletes, one to three simulated games are needed before advancing to game participation with limited pitch count. PS athletes may need 3 to 10 simulated games (1 to 4 weeks) before beginning game participation.

Phase V: Game Progression

Upon successful completion of simulated game activity, the throwing athlete begins full restricted game participation. For starting players, pitch count is limited to 30 to 50 throws, advancing as tolerated. Relievers begin with a 15- to 20-pitch count, again advancing as tolerated. Advancement to full unrestricted game participation is gradual and is based on symptoms.

Phase VI: Maintenance with Return to Play

The ITP is designed to bridge the gap between core rehabilitation and return to unrestricted athletic participation. It is important for the athlete not to abandon the fundamental ROM, flexibility, strength, and endurance training that established the framework for return. The athlete does not maintain the same volume of rotator cuff and scapular strengthening exercises with return to full participation. However, the athlete must maintain adequate strength and flexibility to avoid reinjury.

CONCLUSION

This chapter is intended to provide a general systematic outline of a typical throwing progression. ITPs are individualized for each athlete based on symptoms, physiologic healing, recovery, and tolerance to new physiologic loads.

Implementing this treatment tool combined with astute practical application assists the clinician in returning the throwing athlete to an optimal outcome.

REFERENCES

1. Dillman CJ, Glenn FS, Andrews JR. Biomechanics of pitching with emphasis upon shoulder kinematics. *J Orthop Sports Phys Ther* 1993;18:402–408.
2. Pappas AM, Zawacki RM, Sullivan TJ. Biomechanics of baseball pitching. *Am J Sports Med* 1985;13:216–222.
3. Pappas AR, Zawacki RM, McCarthy CF. Rehabilitation of the pitching shoulder. *Am J Sports Med* 1985;13:223–235.
4. Coleman E, Axe MJ, Andrews JR. Performance profile-directed simulated game: an objective functional evaluation for baseball pitchers. *J Orthop Sports Phys Ther* 1987;9:101–104.
5. Axe MJ, Snyder-Mackler L, Konin JG, et al. Development of a distance-based interval throwing program for little league-aged athletes. *Am J Sports Med* 1996;24:594–602.
6. Wilk KE, Arrigo CA. Interval sports programs for the shoulder. In: Andrews JR, Wilk KE, eds. *The athlete's shoulder*. New York: Churchill Livingstone, 1994;669–671.
7. Fleisig GS, Zheng N, Barrentine SW, et al. Kinematic and kinetic comparison of full-effort and partial-effort baseball pitching. Presented to the American Society of Biomechanics Oct. 17–19, 1996.

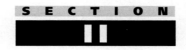

LESIONS OF THE
OVERHEAD SHOULDER

9

INTERNAL IMPINGEMENT

JAMES R. ANDREWS
PATRICK J. CASEY

INTRODUCTION

Overhead athletes subject the shoulder to tremendous forces and stresses during competition. Extreme external rotation with the arm abducted 90 degrees is required to generate the appropriate force to pitch a 90-mph fastball, serve in tennis, or hit a winner in volleyball. In particular, during the late cocking phase of throwing, the arm can require 170 to 180 degrees of external rotation to generate the torque required (1,2) (Fig. 9-1). Moreover, the shoulder is one of the least constrained joints in the human body

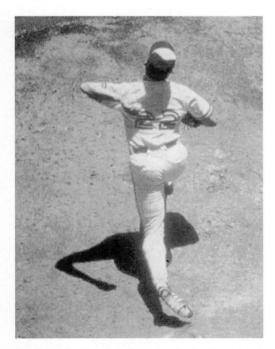

FIGURE 9-1. Professional pitchers routinely place the shoulder in 170 degrees of external rotation during the late cocking phase of throwing. (From Andrews JR, Dugas J. Diagnosis and treatment of shoulder injuries in the throwing athlete: the role of thermal-assisted capsular shrinkage. *AAOS Instruct Course Lect* 2001;50:17–21, with permission.)

with the glenoid and labrum combined surface area totaling only 28% of the humeral articular surface area (3).

During the acceleration phase of pitching, the shoulder joint is exposed to some of the highest forces seen in the body. A throwing athlete often generates 7,000 degrees of angular velocity per second repetitively throughout a performance (1,4). Not only does the shoulder have to generate this angular velocity, it also must dissipate this energy in the deceleration phase of throwing. The arm position and force required to create such acceleration can lead to pathology in the shoulder over the course of a season or career.

Internal impingement is a process by which there is repeated contact between the undersurface of the rotator cuff tendon and the posterosuperior glenoid that leads to injury and dysfunction. Internal impingement pathology is essentially an overuse injury associated with overhead athletics. With rare exception, it is not usually seen in patients unless they are high caliber athletes who perform repetitive abduction and external rotation of the glenohumeral joint. Typically, these patients have symptoms only while playing and are free of symptoms during activities of daily living. Internal impingement has only recently been recognized as a cause of pain and dysfunction in the shoulder (5). Modern understanding of this disease process and its treatment is still in infancy, even though it represents about 80% of the problems seen in the throwing and overhead shoulder in our experience.

HISTORY

Internal impingement has been well recognized as a clinical entity for more than a decade. The major tool that led to its discovery was the arthroscope. Routine arthroscopy has led to improved visualization and understanding of the glenohumeral anatomy, yielding a high amount of information with minimal invasiveness. Visualization of the posterior labrum, posterior glenoid, and undersurface tear of the rotator cuff became much improved with arthroscopy compared with the traditional open procedures.

One of the earliest descriptions of internal impingement was by Barnes and Tullos in 1978 (6). Examining 56 baseball players with shoulder pain, they described the typical symptoms of internal impingement in 24 of them. However, the authors attributed their symptoms to Bennett's lesions (thrower's exostoses) despite normal x-ray studies. Although they may not have appreciated the exact mechanism of injury, this was an important description of posterior shoulder pain in the overhead athlete. During the same time period, Jackson described 10 young pitchers with shoulder pain and the inability to pitch (7). He believed these players were having primary external impingement and performed subacromial decompressions on these patients. His results were fair, with just more than half returning to competition. In retrospect, he too was probably describing internal impingement in these throwing athletes.

Several years later, Andrews and colleagues published his arthroscopic findings of shoulder pathology in the throwing athlete (8,9). In the 35 pitchers who underwent shoulder arthroscopy, they found 73% had partial undersurface tears of the rotator cuff muscles (9). Andrews found this unusual considering these patients were young, healthy athletes with no history of acute traumatic episodes to the shoulder. He hypothesized that repetitive tensile forces, not contact between the posterosuperior glenoid and the rotator cuff muscles, caused these injuries.

Walch was the first clinician to correctly describe the pathogenesis of internal impingement (5). Looking at 17 throwing athletes, he found that 16 had contact between the posterior glenoid and undersurface of the infraspinatus in the abducted and externally rotated position during arthroscopy. All of these patients were young (average age 25 years) and were not thought to be at risk of tearing the rotator cuff tendons. His finding of labral wear and undersurface tearing was the first descriptions that these processes were caused by an impingement within the glenohumeral joint itself. During this same time period, Jobe did cadaveric and clinical studies demonstrating that repetitive contact between the undersurface of the rotator cuff and the posterosuperior glenoid in throwing athletes led to shoulder injury and pathology (3,10).

ETIOLOGY

The shoulder is a complex joint with multiple articulations, ligaments, and tendons involved in its kinematics. These structures generally work in concert with one another; however, if there is dysfunction in one, it may affect other structures of the glenohumeral joint. Internal impingement has an insidious onset that slowly becomes more debilitating with time as more components of the shoulder become involved. In other words, injury begets injury.

Internal impingement is caused by the repetitive contact and microtrauma that occurs to the posterior labrum and the undersurface of the rotator cuff musculature during the throwing motion (Fig. 9-2). Contact between the posterosuperior glenoid and the cuff also occurs in asymptomatic people (11). Therefore, some contact between these structures may be physiologic, but repetitive contact with altered shoulder mechanics is pathologic.

The overhead athlete who develops internal impingement tends to have repeated stress placed on the glenohumeral joint over the course of many years. These stresses often lead to adaptive changes to the surrounding tissue and altered shoulder mechanics. The structures that are most commonly involved in internal impingement include the humeral head, the anterior capsule, the inferior glenohumeral ligament, the posterior capsule, and the rotator cuff muscles.

The humeral head develops, on average, 17 degrees more retroversion in a throwing arm than the nondominant side (12). This is likely secondary to the repetitive torsional stresses seen to the physis during juvenile development. Increased retroversion provides greater external rotation in the abducted position and may be a protective mechanism against internal impingement (13). Increased retroversion does not lead to a greater total arc of motion than on the contralateral side, but it does lead to an "overrotation" of motion, which is more external and less internal rotation in the 90-degree abducted position. Patients with diminished

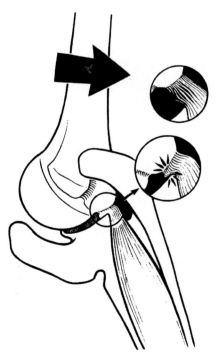

FIGURE 9-2. Diagram showing the contact between the rotator cuff muscles and the posterosuperior glenoid in the throwing position. (From Riand N, Levigne C, Renaud E, et al. Results of derotational humeral osteotomy in posterosuperior glenoid impingement. *Am J Sports Med* 1998;26[3]:453–459, with permission.)

retroversion are more likely to impinge the cuff between the posterosuperior glenoid and the greater tuberosity in the late cocking position (14). The overrotation that develops in a throwing arm allows more external rotation in the abducted position before anterior ligamentous restraint is reached. Baseball players who become pitchers after full skeletal maturity has been reached may be more at risk for development of internal impingement secondary to less retroversion of the humeral head.

The inferior glenohumeral ligament and anterior capsule are static restraints to forward translation of the humeral head in the throwing position. The subscapularis muscle is a dynamic restraint. With repetitive overhead motion, the subscapularis can fatigue and provide less dynamic restraint. The anteroinferior glenohumeral ligament may then be subjected to more force, which over time can lead to plastic deformation and rotational instability. That is, the repetitive throwing or overhead motion stresses the anterior capsule and causes increased laxity (15–21). Laxity of the anterior capsule can lead to both increased translation and external rotation (22). Increased anterior movement of the humeral head may exacerbate the contact between the posterosuperior glenoid and the rotator cuff (23). Normally, in external rotation, there is obligate posterior translation of the humerus that allows for more motion and less contact between the greater tuberosity and posterosuperior glenoid (24). Posterior translation prevents a mechanical block between greater tuberosity and glenoid. With laxity in the anterior capsule and subsequent loss of posterior translation, there is increased contact leading to injury.

Posterior tightness may also develop in throwers (13,25,26). Some authors believe that this posterior tightness originates from a capsule contracture and may lead to a decrease in the needed posterior translation of the humerus during abduction external rotation to avoid cuff impingement (24,27). Both posterior capsule tightness and anterior laxity have an additive effect on diminished humeral posterior translation. Again, this loss of posterior translation of the humeral head exacerbates contact between the undersurface of the infraspinatus and the posterosuperior glenoid, worsening the internal impingement. In our experience, we believe the posterior tightness may also be related to an infraspinatus or teres minor contracture isolated or in combination with the capsule itself. In some recent data from our institution (Wilk KE. *Personal communication,* 2000.), we have found in elite throwing athletes there can be lack of internal rotation in the 90-degree abduction position and concomitant posterior laxity. Whether the posterior tightness is due to capsule contracture, or cuff contracture, or both, the clinical manifestation is the same with diminished posterior translation and resultant posterior superior translation of the humeral head, worsening the internal impingement.

Burkhart and Morgan have suggested that internal impingement is related to repetitive posterosuperior sub-luxation of the humeral head in the throwing position (28,29). When in the abducted and externally rotated position, there is a torsional stress on the biceps anchor, referred to as the peel-back mechanism. Repetitive torsional stresses can lead to the posterosuperior labrum lifting off the glenoid. The end result is pathologic posterosuperior motion of the humeral head. This motion, along with the torsional stresses on the rotator cuff, leads to fatigue and failure. A recent biomechanical model (Tibone JE, MD. *Personal communication.*) has shown that, if a posteroinferior capsule contracture is present, the humeral head demonstrates a resultant posterosuperior subluxation, leading to internal impingement and rotator cuff failure.

The cuff muscles, which function as dynamic stabilizers of the glenohumeral joint, compensate for the changes in static restraint in internal impingement. However, while the rotator cuff tendons perform more work, they are subject to repeated articular-sided injury from internal impingement. This can lead to partial tears, tendonitis, and weakness within the cuff musculature. A cycle develops in which the rotator cuff muscles compensate for capsular changes, but in a fatigued, weakened, or injured state. The result is the injured rotator cuff muscles cannot function maximally and becomes dysfunctional as a dynamic stabilizer.

Other pathology in the shoulder may worsen or contribute to internal impingement. For example, overhead athletes are also at risk for SLAP (superior labrum anterior-to-posterior) lesions. SLAP lesions are not caused by internal impingement, but rather are the result of excess stress and contact on the biceps anchor. SLAP lesions have been found to increase anterior translation of the humeral head up to 6 mm (30). That is, SLAP lesions lead to further loss of static restraint. In one biomechanical study, loss of the biceps anchor resulted in an increase in 100% strain on the inferior glenohumeral ligament (1). This increase in anterior translation may worsen the contact and stresses seen on the posterior labrum and undersurface of the rotator cuff musculature (31).

Internal impingement is related to a number of structures in the shoulder. In essence, repetitive stress leads to secondary changes in the static stabilizers, which leads to pathologic movement and dysfunction of rotator cuff muscles. A cycle develops in which a series of abnormalities reinforce each other and lead to altered mechanics of the shoulder.

DIFFERENTIAL DIAGNOSIS

Shoulder pain in the overhead athlete is a common manifestation. Most overhead and throwing athletes develop some pain at some point during the season. Differentiating between routine soreness and pathologic pain in overhead shoulder pain can be a difficult, but important task. There are a number of diagnoses that must be considered in the overhead athlete. It is critical that an accurate diagnosis be established because treatment protocols differ significantly.

Rotator cuff tendonitis or bursitis is the most common problem seen in the throwing and overhead athlete. This pain is usually worse the day after activity than during the actual event. It is typically described as a deep soreness. Any movement or position of the arm can exacerbate pain. Unlike internal impingement, this pain is more diffuse and not localized to the posterior aspect of the shoulder. Patients complain of having difficulty lifting the arm and localize pain to the greater tuberosity of the shoulder. This pain typically improves with rest and antiinflammatories after a short period of time.

Throwers' exostosis, commonly known as a Bennett's lesion, can mimic internal impingement. Pain is often found in the posterior part of the shoulder and is worse during late cocking. Patients often describe a pinching sensation during throwing. Pain typically ceases with rest. A Bennett's lesion may localize posterior pain more toward the inferior aspect of the glenohumeral joint than the superior aspect. Radiographs differentiate a Bennett's lesion from internal impingement. The Stryker notch view typically shows a calcification at the posteroinferior glenoid rim consistent with an exostosis.

SLAP lesions are another common injury seen in throwing and overhead athletes. Like internal impingement, these patients often have pain during late cocking and early acceleration. Although SLAP lesions can produce pain in a number of locations about the shoulder, there is usually a strong anterior component to it. This is usually different from internal impingement in which the pain is predominantly posterior. Physical examination is the cornerstone to differentiating SLAP injuries from internal impingement. In our experience, O'Brien's test and the "clunk" test usually have a positive response in SLAP tears and are negative for internal impingement. The internal impingement test is usually negative in SLAP lesions and positive in internal impingement. Coronal oblique magnetic resonance (MR) images of the shoulder are another helpful tool in differentiating the two lesions. SLAP tears usually demonstrate contrast tracking under the biceps anchor, whereas internal impingement generally shows an intact labrum.

Isolated posterior labrum tears are the most difficult to differentiate from internal impingement. Both present with posterior shoulder pain, and with pain in the abducted and externally rotated position, and they develop insidiously over time. In our experience, posterior labral tears on imaging studies can be hard to discern. Often times, arthroscopy is necessary to delineate these two lesions.

It is not uncommon for internal impingement to occur concomitantly with other pathology. An astute clinician should always consider the possibility that more than one process is occurring in the injured shoulder, especially in an overhead athlete. All shoulder pathologies need to be addressed to have a successful result and a return to competitive play.

HISTORY AND PHYSICAL EXAMINATION

The history is the first and the most important information obtained from the patient. The history should reveal the chronicity of the injury, the location of the pain, the position that aggravates the pain, and the treatments that have occurred. Typical questions that we ask are as follows:

- Did the pain developed slowly over time or acutely after a certain pitch or motion?
- Is this the first episode of pain in your career or is the pain something you have struggled with over many seasons?
- Have you been "shut down?" If so, for how long?
- Have you had any treatment modalities such as rehabilitation, physical therapy, ultrasound, or cortisone shots and have any been effective?
- During what phase of throwing or overhead motion do you have discomfort?
- Is the intensity of the pain worse during throwing and overhead activity or afterward?
- Are the number of games or innings pitched more than in previous seasons?
- Have you lost control or velocity?

Patients with internal impingement usually describe an insidious onset of pain in the shoulder. Pain tends to increase as the season progresses. Symptoms may have been present over the past couple of seasons, worsening in intensity with each successive year. Originally, rest and physical therapy helped, but became less effective over time. Pain is usually described as dull and aching, and is located in the posterior aspect of the shoulder. The late cocking phase seems to be the most painful, whereas ball release and follow-through are often not troublesome. The patient rarely can remember any traumatic episode that occurred. There is typically an increase in the number of innings or game participation during the season. Loss of control and velocity are often present, secondary to the inability to fully externally rotate the arm without pain. There is often a complaint of diminished stamina.

Examination should always be done in males with their shirt removed. Females should ideally be examined in a sports bra, but if that is not possible, a gown should be used to cover the chest, allowing full view of the shoulder. Inspection is always done first. Starting posteriorly, we look for rotator cuff muscle wasting or atrophy across the scapula. Any asymmetry is noted. Any suggestion of a traumatic injury, such as an area of ecchymosis or swelling is recorded. The shoulder musculature should appear symmetric or with slight increase in size in the dominant extremity. In internal impingement, there is often no abnormality seen during inspection.

Next, we palpate the shoulder. Pain can be elicited over the infraspinatus muscle and tendon. The pain is generally worse posteriorly over the glenohumeral joint than over the greater tuberosity. This is different from rotator cuff tendonitis, where the pain tends to be worse over the greater tuberosity. The anterior part of the shoulder is not painful. The bicipital groove and tendon are palpated and are usually asymptomatic. The acromioclavicular joint is almost always asymptomatic. No bony abnormalities are usually present.

Third, we examine range of motion and stability. Active forward flexion, passive forward flexion, and abduction are noted. Both internal and external rotation with the arm abducted 0 degrees and 90 degrees is recorded. Testing for anterior and posterior stability is done with the patient lying supine and the arm abducted approximately 150 degrees. With the arm in the plane of the scapula, firm pressure is applied to the back and front of the humerus. The amount of translation and firmness of the endpoint is recorded. Inferior laxity is tested with the patient sitting upright and downward traction applied to the elbow.

In internal impingement, patients usually have full range of motion. The dominant arm tends to have 10 to 15 more degrees of external rotation and 10 to 15 degrees less of internal rotation with the arm abducted to 90 degrees compared with the nondominant arm (12). The most common presentation is for the overhead athlete to have 2+ anterior laxity and trace to 1+ posterior laxity.

Inferior laxity is often present (15). The throwing or overhead athlete tends to have a firm endpoint to stability testing.

Provocative tests are performed to elicit pain. The impingement or Neer's test is usually negative, as is the Hawkins test and the cross-arm adduction test. O'Brien's test, unless there is a concurrent SLAP tear, is generally negative. The internal impingement test is usually positive. To perform this test, the patient is placed in the supine position with the involved arm abducted 90 degrees and maximally externally rotated. When pain is experienced in the posterior aspect of the glenohumeral joint by the patient, it is considered a positive test. It has recently been reported to have a 90% sensitivity (25). This test recreates the position of the arm in late cocking when there is contact between the undersurface of the rotator cuff muscle and the posterosuperior glenoid.

The relocation test has been advocated by Jobe as a tool to establish the diagnosis of internal impingement (32). With the patient lying supine or prone, the arm is placed in 90 degrees of abduction and maximal external rotation to mimic the throwing or overhead position. In this position, there is often pain in the posterior aspect of the shoulder secondary to anterior translation of the humeral head and a resultant contact between the rotator cuff muscles and the greater tuberosity. A posteriorly directed force that relieves discomfort is considered a positive test. This is because the posterior force relieves the contact by preventing the infolding of tissue between the cuff and labrum (10,33). This is different from the classic apprehension and relocation tests

for diagnosing anterior instability. The pain and apprehension seen with those tests are located in the anterior, not the posterior, aspect of the shoulder.

Strength of the rotator cuff muscles is tested last. The supraspinatus, infraspinatus, and subscapularis typically have normal strength, symmetrical to the contralateral side. There is generally no pain with strength testing.

INITIAL AND CONSERVATIVE TREATMENT

There are two fundamental requirements to having a healthy throwing or overhead shoulder: (a) a large arc of motion to generate force and (2) adequate stability to withstand the created force. To achieve extremes of external rotation with the arm abducted 90 degrees necessitates some degree of laxity to the static restraints of the shoulder (15,34). The rotator cuff muscles attempt to compensate for this laxity by forming a dynamic restraint to humeral head translation. However, the inherent capsular laxity that develops leads to some degree of instability in the shoulder and potentially dysfunction. These competing qualities have been referred to as the *thrower's paradox* (34,35). Therefore, a fine balance needs to be achieved in the throwing or overhead shoulder between obtaining enough motion and enough stability to function effectively.

When internal impingement presents in an overhead athlete, the initial treatment should *always* consist of rest and rehabilitation. Complete cessation from throwing or overhead motion is the critical first step in our treatment protocol. Light throwing or bullpen tossing or quarter-speed tennis serving invariably leads to aggravation and persistence of symptoms. Continued repetitive contact between the rotator cuff tendons and the posterior superior glenoid rim sustains the inflammation and injury. Most athletes do not understand the importance of total shutdown and continue to throw or continue their overhead motion in some fashion unless specifically instructed otherwise.

Physical therapy is initiated as soon as possible. Once the shoulder has quieted down, the focus should be on restoration of dynamic stability and strength in the rotator cuff musculature. By improving dynamic stability, better glenohumeral joint compressive forces are reestablished and anterior translation of the humeral head is decreased. Stretching is done of the infraspinatus and teres minor muscles to improve flexibility. It is done with stabilization of the scapula and pulling the arm across the body with slight internal rotation. Proprioceptive neuromuscular facilitation (PNF) patterns are gradually implemented. This technique requires the athlete to move the arm through a throwing or overhead arc with constant manual resistance, interrupted with abrupt antagonist forces against which parascapular and rotator cuff muscles must stabilize. Along with PNF, rhythmic stabilization is done with alternating isometric contractions of the shoulder musculature to increase co-

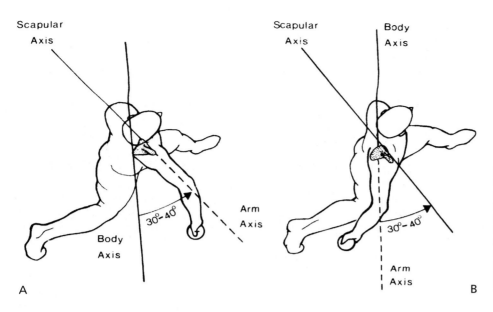

FIGURE 9-3. Example of a pitcher throwing properly with the humerus in the plane of the scapula **(A)** and one throwing with hyperangulation **(B)**. (From Davidson PA, Elattrache NS, Jobe CM, et al. Rotator cuff and posterior-superior glenoid labrum injury associated with increase glenohumeral motion: a new site of impingement. *J Shoulder Elbow Surgery* 1995;4[5]: 384–390, with permission.)

contraction of the cuff. PNF and rhythmic stabilization are done at first with the arm in at the side, gradually moved to 90-90 position, and finally with the arm in endpoint external rotation with the arm abducted 90 degrees (35). The endpoint of physical therapy is to improve dynamic stabilization of the glenohumeral joint, improve posterior flexibility, and increase the strength of the rotator cuff tendons. When this has occurred, the patient's symptoms usually improve. Once these goals have been met, an interval throwing program or similar sport-specific overhead program is started. It is important to study overhead mechanics once throwing, serving, striking, or other motion commences, and athletes should be encouraged or taught to keep the arm in the plane of the scapula and to avoid hyperangulation. Hyperangulation occurs during the late cocking phase when the humerus excessively abducts horizontally leading to internal impingement (36) (Fig. 9-3).

We usually prescribe an antiinflammatory medicine for patients with internal impingement. We have found no study to suggest that corticosteroids have any role in the treatment of internal impingement. In our review of the literature, there is no specific study that addresses how successful rest and rehabilitation are in the treatment of internal impingement. In our clinical experience, we have found that this simple conservative therapy tends to relieve the majority of symptoms and allows for appropriate return to sport.

SURGICAL TREATMENT

When conservative measures do fail and athletes are unable to return to their overhead activities, surgical intervention should be considered. Surgery begins with diagnostic arthroscopy. Using standard posterior and anterior portals,

a systematic examination of the shoulder is performed. The glenoid and humeral articular surfaces are inspected for chondral lesions. The biceps tendon is viewed and its anchor probed to rule out SLAP tears. The labrum is explored with great care taken to rule out a peel-back lesion posteriorly. The capsular volume is assessed by visualization and translational movement of the humeral head. If there is anterior laxity, the humeral head tends to sit on the edge of the anterior glenoid and a drive-through sign is often present. The rotator cuff is visualized along its entire insertion. Partial tearing is usually located on the articular surface and involves the posterior supraspinatus or the infraspinatus (Fig. 9-4). If there is not a complete tear of the rotator cuff, we do not visualize the subacromial space.

Arthroscopic Debridement

Simple arthroscopic debridement of rotator cuff tears and labral fraying was originally described to treat internal impingement (Fig. 9-4). Andrews initially reported on 36 athletes, average age 22 years, who had articular sided partial rotator cuff tears secondary to internal impingement (8). The early results were encouraging: 76% had excellent results, 9% had good results, and 15% had poor results. Eighty-five percent of patients were able to return to their preoperative athletic activity. However, follow-up was only 13 months.

Payne and Altchek looked at a similar group of patients who had internal impingement treated by simple debridement and followed up their cases for an average of 48 months (19). There were only 38% excellent and 28% good results with only 45% returning to preinjury sports activity. The worst group was the overhead athlete who had just debridement in the face of significant anterior laxity, with just 25% having satisfactory results and return to athletics.

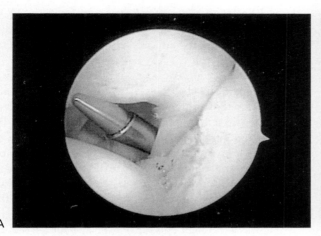 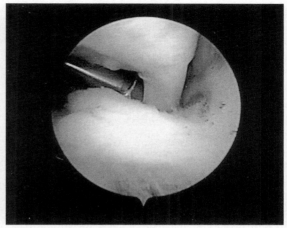

FIGURE 9-4. A,B: Picture of a partial undersurface tear seen in a professional baseball pitcher during arthroscopy.

Altchek also followed up a group of 40 athletes, average age 25 years, who had internal impingement treated with simple labral debridement (37). Even though 72% had relief of symptoms 1 year after surgery, the results deteriorated to only 7% with relief of symptoms at 43 months. Altchek concluded that arthroscopic labral debridement was not an effective long-term solution for internal impingement.

Most recently, Sonnery-Cottet and colleagues published a study with more encouraging results (38). They performed arthroscopic debridement on 28 tennis players with internal impingement and found that, at 4-year follow-up, 50% had returned to preinjury playing level or higher and that 81% were satisfied with the surgery.

Capsulolabral Reconstruction

Another option for treatment of internal impingement is the modified anterior capsulolabral reconstruction. The purpose of this treatment is to address the anterior capsule laxity through imbrication, which, in turn, diminishes the contact between the rotator cuff and the posterosuperior labrum (16,17,32,39,40). The surgery involves the standard deltopectoral approach with transverse splitting of the subscapularis. Without detaching the subscapularis from its insertion, the capsule is visualized and "T'ed" over the anterior glenoid. A superior and inferior flap are created and advanced over one another to decrease the redundant anterior capsule (Fig. 9-5). The results of anterior capsulolabral reconstruction are more encouraging than simple debridement alone.

Jobe was the original surgeon to advocate this procedure (16,17,32,39,40). He operated on 25 overhead athletes with internal impingement and found a 68% excellent and 24% good results after 39 months of follow-up (16). Seventy-two percent of the patients were able to return to their previous level of competition and play for at least one complete season. However, of the pitchers in the study, only

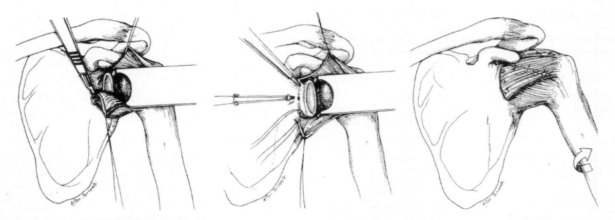

FIGURE 9-5. Anterior capsulolabral reconstruction for internal impingement. (From Meister K. Injuries to the shoulder in the throwing athlete. Part II. *Am J Sports Med* 2000;28[4]:587–601, with permission.)

50% returned to the their previous level, and results were worse for professional pitchers, with only 38% returning.

Several years later, Rubenstein and colleagues reported on a larger cohort of patients with internal impingement that underwent open anterior capsulolabral reconstruction (40). Of the 22 pitchers in the group, 95% had good to excellent results. Seventy-five percent of professional athletes and 100% of the college athletes returned to their previous level of competition.

Finally, Montgomery and Jobe reported on a third group of overhead athletes with internal impingement treated in a similar manner (39). In these 32 patients, there was a 97% good to excellent result with 81% returning to their previous level of competition. Of the professional baseball pitchers, 86% returned to their previous level of competition. These studies have demonstrated that open capsulolabral reconstruction is an effective treatment option in the high demand overhead athlete.

Thermal Capsulorraphy

Another method to reduce the anterior capsular laxity has been the use of thermal energy. Thermal capsulorraphy causes an alteration in the collagen fibrils by promoting increases in cross linkage. The end result is a decrease in col-

lagen length and hence in anterior capsular laxity. Thermal capsulorraphy is usually done in conjunction with debridement of rotator cuff tears and arthroscopic fixation of labral tears.

A recent retrospective study at our institution compared two groups of baseball players who had internal impingement. All had debridement of partial rotator cuff tears and labral or SLAP injuries repaired with suture anchors. However, one group had thermal capsulorraphy to address anterior capsule laxity and another group did not. At 30 months of follow-up, the group with thermal capsulorraphy had an 86% return to the same or higher level of competition, whereas the other group had only a 61% return (20,41). Only one complication occurred in the thermal group, which was a transient episode of axillary neuritis. Similar to the open anterior labral capsulorraphy, thermal capsulorraphy has been shown to be an effective method of reducing anterior capsular laxity and treating internal impingement.

Rotational Osteotomy

While the treatment options mentioned so far have all focused on soft tissue procedures, there has been a recent report involving derotation osteotomy of the humerus. Derotation osteotomy of the humerus addresses the lack of

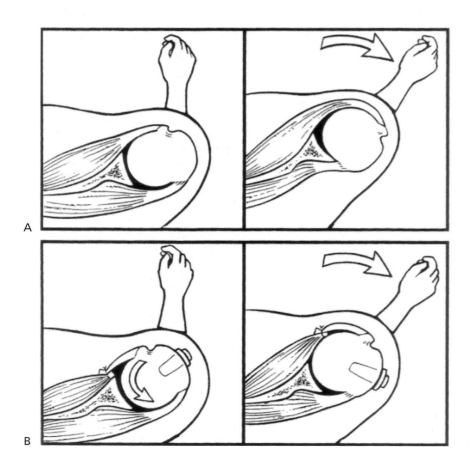

FIGURE 9-6. A: Example of a patient with decreased humeral retroversion that has internal impingement. **B:** Example of how a derotational osteotomy leads to less impingement. (From Riand N, Levigne C, Renaud E, et al. Results of derotational humeral osteotomy in posterosuperior glenoid impingement. *Am J Sports Med* 1998;26[3]:453–459, with permission.)

retroversion in some overhead athletes. By increasing retroversion and shortening the subscapularis muscle, less impingement occurs between the rotator cuff tendon and the posterosuperior glenoid in extremes of external rotation (Fig. 9-6).

A recent study by Riand and colleagues included 20 throwing athletes with internal impingement who were treated with derotation osteotomy and followed up for an average of 46 months (14). Eighty percent had complete resolution of their symptoms and 55% were able to return to the same level of competition. There was one pseudarthrosis, one adhesive capsulitis, and 80% required hardware removal. Although this novel approach has had some limited success, the results have not yet matched the soft tissue procedures for internal impingement and these authors have abandoned the use of the osteotomy procedure.

Subacromial Decompression.

The role of subacromial decompression in overhead athletes with internal impingement remains controversial. Subacromial decompression does not relieve or address the contact between the rotator cuff and the posterior glenoid. Moreover, in our experience, it is unusual for a young athlete to have any hook to the acromion (type II or III) that causes external or outlet impingement.

One study reported that only 22% of throwing athletes with internal impingement returned to the same level of competition after subacromial decompression (42). The authors concluded that "This operation is safe for pain relief, but does not allow an athlete to return to his former competitive status."

The only time that we perform subacromial decompressions in the overhead athlete is when previous arthroscopic surgery (i.e., labral repairs, thermal capsulorraphy with rotator cuff debridement) has not relieved the patient's symptoms and repeat glenohumeral arthroscopy shows no obvious recurrent pathology. In these cases, we do a bursectomy and conservative subacromial decompression as a "last resort" measure.

For a complete description of the senior author's preferred surgical techniques, please refer to Chapter 21.

SUMMARY

Internal impingement is a relatively common problem in the overhead athlete, although a difficult one to treat. Internal impingement is caused by repetitive contact between the undersurface of the rotator cuff and the posterosuperior glenoid. Increased anterior capsular laxity, attenuation of the inferior glenohumeral ligament, diminished retroversion of the humerus, posterior tightness, and dysfunction of the rotator cuff musculature may all play a role in the development of this disease. Rest and physical therapy are the cornerstones of initial treatment. Conservative treatment and rotator cuff strengthening can lead to a resolution of symptoms. If symptoms persist, there are multiple surgical techniques that can be used to treat the condition. The ultimate goal is to obtain a balance between adequate motion and stability of the shoulder joint to allow for the generation and dissipation of the tremendous forces necessary in the overhead athlete.

REFERENCES

1. Fleisig GS, Barrentine SW, Escamilla FR, et al. Biomechanics of overhand throwing with implications for injuries. *Sports Med* 1996;21(6):421–437.
2. Meister K. Injuries to the shoulder in the throwing athlete. Part 1. *Am J Sports Med* 2000;28(2):265–275.
3. Jobe CM, Iannotti JP. Limits imposed on glenohumeral motion by joint geometry. *J Shoulder Elbow* 1995;4(4):281–285.
4. Dillman CJ, Fleisig GS, Andrews JR. Biomechanics of pitching with emphasis upon shoulder kinematics. *JOSPT* 1993;18(2):402–408.
5. Walch G, Boileau P, Noel E, et al. Impingement of the deep surface of the supraspinatus tendon on the posterosuperior glenoid rim: an arthroscopic study. *J Shoulder Elbow Surg* 1992;1:238–245.
6. Barnes DA, Tullos HS. An analysis of 100 symptomatic baseball players. *Am J Sports Med* 1978;6(2):62–67.
7. Jackson DW. Chronic rotator cuff impingement in the throwing athlete. *Am J Sports Med* 1976;4(6):231–240.
8. Andrews JR, Broussard TS, Carson WG. Arthroscopy of the shoulder in the management of partial tears of the rotator cuff: a preliminary report. *Arthroscopy* 1985;1(2):117–122.
9. Andrews JR, Carson WG, McLeod WD. Glenoid labrum tears related to the long head of the biceps. *Am J Sports Med* 1985;13(5):337–341.
10. Jobe CM. Posterior superior glenoid impingement: expanded spectrum. *Arthroscopy* 1995;11(5):530–536.
11. McFarland EG, Hsu CY, Neira C, et al. Internal impingement of the shoulder: a clinical and arthroscopic analysis. *J Shoulder Elbow Surg* 1999;8:458–460.
12. Crockett HC, Gross LB, Wilk KE, et al. Osseous adaptation and range of motion at the glenohumeral joint in professional baseball pitchers. *Am J Sports Med* 2002;30(1):20–26.
13. Tyler TF, Nicholas SJ, Roy T, et al. Quantification of posterior capsule tightness and motion loss in patients with shoulder impingement. *Am J Sports Med* 2000;28(5):668–673.
14. Riand N, Levigne C, Renaud E, et al. Results of derotational humeral osteotomy in posterosuperior glenoid impingement. *Am J Sports Med* 1998;26(3):453–459.
15. Bigliani LU, Codd TP, Connor PM, et al. Shoulder motion and laxity in the professional baseball player. *Am J Sports Med* 1997;25:609–613.
16. Jobe FW, Giangarra CE, Kvitne RS, et al. Anterior capsulolabral reconstruction of the shoulder in athletes in overhand sports. *Am J Sports Med* 1991;19(5):428–434.
17. Jobe FW, Kvitne RS. Shoulder pain in the overhand or throwing athlete. *Orthop Rev* 1989;18(9):963–975.
18. Altchek DW, Dines DM. Shoulder injuries in the throwing athlete. *J Am Acad Orthop Surg* 1995;3(3):159–165.
19. Payne LZ, Altchek DW, Craig EV, et al. Arthroscopic treatment of partial rotator cuff tears in young athletes. *Am J Sports Med* 1997;25(3):299–305.

20. Andrews JR, Dugas J. Diagnosis and treatment of shoulder injuries in the throwing athlete: the role of thermal-assisted capsular shrinkage. *AAOS Instruct Course Lect* 2001;50:17–21.

21. Ellenbecker TS, Mattalino AJ, Elam E, et al. Quantification of anterior translation of the humeral head in the throwing shoulder. *Am J Sports Med* 2000;28(2):161–167.

22. Kuhn JE, Bey MJ, Huston LJ, et al. Ligamentous restraints to external rotation of the humerus in the late-cocking phase of throwing. *Am J Sports Med* 2000;28(2):200–205.

23. Paley KJ, Jobe FW, Pink MM, et al. Arthroscopic findings in the overhand throwing athlete: evidence for posterior internal impingement of the rotator cuff. *Arthroscopy* 2000;16(1):35–40.

24. Harryman DT, Sidles JA, Clark JM, et al. Translation of the humeral head on the glenoid with passive glenohumeral motion. *J Bone Joint Surg (Am)* 1990;72(9):1334–1343.

25. Meister K. Injuries to the shoulder in the throwing athlete. Part II. *Am J Sports Med* 2000;28(4):587–601.

26. Tyler TF, Roy T, Nicholas SJ, et al. Reliability and validity of a new method of measuring posterior shoulder tightness. *J Orthop Sports Phys Ther* 1999;29(5):262–274.

27. Ticker JB, Beim GM, Warner JP. Recognition and treatment of refractory posterior capsular contracture of the shoulder. *Arthroscopy* 2000;16(1):27–34.

28. Burkhart SS, Morgan C. SLAP lesions in the overhead athlete. *Orthop Clin North Am* 2001;32(5):431–441.

29. Burkhart SS, Morgan CD. The peel-back mechanism: its role in producing and extending posterior type II SLAP lesions and its effect on SLAP repair rehabilitation. *Arthroscopy* 1998;14(6):637–640.

30. Pagnani MJ, Deng ZH, Warren RF, et al. Effect of lesions of the superior portion of the glenoid labrum on glenohumeral translation. *J Bone Joint Surg (Am)* 1995;77(7):1003–1010.

31. Morgan CD, Burkhart SS, Palmeri M, et al. Type II SLAP lesions: three subtypes and their relationships to superior instability and rotator cuff tears. *Arthroscopy* 1998;14(6):553–565.

32. Jobe F, Kvitne R, Giangarra C. Shoulder pain in the overhand or throwing athlete. The relationship of anterior instability and rotator cuff impingement. *Orthop Rev* 1989;18:963–975.

33. Tomlinson RJ, Glousman RE. Arthroscopic debridement of glenoid labral tears in athletes. *Arthroscopy* 1995;11(1):42–51.

34. Wilk KE, Arrigo C. Current concepts in the rehabilitation of the athletic shoulder. *J Orthop Sports Phys Ther* 1993;18:365–378.

35. Wilk KE, Meister K, Andrews JR. Current concepts in the rehabilitation of the overhead throwing athlete. *Am J Sports Med* 2002;30(1):136–151.

36. Davidson PA, Elattrache NS, Jobe CM, et al. Rotator cuff and posterior-superior glenoid labrum injury associated with increase glenohumeral motion: a new site of impingement. *J Shoulder Elbow Surg* 1995;4(5):384–390.

37. Altchek DW, Warren RF, Wickiewicz TL, et al. Arthroscopic labral debridement. *Am J Sports Med* 1992;20(6):702–706.

38. Sonnery-Cottet B, Edwards TB, Noel E, et al. Results of arthroscopic treatment of posterosuperior glenoid impingement in tennis players. *Am J Sports Med* 2002;30(2):227–232.

39. Montgomery WH, Jobe FW. Functional outcomes in athletes after modified anterior capsulolabral reconstruction. *Am J Sports Med* 1994;22(3):352–358.

40. Rubenstein DL, Jobe FW, Glousman RE, et al. Anterior capsulolabral reconstruction of the shoulder in athletes. *J Shoulder Elbow Surg* 1992;1(5):229–237.

41. Levitz CL, Dugas J, Andrews JR. The use of arthroscopic thermal capsulorrhaphy to treat internal impingement in baseball players. *Arthroscopy* 2001;17(6):573–577.

42. Tibone JE, Jobe FW, Kerlan RK, et al. Shoulder impingement syndrome in athletes treated by an anterior acromioplasty. *CORR* 1985;198:134–140.

SURGICAL TREATMENT OF PARTIAL THICKNESS ROTATOR CUFF TEARS

JOHN E. CONWAY
STEVEN B. SINGLETON

INTRODUCTION

The most common clinical and surgical findings in the injured shoulder of the overhead athlete include posterior partial thickness articular surface rotator cuff tears, type 2 anterior-to-posterior superior labrum avulsions (SLAP lesions), posterosuperior labrum tears, posteroinferior labrum tears or avulsions, anteroinferior glenohumeral laxity, hypertrophic subacromial bursa, excessive glenohumeral external rotation, deficient glenohumeral internal rotation, and scapular muscle dysfunction (1–3). Although our recognition and understanding of some of the conditions that are responsible for these findings have increased, there is still much about the throwing and overhead shoulder that remains unknown.

Recently, a higher level of awareness, combined with improvements in magnetic resonance imaging (MRI) techniques, has made it possible to document extensive intratendinous delamination of the superior segment of the infraspinatus tendon (4–6). The most appropriate method to surgically manage these *posterior*, *articular* surface, *intra*tendinous rotator cuff tears (PAINT lesions) found in throwing and other overhead athletes is uncertain. It is therefore a challenge for the treating surgeon to maintain reasonable expectations with regard to both the need to restore rotator cuff function and the potential to regain rotator cuff integrity.

PATHOMECHANICS

In 1985, Andrews and colleagues (7) described partial thickness, articular surface rotator cuff tears in a large group of overhead athletes. The occurrence and location of these tears were initially explained by the presence of excessive eccentric forces acting on the articular surface of the posterior rotator cuff during the deceleration segment of the throwing motion (7–9). It is commonly thought that other physiologic and biomechanical processes are also involved.

In the fully cocked overhead throwing position, the humerus is abducted 60 to 70 degrees on the glenoid and is in maximal external rotation. Scapular elevation produces the remainder of arm abduction and glenohumeral extension in the horizontal plane occurs in varying degrees. Arthroscopic, MRI, and cadaver research data have shown that when the shoulder is in this position, the greater tuberosity, the articular surface of the posterior supraspinatus tendon, and the articular surface of the superior infraspinatus tendon are compressed against the posterosuperior edge of the glenoid rim and labrum (4,10–20). This contact between intraarticular bone and soft tissue structures is described by the term *internal impingement* (10–18). Walch (11), Jobe (17), and McFarland (15) have shown that this contact may often be physiologic and occur in the absence of glenohumeral instability. However, excessive anterior glenohumeral laxity, glenohumeral external rotation, and glenohumeral horizontal extension probably increase the internal contact forces when the shoulder is in the late cocking and acceleration segments of the throwing motion (10,17,18,21). A detailed discussion of this condition is contained in Chapter 9.

Whereas internal impingement contact almost certainly contributes to the creation of posterior, articular-surface rotator cuff tears, this contact alone does not completely explain the presence of the rotator cuff tear or the constellation of additional findings in the injured overhead athlete's shoulder. Other factors probably include intrinsic tendon degeneration, local tissue hypovascularity (22), anteroinferior glenohumeral instability (10,23), rotator interval and coracohumeral ligament laxity (21), subacromial outlet impingement (24,25), superior labrum-biceps tendon complex injuries (3,26–29), posterior capsule contracture and internal rotation deficit (14,26,27), humeral retroversion (30), trunk, scapula and shoulder muscle dysfunction (31), excessive eccentric forces (7,8), neurologic conditions, improper mechanics, and far too much throwing or other repetitive overhead activity.

PAINT LESIONS

Over the last decade, the unique partial articular rotator cuff tear pattern recognized in throwers and other overhead athletes has been better defined (1,4,5,10–13,20,32). In our opinion, this is best described as an L-shaped, partial thickness, articular surface tear occurring at the junction of the posterior supraspinatus tendon and the superior infraspinatus tendon (Fig. 10-1). The posterior edge of the tear is typically mobile and often appears as a flap of tendon extending into the joint. The tendon-from-bone segment of the tear is greatest in depth within the posterior supraspinatus tendon; and from this defect, the tear frequently extends well medial into the middle layers of the infraspinatus tendon (Fig. 10-2). This tear pattern differs from partial thickness, articular surface tears associated with primary outlet impingement principally in location. Even though the term *PASTA* (partial articular side tendon avulsion) lesion (33) has been used to describe articular surface tears in an older age patient population, we prefer the term *PAINT lesion* for throwers and other overhead athletes to emphasize the more posterior location and intratendinous involvement of these tears.

Many factors contribute to the articular surface location of these tears. The articular surface of the rotator cuff has fewer arterioles and overall less vascularity than the bursal surface. The articular surface has a higher modulus of elasticity and therefore greater stiffness than the bursal surface. Eccentric forces tend to be concentrated more in the articular surface. Finally, the articular surface has a less favorable stress-strain curve than the bursal sur-

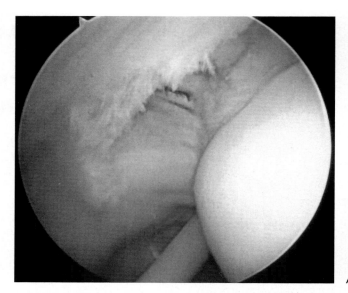

A

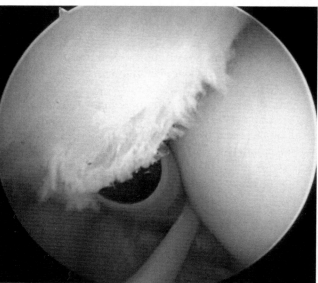

B

FIGURE 10-2. A: Arthroscopic photograph of the typical appearance of a deep articular-surface rotator cuff tear in a thrower. **B:** The intratendinous tear becomes apparent only after placement of an arthroscopic probe into the defect. (Modified from Conway JE. The management of partial thickness rotator cuff tears in throwers. *Oper Tech Sports Med* 2002;10[2]:75–85, with permission.)

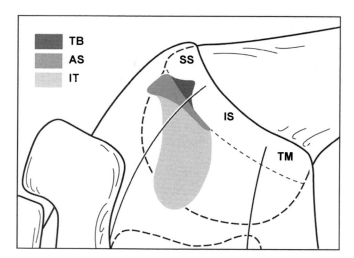

FIGURE 10-1. Diagram demonstrating the unique rotator cuff tear pattern of PAINT lesions seen in overhead athletes. The location of the articular surface tear is posterior, occurring at the junction of the supraspinatus (SS) and infraspinatus (IS) tendons and may extend into the middle layers of the infraspinatus tendon. *TB* defines the area where the tendon is torn from bone; *AS* defines the most common area of the articular surface tear; *IT* defines the possible extent of the intratendinous tear. (From Conway JE. The management of partial thickness rotator cuff tears in throwers. *Oper Tech Sports Med* 2002;10[2]:75–85, with permission.)

face. When combined with the rotator cuff and glenoid contact forces produced by internal impingement, these factors probably explain the occurrence, the location, and the predominance of articular surface rotator cuff tears in overhead athletes (8,10–12,18,20,30,32,34–38). The cause of the intratendinous delamination in these athletes is less clear.

In 1992, Walch and colleagues (13) reported eight rotator cuff tears in 14 throwers and noted that "some tears extend into the depth of the tendon, dissecting into two layers." With improved MR imaging methods, extension of the articular surface tears into the middle layers of the infraspinatus tendon is increasingly recognized in these athletes diagnosed with internal impingement (4–6,35,39). It is likely that the tangentially and perpendicularly opposed vector forces acting on the five-layered architecture of the rotator cuff tendon generate shear stress within the middle layers and thereby create the intratendinous tears (34–36,40). Additionally, the coracohumeral ligament has been shown to blend with the articular surface of the anterior supraspinatus tendon (21). Acting as a primary restraint to external rotation in the late cocking segment of the throwing motion, this ligament probably further increases the shear forces in the middle layers of the posterosuperior rotator cuff tendons.

TREATMENT CONSIDERATIONS

The traditional surgical treatments of the painful overhead athlete's shoulder by arthroscopic rotator cuff and labrum debridement without rotator cuff repair, SLAP repair, or capsular tightening produced fair to good results (7,41–44) that deteriorated with time (2,11,42). Clinically apparent and occult glenohumeral instability may have contributed to the diminished outcomes seen on long-term follow-up. Levitz and colleagues (2) have reported better long-term outcomes in throwers with rotator cuff tears treated additionally with thermal capsulorrhaphy than in similarly injured throwers treated without thermal capsulorrhaphy. However, published and unpublished case reports of capsular ligament insufficiency and transient postoperative axillary nerve injury following thermal capsulorrhaphy have made surgeons appropriately cautious regarding the extent and method of thermal treatment (45–50). Arthroscopic anterior capsule suture plication and rotator interval closure may be other reasonable alternatives for the treatment of concomitant excessive anterior glenohumeral laxity and humeral external rotation.

Craig (51) and Horng-Chaung and colleagues (52) have reported that an insufficient rotator cuff may contribute to increased glenohumeral laxity, and others have demonstrated a glenohumeral stabilizing role for the superior glenoid labrum–biceps tendon complex (3,53,54). In some individuals, repair of the rotator cuff tendons and the superior labrum may be adequate to resolve subtle glenohumeral instability (3). Therefore, the extent of the thermal or suture capsulorrhaphy required, if any, depends on the degree of relative and absolute laxity noted on examination under anesthesia and on the improvement in stability following labrum and rotator cuff repair.

Andrews and colleagues (7) recommended debridement of the torn rotator cuff tendon seen in throwers in order to stimulate a healing response. However, Weber (32) reported that, on second-look, arthroscopy following arthroscopic rotator cuff tear debridement, "healing...was never observed." It is probable that the continued separation of the torn tendon edges, the poor vascularity of the involved tissues (39,55), the formation of a synovial covering within the intratendinous segment of the tear (40,55,56), and the continued contact between the rotator cuff and the glenoid rim during throwing or other overhead motion precludes any potential for spontaneous healing or healing following simple arthroscopic debridement (32,40).

Furthermore, progression of both the depth of the articular surface tear and extent of the intratendinous tear is of considerable concern in the face of continued overhand shoulder motions. Thus, rotator cuff repair may be advisable for the long-term function of the shoulder in some patients (32,37,56–58). However, the percentage depth of the tear that calls for repair, using either open or arthroscopic methods, is controversial. Some authors have suggested that partial rotator cuff tears greater than 50% of the thickness of the tendon should be repaired (37,39,59,60). Others have argued that, in throwers and other overhead athletes, repair potentially increases the morbidity of the procedure and that 75% was a more reasonable depth mitigating for repair (9).

It is also theoretically possible that, in some athletes, the articular surface tear occurs as an adaptation to the imposed demand, allowing greater horizontal extension of the humerus on the glenoid. Repair is therefore susceptible to failure as the athlete returns to maximal effort throwing, serving, and striking. Thus, it may be that those deep tears that are repaired should only be repaired back to a depth of 25% to 40%. The quality of tissue for repair also varies from athlete to athlete. In some athletes, the articular surface segment of the intratendinous tear is so thin that repair seems unreasonable. Debridement alone, even in the presence of deep intratendinous extension, may sometimes be more appropriate. Finally, arthroscopic methods do not allow for closure of intratendinous tears that extend more than 2 cm from the greater tuberosity. For these athletes, debridement or miniopen repair may be a more reliable option.

To address these uncertainties, we are currently following an algorithm for surgical treatment that considers tear depth, pattern, and location as well as tissue quality and athlete's age (Figs. 10-3 and 10-4). We have also proposed an extent of tear score (DWD score) that is based on the depth and width of the articular surface tear and on the extent of the delamination within the tendon (Table 10-1). Measurement for all three elements of the score are taken from preoperative contrast abduction and external rotation (ABER) MRI studies and confirmed at arthroscopy.

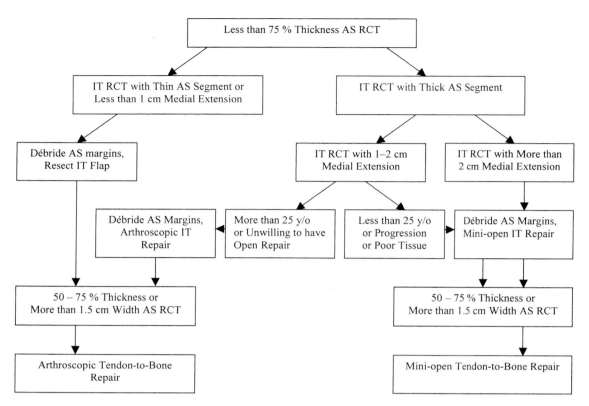

FIGURE 10-3. Treatment algorithm for articular-surface rotator cuff tears less than 75% depth. AS, articular-surface; IT, intratendinous; RCT, rotator cuff tear.

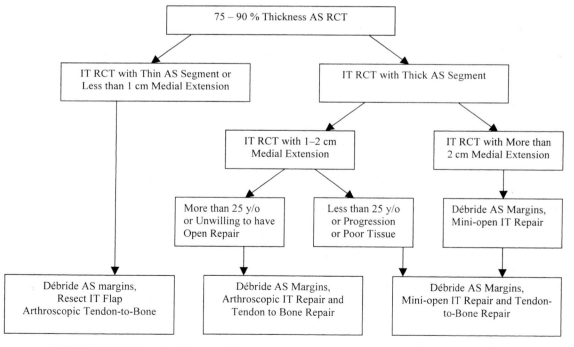

FIGURE 10-4. Treatment algorithm for articular-surface rotator cuff tears more than 75% depth. AS, articular-surface; IT, intratendinous; RCT, rotator cuff tear.

TABLE 10–1. DWD[a] (DEPTH, WIDTH, AND DELAMINATION) GRADING SCALE USED FOR OUTCOME ANALYSIS FOLLOWING SURGERY FOR INTERNAL IMPINGEMENT IN OVERHAND ATHLETES

		Score
Depth	1%–25%	1
	26%–50%	2
	51%–75%	3
	76%–99%	4
Width	>0.0–1.0 cm	1
	>1.0–2.0 cm	2
	>2.0 cm	3
Delamination	>0.0–0.5 cm	1
	>0.5–1.0 cm	2
	>1.0–2.0 cm	4
	>2.0–3.0 cm	6
	>3.0 cm	8
Total possible score		15
Grade	Minimal tear	1–2
	Mild tear	3–6
	Moderate tear	7–11
	Severe tear	12–15

[a]DWD score for PAINT lesions.

MAGNETIC RESONANCE IMAGING

Tirman and colleagues (6) and others (61–63) have advocated the use of MR arthrography performed with the shoulder in both adduction (ADD) and abduction external rotation (ABER) positions and have shown this method to provide clear visualization of the articular surface of the rotator cuff, the superior glenoid labrum, and the anterior inferior capsule labrum complex. Jaovishidha and colleagues (64) demonstrated that exercise before a repeat noncontrast MRI study changed the diagnosis in 23% of patients with the initial MR diagnosis of partial thickness rotator cuff tear. Gadolinium contrast ABER MRI (6,64) combines the advantages of a postexercise arthrogram with MRI and, in our ongoing study, appears to be more sensitive for intratendinous delamination than either contrast MR without ABER images or noncontrast MRI (Fig. 10-5).

AUTHORS' PREFERRED SURGICAL TECHNIQUE (5)

A careful examination of both shoulders under general anesthesia should be repeated until the degree of absolute and relative glenohumeral laxity is clear. The patient is positioned in the 30-degree posterolateral decubitus position with 20 degrees of Fowler's tilt and the arm suspended through a shoulder traction device. During creation of the posterior portal, take care to penetrate the posterior capsule parallel to the glenoid and along the middle of the glenoid rim. A superior or medial portal position limits visualization during rotator cuff repair.

On arthroscopic examination of the glenohumeral joint, observe any apparent "draping" of the articular surface of the infraspinatus tendon because this may represent occult intratendinous delamination. A probe may be used to define the extent of the intratendinous tear (Fig. 10-2B). Assess the mobility of the posterior margin of the articular surface tear with a soft tissue grasping instrument and estimate the relative thickness of the articular segment of the intratendinous tear with a probe. Remove the arm from traction and position the shoulder in abduction and external rotation to determine the extent of posterior superior glenoid contact.

An ordered approach to the debridement and repair process is mandated by the potential to treat multiple injured structures, and we proceed in the manner listed in Table 10-2. Although all of the listed steps are rarely required in a single patient, following this order of treatment restores the anatomy in a sequential manner without compromising any previous or subsequent repair steps.

Where appropriate, limit the extent of tendon debridement to preserve tissue for repair. Glenohumeral abduction separates the torn edge of the rotator cuff tendon away from the humerus and provides better visualization of the tendon insertion site on the greater tuberosity. Because visualization is limited, the debridement of the intratendinous rotator cuff tear is accomplished with caution, but be aware that insufficient debridement of the intratendinous surfaces probably compromise the potential for tendon healing.

Following the PAINT algorithm (Figs. 10-3 and 10-4), there may be three separate segments of the rotator cuff

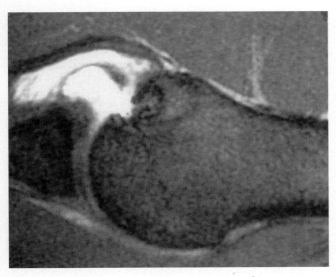

FIGURE 10-5. Abduction, external rotation (ABER) magnetic resonance arthrography documenting an articular surface rotator cuff tear with deep extension into the middle layers of the infraspinatus tendon. (Modified from Conway JE. The management of partial thickness rotator cuff tears in throwers. *Oper Tech Sports Med* 2002;10[2]:75–85, with permission.)

TABLE 10–2. OUTLINE OF AN ORDERED APPROACH[A] TO THE TREATMENT OF MULTIPLY INJURED STRUCTURES IN THE THROWER'S SHOULDER

1. Debride the labrum and glenoid rim.
2. Debride the rotator cuff margins and or resect the articular segment flap.
3. Abrade the greater tuberosity.
4. Repair the posterior and superior labrum.
5. Repair the anterior-inferior labrum.
6. Perform the thermal capsulorrhaphy (rarely) or place anterior capsulorrhaphy sutures.
7. Place the articular-surface rotator cuff tendon-to-tendon sutures.
8. Debride the subacromial space.
9. Place the rotator cuff tendon-to-bone suture anchors and sutures.
10. Tie the articular-surface sutures within the glenohumeral joint.
11. Tie the tendon-to-bone rotator cuff sutures within the subacromial space.
12. Place the intratendinous repair mattress sutures.
13. Tie the intratendinous repair sutures within the subacromial space.
14. Perform the CA ligamentoplasty or limited acromioplasty.

[a]Order of treatment for surgical repair of PAINT lesions.
CA, coracoacromial.

repair: articular surface repair, tendon-to-bone repair, and intra-tendinous repair. The placement of articular surface sutures, when necessary, is performed first. Excessive loss of tissue, either by wear or debridement argues against articular surface closure. The posterior margin of the tear must be thick, mobile, and easily reduced to the anterior margin without creating apparent deformity in the contour of the tendon.

Using a SutureLasso (Arthrex, Inc., Naples, Florida) or similar suture passing instrument, place a no. 2 nonabsorbable suture in the posterior segment of the articular surface flap in such a location as to recreate the angle of the L, in the L-shaped tear, on tendon closure. Pass the free anterior suture limb through the anterior segment of the tear close to the articular margin (Fig. 10-6). When tendon-to-bone repair is required, the suture anchors and tendon-to-bone sutures must be placed before tying the articular surface sutures in order to maintain visualization of the tuberosity and cuff tear margin. The arthroscope is then placed in the subacromial space and debridement of the subacromial space is performed before suture anchor and transcutaneous tendon-to-bone suture placement.

While sustaining arm traction, 30 to 40 degrees of glenohumeral abduction facilitates visualization of, and access to, the supraspinatus insertion site onto the greater tuberosity (Fig. 10-7). This position is useful during both abrasion of the tuberosity and capture of the tendon-to-bone sutures. However, because of the angle to the humeral head, insertion of the suture anchors should be done with

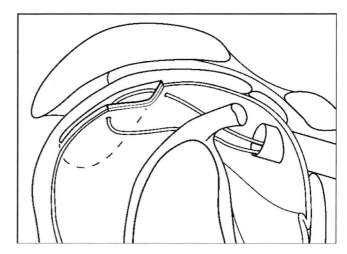

FIGURE 10-6. Diagram of a suture passed through both margins of the articular-surface tear. (From Conway JE. The management of partial thickness rotator cuff tears in throwers. *Oper Tech Sports Med* 2002;10[2]:75–85, with permission.)

minimal glenohumeral abduction. An 18-gauge spinal needle is used to determine the appropriate position for a lateral acromial portal. Incise the skin and then use a no. 11 blade on a no. 7 handle to create a portal through the deltoid and rotator cuff, dividing the tendon in line with its fibers. This step appears to minimize the trauma to the remaining intact fibers of the cuff tendon and a cannula is rarely necessary. Further debridement of the tuberosity with a small curette may be performed through this portal.

One or two suture anchors with a total of two to four sutures may be required for tendon-to-bone cuff repair, and

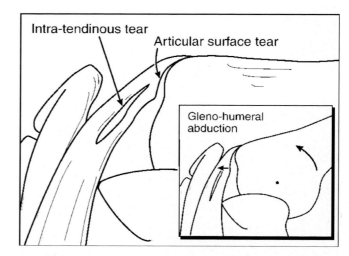

FIGURE 10-7. Diagram of a coronal view of a PAINT lesion with the glenohumeral joint in adduction and abduction demonstrating the improved visualization of the rotator cuff tendon and the greater tuberosity with abduction. (Modified from Conway JE. The management of partial thickness rotator cuff tears in throwers. *Oper Tech Sports Med* 2002;10[2]:75–85, with permission.)

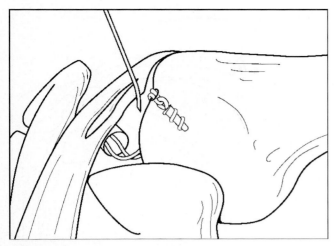

FIGURE 10-8. Diagram showing a suture anchor inserted using a transtendinous method as described in the text. With the tear margin reduced, hollow straight and curved 18-gauge needles are used to retrieve the sutures through the tendon. (From Conway JE. The management of partial thickness rotator cuff tears in throwers. *Oper Tech Sports Med* 2002;10[2]:75-85, with permission.)

we prefer the use of bioabsorbable anchors because they allow better follow-up MRI. Insert the anchors into the cuff footprint, but be aware of the angle of anchor insertion and observe the humeral head for evidence of subchondral penetration.

After anchor placement, abduct the humerus and pull the tendon-to-bone repair sutures out through the anterior portal. Traction on the articular surface repair sutures closes the rotator cuff defect and allows identification of the appropriate location for the tendon-to-bone sutures. In a transcutaneous manner, straight and curved Meniscal Mender II (Instrument Makar, Inc., Okemos, Michigan) needles and a Shuttle Relay (Linvatec, Inc. Largo, Florida) are used to pull the anchor sutures through the cuff tendon in a mattress fashion (Fig. 10-8). The articular surface sutures are tied. Because approximating the edges of the articular surface segment of the tear creates tension on the repair, a sliding knot that locks or clinches the post limb is essential for tight suture loops (Figs. 10-9).

After closure of the articular-surface defect, return the arthroscope again to the subacromial space. Identify, separate, and tie the tendon-to-bone sutures. Return the arthroscope to the glenohumeral joint, inspect the tendon-to-bone repair, and complete the procedure with repair of the intratendinous segment.

The transcutaneous outside-to-inside method for intratendinous tendon repair using straight and curved needles is similar to a method previously described by Snyder (58) for the repair of Snyder classification type A4 anterior articular-surface flap tears (Fig. 10-10). Reinforcing sutures across the articular surface are placed first and the repair process then proceeds into the more posterior and medial segments of the tear. The arthroscope is returned to the subacromial space and all sutures are retrieved and tied through the lateral portal (Fig. 10-11).

In athletes with intratendinous tears that extend medially greater than 2 cm, arthroscopic repair may not be

A
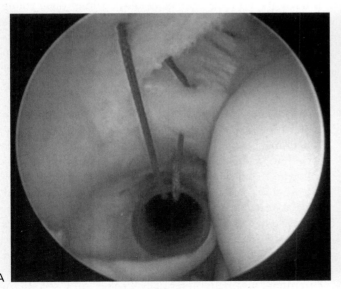

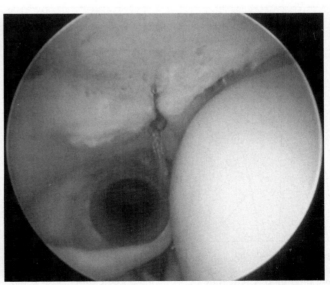
B

FIGURE 10-9. Arthroscopic photographs showing an articular surface rotator cuff tear before **(A)** and after **(B)** closure by tying a tendon-to-tendon loop of suture. (From Conway JE. The management of partial thickness rotator cuff tears in throwers. *Oper Tech Sports Med* 2002;10[2]:75–85, with permission.)

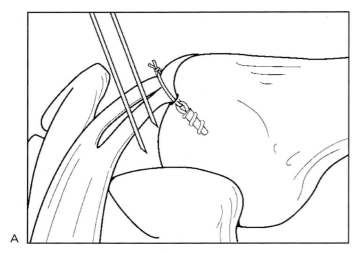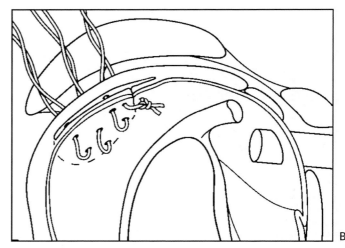

A   B

FIGURE 10-10. Diagram showing a coronal view of the intra-tendinous repair. **A:** Following articular-surface and or and tendon-to-bone repair, hollow 18-gauge needles are used in a tran-scutaneous method to place mattress sutures for intratendinous repair. **B:** The suture placement steps are repeated until enough sutures are placed to close the entire intratendinous defect. (From Conway JE. The management of partial thickness rotator cuff tears in throwers. *Oper Tech Sports Med* 2002;10[2]:75-85, with permission.)

advised and a posterolateral based miniopen approach is preferred. A transcutaneous suture placed through the central region of the tear marks the skin for placement of an incision and a deltoid splitting approach without deltoid origin detachment provides adequate exposure for suture placement. The transcutaneous suture also identifies the point for division of the tendon, in line with its fibers, extending from the tendon insertion to the medial extent of

FIGURE 10-11. Diagram showing a coronal view of a completed rotator cuff tendon repair. The most medial segment of the intra-tendinous tear may be difficult to completely close using this method. (From Conway JE. The management of partial thickness rotator cuff tears in throwers. *Oper Tech Sports Med* 2002;10[2]:75-85, with permission.)

the tear. The surfaces of the intratendinous tear should be abraded with a curette or rasp to remove any synovial lining from the tissue. Tendon-to-bone and intratendinous repair may be accomplished using routine open methods. Because of the relatively poor vascularity of the articular segment of the intratendinous tear, incorporation of a fibrin clot may be a reasonable option (65) (Fig. 10-12).

Supraspinatus outlet impingement symptoms are common in overhead athletes and subacromial decompression should be considered in selected cases. Outlet impingement is rarely the primary cause of shoulder pain in these young overhead athletes (2), and published treatment methods that included acromioplasty failed to yield good results (66–69). Although, subacromial bursectomy is often required, release of the coracoacromial ligament and or acromioplasty in a young thrower or overhead athlete is rarely necessary (70) .

Subacromial decompression may be accomplished in some athletes by simply thinning a hypertrophic coracoacromial ligament with a thermal ablator. However, relative indications for a limited acromioplasty include the following: coracoacromial ligament abrasion, bursal-surface rotator cuff tear, anterior location of the articular surface tear, near full thickness articular surface tear, extensive intratendinous tear, sagittal-oblique MR images demonstrating a prominent anterior edge of the acromion, positive subacromial impingement signs, and age older than 30 years. Because division of the coracoacromial ligament potentially creates of a secondary plane of instability (70–72), the ligament should be preserved when possible.

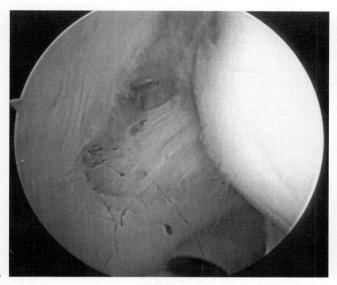
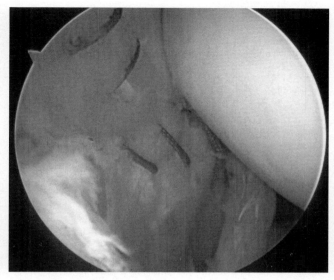

A   B

FIGURE 10-12. Arthroscopic photographs of a rotator cuff tear in a thrower before **(A)** and after **(B)** repair. (From Conway JE. The management of partial thickness rotator cuff tears in throwers. *Oper Tech Sports Med* 2002;10[2]:75–85, with permission.)

Postoperative Protocol

An Ultrasling shoulder immobilizer (DonJoy Orthopedics, LLC, Vista, California) is applied in the operating room and worn for 3 weeks. The immobilizer is removed several times a day for gentle passive motion exercises avoiding horizontal extension and external rotation while the shoulder is abducted. Range of motion is evaluated frequently in the office during the first 2 weeks. Early joint stiffness and motion loss are treated by a physical therapist with gentle stretching exercises. No shoulder rotation above 60 degrees of glenohumeral abduction is allowed until 3 weeks following surgery.

Lower extremity, trunk and scapula exercises are begun immediately. At 3 weeks, passive motion is recovered and a supervised active and strengthening program for the shoulder begins and continues under the direction of a physical therapist or athletic trainer experienced in the care of throwing and overhead athletes. Progress is made toward recovering internal and external rotation strength with the glenohumeral joint adducted before active abduction exercises begin. Following SLAP repair, biceps muscle strengthening is not allowed until 4 weeks after surgery. A throwing program or program specific to the overhead athlete's sport may begin after 3 to 4 months if the following criteria have been met: (a) shoulder motion has been recovered; (b) trunk, scapula, and rotator cuff muscle endurance, balance, and strength have been restored; and (c) there is no pain with activity or during examination.

CONCLUSION

Partial thickness articular surface rotator cuff tears have been recognized in overhead athletes for many years, but the pattern and extent of these tears have only recently become better understood. The reported outcomes following the surgical debridement of this injury have varied. Because the potential for spontaneous healing or healing following simple arthroscopic debridement is limited, repair of the more extensive tears should be considered.

REFERENCES

1. Paley KJ, Jobe FW, Pink, MM, et al. Arthroscopic findings in the overhand throwing athlete: evidence for posterior internal impingement of the rotator cuff. *Arthroscopy* 2000;16:35–40.
2. Levitz CL, Dugas J, Andrews JR. The use of arthroscopic thermal capsulorrhaphy to treat internal impingement in baseball players. *Arthroscopy* 2001;15(6):537–577.
3. Burkhart SS, Parten PM. Dead arm syndrome: torsional SLAP lesions versus internal impingement. *Tech Shoulder Elbow Surg* 2001;2(21):47–84.
4. Conway JE. Arthroscopic repair of partial-thickness rotator cuff tears and SLAP lesions in professional baseball players. *Op Tech Sport Med* 2000;8:281–292.
5. Conway JE. The management of partial thickness rotator cuff tears in throwers. *Oper Tech Sports Med* 2002;10(2):75–85.
6. Tirman PFJ, Bost FW, Garvin GJ, et al. Posterosuperior glenoid impingement of the shoulder: findings at MR imaging and MR arthrography with arthroscopic correlation. *Radiology* 1994;193: 431–436.
7. Andrews JR, Broussard TS, Carson WG. Arthroscopy of the shoulder in the management of partial tears of the rotator cuff: A preliminary report. *Arthroscopy* 1985;1:117–122.
8. Fleisig GS, Andrews JR, et al. Kinetics of baseball pitching with implications about injury mechanisms. *Am J Sports Med* 1995; 23:233–239.
9. Andrews JR. The throwing arm. Kennedy Lectureship. Presented at the 67th AAOS Meeting, Orlando, Florida, February, 2000.
10. Davidson PA, ElAttrache NS, Jobe CM, et al. Rotator cuff and

posterior-superior glenoid labrum injury associated with increased glenohumeral motion: a new site of impingement. *J Shoulder Elbow Surg* 1995;4:384–390.

11. Walch G. Posterosuperior glenoid impingement. In: *Rotator cuff disorders*. 1996;14:193–198.

12. Jobe CM. Current concepts: superior glenoid impingement. *Clin Orthop* 1996;330:98–107.

13. Walch G, Boileau P, Noel E, et al. Impingement of the deep surface of the supraspinatus tendon on the posterosuperior glenoid rim: an arthroscopic study. *J Shoulder Elbow Surg* 1992;1:238–245.

14. Barber FA, Morgan CD, Burkhart SS, et al. Labrum/biceps/cuff dysfunction in the throwing athlete. *Arthroscopy* 1999;15:852–857.

15. McFarland EG, Hsu C-Y, Neira C, et al. Internal impingement of the shoulder: a clinical and arthroscopic analysis. *J Shoulder Elbow Surg* 1999;8:458–460.

16. Edelson G, Teitz C. Internal impingement in the shoulder. *J Shoulder Elbow Surg* 2000;9:308–315.

17. Jobe CM, Sidles M. Evidence for a superior glenoid impingement upon the rotator cuff. *J Shoulder Elbow Surg* 1993;2[Suppl 19](abst).

18. Jobe CM. Posterior superior glenoid impingement. *J Shoulder Elbow Surg* 1995;11:530–536.

19. Edelson G, Teitz C. Internal impingement in the shoulder. *J Shoulder Elbow Surg* 2000;9:308–315.

20. Nakagawa S, Yoneda M, et al. Greater tuberosity notch: an important indicator of articular-side partial rotator cuff tears in the shoulders of throwing athletes. *Am J Sports Med* 2001;29:762–770.

21. Kuhn JE, Bey MJ, et al. Ligamentous restraints to external rotation of the humerus in the late-cocking phase of throwing. *Am J Sports Med* 2000;28:200–205.

22. Lohr JF, Uhthoff HK. The pathogenesis of degenerative rotator cuff tears. *Orthop Trans* 1987;11:237.

23. Montgomery WH III, Jobe FW. Functional outcomes in athletes after modified anterior capsulolabral reconstruction. *Am J Sports Med* 1994;22:352–358.

24. Neer CS II: Impingement lesions. *Clin Orthop* 1983;173:70–77.

25. Neer CS II: Anterior acromioplasty for classic impingement syndrome in the shoulder: a preliminary report. *J Bone Joint Surg (Am)* 1972;50:41–50.

26. Burkhart SS, Morgan CD. The peel-back mechanism: its role in producing and extending posterior type II SLAP lesions and its effect on SLAP repair rehabilitation. *Arthroscopy* 1998;14:637–640.

27. Morgan, C. SLAP lesions in throwing athletes. Presented at 67th AAOS Meeting, Orlando, Florida, February 2000.

28. Andrews JR, Carson WG Jr, McLeod WD. Glenoid labrum tears related to the long head of the biceps. *Am J Sports Med* 1985;13:337–341.

29. Morgan CD, Burkhart SS, Palmeri M, et al. Type II SLAP lesions: three subtypes and their relationships to superior instability and rotator cuff tears. *Arthroscopy* 1998;14:553–565.

30. Walch G, Levigne C. Treatment of deep surface partial-thickness tears of the supraspinatus in patients under 30 years of age. In: *The cuff*. Paris, France: Elsevier, 1997:243–244.

31. Kibler BW. Current concepts. The role of the scapula in athletic shoulder function. *Am J Sports Med* 1998;26:325–337.

32. Weber SC. Arthroscopic debridement and acromioplasty versus mini-open repair in the treatment of significant partial-thickness rotator cuff tears. *Arthroscopy* 1999;15(2):126–131.

33. Snyder SJ. Arthroscopic evaluation and treatment of the rotator cuff. *Shoulder Arthroscopy* 1994;11:133–148.

34. Clark JM, Harryman DT II. Tendons, ligaments, and capsule of the rotator cuff. *J Bone Joint Surg (Am)* 1992;74:713–725.

35. Nakajima T, Rokuuma N, Hamada K, et al. Histologic and biomechanical characteristics of the supraspinatus tendon: reference to rotator cuff tearing. *J Shoulder Elbow Surg* 1994;3:79–87.

36. Fukuda H, Hamada K, Yamada N, et al. Pathology and pathogenesis of partial-thickness cuff tears. In: *The cuff*. Paris, France: Elsevier, 1997:234–237.

37. Gartsman GM, Milne JC. Articular surface partial-thickness rotator cuff tears. *J Shoulder Elbow Surg* 1995;4:409–415.

38. Andrews JR, Angelo RL. Shoulder arthroscopy for the throwing athlete. *Tech Orthop* 1998;3:75–81.

39. Ellman H. Diagnosis and treatment of incomplete rotator cuff tears. *Clin Orthop* 1990;254:64–74.

40. Sonnabend DH, Yu Y, Howlett R, et al. Laminated tears of the human rotator cuff: a histologic and immunochemical study. *J Shoulder Elbow Surg* 2001;10:109–115.

41. Payne LZ, Altchek DW, Craig EV, et al. Arthroscopic treatment of partial rotator cuff tears in young athletes. *Am J of Sports Med* 1997;25:299–305.

42. Altchek DW, Warren RF, Wickiewicz TL, et al. Arthroscopic labral debridement (a three-year follow-up study). *Am J Sports Med* 1992;20:702–706.

43. Tomlinson RJ, Glousman RE. Arthroscopic debridement of glenoid labral tears in athletes. *Arthroscopy* 1995;11:42–51.

44. Martin DR, Garth WP Jr. Results of arthroscopic debridement of glenoid labral tears. *Am J Sports Med* 1995;23:447–451.

45. Anderson K, McCarty EC, Warren RF. Thermal capsulorrhaphy: Where are we today? *Sports Med Arthroscopy Rev* 1999;7:117–127.

46. Fanton GS. Arthroscopic electrothermal surgery of the shoulder. *Oper Tech Sports Med* 1998;6:139–146.

47. Greis PE, Burks RT, Schickendantz MS, et al. Axillary nerve injury after thermal capsular shrinkage of the shoulder. *J Shoulder Elbow Surg* 2001;10:231–235.

48. D'Alessandro, Bradley JP, Conner PM. Prospective evaluation of thermal capsulorrhaphy for shoulder instability: indications and results. Presented AOSSM Specialty Day, 69th AAOS Meeting, Dallas, Texas, 2002.

49. Medvecky MJ, Ong BC, Rokito AS, et al. Thermal capsular shrinkage: basic science and clinical applications. *Arthroscopy* 2001;17(6):624–635.

50. Gryler EC, Greis PE, Burks RT, et al. Axillary nerve temperatures during radiofrequency capsulorrhaphy of the shoulder. *Arthroscopy* 2001;17(6):567–572.

51. Craig, EV. The posterior mechanism of acute anterior shoulder dislocation. *Clin Orthop* 1984;190:212–216.

52. Horng-Chaung H, Zong-Ping L, et al. Influence of rotator cuff tearing on glenohumeral stability. *J Shoulder Elbow Surg* 1997;6:413–422.

53. Pagnani MJ, Speer KP, Warren RF, et al. Effects of the superior portion of the glenoid labrum on glenohumeral translation. *J Bone Joint Surg (Am)* 1995;77:1003–1010.

54. Rodosky MW, Harner CD, Fu FH. The role of the long head of the biceps muscle and superior glenoid labrum in anterior stability of the shoulder. *Am J Sports Med* 1994;22:121–130.

55. Fukuda H, Hamada K, et al. Partial-thickness tears of the rotator cuff. *Int Orthop* 1996;20:257–265.

56. Sonnabend D, Watson E. Structural factors affecting the outcome of rotator cuff repair. *J Shoulder Elbow Surg* 2002;11:212–218.

57. Lyons TR, Savoie FH III, Field LD. Arthroscopic repair of partial-thickness tears of therotator cuff. *Arthroscopy* 2001;17(2):219–223.

58. Snyder SJ. Arthroscopic evaluation and treatment of the rotator cuff. In: *Shoulder arthroscopy.* New York: McGraw-Hill, 1994: 133–178.

59. Paulos LE, Kody MH. Arthroscopically enhanced "mini-approach" to rotator cuff repair. *Am J Sports Med* 1994;22:19–25.

60. Ellman H. Diagnosis and treatment of incomplete rotator cuff tears. *Clin Orthop* 1990;254:64—74.

61. Flannigan B, Kirsunoglu-Brahme S, Snyder S, et al. MR arthrography of the shoulder: comparison with conventional MR imaging. *AJR* 1990;155:829–832.

62. Hodler J, Kirsunoglu-Brahme S, Flannigan B. Injuries of the superior portion of the glenoid labrum involving the insertion of the biceps tendon: MR imaging findings in nine cases. *AJR* 1992;159:565–568.

63. Tirman PFJ, Bost FW, et al. MR arthrographic depiction of tears of the rotator cuff: benefit of abduction and external rotation of the arm. *Radiology* 1994;192:851–856.

64. Jaovishidha S, Jacobson JA, et al. MR imaging of rotator cuff tears: is there a diagnostic benefit of shoulder exercise prior to imaging? *Clinical Imaging* 1999;23:249–253.

65. Thomopoulos S, Soslowsky LJ, et al. The effect of fibrin clot on healing rat supraspinatus tendon defects. *J Shoulder Elbow Surg* 2002;11:239–247.

66. Tibone J. Surgical treatment of tears of the rotator cuff in athletes. *J Bone Joint Surg (Am)* 1986;68:887–891.

67. Roye R, Grana WA, Yates CK. Arthroscopic subacromial decompression: two-to-seven year follow-up. *Arthroscopy* 1995;11: 301–306.

68. Tibone J, Jobe FW, Kerlan RK, et al. Shoulder impingement syndrome in athletes treated by an anterior acromioplasty. *Clin Orthop* 1985;198:135–140.

69. Burns TP, Turba JE. Arthroscopic treatment of shoulder impingement in athletes. *Am J Sports Med* 1992;20:13—16.

70. Payne LZ, Deng XH, et al. The combined dynamic and status contributions to subacromial impingement. a biomechanical analysis. *Am J Sports Med* 1997;25:801–808.

71. Lee TQ, Black AD, Tibone JE, et al. Release of the coracoacromial ligament can lead to glenohumeral laxity: a biomechanical study. *J Shoulder Elbow Surg* 2001;10:68–72.

72. Schneider T, Strauss JM, et al. Shoulder joint stability after arthroscopic subacromial decompression. *Arch Orthop Trauma Surg* 1994;113:129–133.

SUBACROMIAL IMPINGEMENT AND FULL THICKNESS ROTATOR CUFF TEARS IN OVERHEAD ATHLETES

CHAMP L. BAKER
ANDREW L. WHALEY
MARK BAKER

HISTORICAL OVERVIEW

The incidence of shoulder injuries varies with type of sport and the level of the athletic competition. Athletes who participate in overhead sports are particularly susceptible to shoulder injuries. Because of the repetitive, forceful overhead motion in sports such as baseball, swimming, or tennis, unusual stresses occur in the rotator cuff that are not frequently found in the general population (1–4). Because of these stresses, the overhead athlete can sustain cuff tears of varying thickness. Most often, these tears are of partial thickness; full thickness cuff tears are uncommon. In fact, full thickness rotator cuff tears in the general population are uncommon in the first four decades of life, which include the typical ages of the overhead athlete (5–7).

ETIOLOGY OF INJURY

Rotator cuff tears have been traditionally attributed to one of three mechanisms: primary impingement, secondary impingement due to underlying glenohumeral instability, or tensile overload (8). Neer proposed that primary, or subacromial outlet impingement, can result from the impingement of the rotator cuff against the osteophytes on the undersurface of the acromion, at the coracoacromial arch from a congenitally thickened coracoacromial ligament, or from an unstable os acromiale that hinges down and causes impingement (9). Secondary impingement occurs in individuals who have anterior capsular laxity (10). When these individuals place their arms in the overhead position with their shoulders in 90 degrees of abduction and maximal external rotation, the supraspinatus and infraspinatus tendons impinge on or make contact with the posterosuperior aspect of the glenoid and labrum (internal impingement). With repetitive throwing and with the forces generated by the act of throwing,

labral injury and cuff tears can occur. The cuff tears produced by this mechanism of injury are typically partial thickness articular rotator cuff tears. Tensile overload occurs most often with a fall or with a direct blow or force to the shoulder as can occur in contact sports (11). In these situations, the forces across the tendons of the rotator cuff exceed the intrinsic strength of the tendon and it ruptures.

PRESENTATION AND PHYSICAL EXAMINATION

It is important to start the examination of the patient with a careful review of his or her history. Clues to the cause of the problem can be gained by questioning the patient as to whether the pain occurred suddenly or had an insidious onset, where the pain is located, what position the arm is in when the pain occurs, whether the arm ever feels as if it is going "dead," and whether there is any weakness. Patients with a full thickness cuff tear may complain of weakness of the arm, either acutely or of gradual onset. They may also describe pain about the shoulder at night and with activities. A patient with primary impingement reports pain when lifting the arm overhead.

A thorough examination of the extremity for any patient with shoulder pain should include an examination of the cervical spine to rule out a neurologic problem or degenerative disease that can mimic shoulder pathology. If a rotator cuff tear or subacromial impingement is suspected, we then focus our examination and perform specific tests to reproduce the patient's symptoms. Patients with subacromial impingement have reproducible pain with the test described by Hawkins and Kennedy (12). The patient's arm is passively flexed to 90 degrees and forcibly internally rotated (Fig. 11-1). With the Neer test for subacromial impingement (13), the examiner stabilizes the patient's

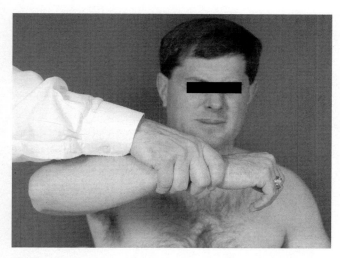

FIGURE 11-1. Hawkins test for impingement. The arm is elevated to 90 degrees and forcibly internally rotated. Pain indicates impingement.

scapula while raising the arm in forward elevation (Fig. 11-2). Both of these tests bring the greater tuberosity, the biceps tendon, and the rotator cuff under the coracoacromial arch and reproduce the painful symptoms.

Patients with full thickness tears of muscles of the rotator cuff exhibit weakness during testing of the particular muscle involved, may have a difference between active and passive

range of motion of the shoulder, and may have atrophy of the muscles involved if it is a chronic tear. During range of motion testing, patients often initially shrug when attempting to abduct their arms if a cuff tear is present because they are using scapulothoracic motion to compensate for the inability of the cuff to abduct the arm. Weakness with abduction or with the shoulder at 90 degrees of abduction and the arm forward flexed 30 degrees with the thumb pointed to the ground would indicate weakness of the supraspinatus (14). Weakness or rupture of the external rotators of the shoulder should also be tested for during the physical examination (Fig. 11-3). Persons with large or massive cuff tears involving multiple tendons are often unable to actively externally rotate their arms. Another way of testing the integrity of the external rotators is to place the arm at the side of the patient with the elbow bent to 90 degrees and the arm passively externally rotated; once the arm is released, it drifts back into internal rotation because of the unopposed action of the subscapularis (external rotation lag sign) (15). Similarly, the inability to actively externally rotate the abducted arm has been termed the *signe de clarion* ("hornblower's sign") because it puts the arm in the position used to blow a bugle (10).

Two tests specifically identify weakness of the subscapularis tendon. The first test is to have the patient attempt to push the wrist off his or her back against resistance, the so-called lift-off test (Fig. 11-4); failure to be able to do so indicates weakness of the subscapularis (16). If patients are unable to reach behind themselves for any reason, we perform a second test, the belly-press test. This test assesses the strength of internal rotation by having the patient place the

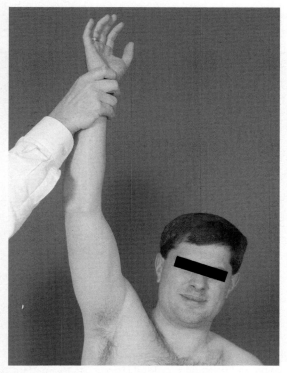

FIGURE 11-2. Neer test for impingement. The arm is raised in forward elevation. Pain near terminal elevation indicates impingement.

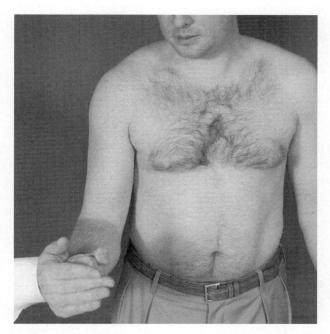

FIGURE 11-3. Weakness with the arm at the side and the elbow to flexed 90 degrees while resisting external rotation indicates weakness or rupture of the external rotators of the shoulder.

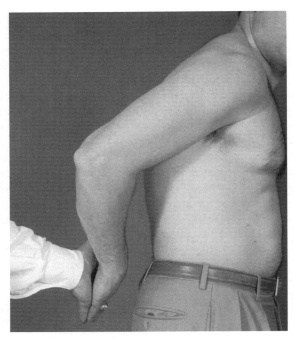

FIGURE 11-4. The lift-off test for subscapularis strength. With the hand behind the back, the patient attempts to push the hand off the back against resistance.

hand of the affected side on the abdomen and then pressing the hand against the abdomen with the elbows in front of the torso. If the subscapularis is not intact, the patient cannot press against the abdomen and the elbow drops behind the torso. Recent work from the Steadman-Hawkins group has demonstrated that, while both the lift-off and the belly-press are valid tests for the integrity of the subscapularis tendon, there are subtle differences (17). The lift-off test is superior for activating the lower portion of the subscapularis, and the belly-press test is superior for activating the upper portion of the subscapularis. Patients with a tear of the subscapularis not only have limited active internal rotation but also have excessive passive external rotation.

If there is a question as to the integrity of the rotator cuff with subacromial impingement, we routinely inject the subacromial bursa with lidocaine, and, after several minutes, we retest the strength of the rotator musculature. If the pain is no longer present but weakness persists, the diagnosis of compromised cuff integrity can be made. If pain is no longer present when the test for impingement is repeated, the diagnosis of subacromial impingement is also made.

RADIOGRAPHIC AND DIAGNOSTIC EVALUATION

We obtain three radiographic views of the involved shoulder in patients with suspected rotator cuff injury. The first is an *anteroposterior view* of the glenohumeral joint in the

scapular plane. This radiograph allows the clinician to examine the glenohumeral joint for evidence of fracture or degenerative disease. Also on this view, one can examine the acromioclavicular joint and assess the acromion for undersurface spur formation or degenerative changes. Additional findings that can be seen on this radiographic view are cal-

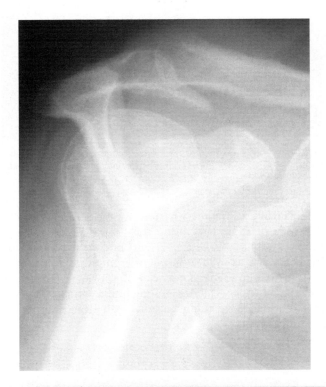

A

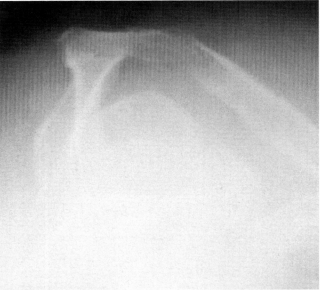

B

FIGURE 11-5. Supraspinatus outlet view shows shape of the acromion and spurs on the distal clavicle. **A:** This patient has a type III acromion because of osteophyte formation that impinges on the rotator cuff. **B:** After arthroscopic subacromial decompression, the same patient has a type I acromion.

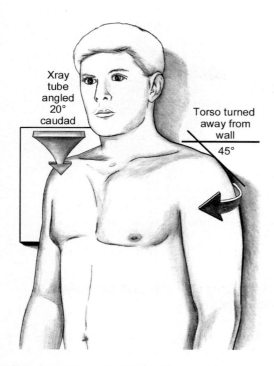

FIGURE 11-6. The ALVIS radiographic view. With the x-ray cassette on the wall and the patient standing, the patient's torso is turned away from the wall 45 degrees, and the x-ray tube is aimed 20 degrees caudad and centered on the joint.

cifications within the cuff tendons and superior migration of the humeral head. Normally, the space available for the cuff tendons between the humeral head and the acromion is estimated to be between 7 and 14 mm (18). With a space of less than 7 mm, there is an increased likelihood of a large rotator cuff tear and a poorer prognosis (19). The second view is the *axillary lateral* radiograph. Not only does this particular view allow one to verify that the shoulder is not dislocated, but it also is used to examine for bony avulsions off the glenoid or the humerus. This view is also used to make the diagnosis of glenohumeral arthritis. An os acromiale is visible on this view. An unstable os acromiale can hinge through the unfused segment and cause impingement symptoms. The third view can be either a *supraspinatus outlet* view (Fig. 11-5) or an *ALVIS*, (*a*nterolateral *v*iew of *i*mpingement *s*ite) view (Figs. 11-6 and 11-7). We use either view to assess the shape of the acromion, bony impingement that might be present, and the space available for the rotator cuff. Of the three acromial shapes visible on these radiographic views—flat (type I), curved (type II), or hooked (type III)—type III acromions a greater association with abnormalities of the rotator cuff (Fig. 11-8) (20).

We obtain additional radiographs as indicated clinically. Nakagawa and associates reported visualizing a notch on the greater tuberosity on the anteroposterior scapular view, the Stryker view, and the 45-degree craniocaudal view in throwing athletes (21). They noted that the presence of a notch was significantly related to the existence of a rotator cuff tear, whereas the size of the notch was significantly related to the depth and width of the tear.

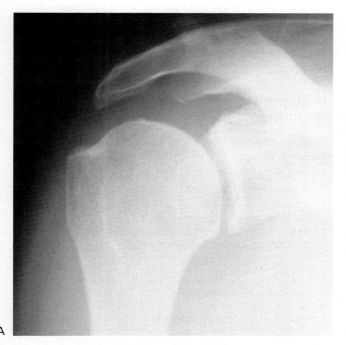

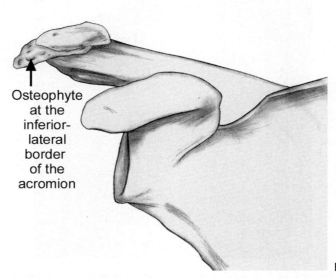

Osteophyte at the inferior-lateral border of the acromion

A   B

FIGURE 11-7. A: ALVIS view shows osteophytes on the lateral border of the acromion. **B:** Drawing shows location of osteophyte that may be source of impingement.

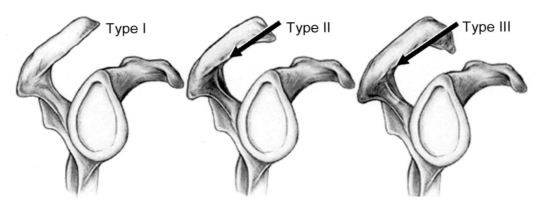

FIGURE 11-8. Three types of acromion: type I, flat; type II, curved; type III, hooked. The arrow indicates the plane of resection for a subacromial decompression.

Magnetic resonance imaging (MRI) is not routinely done unless a question remains regarding the integrity of the cuff or if there is a suggestion of concurrent pathologic anatomy that might need to be addressed at the time of surgery. An MRI scan provides information as to the quality of the tissues of the cuff as well as the size and location of the tears. We order MRI scans with gadolinium contrast because it greatly improves the delineation of cuff disorders and other possible problems, such as labral and bicipital involvement (Fig. 11-9).

CLASSIFICATION OF SUBACROMIAL IMPINGEMENT

Neer classified primary or subacromial impingement into three stages of increasing severity (13) (Table 11-1). Stage I lesions are usually seen in athletes younger than 25 years of age and are characterized by edema and hemorrhage of the subacromial bursa. Stage II lesions are seen in athletes who are typically older than 25 years of age and are characterized by fibrosis and scarring of the subacromial bursa. Stage III impingement is seen in older athletes, usually 40 years or older, and involves the rotator cuff, which is torn to some extent. If impingement is left untreated, it will likely progress through the aforementioned stages, resulting in chronic degeneration and eventually full thickness tears.

TREATMENT OF SUBACROMIAL IMPINGEMENT

Nonoperative Treatment of Subacromial Impingement

In our experience, most patients with subacromial impingement syndrome recover with nonoperative intervention. Prevention and treatment of stage I impingement in athletes can prevent its progression. Icing the shoulder after

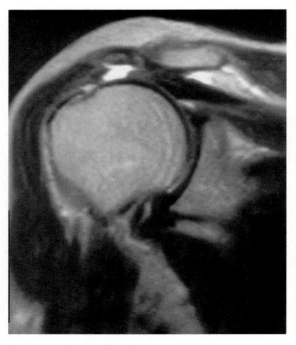

FIGURE 11-9. Magnetic resonance imaging with contrast shows a full-thickness tear of the supraspinatus with contrast leaking into the subacromial space.

TABLE 11–1. NEER CLASSIFICATION OF SUBACROMIAL IMPINGEMENT

Stage	Age
I Edema and hemorrhage	<25 years
II Fibrosis and tendinitis	25–40 years
III Bone spurs and tendon rupture	>40 years

From Meister K, Andrews J. Classification and treatment of rotation cuff injuries in the overhead athlete. *J Orthop Sports Phys Ther* 1993; 18:413–421, with permission.

workouts and nonsteroidal antiinflammatory medications reduce the inflammatory reaction. Ultrasound and transcutaneous nerve stimulation may be helpful in the treatment of athletes with impingement. The nonoperative program should include rest or modification of activities, subacromial injection of steroids, and a physical therapy regimen.

The patient with impingement syndrome should be placed on a program of strengthening exercises. The following program should be adhered to until all strengthening goals are met.

Phase 1 (Protective)

- Heat and ice as needed to help obtain motion
- Achieve staged passive range-of-motion goals in forward elevation
- Achieve staged passive range-of-motion goals in external rotation at 20 and 90 degrees of abduction
- Posterior capsule stretching
- Initiate functional internal rotation and active assisted range of motion as tolerated
- Theraband scapular retractions
- Progressive serratus anterior strengthening (isolated)
- Theraband external rotation and internal rotation strengthening (pain-free, elbow by side)
- Active assisted forward elevation → active forward elevation (pain-free)
- Continue isometric abduction

Cautions:
Do not initiate rotator cuff strengthening until night pain has subsided and overall pain level is low.

- Assure normal scapulohumeral rhythm with active forward elevation.

Phase 2 (Progressive Strengthening)

Goals

- Achieve staged range-of-motion goals
- Eliminate shoulder pain
- Improve strength, endurance, and power
- Increase functional activities
- Scapular stabilization
- Core strengthening

Operative Treatment of Subacromial Impingement

Treatment depends somewhat on the stage of the disease, with stage I and most of stage II impingement being amenable to nonoperative treatment. In general, most athletes with early stages of primary impingement without full thickness rotator cuff tears do well with nonoperative treatment aimed at strengthening the cuff musculature, reducing inflammation,

and regaining range of motion (12,22). When patients do not respond to nonoperative treatment or have advanced stage II or stage III impingement, they are treated surgically with open anterior acromioplasty, resection of coracoacromial ligament, or by arthroscopic subacromial decompression.

Initial reports on the surgical treatment of impingement in athletes were not particularly encouraging. Tibone and co-workers reported their results of open acromioplasty in young athletes (28 overhead athletes) with chronic impingement (23). Overall, 26 of the 34 shoulders (76%) continued to have problems with throwing or overhead activities after surgery, and only 22% of pitchers and throwers had a good result. Fly and associates also reported their results with arthroscopic subacromial decompression in young athletes with chronic impingement (24). Despite excellent relief of pain, only 77% could return to their previous levels of activity. These reports may be misleading. Arroyo and associates asserted that some of the patients in these studies might have had internal impingement leading to failures of surgical treatment (25).

Bigliani and others reported the results of 26 patients (10 recreational athletes, no high-performance athletes) who were younger than 40 years with primary impingement (26). They concluded that open acromioplasty would give good results (81% excellent or good) in patients who had not responded to nonoperative treatment. Although this and other published studies have reported higher satisfaction rates with open or arthroscopic decompressions, usually in the range of 80%, most show only modest improvement in the results of overhead athletes. Roye and associates reported their results of subacromial decompression in 90 shoulders (including 34 throwing athletes and 12 pitchers) with stage II or early stage III impingement at 2 to 7 years of follow-up (27). They found that arthroscopic decompression was comparable to open acromioplasty, regardless of the presence of a cuff tear (93% satisfaction). They did note, however, that throwing athletes might not return to their preinjury levels of functional activity (68% satisfactory results), that reinjury is common, and that pitchers had the worst prognosis (50% satisfactory results). The authors recommended that any instability of the shoulder be treated concomitantly. Despite the better overall patient satisfaction rate in these studies, it seems that it is difficult for the overhead athlete to return to his or her previous level of competition after subacromial decompression.

In cases of primary impingement in which nonoperative treatment has failed to relieve symptoms, it is important to identify the cause of the impingement (the shape of the acromion or presence of osteophytes, a thickened coracoacromial ligament, or os acromiale) and verify that there is no concomitant internal impingement. One should also be cognizant that acromioclavicular arthritis can mimic impingement and should be dealt with accordingly. Neer is credited with identifying the need to resect the offending bony portion of the acromion impinging upon the cuff (9).

Several authors have noted that selective sectioning of the coracoacromial ligament gave good results in the treatment of impingement in the overhead athlete (12,13,22,28). Jackson reported his results in 10 athletes with chronic impingement who underwent an open resection of the coracoacromial ligament (29). Five of the patients had excellent results with no pain and full function, and six of the patients were able to return to their previous levels of competition. Another cause of impingement is an unstable os acromiale, which can hinge through the unfused portion with contraction of the deltoid and impinge on the rotator cuff. Satterlee demonstrated that surgical fusion of an impinging os acromion with internal fixation could alleviate symptoms of impingement (30).

Primary impingement and cuff tears can be interrelated. Although there was no mention of athletes in their study group, Esch and co-workers reviewed their results of arthroscopic subacromial decompression in 71 patients (age range, 17 to 89 years) with stage II or III impingement (31). Using the UCLA rating system, they found satisfactory subjective results in 82% and satisfactory objective results in 78% of their patients with stage II impingement. Of those with stage II impingement without a cuff tear, the objective score was 82%. Patients with stage II impingement and a partial cuff tear had an objective score of 78%. Of those with stage III impingement, they noted that 88% had subjective satisfactory results and 77% had objective satisfactory ratings. The presence of a cuff tear, regardless of thickness, only slightly decreases the subjective and objective results in the general population.

CLASSIFICATION SYSTEM FOR ROTATOR CUFF TEARS

A variety of classification systems for rotator cuff disease exist. Some are applicable for both partial and full thickness cuff tears. Patte described a classification scheme based on the extent of the tear, the topography of the tear in the sagittal and frontal planes, the quality of the tendons, and the status of the biceps tendon (32). Snyder's classification is based on the location of the tear, the tendon involved, and the grade of the tear (Table 11-2) (33). Other ways to describe the type of tear include using descriptive terms: partial or full thickness tear, location and orientation of the tear, and shape of the tear.

Several classification methods based on the size of the tear or number of tendons involved have been described specifically for complete tears. Ellman and co-workers classified full thickness tears as small if they were less than 2 cm, as large if they were between 2 and 4 cm, or as massive if they were greater than 4 cm (19). Post and associates classified small tears as those less than 1 cm, moderate as those between 1 and 3 cm, large as those between 3 and 5 cm, and massive as those greater than 5 cm (34). Others have classified tears that are confined to only the supraspinatus

TABLE 11–2. SNYDER CLASSIFICATION OF ROTATOR CUFF TEARS

Location	Tendon Involved	Grade of Tear
Articular	Supraspinatus	0 = Normal cuff
Bursal	Infraspinatus	1 = Involves bursa and capsule, not tendon
Complete	Rotator interval	2 = <2 cm, minimal tearing of tendon fibers
	Subscapularis	3 = 2 to 3 cm, moderate destruction of tendon fibers
		4 = >4 cm, severe fraying, fragmentation with splits and flap formation

From Kuhn JE, Hawkins RJ. Surgical treatment of shoulder injuries in tennis players. *Clin Sports Med* 1995;14:139–161, with permission.

tendon as small, tears involving two tendons as moderate, and tears involving three or four tendons as large or massive (35). Cofield defined a massive tear as a tear that is larger than 5 cm in maximum diameter (36). Others define massive as disinsertion of at least two complete tendons (36).

Another classification method is based on etiologic factors (Table 11-3) (38). It divides the causes into primary compressive disease, instability with secondary compressive disease, primary tensile overload failure, tensile overload failure secondary to capsular instability, and macrotraumatic failure. Primary compressive disease of the cuff typically occurs in the older individual and is the result of direct compression of the cuff from subacromial impingement. Secondary compressive cuff disease from shoulder instability results in internal impingement and partial articular cuff tears. Primary tensile cuff disease results from repetitive eccentric forces that lead to overload failure of the tendon. Secondary tensile disease results from the overload of the static stabilizers of the shoulder due to repetitive tensile stresses that occur during the overhead throwing motion. The loss of those static stabilizers subsequently results in overstressing and weakening of the cuff, leading to secondary failure of the cuff under tensile forces. Macrotrauma is the result of a single, distinct traumatic event. For an extraneous force to overcome the inherent strength of the cuff, it must surpass the tensile force of the normal tendon. This is particularly rare because the tensile strength of bone is less than that of young healthy tendon.

TABLE 11–3. CLASSIFICATION OF ROTATOR CUFF DISEASE

Type	Classification
I	Primary compressive disease
II	Instability with secondary compressive disease
III	Primary tensile overload failure
IV	Tensile overload failure secondary to capsular instability
V	Macrotraumatic failure

From Meister K, Andrews J. Classification and treatment of rotation cuff injuries in the overhead athlete. *J Orthop Sports Phys Ther* 1993; 18:413–421, with permission.

This type of trauma usually causes a longitudinal tear of the tendon with an avulsion of the greater tuberosity.

OPERATIVE TREATMENT OF FULL THICKNESS ROTATOR CUFF TEARS

Shoulder injuries are common in sports requiring the athlete to use the overhead throwing motion. Although various overhead sports require different techniques, Perry has pointed out that the demands placed on the shoulder in sports such as swimming or tennis are similar to those placed on the shoulder by the overhand throw in baseball (3). However, despite the frequency with which shoulder injuries occur in this population, full thickness rotator cuff tears are, in fact, uncommon.

Hawkins and colleagues (6) report that only 2 of their series of 100 consecutive patients with full thickness cuff tears were less than 40 years of age, and Norwood and co-workers (7) noted only 11 of 103 patients who were younger than 40 years had full thickness cuff tears. These tears are usually the result of primary impingement. This typically occurs in middle-aged overhead athletes—particularly in tennis players who are able to continue playing into their senior years. Rarely, full thickness cuff tears can occur from macrotrauma, such as from a direct blow in contact sports (11), or from traumatic glenohumeral dislocations, usually in athletes older than age 40 years. The mechanism of this type of tear is the result of tensile overloading of the cuff tendons. To attest to the relative rarity of this type of tear, Cofield reported that only 8% of 510 patients who required surgical repair of their cuff reported that the tear occurred from a single traumatic event (39).

Because of the rarity of these lesions in young athletes involved in other overhead sports, most of the peer-reviewed literature on full thickness cuff tears in athletes comes from the results of surgical treatment in tennis players. Tibone and associates reported their results of surgical repair of cuff tears in 45 athletes (40). All patients underwent subacromial decompression and repair of the cuff as indicated. Only 15 of the 45 patients in their series had full thickness tears, and the mean age of this subgroup was 29 years (range, 19 to 40 years). Eight athletes in this subgroup played either baseball or tennis. Two thirds of these overhead athletes with full thickness cuff tears had good results at their final follow-up at a mean of 3.9 years. However, only 56% of all of the athletes returned to their former competitive athletic status, and only 41% of pitchers and throwers returned to their previous level of competition.

Several years later, Bigliani and co-workers reported their results of surgical treatment in 23 tennis players with symptomatic full thickness tears (41). The mean age of the group was 58 years, and only one player was younger than 40 years of age (39 years). Most of the tears were less than 3 cm. Not only were a high percentage of the players able to resume playing (95%), but a large percentage were able to return to

their previous level of competition (83%). In analyzing their results, the investigators also found that the size of the tear affected the end results, with three satisfactory and one unsatisfactory result in patients with a massive cuff tear.

More recently, Sonnery-Cottet and others reported similar results of cuff repair in 51 tennis players with a mean age of 51 years (range, 35 to 67 years) (42). Forty-two of the patients underwent open repair of the cuff and nine patients had debridement with biceps tenotomy. Debridement of the cuff only was indicated if the tear was large and the athlete did not want to undergo extensive postoperative therapy or if the tear was of partial thickness. They found that 80% of the patients were able to return to the sport postoperatively, and most were able to resume the sport at the previous level of competition. Several points should be noted from this study. The authors reported that, when comparing the results of patients on the basis of age at the time of surgery (younger than 50 years versus older than 50 years), there was no significant difference in the length of time before return to tennis or in level of play at return. They also noted that the length of time to return to play after surgery was related to the level of play on return. It is also interesting to note that four of the five patients with full thickness tears who underwent cuff debridement without repair plus biceps tenotomy were able to return to tennis. This result is similar to that of Rockwood and colleagues in their series of irreparable cuff tears treated with debridement of the cuff rather than repair (43).

One may propose that, in general, athletes do better than the general population with regard to postoperative function because they are usually highly motivated and disciplined, and therefore more likely to actively participate in postoperative therapy. Ellman and others later reported their findings in 22 patients (not athletes) with massive, irreparable cuff tears who were treated with subacromial decompression and cuff debridement without repair (44). They noted that they were able to provide pain relief for the patients, but they were not able to improve shoulder function significantly. The difference between the findings of Ellman and colleagues (44) and Sonnery-Cottet and co-workers (42) with regard to debridement of the cuff alone may possibly be attributed to the desire and motivation of athletes, regardless of age, to return to competition in a sport they enjoy.

The reason most of the literature dealing with full thickness cuff tears in overhead athletes comes from surgical treatment of tennis players is most likely due to the fact that tennis players are able to continue their competition well into middle age—a time when the incidence of full thickness tears increases. It may be postulated that, in sports such as baseball, pitchers retire before reaching middle age or some other career-ending injury occurs before a full thickness cuff tear can occur.

In discussing the goals of surgery with the athletic patient, it is important to point out that several factors have been identified as having an influence on the outcome of cuff repairs in the general population. Cofield and colleagues reported that the size of the tear was the single most important factor influencing long-term results (45). Hattrup was able to show that patients older than 65 years of age tend to have poorer results as well as having larger rotator cuff tears (46). Pollock and colleagues reported similar findings in their study of the effect of tear size and long-term results (47). In that study, satisfactory results were obtained in 95% of small, 94% of medium, 88% of large, and 84% of massive tears. Although a large number of patients with large and massive tears had satisfactory results, the results were inferior to those with small or medium tears. Ellman and co-workers demonstrated a correlation between a poor result and preoperative strength and active range of motion (19). They determined that if the patient had grade 3/5 strength or less, or were unable to abduct the shoulder beyond 100 degrees, there was an increased risk of a poor result after cuff repair. Unsatisfactory results in this study were usually related to poor function—not to poor pain relief.

Although technically demanding, arthroscopic repair of full thickness rotator cuff tears has been shown to produce satisfactory results (48). Along with the advantages of the arthroscopic technique, smaller skin incisions, access to the glenohumeral joint for inspection and treatment of intraarticular lesions, no detachment of the deltoid, and less soft tissue dissection, Gartsman and colleagues found that their patients' results were comparable with those obtained with the open method of repair (48). It is also important to note that the final outcome of the cuff repair may not necessarily be directly related to complete healing of the cuff tear. Liu and Baker assessed shoulder function and cuff integrity in 33 patients at an average of 3.7 years who had undergone arthroscopically assisted, miniopen cuff repairs (49). They found that the integrity of the cuff at follow-up examination does not determine the functional outcome of the patient. Calvert and co-workers demonstrated good function, pain relief, and satisfaction despite having a documented dye leak at follow-up shoulder arthrography (50). Other authors have validated this assertion (51).

AUTHORS' PREFERRED TREATMENT ALGORITHMS AND TECHNIQUES

An overhead athlete with complaints of shoulder pain is assessed initially by a history that emphasizes questions about precipitating factors of pain, intensity and duration of pain, and weakness. The examination focuses on detecting restricted motion, weakness, and instability. Diagnostic radiographic studies include anteroposterior, lateral, axillary, and outlet—either supraspinatus or ALVIS—views.

Nonoperative Treatment

If a diagnosis of a full-thickness tear has been made previously, the patient is a surgical candidate. However, if a ten-

tative diagnosis of rotator cuff disease is made, rehabilitation exercises are instituted for range of motion and strengthening of the cuff. Depending on the patient's symptoms and the determination of whether the patient is experiencing primarily weakness or impingement, a subacromial injection is given. The injection eliminates the symptoms related to bursal irritation and weakness due to pain. The shoulder is reexamined after the injection. The patient is most often referred for physical therapy and given a follow-up appointment for 4 to 6 weeks.

If at the follow-up visit, the patient continues to have signs of cuff disease, additional imaging studies, usually without contrast, are ordered. Exercises are continued and antiinflammatory medication may be given. If the patient did not receive a subacromial steroid injection at the initial visit, one may be given at this time.

Operative Treatment

If an athlete has followed the nonoperative treatment regimen described earlier for at least 3 months, continues to have symptoms, and has a positive imaging study or radiographic evidence of bony impingement, surgery is considered. Most of the tears that occur in overhead athletes are small, with minimal retraction. They are best treated by an arthroscopic evaluation under general anesthesia with an interscalene block. First, the glenohumeral joint is examined and then the subacromial bursa. Next, in patients older than 35 years old or in younger patients, if impingement of the cuff is evident, an anterior acromionectomy is done. If the cuff tear is complete, arthroscopic repair is the surgical treatment of choice. The senior author's second choice of surgical technique is a miniopen repair. The miniopen technique is used more often in patients in whom the subscapularis is involved or a biceps tenodesis is indicated.

The need for decompression of the acromioclavicular joint is a preoperative decision based on the patient's symptoms and response to the injection. If the patient is asymptomatic, we believe there is usually no need to remove any portion of the clavicle. However, if a decision has been made to decompress the acromioclavicular joint, the procedure is done using a combination of posterior and anterior portals. The goal of subacromial decompression is to relieve the site of impingement and to improve the amount of room available for the cuff.

Preoperative Preparation. Unless contraindicated, all patients receive a preoperative interscalene block, which has a twofold purpose. It reduces the amount of narcotics needed for effective anesthesia and provides prolonged postoperative pain relief. A general anesthetic is used and patients are sent home several hours after surgery.

Before the patient is positioned for surgery, an examination under anesthesia is done. If restricted motion is detected, gentle manipulation restores the motion. A balance suspension is used to allow abduction of the arm to 45

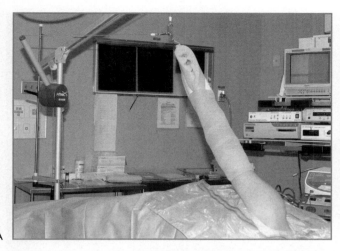
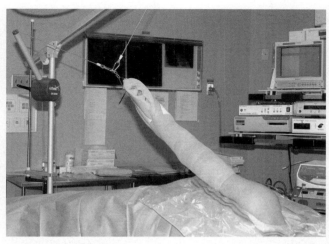

A   B

FIGURE 11-10. A: Patient positioning for arthroscopic surgery of the glenohumeral joint. The arm is in approximately 45 degrees of abduction and slight forward flexion with 10 pounds of traction. **B:** If the subacromial space is to be entered, the arm is lowered to approximately 15 degrees of abduction with 5 pounds of traction.

degrees for easier access to the glenohumeral joint (Fig. 11-10). If a miniopen incision is needed, the arm is lowered approximately 15 degrees.

Portal Placement. The bony landmarks of the shoulder are outlined to identify the acromion, clavicle, acromioclavicular joint, spine articulation, and coracoid process. With the patient in the lateral decubitus position, a *posterior portal* is established by entering the soft spot of the posterior capsule, 2 cm inferior and 1.5 cm medial to the posterolateral corner of the acromion. Under direct visualization using the outside-in technique, the *anterior portal* is created lateral to the coracoid process below the coracoacromial ligament at the level of the acromioclavicular joint. The *direct lateral portal* is routinely used for subacromial decompression and cuff repairs, and this portal is placed lateral and anterior to the middle of the acromion. Occasionally, a fourth portal, the *accessory anterolateral* portal, may be used for placement of a suture anchor and assistance with arthroscopic knot tying.

Diagnostic Arthroscopy. A 4-mm 30-degree angled arthroscope connected to the pump, which is normally set at 40 mm Hg, is inserted through the posterior portal. Epinephrine is used in the initial bag to help reduce bleeding. The anesthesiologist is asked to keep the systolic pressure below 100 mm Hg unless contraindicated by the patient's medical condition.

We thoroughly examine the glenohumeral joint, looking for any other occult pathology. A standard examination begins in the interval between the rotator cuff and subscapularis. An anterior portal is established in this area using an outside-in or inside-out technique. A probe can then be inserted to assist in examination. It is helpful to pull down on the biceps tendon to ensure there is no fibrillation or tear of the tendon in the extraarticular portion. The undersurface of

the rotator cuff in this area is inspected visually and by palpation with the probe. The entire labrum, from the anterosuperior to the anteroinferior to the posteroinferior and back up to the posterosuperior aspect, is examined and probed for tears. The middle and anteroinferior glenohumeral ligaments are visualized and observed for signs of injury. The glenoid surface and the posterior aspect of the humeral head area are also observed for degenerative changes.

Using a switching stick, the scope is placed next in the anterior portal and the probe is inserted posteriorly and the examination is completed. Next, we attempt to characterize the size and location of the cuff tear from inside the glenohumeral joint if one is present (Fig. 11-11). If a partial or complete tear is identified on the articular side, an 18-gauge needle can be used to localize the tear and a polydioxanone (PDS) suture passed through that needle to localize the tear from the articular to the bursal side.

Surgical Procedure. After assessment of the glenohumeral joint is complete, we redirect the scope through the same posterior portal into the subacromial space. If necessary, we perform a bursectomy to allow us to visualize the entire subacromial space and cuff. A lateral portal can be established at this time, and a shaver or a radiofrequency probe (monopolar or bipolar) can be used to clean away the bursal tissue for better visualization.

At this point, we again inspect the entire cuff and try to characterize the cuff tear if one is present and determine whether the cuff is mobile and repairable. We also determine whether there is contact between the cuff and acromion or the coracoacromial ligament that could cause impingement problems.

After the bursectomy is performed and the entire coracoacromial ligament and anterior aspect of the acromion can be visualized, a decision is made to proceed with an acromioplasty, if indicated. From the lateral portal, a

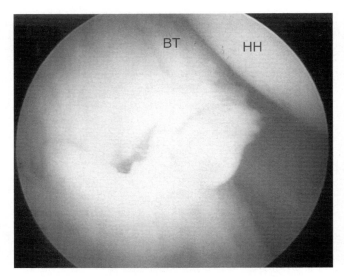

FIGURE 11-11. With the arthroscope in the posterior portal and oriented superiorly toward the rotator cuff, a tear can be visualized in the cuff. BT, biceps tendon; HH, humeral head.

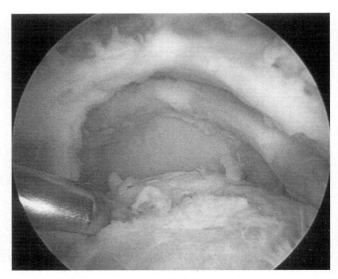

FIGURE 11-12. The humerus is debrided for insertion of suture anchors and reattachment of the cuff.

radiofrequency wand is used to detach the coracoacromial ligament, and a motorized shaver or burr is used at the most anterolateral aspect of the acromion. The scope is then placed laterally and the shaver posteriorly using a cutting-block technique. The anterior edge of the acromion is removed back to the acromioclavicular joint.

If a decision has been made to decompress the acromio-clavicular joint, it is done through the posterior and anterior portals with resection of a total of between 10 and 15 mm of bone taken equally from both sides of the joint.

Evaluation of the cuff tear includes determining the amount of retraction of the tear from the greater tuberosity as well as the size of the tear. Tear mobility and tear quality are also assessed and are important in determining repairability. Crescent-type tears can be repaired directly to the tuberosity with suture anchors. Larger U-shaped tears may be first treated with margin convergence and then a simple repair of the remaining portion of the tear.

Once magnitude, retraction, mobility, and tissue quality of the tear have been assessed, a decision regarding the type of repair can be made. The arthroscope is placed in the lateral portal to give a more panoramic view of the repair site. With a shaver in the posterior portal, the soft tissue footprint of the cuff is debrided to create a bony bed (Fig. 11-12). The frayed edge of the cuff tendon can be debrided conservatively but most of the substance of the tendon itself should be preserved. If the tear is chronic and there is minimal retraction, soft tissue releases can be done along with an intraarticular release adjacent to the glenoid and an excision of adhesions on the bursal side to free the tendon.

Arthroscopic Rotator Cuff Repair

The concept of repair consists of mobilization of the tendon and advancement back to the tuberosity. For massive tears,

retracted tears, or U-shaped tears, side-to-side convergence should be performed initially. The scope is placed through the lateral portal and a suture lasso or a penetrator-type instrument is brought from the anterior portal to grasp the anterior portion of the cuff. It is passed through the posterior portion of the tendon and is grasped with the penetrating instrument. This technique allows a single stitch to come through the tendon and to be then tied through the posterior portal with the knot posterior. As many sutures as are needed are passed to approximate the tear to the small triangle left on the tuberosity. The senior author's (CLB) preference is a nonabsorbable suture, such as the fiberwire suture by Arthrex (Arthrex, Inc., Naples, Florida). Reinspection usually reveals a small triangular portion of cuff available for repair back to the tuberosity. From the lateral portal, an 18-gauge needle is used to approximate the angle. Using a punch or a drill, a guide hole is made and a suture anchor is placed in the tuberosity at a 45-degree angle (Fig. 11-13). The anchors usually have two separate stitches.

Two sutures are retracted so the surgeon is handling only one set of sutures at a time. Next, a penetrating instrument in the anterior portal is brought in through the cuff to grasp one of the sutures and bring it out the front to be tied in a simple knot (Fig. 11-14). Both sutures are passed before the knots are tied. It is best to tie both knots from one suture anchor and then to assess the need for another. If needed, another suture anchor usually can be placed more posteriorly and, in a similar fashion, the stitches are passed through the cuff with the knot tied on top. Most often, the surgeon can use a sliding knot for the first knot and a series of half-hitch knots for the second suture (Fig. 11-15). The repair is inspected to ensure that it is intact and that there is adequate clearance between the cuff and the arch of the acromion. The portals are closed with nylon ligature, and the dressing is applied.

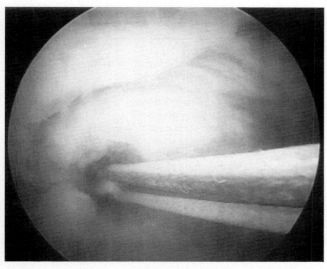

FIGURE 11-13. A suture anchor is inserted into the humerus.

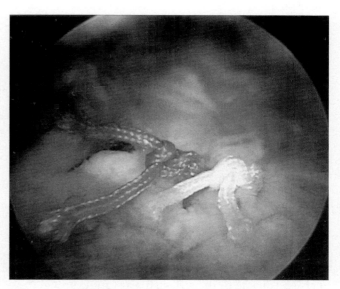

FIGURE 11-15. The repair is complete.

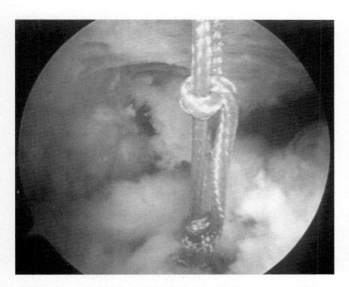

FIGURE 11-14. A knot is tied arthroscopically to reapproximate the cuff to the humerus.

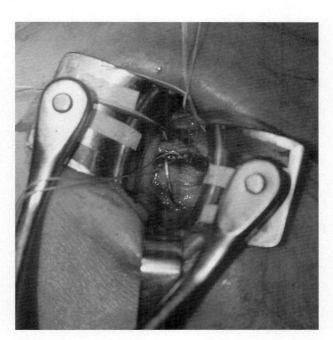

FIGURE 11-16. Rotator cuff tear in a right shoulder is exposed through a miniopen incision. Sutures have been placed in the cuff for the repair.

TABLE 11–4. RANGE-OF-MOTION GUIDELINES FOR POSTOPERATIVE REHABILITATION AFTER ARTHROSCOPIC OR ARTHROSCOPICALLY ASSISTED MINI OPEN ROTATOR CUFF REPAIR

Postoperative Interval	Passive Forward Elevation	Passive External Rotation at 20° of Abduction	Passive External Rotation at 90° of Abduction	Active Assisted Forward Elevation	Active Forward Elevation
Postoperative day 1	90°	0°–20°	NA	NA	NA
Postoperative week 1	120°	20°–30°	NA	NA	NA
Postoperative week 3	140°	45°	45°	90°	NA
Postoperative week 6	WNL	60°	75°	—	120°
Postoperative week 9	WNL	WNL	WNL	—	140°+

WNL, within normal limits.

Arthroscopically Assisted (Miniopen) Technique

If we are not able to accomplish a cuff repair arthroscopically, the repair can be done through a modified, or miniopen, approach. The arm is taken out of traction or brought down closer to the body (Fig. 11-10B).

After the diagnostic arthroscopy and mobilization, we perform an arthroscopic subacromial decompression in the manner described earlier. Once the decompression is complete, we then make a small (less than 5 cm) horizontal incision in Langer's lines parallel to the acromion. We carefully split the deltoid in line with its fibers. The tear can be seen easily at this point (Fig. 11-16). It is helpful to place a stay suture in the torn cuff before the incision is made so the retracted tear can be brought easily into view.

The surgeon can then determine the choice of suture anchors or transosseous tunnels. The preference, in most cases, would be a suture anchor and a simple stitch closure. Once the cuff tear has been repaired, the deltoid muscle is closed with nonabsorbable sutures. The skin is closed and a shoulder immobilizer is applied.

Rotator cuff surgery is done as an outpatient procedure. Protective immobilization of the shoulder is continued for 3 to 4 weeks while regaining passive motion. In the next 3 to 4 weeks, strengthening of the shoulder is begun. At roughly 3 months after surgery, the patient can begin some sport-directed activities. Full recovery usually takes 6 months for an overhead athlete.

Rehabilitation

There are three phases of shoulder rehabilitation for patients who have undergone surgical treatment of rotator cuff disease: phase 1, the immediate postoperative, or *protective*, phase; phase 2, the *progressive strengthening* phase; and phase 3, the *advanced conditioning and return-to-sport* phase. The postoperative rehabilitation programs for the arthroscopic and miniopen rotator cuff repair are essentially the same. In the protocol, we use the range-of-motion guidelines in Table 11-4.

The goals of phase 1 are to minimize pain and inflammatory response, to achieve staged range-of-motion goals, to establish a stable scapula, to initiate pain-free rotator cuff and deltoid strengthening, and to minimize deltoid atrophy. The exercises and modalities listed in Table 11-5 are used in this phase of the rehabilitation program.

Phase 2 rehabilitation goals are to achieve staged range-of-motion goals, to eliminate shoulder pain, to improve strength, endurance, and power, to increase functional activities, to establish a stable scapula, and to continue core strengthening. Table 11-6 lists the exercises used in this phase of rehabilitation (Figs. 11-17 through 11-23).

TABLE 11–5. PHASE 1 REHABILITATION EXERCISES AND MODALITIES

Postoperative Day 1

Elbow, wrist, and hand active range of motion

Passive forward elevation in plane of scapula to tolerance; 10 repetitions (reps), twice a day (passive forward elevation by family member with patient sitting or supine depending on pain tolerance and muscle guarding)

Supine passive external rotation to tolerance with T-stick in 0°–20° flexion and 20° abduction; 15 reps, twice a day (also can be performed with assistance by a family member with patient in sitting or supine position)

Cervical spine active range of motion

Ice

Positioning full time in sling

Cautions: Ensure normal neurovascular status

Postoperative Week 1–3

Continue elbow, wrist, and hand and C-spine active range of motion

Shoulder shrugs and retractions (no weight)

Continue passive forward elevation (when 120° is reached, begin rope and pulley or supine passive forward elevation)

Continue T-bar passive external rotation at 20° abduction and as tolerated at 90° abduction

Isometrics, keeping elbow flexed to 90° (submaximal, pain-free)

Abduction, flexion, external rotation, internal rotation

Manual scapula strengthening[a]

Pain control modalities as needed (ice, high-voltage galvanic stimulation)[a]

Aquatics passive and active range of motion activities (pain-free)[a]

Complications/cautions: If pain level is not dissipating, decrease intensity and volume of exercises.

Postoperative Week 3–6

Heat or ice as needed to help obtain motion

Discontinue sling as comfortable

Achieve staged passive range of motion goals in forward elevation

Achieve staged passive range of motion goals in external rotation at 20° and 90° abduction

Posterior capsule stretching

Initiate functional internal rotation, active assisted range of motion as tolerated

Theraband scapular retractions

Progressive serratus anterior strengthening (isolated)

Theraband external rotation and internal rotation strengthening (pain-free, elbow by side)

Active assisted forward elevation → active forward elevation (pain-free)

Continue isometric abduction

Closed chain approximation activities[a]

Aquatics[a]

Mobilizations as needed[a]

Light proprioceptive neuromuscular facilitation D1, D2, and manual resistance for cuff, deltoid, and scapula (rhythmic stabilization or slow reversal hold)[a]

Trunk stabilization and strengthening[a]

Cautions: Do not initiate rotator cuff strengthening until night pain has subsided and overall pain level is low. Ensure normal scapulohumeral rhythm with active forward elevation

[a]Adjunctive exercises.

TABLE 11–6. PHASE 2 REHABILITATION EXERCISES AND MODALITIES

Postoperative Week 6–9

Continue self stretching in all planes to obtain full passive range of motion

Advance scapular strengthening

Advance Theraband strengthening of cuff below shoulder level

Initiate isotonic dumbbell exercises for deltoid, supraspinatus, up to 3 lb max (when full active forward elevation is nearly achieved)

Mobilizations as needed[a]

Aquatics for strengthening[a]

Close kinetic chain activities for dynamic stability of scapula, deltoid, cuff[a]

Open chain kinesthetic awareness drills (e.g., range of motion replication)[a]

Upper body ergometer[a]

Trunk stabilization and strengthening[a]

Cautions: Strengthening program should progress only without signs of increasing inflammation

Strengthening program should emphasize high repetitions, low weight, and should be performed a maximum of 2 times a day.

Postoperative Week 9–12

Continue stretching as needed

Continue deltoid, cuff, and scapula strengthening as above (5 lb max for isotonic strengthening) with the following progressions:

   Prone isotonic strengthening as needed

   Decreasing amounts of external stabilization provided to shoulder girdle

Integrate functional patterns

   Increase speed of movements

   Integrate kinesthetic awareness drills into strengthening activities

   Decrease rest time to improve endurance

May return to golf and tennis ground strokes after completing strengthening progression (as above)

Progressive closed kinetic chain dynamic stability activities[a]

Impulse[a]

Initiate isokinetic strengthening[a]

Mobilizations as needed[a]

Trunk stabilization and strengthening[a]

[a]Adjunctive exercises.

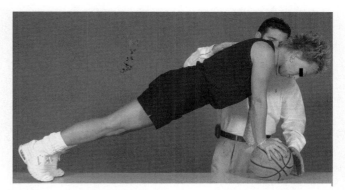

FIGURE 11-18. Closed chain scapular stabilization exercise. The patient balances upper body on ball in 30-second intervals.

The goals of phase 3, the advanced conditioning phase, are to normalize strength, endurance, and power; to return to full activities of daily living and recreational activities, and to return to sport. Table 11-7 lists the exercises used in this phase of rehabilitation (Fig. 17-23). During this phase, the athlete incorporates sport-specific activities into the program to help achieve the ultimate goal of returning to one's sport.

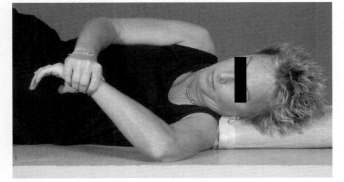

FIGURE 11-17. Positioning for posterior capsular stretch or "sleeper" stretch. Patient is in side-lying position with the affected shoulder in approximately 90 degrees of forward flexion and the elbow in 90 degrees of flexion. Using the contralateral hand, the patient gently brings the wrist into internal rotation until slight stretch is felt.

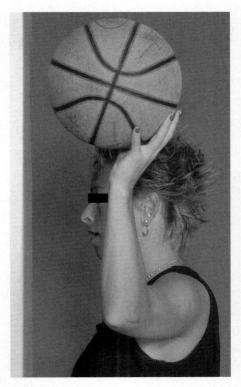

FIGURE 11-19. Overhead open chain endurance-stabilization exercise. With the shoulder in approximately 80 to 90 degrees of horizontal abduction and external rotation, the patient bounces the ball rapidly in 30-second intervals.

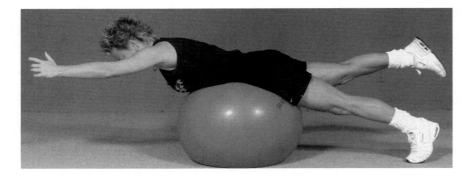

FIGURE 11-20. Lower trapezius-scapular stabilization exercise combined with core strengthening. Patient is positioned with Swiss ball at mid body. Patient elevates affected arm while lifting the contralateral lower extremity and holds for 5 seconds.

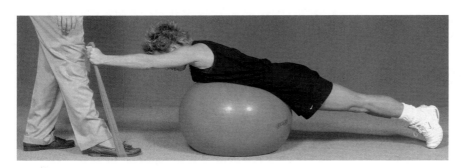

FIGURE 11-21. Prone rotator cuff strengthening over Swiss ball. This exercise combines core strengthening with lower trapezius activation.

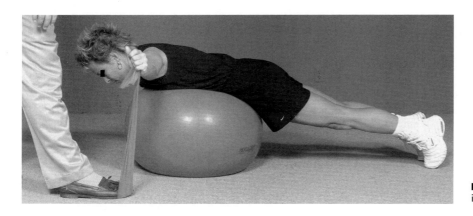

FIGURE 11-22. Prone shoulder strengthening in horizontal abduction over Swiss ball.

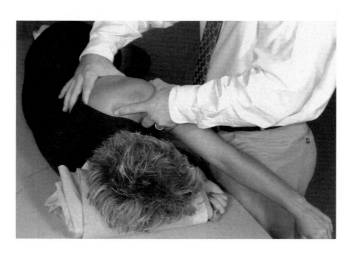

FIGURE 11-23. Posterior-inferior stretch. With the patient in the side-lying position and the humerus elevated to the desired position depending on the capsular end feel, the practitioner stabilizes the patient's arm with his or her body. With a downward rotation, the scapula is mobilized on the humerus.

TABLE 11–7. PHASE 3 REHABILITATION EXERCISES AND MODALITIES

Postoperative Month 3–6

Stretching as needed

Continue deltoid, cuff, and scapula strengthening progression

Transition to maintenance deltoid, cuff, and scapular strengthening program once discharge strength criteria are met

Initiate plyometric program (if needed)

Do not begin until grade 5/5 manual muscle test for rotator cuff and scapula is achieved

Begin with beachball or tennis ball, progressing to weighted balls

    2-handed tosses: waist level, overhead, diagonal

    1-handed stability drills

    1-handed tosses (vary amount of abduction, UE support, amount of protected ER.

May begin interval throwing program after 3–6 weeks of plyometrics

Initiate progressive replication of demanding activities of daily living or work activities

Discharge and return-to-sport criteria

Passive range of motion within normal limits for activities of daily living, work, or sports

Manual muscle test 5/5 shoulder girdle or satisfactory isokinetic test

Complete plyometric program, if applicable

Complete interval return-to-sport program, if applicable

ER, external rotation; UE, upper extremity.

CONCLUSION

In conclusion, overhead athletes are susceptible to shoulder injuries because of the nature of their sport. Although shoulder injuries are common, full thickness cuff tears are not. Primary or subacromial impingement typically occurs in the older athlete engaged in overhead sports. The results of arthroscopic and open subacromial decompression are good as long as the offending structure—thickened coracoacromial ligament, unstable os acromiale, shape of the acromion, or osteophyte—is properly identified. With proper identification and treatment of the cause of the impingement, we believe—and our belief is supported by the literature—that the overhead athlete can often return to his or her sport at the previous level of competition. Because most athletes are by nature dedicated and disciplined and actively participate in postoperative therapy, they often achieve good results from cuff repair. Most literature on this topic examines tennis players, possibly because tennis players can play competitively later into middle age—a time when this type of cuff tear typically occurs. It may also be true that, in other overhead sports, athletes stop competing for some other reason before a full thickness cuff tear occurs.

REFERENCES

1. Pappas AM, Zawacki RM, Sullivan TJ. Biomechanics of baseball pitching: a preliminary report. *Am J Sports Med* 1985;13: 216–222.
2. Jobe FW, Moynes DR, Tibone JE, et al. An EMG analysis of the shoulder in pitching: a second report. *Am J Sports Med* 1984;12: 218–220.
3. Perry J. Anatomy and biomechanics of the shoulder in throwing, swimming, gymnastics and tennis. *Clin Sports Med* 1983;2(2): 247–270.
4. Richardson A, Jobe F, Collins H. The shoulder in competitive swimming. *Am J Sports Med* 1980;8:159–163.
5. Hawkins RJ, Morin WD, Bonutti PM. Surgical treatment of full-thickness rotator cuff tears in patients 40 years of age or younger. *J Shoulder Elbow Surgery* 1999;8:259–265.
6. Hawkins RJ, Misamore GW, Hobeika PE. Surgery for full-thickness rotator cuff tears. *J Bone Joint Surg (Am)* 1985;67: 1349–1355.
7. Norwood LA, Barrack R, Jacobson KE. Clinical presentation of complete tears of the rotator cuff. *J Bone Joint Surg (Am)* 1989; 71:499–505.
8. Rizio L, Uribe JW. Overuse injuries of the upper extremity in baseball. *Clin Sports Med* 2001;20:453–468.
9. Neer CS. Anterior acromioplasty for the chronic impingement syndrome in the shoulder. *J Bone Joint Surg (Am)* 1972;54: 41–50.
10. Walch G, Boileau P, Noel E, et al. Impingement of the deep surface of the supraspinatus tendon on the posterosuperior glenoid rim: an arthroscopic study. *J Shoulder Elbow Surg* 1992;1: 238–245.
11. Blevins FT, Hayes WM, Warren RF. Rotator cuff injury in contact athletes. *Am J Sports Med* 1996;24:263–267.
12. Hawkins RJ, Kennedy JC. Impingement syndrome in athletes. *Am J Sports Med* 1980;8:151–158.
13. Neer CS II. Impingement lesions. *Clin Orthop* 1983;173:70–77.
14. Yocum L. Assessing the shoulder: history, physical, differential diagnosis and special test. *Clin Sports Med* 1983;2:281–289.
15. Bigliani LU, Cordasco FA, McIlveen SJ, et al. Operative treatment of massive rotator cuff tears: long term results. *J Shoulder Elbow Surg* 1992;1:120–130.
16. Gerber C, Krushell RJ. Isolated rupture of the tendon of the subscapularis muscle. *J Bone Joint Surg (Br)* 1991;73(3):389–394.
17. Tokish JM, Decker MJ, Ellis HB, Torry MR, Hawkins RJ. The belly press test for the physical examination of the subscapularis muscle: electromyographic validation and comparison to the lift-off test. *J Shoulder Elbow Surg* 2003;12:427–430.
18. Weiner DS, Macnab I. Superior migration of the humeral head. A radiological aid in the diagnosis of tears of the rotator cuff. *J Bone Joint Surg (Br)* 1970;52(3):524–527.
19. Ellman H, Hanker G, Bayer M. Repair of the rotator cuff. *J Bone Joint Surg (Am)* 1986;68(8):1136–1144.
20. Bigliani LU, Morrison DS, April EW. The morphology of the acromion and its relationship to rotator cuff tears. *Orthop Trans* 1986;10:216.
21. Nakagawa S, Yoneda M, Hayashida K, et al. Greater tuberosity notch: an important indicator of articular-side partial rotator cuff tears in the shoulders of throwing athletes. *Am J Sports Med* 2001;29:762–770.
22. Hawkins RJ, Hobeika PE. Impingement syndrome in the athletic shoulder. *Clin Sports Med* 1983;2:391–405.
23. Tibone JE, Jobe FW, Kerlan RK, et al. Shoulder impingement syndrome in athletes treated by an anterior acromioplasty. *Clin Orthop* 1985;198:134–140.
24. Fly WR, Tibone JE, Glousman RE, et al. Arthroscopic subacromial decompression in athletes less than 40 years old. *Orthop Trans* 1983;7:170.
25. Arroyo JS, Hershon SJ, Bigliani LU. Special considerations in the athletic throwing shoulder. *Orthop Clin North Am* 1997;28:69–78.
26. Bigliani LU, D'Alessandro DR, Duralde XA, et al. Anterior

acromioplasty for subacromial impingement in patients younger than 40 years of age. *Clin Orthop* 1989:246:111–116.

27. Roye RP, Grana WA, Yates CK: Arthroscopic subacromial decompression: two to seven year follow up. *Arthroscopy* 1995;11: 301–306.

28. Ha'eri GB, Wiley AM. Shoulder impingement syndrome: results of operative release. *Clin Orthop* 1982;168:128–132.

29. Jackson DW. Chronic rotator cuff impingement in the throwing athlete. *Am J Sports Med* 1976;4:231–240.

30. Satterlee CC. Successful osteosynthesis of an unstable mesoacromion in 6 shoulders: a new technique. *J Shoulder Elbow Surg* 1999;8:125–129.

31. Esch JC, Ozerkis LR, Helgager JA. Arthroscopic subacromial decompression: results according to the degree of rotator cuff tear. *Arthroscopy* 1988;4:241–249.

32. Patte D. Classification of rotator cuff lesions. *Clin Orthop* 1990; 254:81–86.

33. Snyder SJ. Rotator cuff lesions, acute and chronic. *Clin Sports Med* 1991;10:595–614.

34. Post M, Silver R, Singh M. Rotator cuff tear. Diagnosis and treatment. *Clin Orthop* 1983;173:78–91.

35. Bassett RW, Cofield RH. Acute tears of the rotator cuff. The timing of surgical repair. *Clin Orthop* 1983;175:18–24.

36. Cofield RH. Subscapular muscle transposition for repair of chronic rotator cuff tears. *Surg Gynecol Obstet* 1982;154:667–672.

37. Iannotti JP, Williams GR. *Disorders of the shoulder: diagnosis and management.* New York: Lippincott Williams & Wilkins, 1999:63.

38. Meister K, Andrews JR. Classification and treatment of rotator cuff injuries in the overhand athlete. *J Orthop Sports Phys Ther* 1993;18:413–421.

39. Cofield RH. Rotator cuff disease of the shoulder. *J Bone Joint Surg (Am)* 1985;67:974–979.

40. Tibone JE, Elrod B, Jobe FW, et al. Surgical treatment of tears of the rotator cuff in athletes. *J Bone Joint Surg (Am)* 1986;68: 887–891.

41. Bigliani LU, Kimmel J, McCann PD, et al. Repair of rotator cuff tears in tennis players. *Am J Sports Med* 1992;20:112–117.

42. Sonnery-Cottet B, Edwards TB, Noe E, et al. Rotator cuff tears in middle-aged tennis players: results of surgical treatment. *Am J Sports Med* 2002;30:558–564.

43. Rockwood CA, Williams GR, Burkhead WZ. Debridement of degenerative, irreparable lesions of the rotator cuff. *J Bone Joint Surg (Am)* 1995;77:857–866.

44. Ellman H, Kay SP, Wirth M. Arthroscopic treatment of full-thickness rotator cuff tears: 2 to 7 year follow up study. *Arthroscopy* 1993;9:195–200.

45. Cofield RH, Hoffmeyer P, Lanzar WH. Surgical repair of chronic rotator cuff tears. *Orthop Trans* 1990;14:251–252.

46. Hattrup SJ. Rotator cuff repair: relevance of patient age. *J Shoulder Elbow Surg* 1995;4:95–100.

47. Pollock RG, Black AD, Self EB, et al. Surgical management of rotator cuff disease. *J Shoulder Elbow Surg* 1996;5:S37.

48. Gartsman GM, Khan M, Hammerman SM. Arthroscopic repair of full-thickness tears of the rotator cuff. *J Bone Joint Surg (Am)* 1998;80:832–839.

49. Liu SH, Baker CL. Arthroscopically assisted rotator cuff repair: correlation of functional results with integrity of the cuff. *Arthroscopy* 1994;10:54–61.

50. Calvert P, Packer N, Stoker D, et al. Arthrography f the shoulder after operative repair of the torn rotator cuff. *J Bone Joint Surg (Br)* 1986;68(1):147–150.

51. Packer NP, Calvert PT, Bayley JIL, et al. Operative treatment of chronic ruptures of the rotator cuff of the shoulder. *J Bone Joint Surg (Br)* 1983;65:171–175.

12

UNIDIRECTIONAL ANTERIOR INSTABILITY

RUSSELL F. WARREN
WILLIAM D. PRICKETT

INTRODUCTION AND HISTORICAL REVIEW

The act of throwing places unique demands on the stabilizing structures of the glenohumeral joint, and over 50% of college or professional baseball pitchers report shoulder pain (1). The overhead athlete must maintain precise control of the ball while generating significant stresses upon the bony and soft tissue restraints of the shoulder. These athletes may display a spectrum of instability ranging from asymptomatic translation to symptomatic subluxation. This difference is often subtle, especially considering the relative increased joint laxity present in throwers compared with nonthrowers (2). Instability is defined as a pathologic increase in glenohumeral translation that results in symptoms (3).

Anatomy and Biomechanics

The act of throwing involves a transfer of kinetic energy from the lower extremities and trunk to the upper extremity. The sequence of events in overhand throwing has been well documented and consists of six phases (Fig. 12-1): windup, stride, arm cocking, arm acceleration, arm deceleration, and follow-through (4–6). Throughout the process, the arm is maintained in approximately 100 degrees of abduction with external rotation reaching 175 degrees in the cocking phase and 105 degrees of internal rotation in the follow-through phase (7,8). Dillman and colleagues (4) estimated the speed of ball acceleration to be 7,000 degrees per second, with a torque estimate of 52 Nm in baseball pitchers. Additional analysis has shown that the humeral head experiences an anterior translation force of 40% body weight during the cocking phase and a distraction force equivalent to 80% body weight during follow-through. Given the supraphysiologic loads placed on the surrounding soft tissues of the shoulder, subtle increases in translation may result in marked symptoms in overhead athletes.

Shoulder stability is a function of static and dynamic restraints. The static restraints are primarily the capsuloligamentous structures, with mild contributions from articular congruity and negative intraarticular pressure. The dynamic restraints consist primarily of the periarticular musculature. The anterior capsuloligamentous complex, as described by Flood in 1829 (9), consists of the anterior shoulder capsule with its relatively constant capsular thickenings that comprise the superior, middle, and inferior glenohumeral ligaments. The coracohumeral ligament (CHL), another thickening of the anterior capsule, originates from the base of the coracoid and inserts into the greater and lesser tuberosities (10). The superior glenohumeral ligament (SGHL) originates anterior to the long head of the biceps at the supraglenoid tubercle and inserts slightly anterior to the biceps tendon into the lesser tuberosity (10). The middle glenohumeral ligament (MGHL) originates from the anterior labrum between the 1- and 3-o'clock positions and inserts into the lesser tuberosity with the subscapularis (11). As described by DePalma and co-workers (12), the MGHL has the greatest variation in size of all the ligaments of the shoulder and has two morphologic variations: (a) sheetlike, which is confluent with the inferior glenohumeral labral (IGHL) complex, or (b) cordlike with a sublabral foramen. The IGHL complex consists of an anterior band, posterior band, and an intervening pouch. The anterior band originates from the anteroinferior glenoid labrum and periosteum and inserts into the anteroinferior humeral anatomic neck. The posterior band originates from the posteroinferior glenoid and inserts into the posteroinferior anatomic neck of the humerus. The intervening pouch connects the anterior and posterior bands of the IGHL while cradling the humeral head inferiorly (13).

The individual ligaments of the shoulder become taut at varying degrees of glenohumeral motion. The anterior band of the IGHL complex dampens anterior and inferior humeral translation with increasing amounts of humeral abduction (14,15). At lower levels of abduction, the

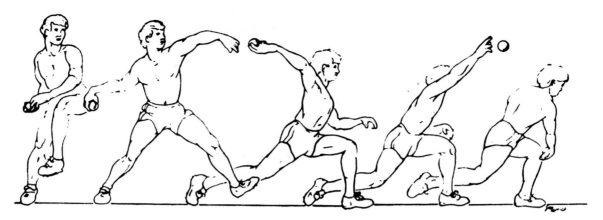

FIGURE 12-1. The five phases of pitching a baseball (from left to right) wind-up, early cocking, late cocking, acceleration, and follow-through. Wind-up or preparation: Preliminary activity dominated by flexion of the upper extremity, with both hands holding the ball. Early cocking: A period of abduction and external rotation of the shoulder that begins as the ball is released from the nondominant hand. Late cocking: Contact of the forward foot with the ground divides this stage from early cocking. Late cocking continues until maximum external rotation at the shoulder is attained. Acceleration: Starts with the posture of maximum abduction and external rotation at the shoulder and continues until release of the ball, as the ball leaves the fingers. Follow-through: The final interval of motion as the arm flexes and internally rotates across the chest and is decelerated. (From Glousman R, Jobe F, Tibone J, et al. Dynamic electromyographic analysis of the throwing shoulder with glenohumeral instability *J Bone Joint Surg [Am]* 1988;70:220–226, with permission.)

MGHL limits anterior humeral translation and when the arm is at the side, the SGHL and CHL resist inferior humeral translation (14,15). The function of the biceps tendon with respect to shoulder stability is controversial. It has been reported to depress the humeral head and decrease the load sustained in the IGHL complex, (16,17) while others have noted essentially no functional role in dynamic stability and only a questionable role as a static restraint to excessive glenohumeral motion (18).

EMG (electromyography) analysis has helped provide insight into the dynamic constraints and firing patterns of the shoulder musculature during the overhead throw (19) (Fig. 12-2). The pitching motion is a complex interplay of several muscles, which combine in precise firing patterns to provide a fluid and forceful overhand throw. The rotator cuff functions to maintain stability and initiate motion, while the other muscles generate force during acceleration and dampen distraction during follow-through (5,20–24).

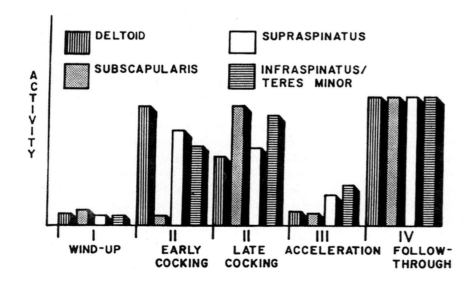

FIGURE 12-2. A summary of the muscle activity during the stages of a throw or pitch. (From Jobe FW, Tibone JE, Perry J, et al. An EMG analysis of the shoulder in throwing and pitching. A preliminary report. *Am J Sports Med* 1983;11:3–5, with permission.)

ETIOLOGY OF INJURY

In the overhead athlete, mild incompetence of the anterior restraints (secondary to repetitive microtrauma or fatigue and dyssynchrony of the dynamic stabilizers) may allow subtle amounts of increased humeral head translation with respect to the glenoid. Normally, with the arm abducted 90 degrees as it is externally rotated, the humeral head translates posteriorly. This coupled posterior translation occurring with external rotation at 90 degrees of abduction may be decreased or anterior translation may occur in the setting of anterior laxity. These altered mechanics may strain the posterosuperior rotator cuff to an increasing degree with resultant rotator cuff tears. This concept has been described by Walch and colleagues (25) and by Jobe and co-workers (26) and has been coined as "internal impingement." The increased contact of the posterior supraspinatus and infraspinatus on the posterosuperior glenoid in the late cocking/early acceleration phase may cause pain and weakness that further accentuate the athlete's underlying anterior microinstability (27).

Shoulder instability in the thrower rarely reaches proportions of frank dislocation unless the athlete experiences an isolated high external load such as a quarterback sack or sliding headfirst into a base. When macroscopic instability occurs, detachment of the IGHL complex from the anterior glenoid is the most common defect noted (28). This injury has been referred to as the *Bankart lesion* (29), although it has been proven to be more than one defect and it exists as a spectrum of lesions that render the IGHL complex incompetent. These defects may occur along the entire course of the anterior IGHL complex, ranging from anterior labroligaruentous periosteal sleeve avulsions (ALPSA) to humeral avulsion of the glenohumeral ligament (HAGL). Bigliani and co-workers (30) loaded the IGHL complex to failure and noted defects at the glenoid insertion (40%), midsubstance (35%), and humeral origin (25%). Importantly, when the complex failed at one location, it underwent significant plastic deformation in other regions. This was clinically evident in Rowe's series (31,32), which showed greater than 50% of patients with instability had abnormal capsular redundancy. Additional studies by Turkel and colleagues (33) and Warren (34) have emphasized the importance of a circumferential injury pattern in the shoulder with macroscopic instability; thus, not only does an anterior dislocation occur with an anterior injury (Bankart lesion) but also some form of posterior injury often exists. The posterior injury may take the form of a capsuloligamentous disruption or a bony injury (posterosuperior humeral impaction fracture).

In addition to the attenuation of the anterior capsulolabral tissue and the articular sided partial thickness rotator cuff tears of the infraspinatus, other structures may also be affected by the increased humeral translation with respect to the glenoid. Abnormal superior elevation of the humeral head may allow for subacromial impingement, and excess distraction during follow-through may place increased tensile stress on the rotator cuff or the long head of the biceps and its origin from the superior glenolabral complex.

PRESENTATION AND PHYSICAL EXAMINATION

The symptoms of shoulder instability in the throwing athlete are usually more subtle than those of the nonthrower. Throwers often present with symptoms of pain, decreased ball velocity, decreased control, occasionally "dead arm" syndrome, and, rarely, actual episodes of subluxation or dislocation. It is unlikely that an elite thrower would present with recurrent gross instability because the athlete would be unable to function at or even near their maximal throwing effort and would thus gravitate to nonthrowing positions.

The location of the athlete's pain and the phase of throwing are important clues as to the etiology of the thrower's symptoms. Internal impingement with anterior capsulolabral stretch typically results in pain at the posterior joint line during the cocking phase and early acceleration phase when the humerus experiences maximal external rotation (25,35). Throwers who note pain during follow-through often have posterior capsulolabral injury because the internal rotation of follow-through stresses the posteroinferior capsulolabral complex (3).

The bench examination begins with observation for soft tissue symmetry and for any evidence of muscular atrophy or previous incisions. Neck range of motion, strength testing, and provocative maneuvers such as Spurling's test (36) may elicit symptoms of a nerve root compression that may cause pain and affect the dynamic restraints of the glenohumeral joint. Additional pain generators such as the long head of the biceps and superior labrum are tested with provocative maneuvers such as Speed's, Yergason's, and "clunk" (37) tests, the anterior slide test of Kibler (38), and the active compression test of O'Brien (39). The acromioclavicular joint is evaluated by direct palpation and cross body adduction. Subacromial pathology may be evaluated with Hawkins (40) and Neer's (41) tests, and periscapular muscular strength is evaluated by manual muscle force testing.

When evaluating shoulder stability, examination and comparison of the asymptomatic shoulder to the symptomatic shoulder is important. Athletes with anterior microinstability may show increased external rotation and limited internal rotation with the arm abducted 90 degrees secondary to contracture of the posterior rotator cuff or posterior capsule, or due to developmental changes in glenohumeral geometry (42). Anecdotally, it has been suggested that a substantial decrease in internal rotation of the dominant shoulder may predispose the athlete to shoulder pain (3).

Active and passive motion are helpful in assessing the overall function of the shoulder; however, they may be limited by patient apprehension as a result of instability. Strength testing of the periarticular musculature is then carried out with an emphasis on the rotator cuff.

Provocative testing may help localize the athlete's pain. With the arm adducted in the neutral position, inferior stress is applied to the humerus and the acromiohumeral "sulcus" is evaluated. Some authors recommend performing this test in neutral (evaluate inferior capsular and rotator interval laxity) and in external rotation (tensions the rotator interval). Thus (a decrease in the sulcus as) one goes from neutral to external rotation *implies inferior* capsular laxity. By contrast, if the sulcus stays constant, this suggests excessive laxity in the rotator interval. The sulcus may be graded as 0 to 3+ (grade 0 = no increased translation, grade 1+ = mild increased translation of less than 1 cm, grade 2+ = 1 to 2 cm of inferior translation, and grade 3+ = greater than 2 cm of inferior translation (8). The load and shift test centers the humeral head on the glenoid, then anterior and posterior translational stresses are applied to the humerus. The amount of humeral translation during the load and shift is also graded as 0 to 3+ (grade 0 = no increased translation, grade 1+ = mild increased translation to the glenoid rim, grade 2+ = distinct subluxation that reduces passively, and grade 3+ = complete dislocation that requires manual reduction) (8). This test may also elicit mechanical symptoms related to labral or articular defects or apprehension as the athlete anticipates glenohumeral subluxation. The examiner should expect a normal thrower's shoulder to display some increased laxity with true instability existing when a 2+ load and shift test is present (3). The quality of the endpoint in the direction tested is also valuable, in that a solid endpoint essentially excludes macroscopic instability. The apprehension and relocation maneuvers are also valuable in evaluating anterior shoulder instability (Fig. 12-3). The apprehension test is performed by placing the humerus in a position of maximal external rotation at 90 degrees of humeral abduction and assessing the athlete's response to feelings of subluxation or dislocation (43). In this apprehensive position, a posteriorly directed load is applied to the shoulder and an assessment of the symptomatic relief (sense of dislocation) is recorded (43). Positive apprehension and relocation tests are markers for anterior instability. However, if in the position of apprehension the athlete notes posterior shoulder pain that is relieved with the relocation maneuver, then the athlete's symptoms may be due to internal impingement with rotator cuff injury (25). Before the completion of the physical examination, signs of generalized ligamentous laxity are evaluated that may provide clues as to a multidirectional component to the thrower's instability. Following the physical examination, in the setting of a complicated clinical scenario, the physician may augment the clinical evaluation with the use of differential injection techniques. Lastly, upon completion of the bench examination, the physician observes and interacts with the athlete while the athlete is throwing. This allows evaluation of the

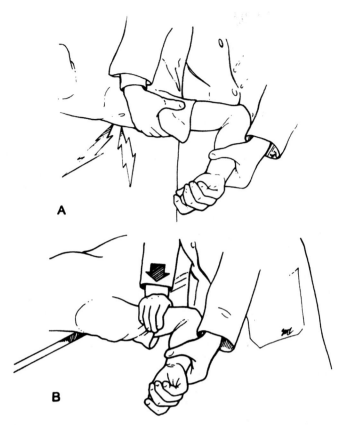

FIGURE 12-3. A: Provocative component of relocation test. Humerus is pulled anteriorly during this part of test. **B:** Posterior force applied to humerus. Positive test is indicated by posterior superior shoulder pain with anteriorly directed force, relieved by subsequent posteriorly directed push. Note maximal external rotation of shoulder throughout both parts of test. (From Davidson PA, Elattrache NS, Jobe CM, et al. Rotator cuff and posterior-superior glenoid labrum injury associated with increased glenohumeral motion: a new site of impingement. *J Shoulder Elbow Surg* 1995;4:384–390, with permission.)

mechanics of the throw and confirms the location of pain during the throwing cycle.

RADIOGRAPHIC AND DIAGNOSTIC EVALUATION

Plain radiographs are an essential supplement to the history and physical examination of the patient with suspected anterior instability. They demonstrate bony integrity, glenohumeral alignment, arthritic changes, loose bodies, and periarticular calcification, and the potential exists to visualize signs of prior subluxations or dislocations. Our standard series includes a true anteroposterior (AP) view in neutral rotation, West Point, outlet, and Stryker notch views. The AP in neutral rotation allows the evaluation of the glenohumeral joint space and large Hill-Sachs lesions may also be evident. The West Point view is especially useful to evaluate

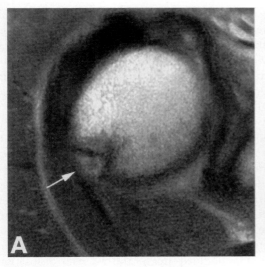
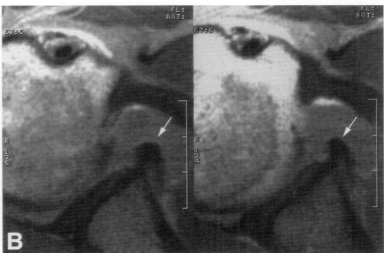
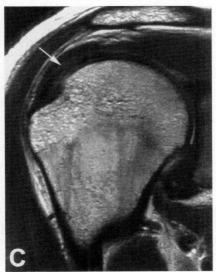

FIGURE 12-4. Axial fast spin-echo sequence in a patient following an acute dislocation demonstrates a defect at the posterolateral aspect of the humeral head (*arrow*) **(A)** and a displaced anterior labral fragment (*arrows*) **(B)** on two consecutive images. **C:** Oblique coronal fast spin-echo sequence demonstrates abnormal signal on the articular side of the rotator cuff (*arrow*). (See corresponding arthroscopic image Fig. 12-8.)

anterior or posterior subluxation or the presence of a bony Bankart lesion. The outlet view confirms humeral location with respect to the glenoid and defines the supraspinatus outlet. The Stryker notch view is used to evaluate the contour of the posterosuperior aspect of the humeral head and evaluate for the presence of a Bennett's lesion due to injury adjacent to the posteroinferior glenoid rim.

Magnetic resonance imaging (MRI) is an invaluable tool in the assessment of the throwing athlete. Using high-quality imaging equipment and software, bony and soft tissue injuries about the throwing shoulder can be evaluated with greater than 90% accuracy (44–46). Precise depiction of the injury pattern using MRI helps with patient education and preoperative planning. Patients may benefit from a more accurate understanding of their injury, prognosis, and, when appropriate, their postoperative expectations. In the throwing athlete with anterior instability, particular attention is directed to the anterior capsulolabral structures, the posterior rotator cuff, and the posterosuperior humeral head (Fig. 12-4).

CLASSIFICATION OF INJURY

Anterior shoulder instability presents as a spectrum of defects, and we have found the classification system of Kvitne and Jobe (43) (Table 12-1) useful. This system allows for an understanding of the pathogenesis and treatment options, and it provides some prognostic information for the athlete. Patients in group I are typically older and display classic subacromial impingement signs. Patients in group II have developed anterior microinstability with subsequent internal impingement. Group III patients present with multidirectional instability, and group IV patients typically have an isolated high external load with resultant glenohumeral dislocation.

TABLE 12–1. CLASSIFICATION OF ANTERIOR SHOULDER INSTABILITY

Group I	Pure impingement No instability
Group II	Primary instability due to chronic labral microtrauma Secondary impingement
Group III	Primary instability due to generalized ligamentous laxity Secondary impingement
Group IV	Pure instability No impingement

From Kvitne RS, Jobe FW. The diagnosis and treatment of anterior instability in the throwing athlete. *Clin Orthop* 1993;107–123, with permission.

NONOPERATIVE TREATMENT, REHABILITATION, AND RESULTS

Rehabilitation of the throwing athlete with anterior shoulder instability is critical. In designing a rehabilitation program, it is important to correctly identify the underlying process and the athlete's goals. Until recently, the mainstay of nonoperative and postoperative treatment of shoulder pain due to instability was strict immobilization. However, improvements in modern understanding of shoulder instability have allowed caregivers to design patient specific programs focusing on strengthening of the periarticular stabilizing muscles (47). Using electromyographic (EMG) analysis in pitchers and nonathletic normal volunteers with anterior instability, Glousman and colleagues (48) demonstrated markedly diminished activity in the pectoralis major, subscapularis, serratus anterior, and latissimus dorsi in the late cocking and acceleration phases of throwing.

This muscular imbalance contributes to and potentially exacerbates anterior instability; based on these deficiencies, a physical therapy program directed to strengthening these muscles may allow for improved success with conservative treatment. This chapter addresses the nonoperative and operative approaches to patients with type II (microscopic) and type IV (macroscopic) instability (43).

In the throwing athlete with internal impingement, an initial period of rest with inflammatory control using nonsteroidal antiinflammatory drugs (NSAIDs) and physical therapy modalities is implemented. The majority of these athletes demonstrate excessive external rotation, limited internal rotation, and posterior capsular tightness. The rehabilitation program initially focuses on a stretching program that includes cross body adduction and abduction with internal rotation. A generalized muscular strengthening program (as outlined later for the traumatic dislocation) is then implemented. Additional, exercise drills such as rhythmic stabilization in mid motion, end-range proprioceptive training, and perturbation training may improve neuromuscular control and augment the dynamic stabilization of the shoulder joint (49,50) .

The athlete with internal impingement may return to a gradual throwing program once there is full motion, normal strength, and an absence of apprehension or impingement signs. To provide proper muscle balance, the external rotator muscles should be at least 65% of the strength of the internal rotators (49). When the athlete begins the interval throwing program, the mechanics should be carefully scrutinized, because some throwers who exhibit internal impingement allow their arm to lag behind the scapula (Fig. 12-5). This "hyperangulation," as described by Jobe and colleagues (51), leads to excessive strain on the anterior capsule and may exacerbate impingement of the posterior rota-

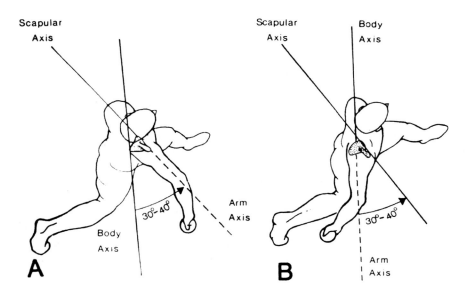

FIGURE 12-5. Angular relationships of body axis, scapula, and upper arm are demonstrated during acceleration phase of throwing. **A:** Normal, with scapula and arm being collinear. Note that both arm and scapular axes are forward of body axis. **B:** Arm lags behind scapula, which would increase angular torques acting on glenohumeral joint. (From Davidson PA, Elattrache NS, Jobe CM, et al. Rotator cuff and posterior-superior glenoid labrum injury associated with increased glenohumeral motion: a new site of impingement. *J Shoulder Elbow Surg* 1995;4:384–390, with permission.)

tor cuff. Muscle endurance exercises are also emphasized in the return to throwing, as numerous studies have shown altered mechanics, proximal humeral migration, and diminished proprioception as fatigue occurs in the throwing athlete (52,53).

The treatment of the throwing athlete with macroscopic instability (type IV) is generally operative. Following an initial episode of a traumatic subluxation or dislocation, an MRI scan is useful to note labral injury; if detachment is seen, then surgical repair is advised. If only capsular stretch is present, protection and rehabilitation may be useful. The early rehabilitation program for the thrower who elects nonoperative treatment focuses on an initial period of immobilization while inflammation is brought under control using NSAIDs and physical therapy modalities. The time allotted for immobilization following an acute dislocation is debated, and a lack of correlation between length of immobilization and recurrence is a common theme (54–58). This lack of correlation may be due to a nonanatomic reapproximation of the Bankart lesion to the anteroinferior glenoid, as well as an interstitial injury sustained by the IGHL complex. However, when a focused rehabilitation program is implemented after an initial period of immobilization, redislocation rates in nonthrowers have decreased (59,60).

After the acute pain of the dislocation resolves, the patient is instructed to begin deltoid isometric contractions and gentle pendulum exercises. The athlete may then progress to isotonic exercises within a pain-free range of motion, using Therabands (Hygienic, Akron, Ohio), surgical tubing, or weights. As the pain and subjective sense of shoulder subluxation resolves, the dynamic glenohumeral stabilizers (rotator cuff, deltoid, pectoralis major, and latissimus dorsi) are strengthened using a set of four exercises as described by Townsend and colleagues (61). The scapular stabilizers consisting of the trapezius, levator scapulae, rhomboid major and minor, and the middle and lower serratus anterior are also addressed using a core group of additional exercises as described by Moseley and colleagues (62). Isokinetic exercises are a useful adjunct, and approximately 4 to 6 months after the shoulder dislocation, a gradual return to a throwing program is commenced. The thrower is allowed to return to competition when range of motion is full, apprehension is eliminated, and strength is comparable to the contralateral shoulder. Athletes must be cautioned against the high rate of recurrence given their age, repetitive provocative arm positioning, and potential for recurrent high external loads to the shoulder.

OPERATIVE TREATMENT, REHABILITATION, AND RESULTS

Operative treatment of anterior shoulder instability is primarily reserved for those athletes who fail conservative treatment or those with a high likelihood of recurrent instability such as the thrower with a traumatic dislocation. Successful operative treatment in these patients lies in establishing the correct diagnosis of a defined lesion in a motivated patient who will comply with a strict postoperative rehabilitation program.

The spectrum of anterior glenohumeral instability and its associated findings may be treated entirely through an open procedure or an arthroscopic approach. The anterior capsulolabral laxity may be treated by repair of avulsed structures (e.g., Bankart lesion), capsulorrhaphy, capsular imbrication, or thermal modification of the tissue. The goal of these approaches focuses on regaining function while alleviating symptomatic anterior laxity.

The most common disorder affecting the overhead thrower is internal impingement resulting from anterior microinstability with or without an associated articular sided partial thickness rotator cuff tear of the infraspinatus. Surgical approaches have included open and, more recently, arthroscopic anterior stabilization procedures. The anterior capsulolabral reconstruction (ACLR) described by Jobe for throwers with anterior instability has stood the test of time (63) (Fig. 12-6). This procedure is performed through a subscapularis muscle–splitting approach and the capsule is divided horizontally from the humeral anatomic neck to the glenoid neck. A T-plasty of the capsule is then performed along the glenoid neck, providing exposure of the anterior labrum and IGHL complex. As per the original description, suture anchors are then placed 2 to 3 mm medial to the intact articular cartilage, and the capsular flaps are tensioned to allow 90 degrees of humeral abduction and 75 to 80 degrees of humeral external rotation. If a Bankart lesion is found, the labrum is divided and elevated with the respective superior and inferior capsular flaps and the tissue is incorporated into the capsular reconstruction. The rehabilitation program begins on the first postoperative day and gradually progresses from gentle range-of-motion exercises to muscle strengthening exercises over the subsequent 6 months. Patients then begin a progressive throwing program once they display 80% strength of the contralateral shoulder. Unrestricted athletic activity is allowed when muscle synchrony, strength, power, and endurance have normalized. The results of this reconstruction have been reported in a large series of elite athletes involved in overhead sports (105 patients: 38 professional, 25 collegiate, 42 recreational) with 68% of professional, 80% of collegiate, and 86% of recreational athletes returning to their prior level of play at an average of 1 year (64). In the subgroup of elite baseball pitchers, 60% returned to their previous level of competition.

A modification of the ACLR by Jobe (63) was described by Altchek and co-workers (65). This modification (Fig. 12-7) eliminates the T-plasty along the glenoid rim and imbricates the horizontal capsulotomy in a pants-over-vest fashion, with the arm in at least 60 degrees of scapular

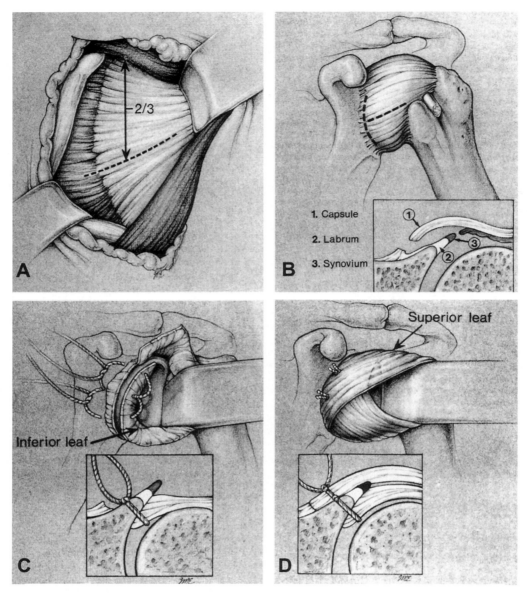

FIGURE 12-6. Anterior capsulolabral reconstruction. **A:** Anterior view of the left shoulder. The incision is made in the "safe" interval at the junction of the middle third and the lowest third of the muscle and tendinous portion of the subscapularis. **B:** Anterior view of the left shoulder showing T-shaped incision in the capsule and synovial lining. **C:** The inferior capsule flap is shifted superiorly to lie within the margin of the joint. **D:** The superior capsular flap is shifted inferiorly outside the joint. (From Jobe FW, Giangarra CE, Kvitne RS, et al. Anterior capsulolabral reconstruction of the shoulder in athletes in overhand sports. *Am J Sports Med* 1991;19:428–434, with permission.)

abduction and 90 degrees of external rotation. This modification attempts to avoid overtightening the anterior structures with resultant loss of external rotation. The postoperative protocol is similar to that described for the ACLR, with return to throwing when strength is approximately 80% of the contralateral extremity.

Arthroscopic treatment of internal impingement has evolved, with a premise that minimizing anterior shoulder dissection will result in fewer postoperative limitations of external rotation. This approach initially focused on isolated debridement of the partial thickness rotator cuff tear, but results have been marginal with respect to return to sport and relief of symptoms. Riand and co-workers (66) reported their results of isolated debridement in 75 overhead athletes with internal impingement, and no elite throwers returned to their previous level of competition and their overall satisfaction rate was 40%. Payne and colleagues also reported their results of isolated debridement in ath-

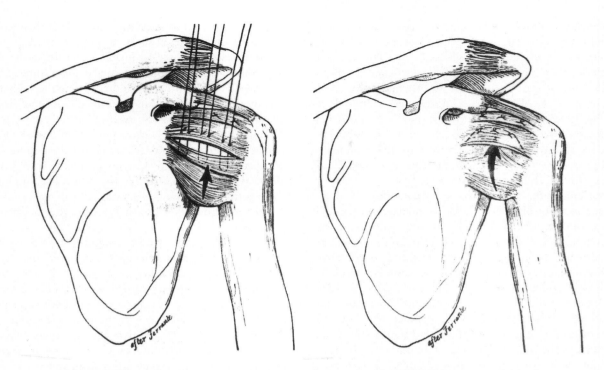

FIGURE 12-7. Technique for capsular repair when there is no labral detachment. **A:** The horizontal capsular incision is plicated using mattress sutures. **B:** The completed capsular plication. (From Altchek DW, Dines DM. Shoulder injuries in the throwing athlete. *J Am Acad Orthop Surg* 1995;3:159–165, with permission.)

letes younger than 40 years old, and their rate of return to sport at the same level of competition ranged from 25% to 64% (67).

Given the poor results of isolated debridement of partial thickness rotator cuff tears due to internal impingement, Levitz and colleagues (68) compared debridement with debridement plus thermal capsulorrhaphy in baseball players. The debridement was performed in standard fashion, and the thermal capsulorrhaphy was performed using the Oratec monopolar radiofrequency probe (Oratec, Menlo Park, California). Radiofrequency energy allows heating of collagenous tissue with resultant collagen denaturization and tissue shrinkage (69–71). The technique of thermal capsulorrhaphy, as described by Levitz and colleagues (68), consisted of slowly "painting" the shoulder capsule initially through the anterior portal beginning at the IGHL and progressing toward the rotator interval. The probe was then switched to the posterior portal and the posterior inferior portion of the IGHL was "painted." Patients in the debridement-only group returned to sport at an average of 7.2 months after surgery, but at 2.5 years only 67% were competing compared with 90% of athletes in the debridement plus thermal capsulorrhaphy group. Patients in this later group displayed a 7-degree asymptomatic loss of external rotation compared with the debridement only group. The experience at our institution with thermal capsulorrhaphy

has been less successful, with a 31% failure rate due to recurrent instability or pain (72).

An alternative surgical approach to internal impingement has focused on the osseous adaptive changes present in the proximal humerus. Riand and colleagues (42) used a proximal humeral derotational osteotomy with a subscapularis myorrhaphy in 20 European throwers who had failed arthroscopic debridement. They reported only 55% of throwing athletes were able to return to their previous level of competition and recommended this surgery only as an option after failure of all other forms of treatment.

A subpopulation of overhead athletes with anterior instability may suffer from a more global instability pattern rather than internal impingement. These athletes display multidirectional instability (MDI) with inferior capsular laxity and more anterior than posterior laxity. Numerous studies have analyzed the results of surgical treatment in these patients; however, results are limited in overhead athletes. Bigliani and colleagues (73) reviewed 68 shoulders in athletes (10 elite overhead throwers) treated with a laterally based capsular shift procedure with overall excellent results; however, only 50% of elite throwers returned to their previous level of competition. Altchek and colleagues (74) described a T-plasty modification of the Bankart procedure for multidirectional instability of the anterior and inferior types. In this modification, the subscapularis is detached laterally and a transverse capsulotomy is made from the humeral neck to the mid glenoid and the capsule is "T'ed" from superior to inferior at the glenoid neck. The superior and inferior flaps are then closed in a pants-over-vest fashion. The overall satisfaction rate in Altchek's series was excellent in 95% of patients (74). However, only three throwing athletes were in this cohort and each noted the inability to throw a ball with as much velocity as before the operation. Arthroscopic modifications to the aforementioned procedures have been used, but their use in overhead athletes with MDI has not been reported.

Occasionally, the overhead athlete may sustain an acute first time anterior dislocation and the management is primarily operative. The likelihood of a successful nonoperative program is unlikely given their numerous risk factors for recurrence, including their age, recurrent provocative arm positioning, and the potential for another forcefully applied external load (54,57–59). Given the paucity of literature, for the overhead athlete who sustains an anterior dislocation, one must turn to the contact athlete for a marker of surgical treatment options and results. There are numerous reports of open shoulder stabilization with excellent results with respect to recurrence (73,75,76). However, given the low tolerance for motion loss, throwers are typically managed with an arthroscopic technique. Arthroscopic Bankart repair has been described using staples, transglenoid sutures, cannulated bioabsorbable implants, and suture anchors. More than 60 studies have reviewed redislocation rates using these techniques with recurrence rates typically ranging from 10% to 20% (77). Laurencin and colleagues noted improved arthroscopic results in patients with a history of traumatic unidirectional instability, a Bankart lesion, a robust IGHL, and minimal bony erosions (78).

COMPLICATIONS

A successful surgical result in the throwing athlete must avoid recurrence of instability while allowing sufficient external rotation to allow the athlete to throw at their preoperative level. This delicate balance is difficult to achieve as is evidenced by the lower return to sport rates of throwers compared with nonthrowers. Common reported complications after anterior shoulder surgery include recurrence of instability and stiffness and, rarely, such problems as neurovascular injury, infection, subscapularis rupture, intraarticular hardware, and postinstability repair arthritis. No recent report of postinstability repair arthritis in overhead throwers has been published and complications such as infection, subscapularis failure, and placement of hardware into the shoulder joint can be eliminated with meticulous attention to surgical detail and postoperative patient compliance. The typical nonthrowing athlete who has no evidence of recurrent anterior instability but lacks 10 to 20 degrees of external rotation may function at their preoperative level and be considered a surgical success, but the throwing athlete would be unable to return to throwing at a previous level and would be considered a surgical failure.

Open shoulder procedures that violate the subscapularis are more at risk to limit motion and overconstrain the shoulder. In the series of overhead throwers reported by Montgomery (64), 69% of all pitchers and 60% of professional pitchers were able to return to their same level of competition. They reported no problems with infection, nerve damage, or hardware migration. The modification proposed by Altchek and colleagues (3) may avoid overtightening of the anterior structures and thus preserve external rotation.

Historically, arthroscopic instability repairs were more likely to develop recurrence of symptoms rather than stiffness. Cole and colleagues (77) reviewed more than 60 recent studies comparing recurrence rates of anterior shoulder instability after arthroscopic anterior capsulolabral reconstruction and consistently found redislocation rates to be approximately 10% to 20%. Many of these studies have recurrence rates that decrease as surgeon experience increases, and most of these arthroscopic repairs are in nonthrowers.

The modification of capsular tissue with thermal energy has gained recent popularity; as with other techniques, complications of this procedure include recurrence of preoperative symptoms. However, Levitz and co-workers reported only a 10% failure rate in elite overhead throwers (68) with internal impingement secondary to anterior microinstability. Anderson and colleagues (79) reported on a larger nonthrowing population and determined specific risk factors for early failure, which included a history of prior shoulder surgery, multiple dislocations, a component of MDI, and a return to contact sports. However, reports of axillary neuritis, capsulitis, and capsular deficiency have been noted during revision surgery for recurrent symptoms following thermal capsulorrhaphy (80). The biomechanical properties of the capsular tissue may also be adversely altered, to an unknown extent, as time of exposure and temperature increase (81,82). This may predispose patients to a recurrence of symptoms and possibly capsular deficiency. We have stopped using the technique of thermal capsulorrhaphy based on an unacceptably high (31%) recurrence rate seen in our patient population with anterior subluxation or dislocation (72).

AUTHORS' PREFERRED TREATMENT

A thorough history, physical examination, and review of imaging studies is performed in the manner described in this chapter. After a diagnosis is reached, a detailed discussion with the athlete and athletic trainer regarding the benefits and complications of nonoperative and operative treatment is undertaken. Overhead athletes with anterior microinstability who have failed conservative treatment and those with macroscopic anterior instability are indicated for surgery.

The operative treatment begins with an interscalene block and positioning in the beach chair position. Examination under anesthesia is performed, testing for passive range of motion and instability. The amount of sulcus, anterior, and posterior translation are graded 0 to 3+. Diagnostic arthroscopy follows the examination under anesthesia. A spinal needle localizes the anterior portal high and lateral in the rotator interval, thus allowing a second portal to be placed more inferior through the rotator interval as needed. Following a complete diagnostic arthroscopy, the arthroscope is placed through the anterior portal to fully evaluate the tissue quality and determine the extent of the anterior capsulolabral attenuation. The final surgical plan is devised upon collaboration of the history, clinical examination, imaging studies, examination under anesthesia, and diagnostic arthroscopy (Table 12-2).

Overhead throwers are treated with an all arthroscopic method unless they display 3+ anterior laxity and/or 3+ inferior laxity, or if they have markedly attenuated anterior capsulolabral tissue. We initially address the partial thickness rotator cuff tear by debriding the articular surface of the rotator cuff with a 4.5-mm curved or straight full radius shaver (Fig. 12-8). If the rotator cuff tear encompasses more than 50% of the thickness of the tendon, we debride the remnant and proceed with arthroscopic rotator cuff repair. Next, we address the anterior capsulolabral complex, viewing from the posterior portal. The athlete with internal impingement typically has an intact but moderately attenuated anterior capsulolabral complex without a classic Bankart lesion. We superficially abrade the anterior labrum and capsular complex with a 4.5-mm shaver. A second rotator interval portal just superior to the subscapularis is estab-

lished using either a 6.25 mm or 8 mm × 7 cm Arthrex clear screw-in cannula (Arthrex, Naples, Florida). We then pass a series of sutures (typically three) through the IGHL and anterior capsule and imbricate the IGHL and capsular tissue to the intact labrum. We start inferior at the 5- or 6-o'clock position on the glenoid and pass the Spectrum hook (Spectrum Tissue Repair System, Linvatec, Largo, Florida) loaded with a 2-0 Prolene suture (polypropylene suture, Ethicon, Somerville, New Jersey) into the IGHL approximately 1 cm away from the labrum and then advance this tissue to the articular margin of the glenoid. The Prolene limbs are then grasped and brought out the high anterior portal. A no. 2 Ethibond suture (Ethibond Excel polyester suture, Ethicon, Somerville, New Jersey) is shuttled through the tissue using the Prolene suture. The limbs are retrieved through the clear cannula and the knots are tied in standard arthroscopic technique imbricating the IGHL complex to the glenoid margin (Fig. 12-9). We rarely imbricate or close the rotator interval in overhead athletes given the propensity to limit external rotation.

Athletes with 3+ instability, Bankart's lesion, and a robust IGHL are also candidates for arthroscopic reconstruction. Standard diagnostic arthroscopy is performed with attention to the documentation of associated injuries such as a Hill-Sachs lesion. As described earlier, our repair technique is similar to that of the capsular imbrication procedure, except we use a biodegradable anchor placed into the glenoid articular margin at a 45-degree angle to the surface. One limb is shuttled around the avulsed tissue and then the sutures are tied using an arthroscopic technique (Fig. 12-10). It is imperative to mobilize the Bankart's lesion before repair, because it often scars inferior and medial to its insertion on the glenoid articular margin. A 4.5-mm shaver or bone rasp is placed through the anterior portal and is positioned between the anterior labrum and the glenoid to debride the bone to a cancellous bleeding

TABLE 12–2. AUTHOR'S PREFERRED TREATMENT ALGORITHM

Clinical Diagnosis	Exam Under Anesthesia[a,b]	Pathology	Tissue Quality	Procedure
Microscopic instability with internal impingement	0/1+ anterior	Capsular laxity +/- PTRCT	Good	Arthroscopic capsular plication (+/-) debride PTRCT
Macroscopic instability	2+/3+ anterior 0/1+/2+ inferior	(+) Bankart lesion	Good	Arthroscopic Bankart repair
	2+/3+ anterior 0/1+/2+ inferior	(+/-) Bankart lesion	Poor	Open capsular shift (+/-) Bankart repair
	2+ anterior 0/1+/2+ inferior	(-) Bankart lesion	Good	Arthroscopic capsular plication
	3+ anterior 0/1+/2+ inferior	(-) Bankart lesion	Good	Open capsular shift (+/-) Bankart repair
	Any anterior 3+ inferior	(+/-) Bankart	Any lesion	Open capsular shift (+/-) Bankart repair

[a]Anterior load and shift: 0 = no translation; 1+ = translation to glenoid rim; 2+ = dislocation with spontaneous reduction; 3+ = locked dislocation.
[b]Sulcus sign: 0 = no sulcus; 1+ = <1 cm; 2+ = 1–2 cm; 3+ = >2 cm.
PTRCT, partial thickness rotator cuff tear.

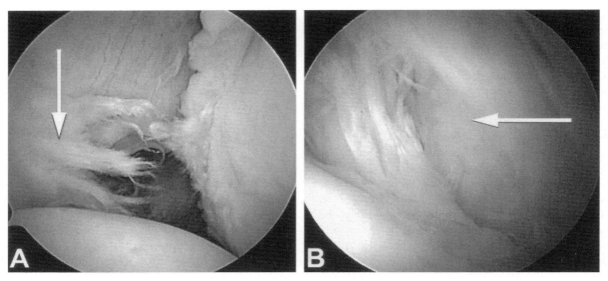

FIGURE 12-8. A: Arthroscopic images of an articular sided partial thickness rotator cuff tear *(arrow)* encompassing less than 50% of the thickness of the tendon insertion. **B:** The same partial thickness tear after debridement *(arrow).*

surface and to fully mobilize the IGHL complex. The Bankart's lesion and attached IGHL are then imbricated to the articular margin.

In the overhead athlete with deficient anterior capsulolabral tissue or marked inferior instability in whom an arthroscopic repair is less likely to be successful, we proceed with an open anterior capsular shift. The shoulder is approached through an anteroinferior incision in the axillary fold. The deltopectoral interval is identified and the cephalic vein is retracted laterally. The clavipectoral fascia is divided and a self-retaining retractor is placed deep to the

deltoid muscle, providing exposure of the subscapularis and anterior humeral circumflex vessels. We then split the muscular portion of the subscapularis in line with its fibers from the humeral insertion to the glenoid neck. The interval between the subscapularis and the capsule is bluntly developed with an elevator. The capsule is the divided in line with the subscapularis split. In the event of gross capsular redundancy with a Bankart lesion, the capsule is T'ed along

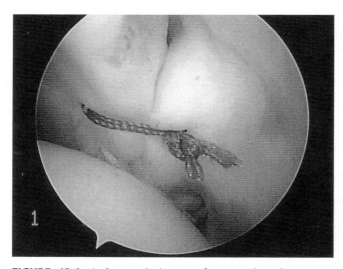

FIGURE 12-9. Arthroscopic image of a capsular plication in which the capsule has been advanced to the intact anterior labrum.

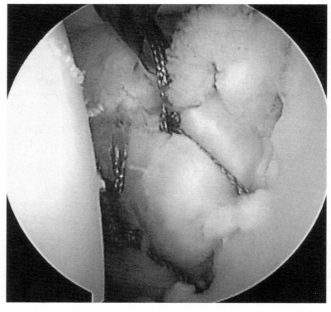

FIGURE 12-10. Arthroscopic image of a Bankart repair in which the inferior glenohumeral labral complex has been sutured to the glenoid margin.

the glenoid margin with subsequent superior advancement of the inferior leaf and imbrication of the superior leaf over the inferior leaf. More commonly in elite throwers, to minimize the risk of postoperative stiffness, the capsule is not T'ed, and the superior and inferior flaps of the transverse capsulotomy are imbricated over one another. If a Bankart repair is necessary, it is visualized and repaired through the horizontal capsulotomy using biodegradable suture anchor fixation into the glenoid articular margin. It is imperative to position the arm in at least 60 degrees of scapular abduction and 90 degrees of external rotation when tensioning the capsular repair. We have found that, by not detaching the subscapularis and not shifting the capsule in a medial lateral direction, athletes have less postoperative motion loss.

Our postoperative protocol involves strict immobilization in a sling for the initial 4 weeks except for gentle pendulum exercises and range of motion and strengthening of the hand, wrist, and elbow. A gradual stretching and strengthening program is then implemented and athletes may begin an interval tossing program approximately 4 to 6 months postoperatively when motion is pain-free and without limitations. Return to sport is dictated by subjective stability and confidence, comparative strength to the contralateral shoulder, and by the athlete's sense of power and control while throwing.

REFERENCES

1. Barnes DA, Tullos HS. An analysis of 100 symptomatic baseball players. *Am J Sports Med* 1978;6:62–67.
2. Bigliani LU, Codd TP, Connor PM, et al. Shoulder motion and laxity in the professional baseball player. *Am J Sports Med* 1997;25:609–613.
3. Altchek DW, Hobbs W. Evaluation and management of shoulder instability in the elite overhead thrower. *Orthop Clin North Am* 2001;32:423–430.
4. Dillman CJ, Fleisig GS, Andrews JR. Biomechanics of pitching with emphasis upon shoulder kinematics. *J Orthop Sports Phys Ther* 1993;18:402–408.
5. Fleisig GS, Andrews JR, Dillman CJ, et al. Kinetics of baseball pitching with implications about injury mechanisms. *Am J Sports Med* 1995;23:233–239.
6. Werner SL, Fleisig GS, Dillman CJ, et al. Biomechanics of the elbow during baseball pitching. *J Orthop Sports Phys Ther* 1993;17:274–278.
7. Dillman CJ, Fleisig GS, Werner SL. Biomechanics of the shoulder in sports: throwing activities. In: Matsen RA, Hawkins RJ, eds. *The shoulder: a balance of mobility and stability.* Rosemont, IL: American Academy of Orthopaedic Surgeons, 1993:621–633.
8. Altchek DW, Dines DM. Shoulder injuries in the throwing athlete. *J Am Acad Orthop Surg* 1995;3:159–165.
9. Flood V. Discovery of a new ligament of the shoulder joint. *Lancet* 1829;1:672–673.
10. Jost B, Koch PP, Gerber C. Anatomy and functional aspects of the rotator interval. *J Shoulder Elbow Surg* 2000;9:336–341.
11. Steinbeck J, Liljenqvist U, Jerosch J. The anatomy of the glenohumeral ligamentous complex and its contribution to anterior shoulder stability. *J Shoulder Elbow Surg* 1998;7:122–126.
12. DePalma AF CG, Bennett GA. Variational anatomy and degenerative lesions of the shoulder joint. *AAOS Instruct Course Lect* 1949;XVI:255–281.
13. O'Brien SJ, Neves MC, Arnoczky SP, et al. The anatomy and histology of the inferior glenohumeral ligament complex of the shoulder. *Am J Sports Med* 1990;18:449–456.
14. Warner JJ, Deng XH, Warren RF, et al. Static capsuloligamentous restraints to superior-inferior translation of the glenohumeral joint. *Am J Sports Med* 1992;20:675–685.
15. Bowen MK, Warren RF. Ligamentous control of shoulder stability based on selective cutting and static translation experiments. *Clin Sports Med* 1991;10:757–782.
16. Rodowsky M, Harner, CD, Fu FH. The role of the long head of the biceps muscle and superior glenoid labrum in anterior instability of the shoulder. *Am J Sports Med* 1994; 22: 121–130.
17. Warner JJ, McMahon PJ. The role of the long head of the biceps brachii in superior stability of the glenohumeral joint. *J Bone Joint Surg Am* 1995;77:366–372.
18. Yamaguchi K, Riew KD, Galatz LM, et al. Biceps activity during shoulder motion: an electromyographic analysis. *Clin Orthop* 1997;122–129.
19. Jobe FW, Moynes DR, Tibone JE, et al. An EMG analysis of the shoulder in pitching. A second report. *Am J Sports Med* 1984;12:218–220.
20. Bradley JP, Tibone JE. Electromyographic analysis of muscle action about the shoulder. *Clin Sports Med* 1991;10:789–805.
21. Feltner MDJ. Dynamics of the shoulder and elbow joints of the throwing arm during a baseball pitch. *Int J Sport Biomech* 1986;2:235–259.
22. DiGiovine NM JF, Pink M, Perry J. An electromyographic analysis of the upper extremity in pitching. *J Shoulder Elbow Surg* 1992;1:15–25.
23. Jobe FW, Tibone JE, Perry J, et al. An EMG analysis of the shoulder in throwing and pitching. A preliminary report. *Am J Sports Med* 1983;11:3–5.
24. Jacobs P. The overhand baseball itch: a kinesiological analysis and related strength-conditioning programming. *National Strength Conditioning J* 1987;9:5–13.
25. Walch GBP, Noel E, Donell ST. Impingement of the deep surface of the supraspinatus tendon on the posterosuperior glenoid rim: an arthroscopic study. *J Shoulder Elbow Surg* 1992;1:238–245.
26. Davidson PA, Elattrache NS, Jobe CM, et al. Rotator cuff and posterior-superior glenoid labrum injury associated with increased glenohumeral motion: a new site of impingement. *J Shoulder Elbow Surg* 1995;4:384–390.
27. Tibone JE. Glenohumeral instability in overhead athletes. In: Bigliani LU, eds. *The unstable shoulder.* Rosemont, IL: American Academy of Orthopaedic Surgeons, 1996:91–98.
28. Lintner SA, Speer KP. Traumatic anterior glenohumeral instability: the role of arthroscopy. *J Am Acad Orthop Surg* 1997;5:233–239.
29. Bankart A. Recurrent or habitual dislocation of the shoulder-joint. *BMJ* 1923;2:1123–1133.
30. Bigliani LU, Pollock RG, Soslowsky LJ, et al. Tensile properties of the inferior glenohumeral ligament. *J Orthop Res* 1992;10:187–197.
31. Rowe CR. Instabilities of the glenohumeral joint. *Bull Hosp Joint Dis* 1978;39:180–186.
32. Rowe CR. Recurrent anterior transient subluxation of the shoulder. The "dead arm" syndrome. *Orthop Clin North Am* 1988;19:767–772.
33. Turkel SJ, Panio MW, Marshall JL, et al. Stabilizing mechanisms preventing anterior dislocation of the glenohumeral joint. *J Bone Joint Surg Am* 1981;63:1208–1217.
34. Warren RF. Instability of shoulder in throwing sports. *AAOS Instruct Course Lect* 1985;34:337–348.

35. Jobe FW, Kvitne RS, Giangarra CE. Shoulder pain in the over-hand or throwing athlete. The relationship of anterior instability and rotator cuff impingement. *Orthop Rev* 1989;18:963–975.

36. Kelly JDI. Brachial plexus injuries: evaluating and treating "burners." *J Musculoskel Med* 1997;14:70–80.

37. Andrews JR, Gidumal RH. Shoulder arthroscopy in the throwing athlete: perspectives and prognosis. *Clin Sports Med* 1987;6: 565–571.

38. Kibler WB. Specificity and sensitivity of the anterior slide test in throwing athletes with superior glenoid labral tears. *Arthroscopy* 1995;11:296–300.

39. O'Brien SJ, Pagnani MJ, Fealy S, et al. The active compression test: a new and effective test for diagnosing labral tears and acromioclavicular joint abnormality. *Am J Sports Med* 1998;26:610–613.

40. Hawkins RJ, Kennedy JC. Impingement syndrome in athletes. *Am J Sports Med* 1980;8:151–158.

41. Neer CS, 2nd. Impingement lesions. *Clin Orthop* 1983;70–77.

42. Riand N, Levigne C, Renaud E, et al. Results of derotational humeral osteotomy in posterosuperior glenoid impingement. *Am J Sports Med* 1998;26:453–459.

43. Kvitne RS, Jobe FW. The diagnosis and treatment of anterior instability in the throwing athlete. *Clin Orthop* 1993;107–123.

44. Legan JM, Burkhard TK, Goff WB 2nd, et al. Tears of the glenoid labrum: MR imaging of 88 arthroscopically confirmed cases. *Radiology* 1991;179:241–246.

45. Gusmer PB, Potter HG, Schatz JA, et al. Labral injuries: accuracy of detection with unenhanced MR imaging of the shoulder. *Radiology* 1996;200:519–524.

46. Connell DA, Potter HG, Wickiewicz TL, et al. Noncontrast magnetic resonance imaging of superior labral lesions. 102 cases confirmed at arthroscopic surgery. *Am J Sports Med* 1999;27: 208–213.

47. Davis A. The conservative treatment for habitual dislocations of the shoulder. *JAMA* 1936;107:1012–1015.

48. Glousman R, Jobe F, Tibone J, et al. Dynamic electromyographic analysis of the throwing shoulder with glenohumeral instability. *J Bone Joint Surg Am* 1988;70:220–226.

49. Wilk KE, Arrigo CA, Andrews JR. Current concepts: the stabilizing structures of the glenohumeral joint. *J Orthop Sports Phys Ther* 1997;25:364–379.

50. Wilk KE, Meister K, Andrews JR. Current concepts in the rehabilitation of the overhead throwing athlete. *Am J Sports Med* 2002;30:136–151.

51. Jobe CM. Superior glenoid impingement. *Orthop Clin North Am* 1997;28:137–143.

52. Voight ML, Hardin JA, Blackburn TA, et al. The effects of muscle fatigue on and the relationship of arm dominance to shoulder proprioception. *J Orthop Sports Phys Ther* 1996;23:348–352.

53. Chen SK WT, Otis JC, et al. Glenohumeral kinematics in a muscle fatigue model: a radiographic study. *Orthop Trans* 1994;18:1126.

54. Rowe C. Prognosis in dislocations of the shoulder. *J Bone Joint Surg (Am)* 1956;38:957–976.

55. McLaughlin HL CW. Primary anterior dislocation of the shoulder. *Am J Surgery* 1950;615.

56. Henry JH, Genung JA. Natural history of glenohumeral dislocation—revisited. *Am J Sports Med* 1982;10:135–137.

57. Hovelius L, Augustini BG, Fredin H, et al. Primary anterior dislocation of the shoulder in young patients. A ten-year prospective study. *J Bone Joint Surg Am* 1996;78:1677–1684.

58. Simonet WT, Cofield RH. Prognosis in anterior shoulder dislocation. *Am J Sports Med* 1984;12:19–24.

59. Yoneda B WR, McIntosh DL. Conservative treatment of shoulder dislocation in young males. *J Bone Joint Surg (Br)* 1982;64: 254–255.

60. Aronen JG, Regan K. Decreasing the incidence of recurrence of first time anterior shoulder dislocations with rehabilitation. *Am J Sports Med* 1984;12:283–291.

61. Townsend H, Jobe FW, Pink M, et al. Electromyographic analysis of the glenohumeral muscles during a baseball rehabilitation program. *Am J Sports Med* 1991;19:264–272.

62. Moseley JB Jr, Jobe FW, Pink M, et al. EMG analysis of the scapular muscles during a shoulder rehabilitation program. *Am J Sports Med* 1992;20:128–134.

63. Jobe FW, Giangarra CE, Kvitne RS, et al. Anterior capsulolabral reconstruction of the shoulder in athletes in overhand sports. *Am J Sports Med* 1991;19:428–434.

64. Montgomery WH 3rd, Jobe FW. Functional outcomes in athletes after modified anterior capsulolabral reconstruction. *Am J Sports Med* 1994;22:352–358.

65. Altchek DW, Simonian PT. Special considerations in the treatment of shoulder instability in the throwing athlete. In: Warren RF, Craig EV, Altchek DW, eds. *The unstable shoulder.* Philadelphia: Lippincott-Raven, 1999:232.

66. Riand N, Boulahia A, Walch G. (Posterosuperior impingement of the shoulder in the athlete: results of arthroscopic debridement in 75 patients). *Rev Chir Orthop Reparatrice Appar Mot* 2002;88: 19–27.

67. Payne LZ, Altchek DW, Craig EV, et al. Arthroscopic treatment of partial rotator cuff tears in young athletes. A preliminary report. *Am J Sports Med* 1997;25:299–305.

68. Levitz CL, Dugas J, Andrews JR. The use of arthroscopic thermal capsulorrhaphy to treat internal impingement in baseball players. *Arthroscopy* 2001;17:573–577.

69. Allain JC, Le Lous M, Cohen S, et al. Isometric tensions developed during the hydrothermal swelling of rat skin. *Connect Tissue Res* 1980;7:127–133.

70. Flory PJ GR. Phase transition in collagen and gelatin systems. *J Am Chem Soc* 1958;80:4836–4845.

71. Verzar F, Nagy IZ. Electronmicroscopic analysis of thermal collagen denaturation in rat tail tendons. *Gerontologia* 1970;16:77–82.

72. Toth A, Petrigliano F, Doward D, et al. Radiofrequency thermal-assisted capsular shrinkage for shoulder instability: Minimum two-year follow-up. Presented at The American Orthopaedic Society for Sports Medicine Annual Meeting, Orlando, Florida, 2002.

73. Bigliani LU, Kurzweil PR, Schwartzbach CC, et al. Inferior capsular shift procedure for anterior-inferior shoulder instability in athletes. *Am J Sports Med* 1994;22:578–584.

74. Altchek DW, Warren RF, Skyhar MJ, et al. T-plasty modification of the Bankart procedure for multidirectional instability of the anterior and inferior types. *J Bone Joint Surg Am* 1991;73: 105–112.

75. Cooper RA BJ. The inferior capsular-shift procedure for multidirectional instability of the shoulder. *J Bone Joint Surg (Am)* 1992;74:1516–1521.

76. Lusardi DA, Wirth MA, Wurtz D, et al. Loss of external rotation following anterior capsulorrhaphy of the shoulder. *J Bone Joint Surg (Am)* 1993;75:1185–1192.

77. Cole BJ WJ. Arthroscopic versus open Bankart repair for traumatic anterior shoulder instability. *Clin Sports Med* 2000;19: 19–48.

78. Laurencin CT SS, Warren RF, Altchek DA. Arthroscopic Bankart repair using a degradable tack. A followup study using optimized indications. *Clin Orthop* 1996;332:132–137.

79. Anderson K, Warren RF, Altchek DW, et al. Risk factors for early failure after thermal capsulorrhaphy. *Am J Sports Med* 2002; 30:103–107.

80. Ruotolo C, Nottage WM, Flatow EL, et al. Controversial topics in shoulder arthroscopy. *Arthroscopy* 2002;18:65–75.

81. Naseef GS 3rd, Foster TE, Trauner K, et al. The thermal properties of bovine joint capsule. The basic science of laser- and radiofrequency-induced capsular shrinkage. *Am J Sports Med* 1997;25:670–674.

82. Wall MS, Deng XH, Torzilli PA, et al. Thermal modification of collagen. *J Shoulder Elbow Surg* 1999;8:339–344.

13

UNIDIRECTIONAL POSTERIOR INSTABILITY

THOMAS A. JOSEPH
SUMANT G. KRISHNAN

HISTORICAL OVERVIEW

The most common instability pattern encountered in the overhead athlete is subtle anterior instability secondary to repetitive microtrauma to the anterior capsule. Since Jobe's initial description of this entity in baseball pitchers, the concept has been carried over to other sports in which the shoulder is repetitively challenged by an anterior joint reactive force (1). One must, however, maintain a high index of suspicion for all instability patterns in overhead athletes, in that any busy shoulder or sports medicine specialist will encounter patients with multidirectional or unidirectional posterior instability. Table 13-1 lists athletic activities that may repetitively stress the posterior capsule. Because isolated posterior instability is rare in the overhead athlete, little is written pertinent to this group of patients. This chapter integrates basic science, historical treatment approaches, and modern rehabilitative and arthroscopic experience in managing overhead athletes with posterior instability. In addition, the importance of maintaining a balance of mobility and stability is emphasized in the treatment approaches discussed for overhead athletes with posterior instability.

TABLE 13–1. ATHLETIC ACTIVITIES THAT MAY REPETITIVELY STRESS THE POSTERIOR CAPSULE

Activity	Motion
Weight lifting	Bench press, push-ups
Pitching	Follow-through phase
Swimming	Butterfly and freestyle strokes
Boxing	Axial load with punching
Gymnastics	Parallel bars, rings
Racquet sports	Backhand strokes
Batting	Motions of lead arm
Golf	Motions of lead arm
Football	Offensive lineman maneuvers
Archery	Motions of both arms
Volleyball	Follow-through phase of serve

From Joseph TA, Brems JJ. Multidirectional and posterior instability. In: Norris T, ed. *OKU-2: Shoulder and elbow,* 2nd ed. American Academy of Orthopaedic Surgery, 2002:97, with permission.

ANATOMY AND BIOMECHANICS

A thorough understanding of shoulder anatomy and sport-specific biomechanics is necessary when attempting to diagnose and treat this group of patients with precision. Several basic science studies have helped to define the roles of various anatomic structures in maintaining glenohumeral stability. In addition, throwing mechanics have been studied extensively through clinical observation, the use of video cinematography, and electromyography (EMG). Other overhead activities that have been biomechanically analyzed include throwing a football, various swimming strokes, the golf swing, tennis swings, and volleyball serves (2–11).

A comprehensive knowledge of the basic science of instability and the biomechanics of sport assists diagnostically in targeting the offending phase of physical activity and therapeutically in precisely designing a rehabilitative or surgical plan. Both compromised soft tissue restraints and abnormal scapulohumeral anatomy may contribute to posterior instability. Osseous architectural variants that have been described in association with posterior instability include excessive glenoid or humeral retroversion, glenoid hypoplasia, and diminished tilting angles and concavity of the inferior glenoid (12–17). These abnormalities are extremely rare in the athletic population. By far, most symptomatic overhead athletes demonstrate occult posterior subluxation, most commonly due to posterior capsular laxity. There have only been a select few studies defining the primary soft tissue restraints to posterior translation (18–24). In a cadaveric sectioning study, Ovesen and Nielsen showed that the infraspinatus and teres minor muscle-tendons stabilized the glenohumeral joint for internal rotation in the first half of abduction, whereas the lower half of the posterior capsule became more important beyond 40 degrees of abduction (18). The work of Debski and co-workers suggest that passive tension in the rotator cuff plays a more significant role than other soft tissue structures in resisting posterior loads at 30, 60, and 90 degrees of abduction (19). More specifically, Blasier and colleagues found the subscapularis to be the most significant active restraint to posterior humeral subluxation at 90 degrees of abduction (20). Of the passive restraints, the coracohumeral ligament contributed most with the arm in neutral rotation, whereas the inferior glenohumeral ligament (IGHL) complex contributed most in internal rotation. The contribution of the posterior capsule superior to the posterior band of the IGHL was less significant and decreased with greater displacement of the humeral head. O'Brien found the IGHL complex (with associated posteroinferior capsule) to be the primary static stabilizer against posterior instability with the arm in 90 degrees of abduction (21). Several other studies have shown that the rotator interval structures (superior glenohumeral ligament and coracohumeral ligament) limit inferior translation and serve as secondary restraints to posterior translation (25–28). Although the importance of the anteroinferior labrum as an anchor for the anterior band of the inferior glenohumeral ligament is well recognized, damage to the posterior labrum may also contribute to instability. From a quantitative standpoint, the labrum has been shown to deepen the glenoid socket by 50% and contribute up to 20% to the stability ratio in the inferior and posteroinferior directions (29,30). Weber and Caspari created posterior dislocations in nine cadaver shoulders and found posterior Bankart or capsular tears in all specimens. No anterior pathology was seen (24). This is in contrast to Warren's work, which noted that damage to both the anterior and posterior capsule was necessary to experimentally produce a posterior dislocation (23).

In addition to describing the primary and secondary stabilizing effects of various regions of the glenohumeral capsule, several studies have sought to determine the effects of surgical alteration of these same regions. A recent study by Gerber and colleagues quantified the effect of selective capsulorrhaphy on passive range of motion of the glenohumeral joint (31). This information may be used to more specifically target pathologic zones of capsule in the form of surgical plication or releases. Tibone and co-workers studied the effects of arthroscopic thermal capsuloplasty using a radiofrequency probe on anterior and posterior glenohumeral translation. They found that both laser and thermal shrinkage of the anteroinferior capsular structures resulted in a significant reduction in anterior and posterior translation (32,33). Conversely, thermal shrinkage of the posterior capsule using a radiofrequency probe failed to result in a significant decrease in either posterior or anterior translation using the same model (34). This may be due to the fact that the posterior capsule is generally thinner and stiffer, and has a lower strain to failure than its anterior counterpart (35,36). Selecky and co-workers used the same model to demonstrate a significant reduction in both anterior and posterior glenohumeral translation following rotator interval thermal capsuloplasty (37). The effects were slightly more significant with respect to posterior translation. These studies lend support to the surgical philosophy

of addressing the thicker, more robust anterior capsular tissues to achieve a posterior tensioning effect via the "circle concept."

ETIOLOGY OF INJURY AND CLASSIFICATION

The evaluation of a patient with shoulder instability should seek to identify any contributing major traumatic event, repetitive microtrauma, or voluntary history. In patients with an atraumatic history, the role of repetitive microtrauma and generalized ligamentous laxity must each be considered. Although congenital posterior instability has been described in patients with abnormal osseous architecture such as glenoid dysplasia and excessive humeral retroversion, the majority of competitive overhead athletes presenting with an atraumatic picture either have generalized ligamentous laxity that places them at increased risk for developing symptoms or have stretched out their ligamentous restraints due to the cumulative microtrauma of sport. Some sport-specific movements exert a direct posterior joint reactive force whereas others impart tractional stress due to muscular pull and momentum. The shoulders of football linemen and boxers, for example, are repetitively subjected to forceful posterior loads. Mair and co-workers recently reported on nine contact athletes with posterior labral detachment resulting in pain without instability (38). It is during the follow-through phase of overhead activity (pitching, swimming, tennis, volleyball) that the integrity of the posterior capsule is challenged by distraction and stretch. A similar mechanism has recently been described in the lead arm of golfers at the top of the backswing (39). The same phenomenon may occur during backhand movements while batting or participating in racquet sports.

Although many instability classification systems have been described, none are comprehensive or absolute. Joseph and colleagues recently described an etiology based classification system for multidirectional instability, which may also be used to better characterize posterior instability (40). Patients with congenital or type I instability exhibit inherited generalized ligamentous laxity. They tend to first present at an early age and frequently become symptomatic with normal activities of daily living or routine light athletic activity. Structurally, their soft tissue restraints are intact but lax. Patients with type II or acquired instability become symptomatic as a direct result of repetitive microtrauma from their offending sport. These patients usually lie within the middle of the connective tissue spectrum, with collagen that undergoes plastic deformation and stretch in response to cumulative loading. Common offending activities include gymnastics, weightlifting, swimming, and throwing sports. This group of patients differs from those with congenital laxity in that they do not possess gross generalized ligamentous laxity. Laxity is primarily found in the joints subjected to repetitive stretch. Within the group of patients with acquired instability due to repetitive microtrauma exists a subset of patients with bidirectional (anterior and posterior) instability without inferior instability. Type III (posttraumatic) instability follows a specific traumatic event. There should be a higher index of suspicion for structural abnormalities such as labral disruption in these patients. In our experience, pain was also a more consistent component of symptoms in these patients (40). Antoniou and colleagues described four distinct anatomic lesions discovered arthroscopically in patients with posteroinferior instability. Seventy-eight percent of their patients had a traumatic etiology. Arthroscopic findings included labral detachment (12%), chondral or labral erosion (17%), synovial or capsular stripping (22%), and labral split or flap tears (32%) (41).

In addition to subclassifying based on etiology, the presence of voluntary activity should be sought in all cases, because this influences one's treatment approach, both diagnostically and therapeutically. We routinely ask patients whether or not they are able to demonstrate what happens with their shoulder. This reinforces diagnostic accuracy and often defines the "position at risk." It is important to then discourage this behavior. Although voluntary instability has been traditionally regarded as a "red flag," it has come to be well accepted that different voluntary patterns exist (habitual, positional, neuromuscular) and that some of these patients may still benefit from surgical treatment (42).

PRESENTATION AND PHYSICAL EXAMINATION

Because many patients with posterior instability may present with pain as their chief complaint, responsibility often rests with the physician to make an accurate diagnosis based on history and physical examination findings. Most overhead athletes can specifically describe the offending position or action that reproduces their symptoms. In addition, some may be able to voluntarily demonstrate subluxation. Although this behavior should be discouraged, seeing it at least once in the clinical setting can be extremely helpful diagnostically (Fig. 13-1). An opportunity to examine any patient with instability on multiple occasions before surgical intervention is paramount.

Regardless of the suspected instability pattern, the instability examination includes the same inventory in all patients. First the patient is examined for signs of generalized ligamentous laxity. After a cursory cervical spine examination, the patient is asked to actively elevate and lower both arms. Inspection is performed from the front and the back, specifically looking for any asymmetry, dyskinesia, or dynamic scapular winging. Bilateral active and passive range of motion is recorded. Sulcus testing is performed with the patient seated and the arm in neutral and external rotation. For load-

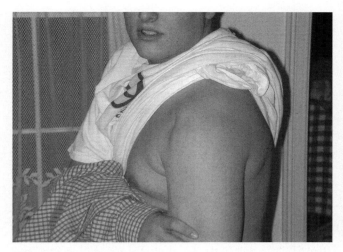

FIGURE 13-1. Voluntary posterior instability. This patient was able to voluntarily subluxate his shoulder posteriorly with muscular contraction while the arm was positioned at his side.

and-shift testing, it is helpful to examine the contralateral shoulder first, with the patient supine to facilitate relaxation. While supine, apprehension and relocation maneuvers and posterior stress tests may be performed. The patient is then seated and confirmatory tests such as "the jerk test" for posterior instability, the active compression test, and other labral tests may be performed. It is important in performing the jerk test to start with a light posterior directed force, because patients with significant posterior laxity may forcefully relocate with this maneuver, causing discomfort and subsequent guarding. The examination then proceeds through the usual areas of palpation, other specific shoulder tests, and neurovascular assessment. In any patient who comes to require surgical treatment, the load-and-shift examination is repeated with the patient under anesthesia and compared with the contralateral extremity.

RADIOGRAPHIC AND DIAGNOSTIC EVALUATION

For most overhead athletes with posterior instability, plain radiographs are of little diagnostic value. Nevertheless they should always be ordered to rule out tumor, skeletal anomalies, and impression defects or fractures. The typical shoulder series includes a true or "scapular" anteroposterior (AP) supraspinatus outlet view to assess acromial morphology and a West Point or axillary view. It is helpful to routinely assess the position of the humeral head relative to the glenoid on both AP and axillary views.

For this group of patients, the use of magnetic resonance imaging (MRI) may be of some benefit, especially if surgical treatment is under consideration. The importance of diagnostic precision is well recognized and clinical presentations can often be confusing. Whether or not gadolinium enhancement is used depends on the preference of the reading physician in cases of suspected labral detachment. When dealing with elite athletes who fail to improve with conservative treatment measures, an MRI scan is often requested, if not expected, by the athlete or agent, and the information and reassurance that it provides makes it well worth the additional cost.

NONOPERATIVE TREATMENT, REHABILITATION, AND RESULTS

For most overhead athletes with posterior instability, nonoperative treatment options should be exhausted before considering surgical intervention. Nonoperative options include rest, medications, injections, physical therapy, and occasionally immobilization. It is important to accurately pass on to the treating physical therapist the exact instability pattern, offending actions, and positions of risk. Physical therapy protocols are helpful but must often be tailored to the individual.

If scapular winging is present, this must be targeted to achieve a successful result. Once primary scapular winging has been ruled out, muscle retraining and biofeedback should be employed to restore normal glenohumeral and scapulohumeral mechanics. In the case of secondary scapular winging, abnormal muscle firing patterns (activation and suppression) occur in an attempt to move the glenoid relative to the humeral head. With posterior instability, the most commonly observed pattern of winging is that of serratus dysfunction, whereby scapular abduction increases stress to the posterior capsule.

In general, physical therapy programs are often an effective way of managing atraumatic posterior instability. Traditionally, most programs have focused on strengthening of the posterior cuff muscles (infraspinatus and teres minor) as well as the scapular stabilizers. In the at-risk position of 90 degrees of forward elevation, Blasier and colleagues found that, of the active stabilizers, the subscapularis provided the most resistance to posterior subluxation of the humerus (20). Clinically, this was thought to suggest that strengthening of the subscapularis may augment posterior instability of the shoulder. In patients with a traumatic history, the results have been less favorable. In Burkhead and Rockwood's series, only 4 of 11 patients with traumatic posterior instability responded well to an exercise program (43). Misamore and Facibene have shared a similar experience (44). Pande and colleagues performed EMG studies in four patients with voluntary posterior instability and were able to describe two distinct patterns of abnormal muscle firing patterns (45). Although it may be impractical to perform EMG studies in all patients before writing a physical therapy prescription, this information is extremely valuable in that it highlights the importance of selective rehabilitative efforts. Indiscriminate rehabilitative programs may aggravate or accentuate symptoms. Beall and co-workers implemented an EMG biofeedback program to successfully treat three patients with voluntary posterior instability through reeducation of muscle contraction-relaxation patterns (46). In addition to formal rehabilitative supervision, it is also helpful to communicate with the athletic trainers or pitching coaches who work with the athlete regularly. Small changes in fundamental throwing mechanics can often make a significant difference.

OPERATIVE TREATMENT, REHABILITATION, AND RESULTS

When nonoperative treatment fails, we are faced with the challenge of restoring stability without sacrificing the motion that overhead athletes rely on to perform their sport. Most team physicians would agree that this is best accomplished arthroscopically. This opinion is not universal, however, and several studies have demonstrated good results following open surgical procedures in athletes (35,42,44,47–50). Although instability symptoms were alleviated in a high percentage of patients, the rate of return to sport in many of these studies was low (47,49,50). In the overhead athlete, this concern is amplified.

Within the past 5 years considerable progress has been made with arthroscopic instability surgery. Indications, techniques, and surgical instrumentation have been refined such that capsular and labral pathology may be precisely addressed without the added scar response of an open procedure. Several studies have demonstrated excellent restoration of stability without the added concerns of contracture and motion loss (41,51–56). Williams and colleagues recently reported successful results in 24 of 26 patients (92%) with posterior "reverse Bankart" lesions following arthroscopic repair with bioabsorbable tacks (53). Twenty of these patients sustained injuries during athletic activity and no patient in the study lost range of motion postoperatively.

Much has been learned through basic science research about the roles various tissues play in maintaining glenohumeral instability and the effects of surgical intervention on these structures. Anecdotal experience with thermal or laser capsulorrhaphy alone for the treatment of posterior instability has been less than satisfactory. There have been no published outcomes reviewing the use of these techniques in athletes with unidirectional posterior instability. Postsurgical care following arthroscopic stabilization plays an important role in achieving successful results and is discussed in detail with the authors' preferred method of treatment.

AUTHORS' PREFERRED TREATMENT ALGORITHMS AND TECHNIQUE

As emphasized earlier, any patient that comes to require surgical treatment should be reexamined under anesthesia to reinforce, confirm, or refute prior diagnostic impressions, keeping in mind that there is a wide range of posterior laxity in asymptomatic individuals (57–59). This should not be surgically addressed in the absence of instability symptoms.

The patient may be placed in the lateral decubitus or beach chair position. Our preference is to perform arthroscopic posterior instability surgery in the lateral decubitus position because it offers the distinct advantage of being able to apply both lateral and longitudinal traction in order to access the posteroinferior axillary quadrant. Commercially available systems with pulley capabilities for lateral traction magnify the "drive-through sign," facilitating intraarticular work, particularly inferior to the equator of the glenoid.

A standard diagnostic examination of the glenohumeral joint is performed through a posterior portal placed just above the equator of the glenoid because it will later serve as the working portal. Particularly close attention is paid to the integrity of the rotator interval tissues, the inferior glenohumeral ligaments and pouch, and the labrum circumferentially. In patients with a patulous posterior capsule, a "stage sign" may be noted as the scope is withdrawn beyond the posterior glenoid lip (Fig. 13-2). A small 5.5-mm cannula is then established low in the rotator interval just above the subscapularis tendon using an outside-in technique. A second rotator interval portal can be established superiorly to facilitate suture management. As long as no capsular plication is to be performed anteriorly, both of these cannulae may be of small diameter. We find it helpful to use a spinal needle to facilitate portal placement.

By using only a single posterior cannula, trauma to the thin posterior capsule is minimized. Switching sticks are then introduced through both cannulae and the scope is placed anteriorly. With the scope anterior, the entire poste-

rior capsule and labrum can be inspected. If the use of suture hooks is anticipated, a larger cannula is required posteriorly (approximately 8 mm) and is best placed under direct visualization over a metal switching stick. If a posterior Bankarts lesion is present, a grasper is introduced to assess tissue mobility. Any intervening fibrous tissue between the capsulolabral tissue and the glenoid rim must be released so that the detached labral tissue edge and subadjacent capsule may be easily mobilized to the glenoid rim. A shaver or burr is then used to abrade the posterior glenoid neck to create a bleeding surface of bone for tissue healing. In addition, the posterior capsule is scored with a microfracture awl adjacent to zones of plication to stimulate a healing response. Anchors are then placed 1 to 2 mm onto the posterior face of the glenoid, one at a time.

A 45-degree suture hook (Linvatec) is then loaded with either a no. 1 PDS suture or a suture shuttle and is passed first through the capsule and then the labral edge in a pinch-and-tuck fashion. This not only serves to repair the labrum but also provides a posterior capsular shift. The suture or shuttle is then retrieved and used to shuttle one limb of the anchor suture through the detached tissue and out the posterior cannula. After retrieving the second limb of anchor suture out the posterior cannula, the suture is tied down with a knot pusher. The posterior suture limb (i.e., the limb that passes through the labrum and capsule) is the post, because this facilitates creating a "bumper effect" by bunching the tissue up onto the glenoid rim as the knots are secured (Fig. 13-3). As long as the posterior cannula has been placed above the glenoid equator, at least two or three anchors can usually be placed and the entire posterior band of the inferior glenohumeral ligament retensioned.

After completing the posterior repair, the scope is then switched back to the posterior portal over a switching stick.

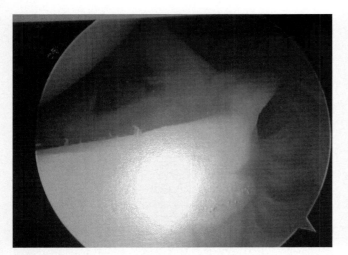

FIGURE 13-2. Arthroscopic view demonstrating excessive posterior capsular laxity. In patients with excessive posterior capsular laxity, the capsule distends away from the glenoid allowing tremendous viewing capacity ("stage sign").

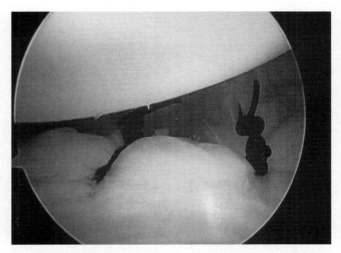

FIGURE 13-3. Posterior capsular plication with recreation of 9the bumper effect.9 By using the capsular limb as a post, soft tissue tensioning may be accomplished while creating a "bumper effect" at the labral edge.

At this point, the rotator interval is systematically closed with absorbable no. 1 PDS suture (usually two to three sutures), plicating the superior glenohumeral ligament to the middle glenohumeral ligament. A short crescent hook is used to pass the PDS through the middle glenohumeral ligament, and a penetrator retrieves the suture through the superior glenohumeral ligament. After all sutures are passed, the sutures are tied in an extracapsular fashion in the subacromial space.

Tibone and colleagues have shown that significant reductions in both anterior and posterior translation can be achieved with thermal treatment of the anteroinferior capsuloligamentous structures (32–33). Conversely, no statistically significant change in posterior translation was affected by thermal treatment of the thin posterior capsule (34). Hence, in select cases with components of inferior or multidirectional instability, we consider "balancing" the joint by lightly addressing the anterior band of the inferior glenohumeral ligament in a "cornrow" fashion with a thermal probe. We do not use thermal devices on the posterior capsule, and our indication for the use of thermal devices in general is extremely limited.

For the patient with posterior instability and an intact posterior labrum, a similar approach is used. However, instead of using anchors, the posterior capsule is plicated to the intact labrum in a pinch-and-tuck fashion using 45-degree suture hooks (Fig. 13-4). This typically starts inferiorly (around the 6-o'clock position) and works superiorly up to the level of the cannula. The intact capsule is first pierced in multiple locations with a microfracture awl to stimulate a healing response. The amount of capsule that is plicated with each pass of the suture hook can be tailored to the individual depending on the degree of instability present. On average, a single pass of the suture hook plicates about 1 cm of capsule. Again, it is important to make the suture limb that passes through the capsule the post in order to achieve a "bumper effect" with the tissue. Theoretically this deepens the glenoid and may serve to better contain the humeral head through a concavity-compression mechanism. In cases of dramatic posterior instability or laxity that is present with the humerus below 90 degrees of forward elevation when performing a "jerk test," we also plicate above the posterior cannula portal and close the posterior portal arthroscopically on the way out (Fig. 13-5). Again, as described previously, we systematically close the rotator interval in these patients.

Despite the perceived advantages of accelerated rehabilitation and earlier return to sport following arthroscopic treatment, we do not move these patients any quicker than we would following an open surgical approach. To avoid any tension on the posterior capsule during the early healing stages, a "gunslinger" brace is used to maintain the arm in a neutral to slightly externally rotated position for 6 weeks (Fig. 13-6). The patient is also instructed to sleep in a recliner. At the time of the first postoperative visit (approximately 10 days postoperatively), the patient is shown how to remove the brace once a day for elbow range of motion. Patients are seen again at 6 weeks postoperatively, at which point they are given a sling to use "as needed" for the next week. Shoulder range of motion is initiated at that visit. Internal rotation is initially restricted to the belt line and is gradually increased over the next 6 weeks. Active cross body adduction is permitted at the ninth week, but passive and active-assisted stretching in this position is discouraged. Strengthening begins 3 weeks after initiating shoulder range of motion. The patient begins with isometrics and progresses to cord or band resistance exercises as tolerated. As strength improves, proprioceptive training is added. Light weight training is permitted after 16 weeks; however, exercises that produce posterior capsular stress (push-ups, bench presses, dips) are avoided for at

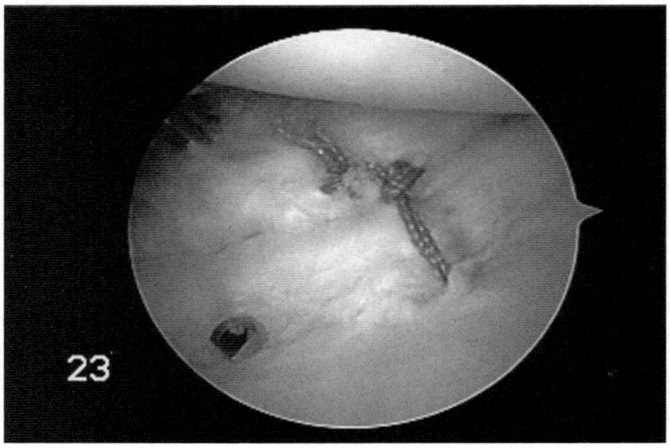

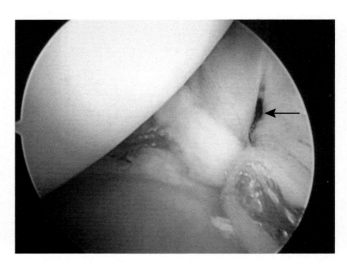

FIGURE 13-4. Pinch and tuck method of capsular plication. Using a 45-degree suture hook, a no. 1 PDS suture or suture shuttle is passed first through capsule and then through the labrum.

FIGURE 13-5. Posterior portal closure. With the scope in the anterior portal, an additional suture (*arrow*) may be passed to close the posterior portal created by the 8-mm cannula.

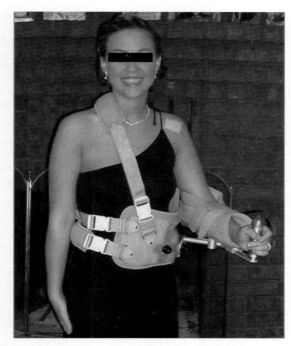

FIGURE 13-6. "Gunslinger" brace. This device maintains the arm in neutral to slight external rotation for 6 weeks.

least 6 months. Typically, return to sport is permitted at 6 months.

COMPLICATIONS

The decision to operate on a symptomatic athlete must include a thorough risk-benefit analysis. Any surgical intervention carries with it the remote possibility of a career-ending complication. For this reason, the use of arthroscopic surgery in athletes holds additional appeal, so long as outcomes are as good or better than more invasive approaches. Adverse surgical outcomes following open posterior instability surgery have included high recurrence rates, problems with hardware, postsurgical degenerative changes, and postsurgical stiffness (35,42,49,50,60–63). Additional complications of inadvertent intraarticular fracture and subcoracoid impingement have been reported in association with glenoid osteotomy (64,65).

Arthroscopic approaches also carry complications unique to technique. Earlier transglenoid methods of passing and tying sutures posteriorly over muscle fascia have been largely replaced by purely intraarticular methods that lessen the risk of suprascapular nerve injury and subcutaneous knot irritation. When performing intraarticular repairs, the use of bioabsorbable suture anchors has also come into favor due to concerns with metal implants. Applications of thermal methods have also been refined to reflect more specific indications and to avoid complication.

Wong and Williams recently conducted a survey of 379 surgeons to evaluate the prevalence of complications related to the use of thermal energy for the treatment of glenohumeral instability (66). They reported a 1.4% incidence of axillary nerve injury, most of which resolved spontaneously. The majority (93%) of these injuries were pure sensory and lasted an average of 2.3 months. Combined sensory and motor deficits (7%) lasted an average of 4 months. Greis and colleagues reported on a small case series of four patients with axillary nerve injury following thermal capsulorrhaphy (67). Two patients had pure sensory deficits and two manifested both motor and sensory loss. In a cadaveric study, Gryler and colleagues recorded temperatures along the axillary nerve of nine cadaveric shoulders using thermocouples. In two specimens, maximum temperatures greater than the 67°C setpoint of the device were recorded, confirming that potentially harmful heating of the axillary nerve may occur during thermal capsulorrhaphy (68).

Concern regarding the proximity of the axillary nerve to the inferior capsule may also come into play when passing suture arthroscopically. Several studies have shown the nerve to lie closest to the anterior inferior capsule, between the 5- and 7-o'clock positions (69–72). The axillary nerve lies closer to the humeral capsular insertion than the glenoid capsular insertion. In addition, this distance has been shown to increase with abduction, external rotation, and the use of perpendicular traction (69,70). In a cadaveric study, Bryan et al. found the axillary nerve to lie an average of only 3 mm from the inferior capsule (71). Eakin and colleagues performed anatomic dissections following arthroscopic capsular plication and found the average distance from the nerve to the suture to be 12.5 mm at the anteroinferior position, 14.4 mm at the inferior position, and 24.1 mm at the posteroinferior position (72). Their study demonstrated a relatively safe margin for arthroscopic suture placement when plication was initiated approximately 1 cm from the glenoid rim.

Concern regarding post-thermal capsular fibrosis and deficiency have led some to recommend leaving interval areas of capsule unaddressed by shrinking tissue in a cornrow or grid pattern (40). In patients undergoing revision surgery following failed thermal or laser capsular shrinkage, there has been a high incidence of reported capsular attenuation (66). Capsular fibrosis and motion restriction has also been reported (73). In our hands, the select use of thermal shrinkage is indicated only to augment arthroscopic stabilization performed with suture anchors or plication sutures. When we do use thermal energy, we use a cornrow pattern, leaving areas of normal capsule and taking care to continuously keep the probe moving while shrinking tissue. Because the posterior capsule is thin and less responsive to thermal shrinkage, we do not use the probe is this area.

In addition to complications related to surgical technique, it is important to pay close attention to patient positioning and intraoperative care. With patients in the lateral position, an axillary roll should be placed beneath the down side and the common peroneal nerve should be protected with blankets or foam padding. Arthroscopic work should proceed systematically and in a timely fashion so as to minimize fluid extravasation into local tissues and secondary pulmonary complications. It is the surgeon's responsibility to be present as the patient is awakened to support the extremity and assist in brace application. During the postoperative period of brace wear, careful attention should be paid to areas of constant skin-brace contact. Padding may need to be added or adjustments made to improve comfort and alleviate contact pressure.

REFERENCES

1. Jobe FW, Giangara CE, Kvitne RS et al. Anterior capsulolabral reconstruction of the shoulder in athletes in overhead sports. *Am J Sports Med* 1991;19:428–434.
2. Kelly BT, Backus SI, Warren RF, et al. Electromyographic analysis and phase definition of the overhead football throw. *Am J Sports Med* 2002;30:837–844.
3. Scovazzo ML, Browne A, Pink M, et al. The painful shoulder during the freestyle stroke. *Am J Sports Med* 1991;19:577–582.
4. Pink M, Jobe FW, Perry J, et al. The painful shoulder during the butterfly stroke. *Clin Orthop* 1993;288:60–72.
5. Pink M, Jobe FW, Perry J, et al. The normal shoulder during the backstroke: an EMG and cinematographic analysis of twelve muscles. *Clin J Sports Med* 1992;2:6–12.
6. Pink M, Perry J, Jobe FW, et al. The normal shoulder during freestyle swimming: an EMG and cinematographic analysis of twelve muscles. *Am J Sports Med* 1991;19:569–575.
7. Pink M, Jobe FW, Perry J. Electromyographic analysis of the shoulder during the golf swing. *Am J Sports Med* 1990;18:137–140.
8. Kao JT, Pink M, Jobe FW, et al. Electromyographic analysis of the scapular muscles during a golf swing. *Am J Sports Med* 1995;23:19–23.
9. Chow JW, Carlton LG, Lim YT, et al. Muscle activation during the tennis volley. *Med Sci Sports Exerc* 1999;31:846–854.
10. Kibler WB. Biomechanics of the shoulder during tennis activities. *Clin Sports Med* 1995;14:79–85.
11. Rokito AS, Jobe FW, Pink M, et al. Electromyographic analysis of shoulder function during the volleyball serve and spike. *J Shoulder Elbow Surg* 1998;7:256–263.
12. Brewer BJ, Wubben RC, Carrera GF. Excessive retroversion of the glenoid cavity. A cause of non-traumatic posterior instability of the shoulder. *J Bone Joint Surg Am* 1986;68:724–731.
13. Graichen H, Koydl P, Zicher L. Effectiveness of glenoid osteotomy in atraumatic posterior instability of the shoulder associated with excessive retroversion and flatness of the glenoid. *Int Orthop* 1999;23:95–99.
14. Surin V, Blader S, Markhede G, et al. Rotational osteotomy of the humerus for posterior instability of the shoulder. *J Bone Joint Surg (Am)* 1990;72:181–186.
15. Hurley JA, Anderson TE, Dear W, et al. Posterior shoulder instability: Surgical versus conservative results with evaluation of glenoid version. *Am J Sports Med* 1992;20:396–400.
16. Edelson JG. Localized glenoid hypoplasia. An anatomic variation of possible clinical significance. *Clin Orthop* 1995;321:189–195.
17. Inui H, Sugamoto K, Miyamoto T, et al. Glenoid shape in atraumatic posterior instability of the shoulder. *Clin Orthop* 2002;403:87–92.
18. Ovesen J, Nielsen S. Posterior instability of the shoulder. A cadaver study. *Acta Orthop Scand* 1986;57:436–439.
19. Debski RE, Sakane M, Woo SYL, et al. Contribution of the passive properties of the rotator cuff to glenohumeral stability during anterior-posterior loading. *J Shoulder Elbow Surg* 1999;8:324–329.
20. Blasier RB, Soslowsky LJ, Malicky DM, et al. Posterior glenohumeral subluxation: active and passive stabilization in a biomechanical model. *J Bone Joint Surg* 1997;79(3):430–433.
21. O'Brien SJ, Schwartz RE, Warren RF, et al. Capsular restraints to anterior/posterior motion of the shoulder. *Orthop Trans* 1988;12:143.
22. Harryman DT, Sidles JA, Clark JM, et al. Translation of the humeral head on the glenoid with passive glenohumeral motion. *J Bone Joint Surg (Am)* 1990;72:1334–1343.
23. Warren RF, Kornblatt IB, Marchand R. Static factors affecting posterior shoulder instability. *Orthop Trans* 1984;8:89.
24. Weber SL, Caspari RB. A biomechanical evaluation of the restraints to posterior shoulder dislocation. *Arthroscopy* 1989;5:115–121.
25. Basmajian J, Bazant F. Factors preventing downward dislocation of the adducted shoulder joint in an electromyographic and morphological study. *J Bone Joint Surg Am* 1959;41:1182–1186.
26. Harryman DT, Sidles JA, Harris SL, et al. The role of the rotator interval capsule in passive motion and stability of the shoulder. *J Bone Joint Surg Am* 1992;74:53–66.
27. Jost B, Koch PP, Gerber C. Anatomy and functional aspects of the rotator interval. *J Shoulder Elbow Surg* 2000;9:336–341.
28. Warner J, Deng X, Warren RF, et al. Static capsuloligamentous restraints to superior-inferior translation of the glenohumeral joint. *Am J Sports Med* 1992;20:675–685.
29. Howell SM, Galinat BJ. The glenoid-labral socket. A constrained articular surface. *Clin Orthop* 1989;243:122–125.
30. Lippitt SB, Vanderhooft JE, Harris SL, et al. Glenohumeral stability from concavity-compression: a quantitative analysis. *J Shoulder Elbow Surg* 1993;2:27–35.
31. Gerber C, Werner CML, Macy JC, et al. Effect of selective capsulorrhaphy on the passive range of motion of the glenohumeral joint. *J Bone Joint Surg Am* 2003;85(1):48–55.
32. Tibone JE, Lee TQ, Black AD, et al. Glenohumeral translation after arthroscopic thermal capsuloplasty with a radiofrequency probe. *J Shoulder Elbow Surg* 2000;9:514–518.
33. Tibone JE, McMahon PJ, Shrader TA, et al. Glenohumeral joint translation after arthroscopic, nonablative thermal capsuloplasty with a laser. *Am J Sports Med* 1998;26:495–498.
34. Tibone JE, Lee TQ, Black AD, et al. Glenohumeral translation after arthroscopic thermal capsuloplasty with a radiofrequency probe. *J Shoulder Elbow Surg* 2000;9:514–518.
35. Bigliani LU, Pollack RG, McIlveen SJ, et al. Shift of the posteroinferior aspect of the capsule for recurrent posterior glenohumeral instability. *J Bone Joint Surg (Am)* 1995;77:1011–1020.
36. Ciccone WJ, Hunt TJ, Lieber R, et al. Multiquadrant digital analysis of shoulder capsular thickness. *Arthroscopy* 2000;16:457–461.
37. Selecky MT, Tibone JE, Yang BY, et al. Glenohumeral joint translation after arthroscopic thermal capsuloplasty of the rotator interval. *J Shoulder Elbow Surg* 2003;12:139–143.
38. Mair SD, Zarzour RH, Speer KP. Posterior labral injury in contact athletes. *Am J Sports Med* 1998;26:753–758.
39. Hovis WD, Dean MT, Mallon WJ, et al. Posterior instability of the shoulder with secondary impingement in elite golfers. *Am J Sports Med* 2002;30(6):886–890.
40. Joseph TA, Williams JS Jr, Brems JJ. Laser capsulorrhaphy for multidirectional instability of the shoulder: an outcomes study and proposed classification system. *Am J Sports Med* 2003;31:26–35.

41. Antoniou J, Harryman DT 2nd. Arthroscopic posterior capsular repair. *Clin Sports Med* 2000;19(1);101–114.

42. Fuchs B, Jost B, Gerber C. Posterior-inferior capsular shift for the treatment of recurrent, voluntary posterior subluxation of the shoulder. *J Bone Joint Surg (Am)* 2000;82(1):16–25.

43. Burkhead WZ Jr, Rockwood CA Jr. Treatment of instability of the shoulder with an exercise program. *J Bone Joint Surg (Am)* 1992;74:890–896.

44. Misamore GW, Facibene WA. Posterior capsulorrhaphy for the treatment of traumatic recurrent posterior subluxations of the shoulder in athletes. *J Shoulder Elbow Surg* 2000;9:403–408.

45. Pande P, Hawkins R, Peat M. Electromyography in voluntary posterior instability of the shoulder. *Am J Sports Med* 1989;17:644–648.

46. Beall MS, Diefenbach G, Allen A. Electromyographic biofeedback in the treatment of voluntary posterior instability of the shoulder. *Am J Sports Med* 1987;15:175–178.

47. Hawkins RJ, Janda DH. Posterior instability of the glenohumeral joint: a technique of repair. *Am J Sports Med* 1996;24:275–278.

48. Wirth MA, Groh GI, Rockwood CA Jr. Capsulorrhaphy through an anterior approach for the treatment of atraumatic posterior glenohumeral instability with multidirectional laxity of the shoulder. *J Bone Joint Surg* 1998;80(11):1570–1578.

49. Fronek J, Warren RF, Bowen M. Posterior subluxation of the glenohumeral joint. *J Bone Joint Surg (Am)* 1989;71:205–216.

50. Tibone JE, Bradley JP. The treatment of posterior subluxation in athletes. *Clin Orthop* 1993;291:124–137.

51. Harryman DT III, Duckworth DG. The efficacy of capsulolabral augmentation for managing pathologic findings and symptoms of primary postero-inferior instability. *J Shoulder Elbow Surg* 1998;7:314.

52. McIntyre LF, Caspari RB, Savoie FH III. The arthroscopic treatment of posterior shoulder instability: two-year results of a multiple suture technique. *Arthroscopy* 1997;13:426–432.

53. Williams RJ, Strickland S, Cohen M, et al. Arthroscopic repair for traumatic posterior shoulder instability. *Am J Sports Med* 2003;31(2):203–209.

54. Wolf EM, Eakin CL. Arthroscopic capsular plication for posterior shoulder instability. *Arthroscopy* 1998;14:153–163.

55. Savoie FH, Field LD. Arthroscopic management of posterior shoulder instability. *Oper Tech Sports Med* 1997;5:226–232.

56. Gartsman GM, Roddey TS, Hammerman SM. Arthroscopic treatment of bidirectional glenohumeral instability: two to five year follow-up. *J Shoulder Elbow Surg* 2001;10:28–36.

57. Hawkins RJ, Schutte JP, Janda DH, et al. Translation of the glenohumeral joint with the patient under anesthesia. *J Shoulder Elbow Surg* 1996;5:286–292.

58. Harryman DT, Sidles JA, Harris SL, et al. Laxity of the normal glenohumeral joint: a quantitative *in vivo* assessment. *J Shoulder Elbow Surg* 1992;1:66–76.

59. McFarland EG, Campbell G, McDowell J. Posterior shoulder laxity in asymptomatic athletes. *Am J Sports Med* 1996;24:468–471.

60. Tibone J, Ting A. Capsulorrhaphy with a staple for recurrent posterior subluxation of the shoulder. *J Bone Joint Surg* 1990;72:999–1002.

61. Zuckerman JD, Matsen FA III. Complications about the glenohumeral joint related to the use of screws and staples. *J Bone Joint Surg (Am)* 1984;66:175–180.

62. Warner JJ, Ianotti JP. Treatment of the stiff shoulder after posterior capsulorrhaphy: a report of 3 cases. *J Bone Joint Surg (Am)* 1996;78:1419–1421.

63. Hawkins RJ, Koppert G, Johnston G. Recurrent posterior instability (subluxation) of the shoulder. *J Bone Joint Surg (Am)* 1984;66:169–174.

64. Johnston GH, Hawkins RJ, Haddad R, et al. A complication of posterior glenoid osteotomy for recurrent posterior instability. *Clin Orthop* 1984;187:147–149.

65. Gerber C, Ganz R, Vinh TS. Glenoplasty for recurrent posterior shoulder instability. *Clin Orthop* 1987;216:70.

66. Wong KL, Williams GR. Complications of thermal capsulorrhaphy of the shoulder. *J Bone Joint Surg (Am)* 83[Suppl 2, Pt 2]:151–155.

67. Greis PE, Burks RT, Schickendantz MS, et al. Axillary nerve injury after thermal capsular shrinkage of the shoulder. *J Shoulder Elbow Surg* 2001;10:231–235.

68. Gryler EC, Greis PE, Burks RT, et al. Axillary nerve temperatures during radiofrequency capsulorrhaphy of the shoulder. *Arthroscopy* 2001;17:567–572.

69. Uno A, Bain GI, Mehta JA. Arthroscopic relationship of the axillary nerve to the shoulder joint capsule: an anatomic study. *J Shoulder Elbow Surg* 1999;8:226–230.

70. Jerosch J, Filler TJ, Peuker ET. Which joint position puts the axillary nerve at lowest risk when performing arthroscopic capsular release in patients with adhesive capsulitis of the shoulder? *Knee Surg Sports Traumatol Arthrosc* 2002;10:126–129.

71. Bryan WJ, Schauder K, Tullos HS. The axillary nerve and its relationship to common sports medicine procedures. *Am J Sports Med* 1986;14:113–116.

72. Eakin CL, Dvirnak P, Miller CM, et al. The relationship of the axillary nerve to arthroscopically placed capsulolabral sutures: an anatomic study. *Am J Sports Med* 1998;26:505–509.

73. Fanton GS. Arthroscopic electrothermal surgery of the shoulder. *Oper Tech Sports Med* 1998;6:139-146.

14

MULTIDIRECTIONAL INSTABILITY

GARY MISAMORE
PETER SALLAY
BRENT JOHNSON

HISTORICAL OVERVIEW

In reviewing the literature on multidirectional instability (MDI) of the shoulder, it is very difficult to draw any objective conclusions. There are only a handful of studies published on this topic and the majority of them are retrospective. The most difficult problem in analyzing the literature is determining specifically what type of instability is being reviewed, because there is no mutually accepted precise definition for MDI. This lack of a precise definition results in varied patient populations being evaluated in the literature, which makes comparisons of these studies difficult.

Lippitt and colleagues (1) and Thomas and Matsen (2) have described the traditional classification of shoulder instability described by the acronyms TUBS and AMBRI. TUBS stands for *t*raumatic etiology, *u*nidirectional instability, *B*ankart lesion, and a need for *s*urgery to achieve stability; AMBRI describes instability that is *a*traumatic, *m*ultidirectional, often *b*ilateral, responds well to *r*ehabilitation, and when treated surgically requires an *i*nferior capsular shift. This classification is useful in describing the generalities of the different ends of the spectrum of shoulder instability, but does not capture all of the variations between.

The most important step in reviewing the literature is to critically look at the patient population. Is there a history of a traumatic event? What are the age and activity levels of the patients? How are these results analyzed? Without a clear and precise definition for MDI, one must read reports on its treatment critically. Are the authors truly discussing AMBRI patients or are they describing TUBS patients in whom secondary laxity has developed after an initial traumatic event? Or, do the cases fall somewhere in between?

A definition of MDI should include excessive laxity in multiple directions with reproduction of the patient's feeling of instability. It also should exclude patients with a traumatic onset to the instability, unidirectional instability, and radiographic evidence of bony injury. It is difficult to find a patient population this well defined in the literature.

Nonoperative Treatment

Nonsurgical management of the symptomatic shoulder with MDI is the initial step in treatment, consisting of extensive patient education and physical therapy. It has been the prevailing thought that most patients could be treated successfully by patient education, rotator cuff and shoulder girdle strengthening exercises, and activity modification. In 1956, Rowe (3) reported that a majority of patients with atraumatic shoulder instability did well with physical therapy during short-term follow-up. In 1992, Burkhead and Rockwood (4) reported good or excellent results in 88% of patients treated for MDI with physician-directed rehabilitation at an average follow-up of 48 months. However, in their report, it is not possible to determine any specific details about the MDI patients such as age, specific symptoms, duration of symptoms, and magnitude of shoulder laxity. More recently, in a much more defined population, Misamore and co-workers (5) have shown that only 17 of 57 patients had satisfactory outcomes from the nonsurgical management based on stability and Rowe scores at 7- to 10-year follow-up.

Open Surgical Treatment of Multidirectional Instability

Neer and Foster (6) were the first to report on the inferior capsular shift for MDI in 1980. They reported on 40 shoulders in 36 patients. In their group 26 of 29 patients reported a moderate or severe traumatic event with their initial dislocation. Five of their patients that were included had Bankart lesions. The patient population varied from age 15 to 55 years, and only 17 of the patients were described as having generalized ligamentous laxity. Some of these patients appeared to fit the definition of MDI, but not all of them. They reported only one unsatisfactory result in 32 shoulders that were followed up for more than 1 year. Nine patients in their group returned to competitive sports. Three patients suffered axillary nerve injury.

In 1991, Altcheck and colleagues (7) reported on the surgical treatment of 40 patients for MDI. In this group 39 of 40 patients suffered a traumatic onset with 36 patients suffering a frank dislocation. Thirty-eight of 40 shoulders had a Bankart lesion and 24 had a Hill-Sachs lesion. This group of patients does not seem to fit the definition of MDI. Thirty-six of the 40 patients with at least 2-year follow-up had relief of instability. They also reported that 33 of 40 patients had a full return to sports; although they did not describe or quantify their activity level.

Cooper and Brems (8) reported on 43 shoulders in 38 patients over 6 years. Thirty-two of 43 shoulders had no history of trauma of a magnitude normally associated with dislocation, although for 18 the onset of painful instability could be traced to relatively minor trauma. Twenty-eight of 36 patients had laxity in the opposite shoulder and 29 patients had generalized ligamentous laxity. In this group only seven patients were found to have Bankart lesions. This group of patients more closely represents an MDI population. Thirty-nine shoulders (91%) functioned well with no recurrence of instability. Of these patients, 29 shoulders were thought to be stable enough to allow the patient to return to the same or a more physically demanding job. Sixteen shoulders were stable enough for the patients to return to the same sport and play at the same or a reduced level of activity. However, none of these patients had been elite athletes.

Lebar and Alexander (9) reported on 10 patients surgically treated for MDI over 10 years. In their group, all patients had inferior laxity but only three had generalized ligamentous laxity. Four patients in this group had an initial traumatic onset. At surgery, three Bankart and two Hill-Sachs lesions were found. Also six patients had undergone previous shoulder surgery with four having procedures to address instability. From this information, it is difficult to determine what type of instability these patients had. Eight of 10 patients at 1-year follow-up were happy with their surgery, reporting an overall improvement. One half of the patients received a medical discharge from the military with a disability. Additionally, of the five patients who returned to active duty, only two patients could function without restrictions.

Pollock and co-workers (10) reported on a longer term follow-up for the capsular shift procedure as a treatment of MDI. This study included 52 shoulders in 49 patients. The follow-up ranged from 24 to 132 months, over an average of 61 months. Average age of the patients was 23 years (range 16 to 42). Twenty-five shoulders had a history of a major episode of trauma with their onset of instability and there were 10 Bankart lesions and two anterior glenoid rim fractures identified at the time of surgery. Forty-six shoulders (96%) had good/excellent results. Forty-seven shoulders (96%) remained stable at their most recent follow-up. Recurring anterior instability developed in two shoulders within the first year after surgery. Thirty-one shoulders (86%) were able to return to participation in their premorbid sports activities; however, only 25 shoulders (69%) were able to return at the same level. With longer term follow-up and the activity level of this group of patients, there were no late failures demonstrating that an open capsular shift is a durable procedure.

Bak and co-workers (11) attempted to look at a population of strictly athletes surgically treated with capsular shift for MDI. Their study included 26 shoulders in 25 athletes evaluated at an average follow-up of 54 months (range 25 to 113). Their ages ranged from 16 to 35 years with a median age of 23. In this group, 16 shoulders had symptoms that were initiated by trauma, with one patient having an incomplete Bankart lesion at the time of surgery. Twenty-one patients (84%) returned to their preinjury sport at the same level. Of 21 patients involved in sports utilizing overhead motions, 16 (76%) returned to their previous sport, but there was no comparison made to their preoperative ability. Five shoulders were unstable at follow-up and 2 (8%) were considered failures.

In summary, it would appear that satisfactory results were obtained in approximately 90% of cases (Neer and Foster (6), 97%; Altchek and colleagues (7), 90%; Cooper and Brems (8), 91%; Lebar and Alexander (9), 80%; Pollock and co-workers (10), 96%; Bak and colleagues (11), 84%). However, even with this high percentage of successful results, it does still not seem that many shoulders were functioning well enough to allow a return to stressful activity. Although these reports of surgical treatment of MDI with an inferior capsular shift describe satisfactory results in approximately 90% of patients, the results are difficult to interpret because of varied patient populations. Also, the criteria for satisfactory results are not clearly defined or consistent. Because of this, the limited reports on the surgical treatment of MDI must be viewed cautiously and critically.

Arthroscopic Surgical Treatment of Multidirectional Instability

The literature on arthroscopic treatment of MDI is limited with only short-term results. The arthroscopic treatment of MDI includes two different techniques consisting of capsular plication with sutures and thermal capsulorrhaphy.

Duncan and Savoie (12) published a report on arthroscopic treatment utilizing a transglenoid suture technique. Ten consecutive patients were evaluated with 1- to 3-year follow-up. Although MDI had been diagnosed by the authors, 9 of 10 patients had previous dislocations and four Bankart lesions were identified at the time of surgery, suggesting they were not typical MDI. They reported an average Bankart score of 90 (range 75 to 95) and all patients resumed activities of daily living without discomfort. Four patients were able to return to sporting activities at their preinjury levels.

Treacy and co-workers (13) reported on 25 patients with an average follow-up of 60 months (range 36 to 80) using the same technique. The average age of this patient group was 26.4 years (range 15 to 39). Eleven patients had sustained a prior dislocation, 14 patients had a Bankart lesion identified at the time of surgery, and five patients had evidence of generalized ligamentous laxity. The average Bankart score was 95 (range 50 to 100) and 21 patients (88%) had a satisfactory result according to the Neer system. Three of the patients had episodes of recurrent instability and required further surgical treatment.

McIntyre and colleagues (14) also described a transglenoid suture technique but placed sutures anteriorly as well as posterior to the glenoid. This series consisted of 19 consecutive shoulders treated for MDI. Their average age was 23 years (range 15 to 52). Fourteen of the 19 patients were initially injured during athletic activity. At the time of surgery, seven patients were identified who had both an anterior and posterior Bankart lesion, two had an anterior Bankart lesion, and one had posterior labral fraying. Six patients were identified to have an anterior or posterior Hill-Sachs lesion. At an average follow-up of 34 months postoperatively, the average outcome score was 91 of 100. There were 13 excellent, five good, and one fair result. One patient had repeated episodes of instability that required a repeat arthroscopic capsular shift.

Gartsman and colleagues (15) prospectively evaluated 47 patients treated with an arthroscopic capsular shift for MDI. Their technique consisted of an anatomic repair of the labrum and a capsular plication of the glenohumeral ligaments to the labrum. No transosseus sutures were used. The average age of the patients was 30 years (range 15 to 56). Twenty-seven patients had a history of recurrent subluxation and 20 patients had recurrent dislocation before surgery. Instability after a single traumatic event developed in 21 patients and instability without trauma developed in 26. At the time of surgery, there were 10 Bankart and five Hill-Sachs lesions identified. At an average follow-up of 35 months (range 26 to 67), 44 of 47 shoulders were rated as excellent according to the Rowe score. One patient had episodes of recurrent instability and required a second operative procedure. Twenty-two of 26 patients were able to return to their desired level of athletic participation.

Lyons and colleagues (16) reported on a group of 27 shoulders in 26 patients treated with a combination of laser-assisted capsulorrhaphy and rotator interval suture plication. The average age of the patients was 25 years (range 16 to 46). Four of the patients developed instability from a single traumatic event. Patients who were found to have labral pathology requiring repair were excluded from the study. The follow-up averaged 27 months (range 24 to 35). Twenty-six of 27 shoulders remained stable. Three patients (12%) had an unsatisfactory rating using the Neer criteria and one patient required a reoperation. No perioperative complications were noted.

Fitzgerald and colleagues (17) used thermal capsulorrhaphy without suture plication in the treatment of 33 shoulders for MDI. The mean age of the patients was 27 years (range 17 to 41), and 90% were on active military duty. No Bankart lesions were identified at the time of surgery. At a mean follow-up of 33 months (range 24 to 40), three patients were rated as excellent, 20 good, and seven poor according to the UCLA rating scale.

Favorito and co-workers (18) examined the results of laser-assisted capsular shift. They looked at 30 shoulders in 28 patients with MDI. The mean patient age was 26.4 years (range 12 to 38) with a mean follow-up of 28 months (range 12 to 38). None of the patients had a single traumatic event as inciting their shoulder pain. Twenty-two shoulders were considered successes and had an average UCLA score of 31.91 (range 27 to 35). Five patients were considered failures with a mean UCLA score of 23.6 (range 11 to 33) and required subsequent open capsular shifts.

In summary, the results from the few published reports on arthroscopic treatment of MDI appear to compare favorably with the results from the literature on the open capsular shift. The arthroscopic techniques appear to have a similar success rate around 90%. The recurrence and complication rates also compare favorably. The arthroscopic literature on the treatment of MDI also suffers from the fact that there is no concise definition of the condition, making comparisons and drawing clear conclusions from the literature difficult. One must remember that the aforementioned results concerning open and arthroscopic treatment of MDI are being reported by experienced shoulder surgeons who routinely deal with difficult shoulder problems.

DIAGNOSIS

Typically patients with MDI are younger than 30 years of age. In contrast to traumatic instability, there is a higher percentage of women than men with MDI. Patients often have laxity in their opposite shoulder, which may or may not be symptomatic. They also often have generalized ligamentous laxity. In addition to their complaints of instability, they often complain of a chronic insidious aching in the shoulder. The instability can be severe enough in some cases to allow the shoulder to continuously sublux with activities of daily living. This can result in a continuous aching in the shoulder, in contrast to patients with traumatic unidirectional instability who typically experience infrequent but more intense episodes of pain with subluxation or dislocation.

Because of the generalized aching often associated with MDI, identifying the instability on examination can be difficult. The patients often voluntarily guard during the examination to avoid discomfort or pain. It is not uncommon for these patients to initially have a diagnosis of and undergo treatment for rotator cuff tendonitis or impingement syndrome. It is often not until their shoulder pain subsides that the instability can be demonstrated on subsequent examinations. The details of examination for instability are discussed previously.

The diagnosis of MDI of the shoulder must be confirmed by instability in at least two directions. A typical component of this is inferior instability, demonstrated by the sulcus sign. It is often difficult initially to clearly define the instability pattern. Overhead athletes with MDI can present with various complaints. These include vague chronic pain, dysesthesias, or a "dead arm." Onset of symptoms may have been insidious, may have been initiated by a traumatic event, or may simply have occurred during activities of daily living. All these different histories may represent subtle different types of MDI.

SURGICAL TREATMENT

When physical therapy fails for MDI, surgery can be considered to decrease the redundant capsular tissue. The laxity of the static restraints (capsule) can place a greater demand on the dynamic restraints, resulting in fatigue and injuries to the rotator cuff and scapular stabilizers. Bowen and Warren (19) have hypothesized that redundant capsule with its resulting increased joint volume may result in the development of smaller intraarticular negative pressures and thus circumvent one of the shoulders important restraints, allowing greater translation to occur.

The goal of surgery is to attain a global tightening of the capsule. In most cases, this is attained through an open anterior inferior capsular shift. Even when there is a significant component of posterior instability, this can often be eliminated by an anterior approach in which the rotator cuff interval and anterior superior capsule are imbricated while the anterior, inferior, and posterior capsule are shifted to attain global tightening. By extensive release of the capsular tissues from the humeral neck, even most of the posterior capsule can be adequately mobilized such that an adequate global tightening of the capsule can be performed from an anterior approach to the shoulder. We typically perform a posterior capsular shift for those patients with isolated posterior or posteroinferior instability, or rarely when we feel the instability is so great that posterior capsular shift needs to be combined with an anterior capsular shift.

Open Inferior Capsular Shift

An examination of the shoulder is performed under anesthesia to confirm the pattern and magnitude of instability and document range of motion to reference following the capsular shift. Prior to the open capsular shift, a diagnostic shoulder arthroscopy is usually performed. This allows confirmation of the suspected diagnosis, as well as identifica-

tion and treatment of other pathology. Bankart lesions, partial rotator cuff tears, and SLAP (superior labrum anterior-to-posterior) lesions may be encountered. If identified, these may sometimes be addressed arthroscopically.

The patient is positioned supine with the head of the bed elevated 20 degrees and a bump placed under the scapula to elevate the shoulder off the bed. The patient is positioned off to the side, so the shoulder is off the edge of the table. An arm board is used to support the elbow to prevent extension of the shoulder that could sublux the humeral head anteriorly, making the repair of the capsule anteriorly more difficult. The upper extremity and shoulder are draped to allow access to the anterior and posterior aspects of the shoulder, as well as allow a full range of motion of the upper extremity.

We place our incision in the anterior axilla for cosmetic reasons. The incision is placed in the most prominent skinfold that extends up from the axilla. It begins in the axilla and extends superiorly as needed. The skin and subcutaneous tissue are undermined to identify the deltopectoral interval. A generous amount of subcutaneous tissue mobilization is required when using an axillary incision (Fig. 14-1).

The cephalic vein is identified in the interval and retracted laterally with the deltoid. The pectoralis is retracted medially. The clavipectoral fascia is opened longitudinally lateral to the conjoined tendon, and this is then retracted medially with the pectoralis. The circumflex vessels are exposed, clamped, and coagulated to allow adequate exposure of the inferior capsule at the time of the shift. The subscapularis tendon is incised near its attachment into the lesser tuberosity, leaving adequate tissue for repair. A combination of sharp and blunt dissection is used to separate it from the capsule. The capsular foramen is identified superi-

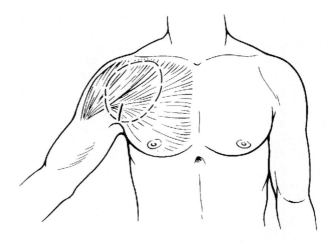

FIGURE 14-1. Anterior capsular shift. Placement of the anterior axillary incision is indicated. The tissues must be undermined superiorly to expose the deltopectoral interval. (From Hawkins RJ, Misamore GW. *Shoulder injuries in the athlete: surgical repair and rehabilitation.* Philadelphia, PA: Elsevier, 1996:192–197, with permission.)

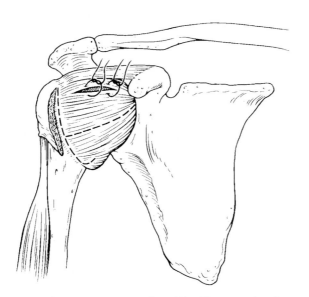

FIGURE 14-2. Anterior capsular shift. The capsular foramen superiorly is closed with sutures. Inferior and superior flaps are created by a T incision in the capsule with the vertical incision placed near the humeral insertion of the capsule. (From Hawkins RJ, Misamore GW. *Shoulder injuries in the athlete: surgical repair and rehabilitation.* Philadelphia, PA: Elsevier, 1996:192–197, with permission.)

orly between the superior and middle glenohumeral ligaments and closed with nonabsorbable sutures.

A capsulotomy is made transversely across the equator of the joint extending from the humerus to the glenoid labrum (Fig. 14-2). Special care is taken not to damage the

articular surface or the labrum. If a Bankart lesion is identified, it can be treated in one of two manners. One option is to repair the Bankart lesion to the glenoid and continue with the capsular shift on the humeral side. The other choice is to perform both the Bankart repair and the capsular shift on the glenoid side. It has been our experience that greater mobilization of the inferior capsule can be performed when it is released on the humeral side. Performing both the Bankart repair and capsular shift on the glenoid side has been useful when treating primarily anteroinferior instability rather than MDI.

The vertical limb of the capsulotomy is made laterally, leaving 1 cm of the capsule attached to the humerus for later repair. A tag suture is placed in the superolateral corner of the inferior capsular flap to aid in orientation at the time of repair. Additionally, the level of the transverse capsulotomy is marked on the humerus with electrocautery to aid in determining the amount of capsular advancement.

The key to accomplishing an appropriate capsular shift for MDI is to ensure that the capsule is released inferiorly and posteriorly as necessary. A blunt retractor or finger can be placed under the inferior margin of the capsule to protect the axillary nerve as it is being released. The humerus is externally rotated and the capsule is carefully released inferiorly and posteriorly (Fig. 14-3). This is only accomplished safely when all soft tissue has been carefully dissected off the inferior aspect of the capsule. The capsular release is performed under direct visualization using a combination of blunt and sharp dissection. Great care must be taken in this area as a result of the proximity of the axillary nerve. Fail-

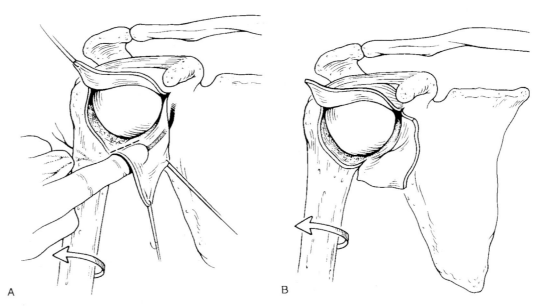

A   B

FIGURE 14-3. Anterior capsular shift. **A:** The capsular incision extends inferior and posterior. **B:** Posterior exposures achieved by external rotation of the arm. (From Hawkins RJ, Misamore GW. *Shoulder injuries in the athlete: surgical repair and rehabilitation.* Philadelphia, PA: Elsevier, 1996:192–197, with permission.)

ure to adequately release the capsule posteriorly can lead to loss of external rotation, yet still leave the patient with anterior inferior instability.

The amount of capsular advancement must be individualized depending on the patient's overall laxity and the quality of the tissue. The inferior flap is advanced superiorly and laterally to reduce the capsular redundancy. The inferior capsular flap is then sutured back to the stump of remaining capsular tissue on the neck of the humerus (Fig. 14-4). This is done with multiple number 2 nonabsorbable sutures. After being tied, these sutures are tagged and are

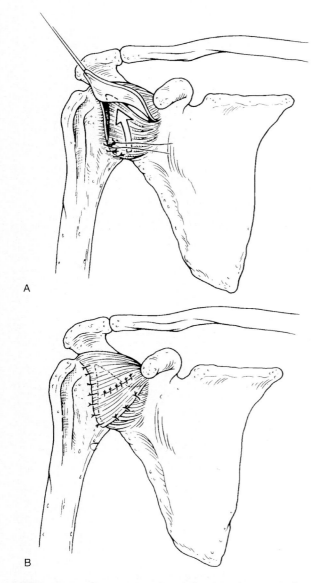

FIGURE 14-4. Anterior capsular shift. Capsular repair is performed by superior and lateral advancement of the inferior flap and inferior and lateral advancement of the superior flap. (From Hawkins RJ, Misamore GW. *Shoulder injuries in the athlete: surgical repair and rehabilitation.* Philadelphia, PA: Elsevier, 1996: 192–197, with permission.)

subsequently used for repair of the superior capsular flap as well. The superior flap is advanced inferiorly and laterally to reinforce the inferior capsular flap. The transverse incision in the anterior capsule is then sutured in an imbricated fashion. There is typically a moderate amount of overlap as both flaps are advanced quite significantly.

Positioning of the arm at the time of capsular closure allows improved visualization and judgment of suture placement for capsular tensioning. Altchek and colleagues (7) recommend holding the arm at 45 degrees of external rotation and 45 degrees of abduction at the time of capsular shift. We have discovered that the tension of our shift is primarily dependent on the suture placement in the capsule as well as the extent of the release, and that the arm position is not a significant factor. There is no formula for proper tensioning of the capsule; one must use sound judgment at the time of surgery.

Following repair the capsular shift is evaluated. Many variables need to be considered, including the patient's age, the degree of generalized ligamentous laxity, and the ultimate goals of the patient (sports, occupation, or activities of daily living). The passive inferior, anterior, and posterior translation as well as range of motion can be compared to the preoperative shoulder. There should be no or little passive translation present following the shift. Generally, the external rotation is moderately decreased but this is quite variable.

The subscapularis tendon is then anatomically repaired with nonabsorbable sutures. The deltoid and pectoralis muscles are allowed to fall together and the subcutaneous tissues and skin are closed in standard fashion. In most cases, hemostasis is not a problem and a drain is not necessary.

Posterior Capsular Shift

In a small percentage of our patients with atraumatic MDI that fail conservative treatment, a pattern is identified in which posterior instability is most predominant and symptomatic direction of laxity. In these cases, we proceed with a capsular shift approached posteriorly. We briefly describe our surgical technique for the posterior capsular shift.

We perform the surgery with the patient in the lateral decubitus position with the affected shoulder up. The skin incision is made vertically from just medial to the posterolateral corner of the acromion inferiorly toward the posterior axillary fold approximately 7 cm long centered over the posterior glenohumeral joint. The deltoid muscle is split in line with its fibers and a deep self-retaining retractor is placed (Fig. 14-5). Normally the tendons and muscle fibers separate off the posterior capsule without much difficulty. The quality of capsular tissue is better on the glenoid side and for that reason we release and repair the capsule to the glenoid. The superior and inferior flaps are created in similar fashion to the anterior approach, except that the vertical

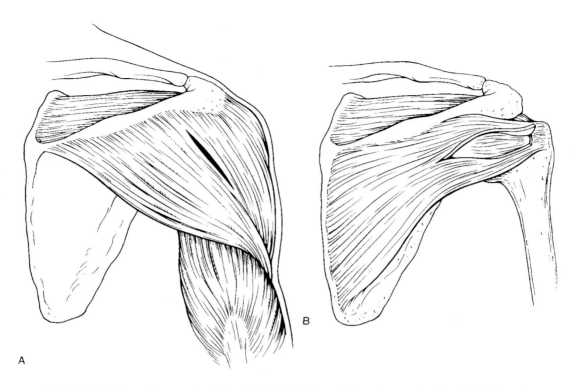

FIGURE 14-5. Posterior capsular shift. **A:** The deltoid is split directly over the joint in the line of the muscle fibers. **B:** The infraspinatus is split directly over the midlevel of the joint in line of the muscle fibers. A short vertical incision in the tendon near its humeral insertion may be added to improve exposure of the capsule. (From Hawkins RJ, Misamore GW. *Shoulder injuries in the athlete: surgical repair and rehabilitation.* Philadelphia, PA: Elsevier, 1996:192–197, with permission.)

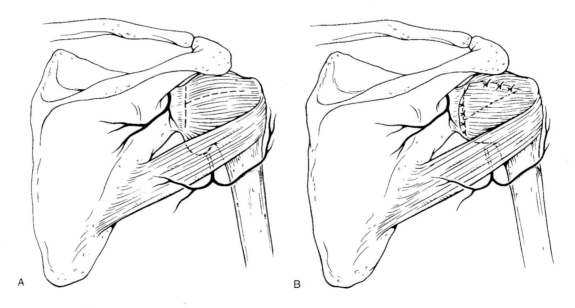

FIGURE 14-6. A: Posterior capsular shift. A T-capsulotomy is made in the posterior capsule with the vertical incision near the glenoid labrum. **B:** Posterior capsular shift. Capsular repair is performed by superior and medial advancement of the inferior flap and inferior and medial advancement of the superior flap. (From Hawkins RJ, Misamore GW. *Shoulder injuries in the athlete: surgical repair and rehabilitation.* Philadelphia, PA: Elsevier, 1996:192–197, with permission.)

component of the capsulotomy is made adjacent to the glenoid (Fig. 14-6). The capsule is incised lateral to the labrum, leaving the glenoid and labral attachment intact. Only infrequently is detachment of the posterior labrum found; therefore the capsule can usually be repaired by suturing it to the labrum. With the posterior approach, it is fairly difficult to tighten the capsule globally.

Arthroscopic Techniques

In certain patients, we attempt to address the capsular redundancy arthroscopically. These patients tend to have less severe instability on examination and not be involved in collision sports.

A routine diagnostic arthroscopic examination of the shoulder is performed initially. Our technique for an arthroscopic capsular shift is similar to the one described by Wichman and Snyder (20). The anterior superior portal is placed slightly more superiorly on instability cases to allow more room for anterior mid glenoid portal. Following this, the anterior mid glenoid portal is established approximately 2 cm lateral and 3 cm distal to the superior portal. A screw in translucent cannula is used.

When starting with the anterior plication, a suture hook is inserted through the anteromedial portal. This is then passed through the anteroinferior capsule and advanced through the anteroinferior portion of the labrum or paralabral capsular tissue, making sure to adequately advance the capsule superiorly. A suture relay is then used to pass a nonabsorbable braided suture through the capsule and labrum. The suture ends are retrieved out of the anterior medial portal and a simple suture is placed, snugging the capsule up to the labrum (Fig. 14-7). This process is repeated as necessary, advancing the capsule superiorly along the anterior edge of the labrum. This typically requires 3 to 4

sutures. The same procedure can be used to address posterior instability. If using the lateral decubitus position, only minimal traction should be used on the arm; otherwise, performing an adequate capsular shift is difficult. At the conclusion of the procedure, the translation of the shoulder is assessed to determine the amount of capsular tightening. If it is thought to be inadequate, further sutures are placed. Following arthroscopic plication, the same postoperative protocol is used as in the open capsular shift.

The use of thermal capsulorraphy to achieve reduction of capsular volume is also used in select patients. Initially, thermal capsulorraphy used a laser, but, because of cost constraints and improved understanding of the basic science of thermal capsulorraphy, radiofrequency heat probes are now used. Patients selected for this technique have less severe instability on examination. A diagnostic arthroscopy is initially performed with standard portals. To shrink the anterior capsule, the probe is inserted through the anterior portal and capsular shrinkage is started at the 6-o'clock position next to the glenoid. A 5-mm strip of capsule is tightened from the area of the glenoid attachment laterally to the humeral attachment of the capsule. This is then repeated anteriorly, creating successive bands and leaving bands of normal capsular tissue between them. This same technique is then used to shrink the posterior capsule. To reach the inferior axillary pouch and the posterior capsule, a posterior inferior accessory portal can be used. It is especially important in the inferior axillary pouch to limit the contact time of the probe with the capsule to avoid thermal injury to the axillary nerve. If the response of the capsule to thermal shrinkage is deemed inadequate, plication sutures are placed rather than repeating or prolonging thermal shrinkage of capsular tissues. These patients also follow the same postoperative protocol as the open capsular shift patients.

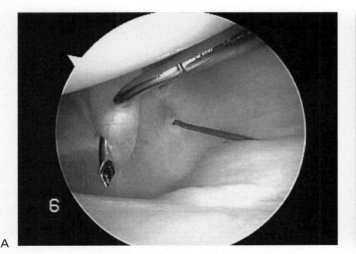 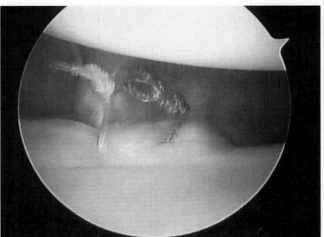

A   B

FIGURE 14-7. Arthroscopic capsular shift. **A:** Suture hook placed through anterior inferior capsule and labrum. **B:** Multiple sutures placed through anterior inferior capsule and labrum.

POSTOPERATIVE CARE

After surgery, each patient is placed in a protective orthosis before leaving the operating room. We prefer a gunslinger prefabricated orthosis (Seattle Systems, Pasadena, CA). The orthosis places the shoulder in slight abduction and external rotation (Fig. 14-8). This position can be modified depending on the instability pattern and the type of repair performed. Typically, patients with principally posterior instability are placed in greater external rotation to prevent stress on the posterior capsule. These procedures are typically performed on an outpatient basis. We believe that the use of a prefabricated orthosis is crucial to the success of the surgery for several reasons. The orthosis supports the arm in a superior direction, helping to prevent postoperative inferior subluxation and stretching of the capsule. These orthoses are also much easier to apply and are tolerated much better than casts. Finally, the orthosis places the upper extremity in a more optimal position, which allows the capsular repair not to receive excessive stretch.

Once wound healing has been demonstrated, the patients are evaluated at monthly intervals to assess their stability, motion, and muscle control. Examination is done gently for the first several months to avoid placing strain on the repair. The length of immobilization varies greatly, depending on several factors. There is no definitive proto-col that is followed postoperatively. Most commonly, the length of full-time immobilization in an orthosis is 4 to 6 weeks. Afterward, we typically have the patients continue to use the orthosis when sleeping for the next 2 to 3 weeks.

When the healing of the capsular tissues is thought to be adequate, the orthosis is discontinued and the patient is placed in shoulder swathe part time for comfort. The patient is permitted to use the shoulder to perform activities of daily living cautiously over the next 3 to 4 weeks as tolerated. Typically patients wean themselves from the swathe over a 2- to 3-week period as their symptoms allow and their strength begins to return. At this time, most patients are ready to begin a formal physical therapy program. If evaluation at this time reveals the shoulder irritability to be resolved and the stability to be good, a program is initiated that focuses on improving range of motion and gentle strengthening. As the shoulder function improves, the intensity of the therapy can be slowly progressed. In general, the patient can be given exercises and the therapy performed at home.

It is crucial throughout the rehabilitative process to closely monitor the patient's symptoms and stability. The rehabilitation must be individualized for each patient. A patient with only subtle instability and an excellent surgical repair can have a period of immobilization shortened and the aggressiveness of their rehabilitation increased. By contrast, when the capsular tissues are poor and the surgical repair tenuous, the immobilization time period needs to be increased and the progress of rehabilitation slowed. There is no typical postoperative protocol for the surgical treatment of MDI. Each patient's progress must be adjusted based on the ongoing clinical assessment of the physician.

Return to activities must also be made on an individual basis. Time to return to sports that require strenuous use of the arm varies from 6 to 12 months. Most patients, however, usually require 9 to 12 months to make a full recovery.

PROGNOSIS

From looking at our experience of the surgical treatment of MDI with an inferior capsular shift, nearly 90% of patients achieve good results with good stability and are able to perform activities of daily living without a problem. Of this group, approximately 66% are able to return to sporting activities, but less than 50% are able to return to a high level of overhead sports participation.

SURGICAL FAILURES

Any time a revision surgery is attempted, the reason for the initial failure must be ascertained to avoid repeating any mistakes. The determination of the most symptomatic direction of instability (anterior or posterior) can typically

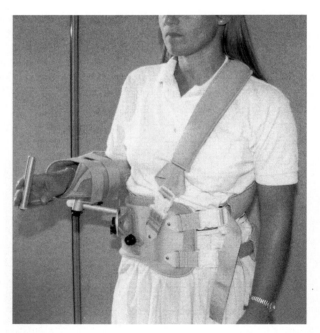

FIGURE 14-8. A prefabricated orthosis immobilizes the arm after surgery. Usually the arm is positioned in neutral rotation, but after a posterior capsular shift, more external rotation may be desired. Note that the orthosis lifts the affected extremity to prevent inferior stress on the capsular repair. (From Hawkins RJ, Misamore GW. *Shoulder injuries in the athlete: surgical repair and rehabilitation.* Philadelphia, PA: Elsevier, 1996:192–197, with permission.)

be made by careful history-taking and repeated physical examinations on subsequent office visits. It is not uncommon for surgery for traumatic anterior instability to have failed because the injury was actually an MDI.

One possible reason for failure may be that the time of immobilization was too short to adequately allow the capsular shift to heal or the rehabilitation was too aggressive. On the other hand, the surgical repair may have been too tight and then compounded by an excessive length of immobilization.

Revision surgery for MDI is no different from other types of revision surgery in orthopedics. The tissue planes are more difficult to cleanly develop and, in some cases, must be performed by sharp dissection. The anatomy can be slightly distorted, which is important when attempting an inferior capsular release because of the proximity of the axillary nerve. In Neer and Foster's (6) original description of the procedure, they reported three patients who suffered an axillary neuropraxia, but did not state whether these were revision cases. Zabinski and colleagues (21) reviewed the results of revision surgery for a subgroup of 21 shoulders with multiple directions of instability. Many different revision procedures were performed and at an average of 61.5 months of follow-up there were only 39% good or excellent results compared with 78% good or excellent results for revision surgery for anterior instability.

SUMMARY

MDI of the overhead shoulder is a difficult entity to correctly diagnose. Some athletes improve with physical therapy and do not require surgery. When therapy fails, surgical reconstruction can provide good to excellent results for activities of daily living but highly variable results for an athlete trying to get back to a high level of competition.

REFERENCES

1. Lippitt SB, Harryman DT, Sidles JA, et al. Diagnosis and management of AMBRI syndrome. *Techniques Orthop* 1991;6:61.
2. Thomas SC, Matsen FA. An approach to the repair of avulsion of the anterior glenohumeral ligaments in the management of traumatic anterior glenohumeral instability. *J Bone Joint Surg (Am)* 1989;71:506.
3. Rowe CR. Prognosis in dislocations of the shoulders. *J Bone Joint Surg (Am)* 1956;62:957.
4. Burkhead WZ Jr, Rockwood CA Jr. Treatment of instability of the shoulder with an exercise program. *J Bone Joint Surg (Am)* 1992;74:890.
5. Misamore GW, Sallay PI, Didelot W. A longitudinal study of patients with multidirectional instability of the shoulder with seven to ten year follow up. (*In press.*)
6. Neer CS, Foster CR. Inferior capsular shift for involuntary inferior and multidirectional instability of the shoulder. A preliminary report. *J Bone Joint Surg (Am)* 1980;62:897.
7. Altcheck DW, Warren RF, Skyhar MJ, et al. T-plasty modification of the Bankart procedure for multidirectional instability of the anterior and inferior types. *J Bone Joint Surg (Am)* 1991;73:105.
8. Cooper RA, Brems JJ. The inferior capsular-shift procedure for multidirectional instability of the shoulder. *J Bone Joint Surg (Am)* 1992;74:1516.
9. Lebar RD, Alexander AH. Multidirectional shoulder instability. *Am J Sports Med* 1992;20:193.
10. Pollock RG, Owens JM, Flatow EL, et al. Operative results of the inferior capsular shift procedure for multidirectional instability of the shoulder. *J Bone Joint Surg (Am)* 2000;82:919.
11. Bak K, Spring BJ, Henderson IJP. Inferior capsular shift procedure in athletes with multidirectional instability based on isolated capsular and ligamentous redundancy. *Am J Sports Med* 2000;28:466.
12. Duncan R, Savoie FH. Arthroscopic inferior capsular shift for multidirectional instability of the shoulder: a preliminary report. *Arthroscopy* 1993;9:24.
13. Treacy SH, Savoie FH, Field LD. Arthroscopic treatment of multidirectional instability. *J Shoulder Elbow Surg* 1999;8:344.
14. McIntyre LF, Caspari RB, Savoie FH. The arthroscopic treatment of multidirectional shoulder instability: two year results of a multiple suture technique. *Arthroscopy* 1997;13:418.
15. Gartsman GM, Roddey TS, Hammerman SM. Arthroscopic treatment of multidirectional glenohumeral instability: 2- to 5-year follow-up. *Arthroscopy* 2001;17:236.
16. Lyons TR, Griffith PL, Savoie FH, et al. Laser-assisted capsulorrhaphy for multidirectional instability of the shoulder. *Arthroscopy* 2001;17:25.
17. Fitzgerald BT, Watson BT, Lapoint JM. The use of thermal capsulorrhaphy in the treatment of multidirectional instability. *J Shoulder Elbow Surg* 2002;11:108.
18. Favorito PJ, Langenderfer MA, Colosimo AJ, et al. Arthroscopic laser assisted capsular shift in the treatment of patients with multidirectional shoulder instability. *Am J Sports Med* 2002;30:322.
19. Bowen MK, Warren RF. Ligamentous control of shoulder stabilization selective cutting and static translation experiments. *Clin Sports Med* 1991;10:757.
20. Wichman MT, Snyder SJ. Arthroscopic capsular placation for multidirectional instability of the shoulder. *Oper Tech Sports Med* 1997;5:238.
21. Zabinski SJ, Callaway GH, Cohen S, et al. Revision shoulder stabilization: 2- to 10-year results. *J Shoulder Elbow Surg* 1999;1:58.

15

DISORDERS OF THE BICEPS TENDON

DAVID W. ALTCHEK
BRIAN R. WOLF

INTRODUCTION

Any overhead athlete places a tremendous amount of stress on the mechanical properties of the shoulder. Excessive stresses may lead to disorders of the biceps tendon and its anchor, ranging from inflammation and instability to degeneration or rupture. Diagnosis of disorders of the long head of the biceps and associated superior labral lesions can be problematic. This results from the often concomitant problems that are present in addition to the biceps lesion, as well as from difficulty in clinically and radiographically confirming biceps pathology. A significant amount of debate surrounds the long head of the biceps tendon with regard to its function in the shoulder. Similarly, some controversy clouds the clinical management of biceps tendon disorders. Although debate remains, there continues to be increasing interest in the role of the biceps within the spectrum of shoulder problems afflicting overhead athletes. Significant advances in technology and techniques have influenced management of biceps disorders. This chapter explores the anatomy and function of the long head of biceps at the shoulder. A discussion of the pathologic disorders that can occur involving the biceps and their proper management with specific attention to the overhead athlete follows. These disorders include inflammatory and degenerative conditions, instability of the biceps tendon, and superior labrum anterior-to-posterior (SLAP) lesions.

ANATOMY AND FUNCTION OF THE LONG HEAD OF THE BICEPS

The biceps brachii muscle has two origins: the long head and the short head. The short head originates from the coracoid process and joins the long head medially at approximately the level of the deltoid tuberosity. The long head arises from the superior aspect of the glenoid and is intimately related to the glenohumeral joint. Previous work has shown that 48% of the time, the long head arises primarily from the posterosuperior labrum, 20% from the superior glenoid tubercle, and 28% from both (1). A separate cadaver study reported approximately 50% originating from the superior labrum and the remainder from the superior glenoid tubercle, with four variations of biceps origin identified (2). The mobility of the origin of the long head of the biceps is variable, and a large amount of mobility can be normal in some shoulders (3).

The long head of the biceps traverses the glenohumeral joint from its origin at the posterosuperior labrum and superior glenoid tubercle, through the rotator interval beneath the coracohumeral ligament, to the intertubercular sulcus between the greater and lesser tuberosities. The tendon is intraarticular but is lined by synovium, making it extrasynovial (3). The tendon turns under the "pulley" of the soft tissues that insert at the articular end of the sulcus (Fig. 15-1). These restraints include the superior glenohumeral ligament, the coracohumeral ligament, and the superior portion of the subscapularis tendon. Once in the groove, the tendon passes beneath the transverse humeral ligament that spans the groove. The groove has an average depth of 4.1 to 4.3 mm and average medial wall angle of 56 degrees (4,5). The tendon is widest at its origin and narrows distally in the arm to form a muscle belly. The blood supply to the tendon is the ascending branch of the anterior circumflex humeral artery, which runs with the tendon in the sulcus. The origin of the tendon also receives arterial supply from labral branches of the suprascapular artery (6). The musculocutaneous nerve supplies innervation.

The function of the long head of the biceps at the shoulder is controversial and not entirely understood. The biceps seems to function as a static anterior and superior restraint for the humeral head, and evidence for a dynamic role has also been reported. Neer proposed that the tendon served as a humeral head depressor and emphasized the importance of maintaining the tendon (7). Electrical stimulation of the long head of the biceps in five patients undergoing arthroscopy was shown to result in compression of the humeral head into the glenoid (8). In a study using 15 cadaveric shoulders in a hanging arm model, superior migration was seen following intraarticular biceps teno-

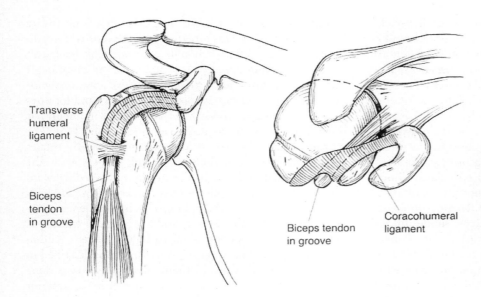

FIGURE 15-1. From its origin at the superior labrum and supraglenoid tubercle, the long head of the biceps tendon passes at approximately a 30-degree angle toward the bicipital groove. It passes through the rotator interval beneath the coracohumeral ligament, which helps provide stability to the tendon within the groove. (From Eakin CL, Faber KJ, Hawkins RJ, et al. Biceps tendon disorders in athletes. *J Am Acad Orthop Surg* 1999;7[5]:300–3110, with permission.)

tomy (9). These authors concluded that the long head of the biceps stabilizes upward humeral migration during powerful biceps contraction. Similarly, superior migration during shoulder abduction in the scapular plane was shown dynamically in seven patients with isolated long head of biceps tears when compared with the intact contralateral shoulder (10). Yet, evidence exists that contradicts any major role of the biceps tendon at the shoulder. In most patients with massive rotator cuff tears not amenable to repair, whose long head of the biceps tendon has ruptured spontaneously or who have undergone a biceps tenotomy during surgical management, it is uncommon to see superior migration of the humeral head. Additionally, electromyographic (EMG) analysis in studies that have controlled for elbow motion has shown no biceps tendon activity at the shoulder in patients with either intact or torn rotator cuffs (11,12).

Several biomechanical studies in cadaveric specimens have examined the role of the biceps tendon in glenohumeral joint stability (13–15). The long head of the biceps has been shown to significantly decrease humeral head translation in the superior, anterior, and inferior directions with increased tension placed in the tendon (14,15). Contraction of the long head of the biceps with the shoulder abducted and externally rotated produces torsional stability of the anterior capsule, which could limit force transmission to the inferior glenohumeral ligament (13). Additionally, injury to the superior labrum biceps origin complex results in increased strain on the inferior glenohumeral ligament (13) and significant increases in anterior inferior glenohumeral joint translation (16).

Evaluation and treatment of the overhead athlete requires some understanding of the physiologic muscle activation patterns seen in overhead activities. Most overhead athletic activities, such as pitching and the tennis serve,

include phases of cocking, acceleration, and follow-through. EMG analysis during pitching has shown biceps function to mainly involve motion at the elbow (17–19). Moderate biceps activity is present during the cocking phase because the elbow usually is flexed in preparation for acceleration. During the acceleration phase, minimal biceps activity is seen. An increased EMG response in the long head of the biceps has been seen in throwers with instability-related symptoms as compared to those without instability symptoms (17). Significant biceps activity is seen during follow-through as the forearm is decelerated to prevent hyperextension at the elbow. It has been postulated that this high-tension period of follow-through results in SLAP lesions in some throwers (8). In analysis of professional versus amateur throwers, professional pitchers were found to use less biceps activity during both acceleration and follow-through phases (18). This implies that the elite athletes, usually with increased skill and optimal form, may use technique that lessens stress on the biceps tendon (20). An alternative "peel-back" mechanism has also been implied to result in superior labral lesions in throwers (21). In extreme abduction and external rotation, the vector of the biceps tendon changes from relatively horizontal and anterior to posterior and vertical. This vector change can result in a torsional injury, or a peeling back, of the superior biceps anchor and labrum complex. Once such an injury is present, repetitive throwing may result in propagation of the lesion.

CLINICAL EVALUATION FOR DISORDERS OF THE BICEPS TENDON

As with all shoulder conditions, a thorough history is necessary to define the nature of a patient's symptoms. Specifics on the onset of symptoms, progression of pain or disability, aggravating activities especially as it relates to athletics, and any treatment to date are crucial information to obtain at the onset of the evaluation. Biceps tendon pain is usually located anteriorly over the region of the intertubercular groove. This pain may migrate inferiorly into the biceps muscle region. Any popping, grinding, clicking, or feeling of subluxation or apprehension should be documented. However, biceps pain can be vague and nonspecific, often presenting in a similar fashion to impingement symptoms, labral pathology, or instability. Often biceps-related disorders occur in conjunction with other pathologic conditions, creating an overlap of symptoms. The different pathologic conditions of the biceps tendon often have subtle differences in terms of symptoms and patients' complaints. Tenosynovitis or degenerative lesions of the biceps tendon often have anterior shoulder pain, which can sometimes be focal. Most of these patients have associated symptoms consistent with impingement. Biceps instability may develop after a traumatic event, with the patient complaining of "snapping" or "popping." A painful clicking within the shoulder can hallmark a SLAP lesion or other labral disorder.

PHYSICAL EXAMINATION

It is important to perform a thorough examination of the shoulder to define any pathology that may be present. The shoulder should be examined for symmetry compared to the unaffected side. Tenderness related to the biceps tendon is often located anteriorly over the intertubercular groove, located approximately 4–7 cm distal to the anterior edge of the acromion. Confirmation that this pain is related to the biceps is achieved by eliciting tenderness over the groove with the shoulder in slight internal rotation. This brings the groove directly anterior in the shoulder. Biceps tendon pain rotates laterally with external rotation of the arm, whereas pain related to the deltoid or other static anterior structures do not change location. Assessment of range of motion should be performed. Overhead throwers often lack some internal rotation compared with the nondominant arm. Biceps pathology can result in some motion loss over time related to pain and resultant stiffness. Impingement testing using Hawkins and Neer tests is usually positive with biceps lesions. Rotator cuff strength testing should be performed. This includes a thorough evaluation of the subscapularis, because biceps tendon pathology is often associated with lesions of the subscapularis insertion on the lesser tuberosity. The lift-off test and the belly-press test best reveal whether an intact subscapularis is present (22). Stability testing using the crank test and the load and shift test are used to evaluate for glenohumeral instability. Overhead athletes with biceps pathology related to subtle instability may present with pain only and not apprehension during these

provocative maneuvers (23). Yergason's test can isolate biceps tendon pain. This is performed with resisted forearm supination (24). Anterior shoulder pain with this maneuver is a positive result. Speed's test is performed by elevation of the supinated arm against resistance. Again, anterior shoulder pain over the groove is considered positive and localizes pain to the biceps tendon. Detecting labral pathology is done with the use of the active compression test (25). The patient elevates the arm 90 degrees and internally rotates the shoulder approximately 10 to 15 degrees with the thumb pointed to the floor. The patient resists a downward pressure. If pain is produced, then the test is repeated with the thumb pointed to the ceiling. This is considered a positive finding if pain resolves, and the positive finding is often related to superior labral pathology. Biceps tendon instability is difficult to isolate. A test has been described in which the patient is placed supine, and palpation is done over the anterior aspect of the shoulder near the anterior acromion and intertubercular groove. The arm is abducted to 90 degrees and externally rotated to 90 degrees. A palpable snap may reveal the subluxation of the biceps tendon out of its groove (26). Differential diagnostic injections are often of benefit when considering biceps tendon pathology. Subacromial injection can improve impingement-related pain but does not improve biceps pain unless a full thickness rotator cuff tear is present. Biceps tenosynovitis or degenerative lesion pain over the anterior shoulder should be improved with an intraarticular injection or an ultrasound-guided biceps sheath injection. This can be confirmed with provocative testing done before and following injection.

IMAGING

Imaging of patients suspected to have pathology related to the biceps tendon should begin with standard x-ray studies of the shoulder including a true anteroposterior (AP), axillary, and outlet view. Lesions of the acromioclavicular joint, osteoarthritis, and a hooked acromion can be found in association with underlying biceps lesions. Degenerative lesions in the biceps related to arthritis of the groove have been described (4,27). A "groove view" is obtained by placing the cassette at the apex of the shoulder and angling the beam slightly medial to the long axis of the humerus (4). This allows for analysis of the depth of the groove and reveals any arthritic changes in the groove. Ultrasound has been advocated by many as a noninvasive and relatively inexpensive modality to evaluate the biceps tendon, sheath, and rotator cuff (28,29). Ultrasound has a reported sensitivity of 0.8 and accuracy of 0.95 in diagnosing bicipital tendinitis (5). A sensitivity of 0.75 and accuracy of 0.98 was found when ultrasound was used to diagnose biceps tendon rupture (5). Tendon dislocation or subluxation can be documented with manipulation of the shoulder during the ultrasound. The imaging modality of choice for biceps tendon pathology is magnetic resonance imaging (MRI) (30,31). MRI can define tendon subluxation, rotator interval lesions, and superior labral pathology in detail. Any associated tears of the rotator cuff are also best defined by MRI. Consideration, however, must always be given to normal anatomic variants, especially when looking for superior labral lesions (3,32). Despite the tremendous improvement in imaging available for lesions of the biceps tendon and associated disorders, there still remains some difficulty with nonspecificity in many cases later found to have biceps pathology at arthroscopy. Imaging findings should always be considered in conjunction with symptoms and clinical findings when considering the optimal treatment course for a patient.

PATHOPHYSIOLOGY OF BICEPS TENDON INJURIES

Most injuries to the biceps tendon and its origin can be separated into one or more of three different categories. These include inflammatory or degenerative lesions, tendon instability, and SLAP lesions (7,33,34). Often, injuries fall into two or more categories, as in the athlete with a SLAP lesion and tendon degeneration. In other cases, one injury can predispose to another, as in the case of a traumatic injury leading to tendon instability and possibly to tenosynovitis or tendon degenerative changes. Thus, there is a wide spectrum or interrelation among the diagnoses related to the long head of the biceps tendon. It is the role of the physician taking care of the overhead athlete to determine the primary cause of the pathology present and to restore optimal function to the shoulder.

TENDON INFLAMMATION AND DEGENERATIVE CHANGES

Injury to the biceps tendon produces a spectrum of disorders ranging from inflammation of the tendon sheath to various stages of degenerative change of the tendon itself. Tendinitis, or inflammation of the tendon, is a misnomer in regard to the long head of the biceps. As is the case with similar maladies involving the lateral elbow and Achilles tendon, inflammatory changes do not typically occur involving the tendon itself. Rather, inflammation of the synovial sheath of the tendon may result in tenosynovitis. Degenerative change of the biceps tendon, frequently referred to as tendinitis, is more appropriately termed *tendinosis* because degenerative change of the substance of the tendon occurs without evidence of inflammatory changes on a histologic level (35). Early in the process of tendon injury, the tendon remains mobile but becomes swollen. In later stages, the sheath of the tendon becomes thickened and can render the inflamed and irregular tendon immo-

bile. Ultimately, a degenerative frayed tendon loses its gliding ability, may become scarred down, and, ultimately, can result in rupture. The overall incidence, and incidence amongst overhead athletes, of bicipital tenosynovitis or tendinosis is unknown. In patients younger than 50 years of age at the time of death, the incidence of degenerative lesions involving the long head of the biceps tendon was 12% in one cadaver study (36). None of these specimens had associated rotator cuff lesions. When evaluating a patient with inflammatory or degenerative changes of the biceps, a determination must be made regarding the cause of the pathology present. This includes a determination of whether the biceps tendon injury is secondary to some other disorder, such as impingement or instability, or is an isolated lesion within the shoulder. Most authors have considered most biceps tendon injuries as secondary lesions to other causes (7,37).

Neer described tenosynovitis of the long head of the biceps as it occurred in relation with rotator cuff injury secondary to impingement (7). Tendon injury and later rupture have been described occurring in conjunction with supraspinatus or subscapularis injury or tear in the vast majority of cases (38). The initial inflammation and later degeneration of the biceps tendon results from impingement of the tendon under the coracoacromial arch. The anterior location of the biceps tendon predisposes it to compression with activities of arm flexion and abduction. Additionally, there is a medial displacing force on the tendon, toward the lesser tuberosity, as it enters the shoulder joint and then traverses at an angle of approximately 30 degrees to the origin at the superior glenoid and labrum (39,40). This potentially adds a mechanical cause for inflammatory or degenerative changes as the tendon abrades against the medial wall of the bicipital groove. Arthritic changes in the bicipital groove have been associated with degenerative tendon changes (41).

Specific translations of the humeral head on the glenoid have been directly related to specific shoulder motions, including anterior and superior translation with flexion and internal rotation of the arm (42). Hence the follow-though phase of overhead throwing or hitting, with the arm in the flexed and internally rotated position, also is associated with this anterior and superior translation of the humeral head. This places anterior shoulder structures, such as the biceps and rotator cuff, at risk for injury from impingement on the coracoacromial arch. Many throwers also exhibit decreased internal rotation thought to be secondary to an acquired tight posterior capsule. A tight posterior capsule also results in superior and anterior head translation (42), again placing the biceps at risk. Kinematic comparisons have found baseball pitchers to be at increased risk for this anterior impingement compared to football quarterbacks (43).

Jobe and colleagues were the first to describe impingement in the overhead athlete related to subtle glenohumeral instability (44) (Fig. 15-2). With overuse, the anterior sta-

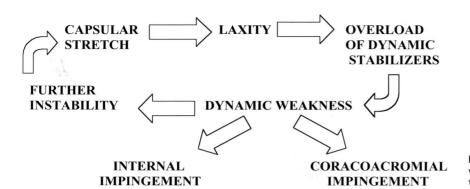

FIGURE 15-2. Diagram illustrating the vicious cycle that may occur in overhead throwers with subtle instability.

bilizing structures of the shoulder can be overloaded and may become stretched, leading to injury to the rotator cuff, superior labrum, and biceps tendon. As the static restraints anteriorly in the shoulder become lax and weak, increased humeral head translation can occur. Subsequently, potential impingement with the coracoacromial arch can involve the rotator cuff and biceps tendon anteriorly. Eventually, the tensile limits of the anterior soft tissue structures and the biceps tendon can be overwhelmed, leading to a tendinopathy from collagen fiber damage (Fig. 15-2). In this scenario of overuse and excessive strain, the intraarticular tendon may be overtly damaged or can appear fine with the damage occurring to the tendon located in the groove anteriorly. This may or may not be related to additional degenerative changes or abnormalities in the bicipital groove (26). Alternatively, increased translation anteriorly can result in "internal impingement" of the posterior rotator cuff on the posterosuperior glenoid labrum when the shoulder is maximally abducted and externally rotated, the cocking position for throwers (23). This may result in posterosuperior labral pathology and articular sided rotator cuff injury.

Nonoperative Treatment

Treatment for suspected tenosynovitis or degenerative biceps lesions begins after accurate diagnosis of the pathology present. It also requires a decision on the primary etiology of symptoms. Possibilities include primary tendon inflammation or degeneration, or secondary tendon injury related to underlying impingement, instability, or recent trauma. Secondary biceps tendon pathology does not improve without proper management of the primary disorder present. Initial treatment for tenosynovitis and degenerative lesions begins with rest, withdrawal of aggravating activities, icing of the shoulder, and a short period of anti-inflammatory medication. Treatment also includes formal rehabilitation of the shoulder. This rehabilitation is similar to that used for impingement type symptoms and rotator cuff disease emphasizing a global shoulder and periscapular muscle strengthening program. This includes strengthening of the internal and external rotators of the shoulder. Addi-

tionally, the trapezius and serratus anterior muscles provide scapular motion that rotates the scapula to avoid impingement anteriorly. Again, weakness of these muscles may cause scapular lag and allow impingement of the anterior soft tissues, including the biceps. Hence a comprehensive shoulder strengthening program is needed.

Initially, until the acute painful phase is passed, therapy should focus on range-of-motion exercises, stretching, and modalities. Strengthening begins once pain is minimized and should include external and internal rotator strengthening and periscapular exercises. In addition, eccentric loading exercises of the biceps itself can be instituted with the strengthening program followed by a gradual return to overhead activities. Improvement should be monitored closely. Physical therapy is instituted for a minimum of 6 weeks. If significant improvement is not occurring at this point, one could consider an injection either intraarticularly or directly into the tendon sheath (45). This should be considered cautiously because adverse effects on healing have been reported with corticosteroids (46). If nonoperative means are deemed a failure after a dedicated effort by all those involved, then consideration of a surgical intervention is appropriate.

SURGICAL TREATMENT

Arthroscopic Evaluation of the Biceps Tendon

Once the patient is in the operating room, a thorough examination under anesthesia is performed. This includes assessment of range of motion and laxity of the shoulder, which should be carefully documented. A standard arthroscopy of the glenohumeral joint should be performed using a posterior viewing portal and a standard anterior rotator interval working portal. A full diagnostic evaluation of the joint is performed with careful inspection of all structures. Special attention is paid to the intraarticular portion of the biceps tendon and its insertion for a complete arthroscopic inspection (47). The biceps sheath is examined for any thickening, fraying or degenerative changes. The tendon itself should be drawn into the joint using a probe to fully examine that portion of the tendon that normally resides in the groove (48) (Fig. 15-3A). This is facilitated by flexing the elbow and supinating the forearm with slight external rotation and abduction of the shoulder (48). An additional 3 to 4 cm of tendon can be viewed in this fashion and may expose occult tendon injury (47). If present, the percentage and extent of degenerative change of the tendon is evaluated. The rotator interval is carefully evaluated and probed for any abnormal laxity, especially around the entrance to the bicipital groove. The bicipital groove can be closely examined through the arthroscope from above and below the biceps tendon (see Fig. 15-3B). The arm can be taken through a range of motion to evaluate for any subluxation of the tendon out of the groove during motion. The insertion of the subscapularis is closely inspected for any degenerative lesions, tearing, or fraying that may be present, particularly the attachment to the lesser tuberosity (see Fig. 15-3C). Looking laterally through the arthroscope

in the anterior aspect of the joint, with the arm in slight internal rotation, allows the best evaluation of the subscapularis. The origin of the biceps is probed to evaluate for any disruption of the anchor or superior labral lesions, recognizing the spectrum of normal variants that can be present (2). The arm is then elevated in the plane of the scapula to fully visualize the articular surface and insertion of the rotator cuff. A thorough evaluation for any excess laxity is done. This includes the presence of a drive-through sign, excessive capsular laxity, or signs of internal impingement. Last, the arthroscope is redirected into the subacromial space, looking for bursal thickening and signs of impingement. The bursal surface of the rotator cuff is carefully inspected.

Bicipital Tenosynovitis and Degenerative Lesions

When lesions of the biceps tendon are known or anticipated preoperatively, a thorough discussion should be undertaken with the patient regarding treatment options,

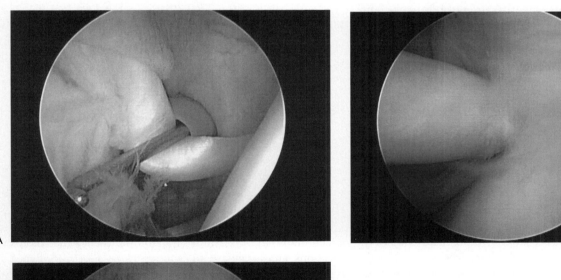

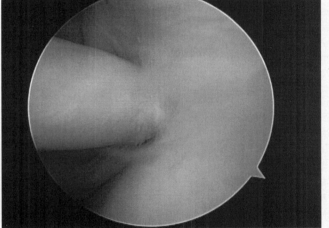

FIGURE 15-3. A: Biceps tendon drawn into the joint to fully examine the portion that normally resides within the bicipital groove. **B:** Biceps tendon entering bicipital groove. **C:** Subscapularis insertion onto lesser tuberosity.

including debridement, tenodesis, and tenotomy. This is especially important when dealing with the overhead athlete. When the biceps is inflamed, removal of synovitis around the tendon is performed using an arthroscopic shaver. Occasionally, a longitudinal split is seen in the tendon that may be amenable to repair arthroscopically. Percutaneously, a spinal needle is placed across the tear using a degradable suture such as number 2-0 polydioxane (PDS). The two ends of the suture are then retrieved though the anterior cannula and arthroscopic knots are tied. Athletes with biceps pathology frequently also have symptoms related to impingement. In this situation, subacromial decompression should be performed in addition to treatment of the biceps tendon itself. In younger athletes, a soft tissue decompression consisting of a bursectomy and coracoacromial decompression is performed. In older athletes, an acromioplasty is performed if the subacromial space is arthroscopically narrowed on examination, or when a large spur or type III acromion is present. In most cases, this resolves tenosynovitis related to impingement. No study has looked solely at the results of debridement of the partially involved biceps tendon. Results of treatment for biceps inflammation or degenerative disease have been reported in conjunction with impingement syndrome and rotator cuff lesions. Neer found that only 30% of patients with a preoperative diagnosis of biceps tenosynovitis had disease at operative inspection (7). They improved with acromioplasty and subacromial decompression.

If a significant portion (greater than 25%) of the tendon is degenerative, or if rupture appears imminent, then a biceps tenodesis should be performed. The cited indications for tenodesis include the following: greater than 25% to 50% partial thickness tears of the tendon, subluxation, disruption of the bicipital groove or soft tissue stabilizers, chronic atrophy of the tendon, and biceps disease in the setting of failed prior acromioplasty for impingement or rotator cuff tendinitis (45,49). Tenodesis can be performed open (37,49,50) or arthroscopically (51–53). If tenodesis is to be performed open, then we advocate arthroscopically tagging the biceps tendon at the level where desired tenodesis will occur before releasing the tendon just distal to its origin. Open tenodesis is performed through a limited anterior approach over the bicipital groove (37,50). The deltoid is split longitudinally or the deltopectoral interval is used. The long head of the biceps is palpated and the transverse ligament and tendon sheath is split, exposing the tendon. The cut tendon can then be retrieved out the wound. There are several methods of securing the tenodesis. These include sewing the tendon into the adjacent soft tissues, including the transverse humeral ligament, using suture anchors or drill holes, or using a keyhole technique with an interference screw. Our preference is to use suture anchors. The bony groove is prepared for tenodesis using a burr or curette. The tendon is amputated at the predetermined level where the tendon is marked. A minimum of two suture anchors are placed into the prepared groove and the tendon is tied down into the groove. The tendon may then also be additionally sewn to adjacent soft tissues. The residual intraarticular portion of the tendon is amputated.

We currently perform most tenodeses arthroscopically using suture anchor fixation (51), although keyhole techniques using interference screws have been described (52,53). If the rotator cuff is intact, the procedure is performed within the joint. A standard posterior portal and a low anterior working portal are used. Additionally, using spinal needle localization, a high anterolateral rotator interval portal is created where a large working cannula is placed. The biceps tendon is again tagged with a suture just proximal to the area where the tendon is exiting the joint and entering the groove. The area of the proximal groove is visualized from the posterior portal and a shaver is introduced through the anterolateral portal to debride any soft tissue and prepare the bone for tenodesis. Two suture anchors are then placed through the anterolateral portal with one set of sutures shuttled out the anterior cannula. A tissue penetrator is then placed through the anterolateral portal and through the biceps tendon just distal to where the tendon is marked. One end of suture is then retrieved through the biceps tendon. This is repeated for each suture of the suture anchors. Arthroscopic knots are then tied, securing the tenodesis. The tendon is then cut proximal to the tenodesis site and released from its origin with the excess remaining portion of tendon removed by the tagging suture.

Results of biceps tenodesis have been reported in several series. Becker and Cofield (50) reviewed 54 cases of tenodesis in the setting of chronic tenosynovitis without an associated acromioplasty having been done. Twenty-two of 54 patients continued to have moderate to severe symptoms after tenodesis and 29 required additional treatment. Fifty percent of patients with long-term follow-up still had moderate pain, mostly located at the anterolateral shoulder. The authors advised against tenodesis without an associated acromioplasty. This study supports the theory that biceps lesions are secondary to impingement. Post and Benca reported on 17 patients who underwent isolated tenodesis without acromioplasty for primary tendinitis, and achieved 92% good to excellent results (47). Patients were excluded from the study if any confounding factors were present such as instability, rotator cuff tear, or overt impingement. These authors concluded that isolated biceps tendinitis can occur and good results achieved with tenodesis if other diagnoses are ruled out. Neviaser and co-workers reported 86% complete pain relief following tenodesis and associated acromioplasty for lesions of the biceps tendon (38).

Spontaneous biceps tendon rupture may occur in the setting of chronic biceps tendon disease and is often associated with resolution of previous shoulder pain. This is often the case in overhead athletes (20). Functional losses after tendon rupture have been reported to be a loss of supination strength of 10% to 21% and loss of elbow flexion strength of 0% to 8% (54,55). Mariani and colleagues compared 26 patients who underwent early tenodesis and a group of 30 patients who were treated nonoperatively (54). No difference in pain or elbow flexion strength was found between the two groups. The surgical group lost 8% supination strength compared to 21% for the nonoperative group. The nonsurgical patients returned to work faster than the patients who underwent tenodesis. The treatment of spontaneous rupture should be nonoperative in most situations in that minimal functional deficit occurs and most athletes report improved shoulder comfort level after it occurs. Rupture occurs in a setting of a chronically degenerated tendon with minimal function in the shoulder. Rupture does result in a cosmetic difference and patients should be counseled regarding this. If a cosmetic defect is unacceptable to the athlete, then tenodesis should be advised.

An additional option to debridement or tenodesis for the degenerative biceps tendon is simple tenotomy. A series of 30 patients who underwent biceps tenotomy for instability, tendon degeneration, or recalcitrant tenosynovitis has been reported (56). One patient was a professional athlete and 12 participated in recreational athletics at least 4 days per week. Only two of the patients underwent concurrent subacromial decompression. Ninety-seven percent were pain free at an average of 19 months of follow-up, and 90% returned to their previous athletic activity level. Concerns with biceps tenotomy are the possible cosmetic deformity of the muscle belly, the "popeye" deformity, and biceps cramping that can occur following tendon release. In the aforementioned series, the complication rate was 13%, with one patient being unsatisfied with the cosmetic deformity and one patient having persistent biceps pain. In a separate series of 30 patients who had suffered a spontaneous rupture of the biceps tendon, 20% had moderate pain with vigorous activities (54). The deformities after rupture were described as mild in seven, moderate in 21, and severe in two.

BICEPS TENDON INSTABILITY

Biceps tendon instability may present as either static or dynamic tendon subluxation or dislocation. As mentioned previously, the tendon angles 30- to 40-degrees from its origin to the bicipital groove, which places medial displacing forces on the tendon (39,40). Additionally, during throwing when the shoulder is in abducted and externally rotated cocking position, increased medial forces on the biceps tendon are present. In contrast, during follow-through phase of internal rotation and flexion, forces on the tendon are directed in a lateral direction (57). A shallow bicipital groove may predispose and contribute to subluxation or dislocation. The cause of this disorder in athletes is unknown although it has been reported in young throwers

(57,58). The stability of the biceps tendon within the groove is secured by the soft tissue sling created by the coracohumeral ligament and the superior glenohumeral ligament within the rotator interval, the upper portion of the subscapularis, and, to a lesser extent, the groove itself (59,60). The transverse humeral ligament provides minimal restraint to the tendon. Biceps tendon subluxation or dislocation is most commonly associated with a rotator cuff injury, frequently involving the subscapularis (39,40) (Fig. 15-4). However, medial subluxation of the tendon can also occur without frank injury to the rotator cuff tendons when the rotator interval is deficient or degenerative (57,59). Subtle subluxation across the superior aspect of the lesser tuberosity can be missed during open surgery or during arthroscopy because the minimal medial displacement is easily overlooked and the superior aspect of the tendon appears intact (60).

Subluxation is usually irreducible and associated with fraying and degenerative changes of the inferior surface of the biceps tendon (60). Dislocation presents with the tendon interposed between the humeral head and glenoid or displaced medially in the superior aspect of the subscapularis tendon (60). In this case, the tendon is usually frayed and degenerative with loss of its normal synovial lining and shape. Four types of dislocation have been described (Table 15-1). If there is a tear into the substance of the subscapularis while the insertions of both the anterior subscapularis fascia and the deep subscapularis fibers remain intact on the lesser tuberosity, then the biceps tendon may dislocate over the lesser tuberosity and into the subscapularis tendon itself (39,60). The biceps may dislocate into the joint with a

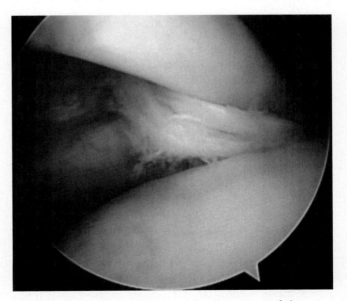

FIGURE 15-4. Arthroscopic photo showing a tear of the superior aspect of the subscapularis tendon and supporting soft tissue structures at the lesser tuberosity. This has allowed medial subluxation of the long head of the biceps tendon.

TABLE 15–1. TYPES OF LONG HEAD OF THE BICEPS TENDON DISLOCATION (60)

Type I	Biceps tendon dislocates "inside" into internal split in subscapularis tendon
Type II	Intraarticular biceps tendon dislocation associated with complete tear of subscapularis muscle and stabilizing ligaments tearing but with intact anterior fascia
Type III	Intraarticular biceps tendon dislocation associated with complete tear of subscapularis tendon, ligaments, and anterior fascia
Type IV	Anterior dislocation of biceps tendon over intact subscapularis tendon secondary to tear of anterior fascia alone

complete tear of the deep insertion of the subscapularis. Intraarticular dislocation may also occur with complete disruption of the entire subscapularis tendon, including the anterior fascia (61). Last, the tendon may dislocate anterior to the subscapularis tendon with isolated anterior fascia and transverse humeral ligament disruption, usually traumatic in nature (40,60).

O'Donoghue reported subluxation of the biceps tendon in a series of young throwers with no apparent injury to the rotator cuff structures (57). Characteristic symptoms included pain on throwing with a palpable snap at a certain point in the arc of motion. Pain was relieved with rest and palpable tenderness over the bicipital groove was present. Subluxation or dislocation was found in 71 patients in a large retrospective series, all with rotator cuff tears of some nature (60). Approximately 15% to 20% of patients with rotator cuff tears have concomitant biceps subluxation or dislocation (40,60). Most agree that it is extremely uncommon to see biceps instability without some injury to the rotator cuff (20,45,60).

Treatment of Biceps Tendon Instability

The primary tenets of treating subluxation of the biceps are identifying the cause of the tendon instability and identifying the amount of damage done to the tendon from its displacement. A chronically subluxated or dislocated tendon will likely show signs of advanced inflammation or degeneration. The tendon also may not be able to be mobilized from its new position. In cases of advanced degenerative changes, or fixed dislocation or subluxation, a tenodesis within the groove should be performed. An attempt at relocation is possible when the tendon remains mobile and severe changes have not yet occurred. Maintaining relocation involves repair and tightening of the rotator interval. Suture repair of the subscapularis tendon to the supraspinatus at the point of exit for the biceps tendon can reduce a redundant rotator interval. Care should be taken to ensure that the biceps tendon is well centered within the groove at the time of repair and stable there throughout a range of motion.

O'Donoghue reported on a small series of throwers with isolated tendon subluxation (57). Effective resolution of symptoms was achieved with tenodesis in these throwers. When impingement of the rotator cuff and rotator interval soft tissues is the cause for tendon instability, then the management is twofold. Treatment includes subacromial decompression and acromioplasty in addition to possible rotator cuff repair and possible biceps tendon tenodesis, or relocation and stabilization within the groove. Last, with tears of the subscapularis insertion on the lesser tuberosity biceps tendon, dislocation or subluxation may result. The subscapularis repair should be performed either through an open deltopectoral approach or, in cases of partial tears of the deep superior aspect of the subscapularis, arthroscopically. Again, recentralization of the intact but displaced biceps tendon at the time of subscapularis repair can be attempted but may be difficult (59).

SLAP LESIONS

Snyder first described the spectrum of injuries to the origin of the biceps tendon in 1990 following a review of 700 shoulder arthroscopies (62). This led to the most widely used descriptive classification system, which places these injuries into one of four types. Type I is a degenerative fraying of the superior labrum with an intact anchor of the biceps tendon. Type II injury is a detachment of the biceps anchor from the superior glenoid attachment site and is the most common injury type, accounting for greater than 50% of SLAP lesions. Type III injury is a bucket-handle tear of the superior labrum with an intact biceps anchor insertion. Type IV injuries involve a bucket-handle tear that extends into the biceps tendon itself. Type II injuries have subsequently been subdivided into three types: anterior, posterior, and anteroposterior (63) (Table 15-2). In addition, three subsequent categories of SLAP lesions have also

TABLE 15–2. SUPERIOR LABRUM ANTERIOR POSTERIOR LESIONS (62–64)

Type I	Fraying of superior labrum, intact biceps anchor
Type II	Detachment of superior labrum and biceps anchor from superior glenoid
	IIA Anterior
	IIB Posterior
	IIC Anterior and posterior
Type III	Bucket-handle tear of superior labrum
Type IV	Bucket-handle tear of superior labrum, which extends into biceps tendon
Type V	Anterior-inferior Bankart lesion that extends superiorly to involve the superior labrum
Type VI	Superior labral detachment, similar to type II, with associated flap tear
Type VII	Superior labral detachment, similar to type II, which extends anteriorly beneath the middle glenohumeral ligament

been proposed: types V, VI, and VII (64). Type V is an anteroinferior Bankart lesion that extends superiorly to involve the superior labrum. Type VI is a superior labral detachment with an associated unstable flap tear. Type VII is a superior labral detachment that extends anteriorly beneath the middle glenohumeral ligament. These injuries are related to traction, compression, or shear injury of the humeral head against the superior glenoid rim (62,63). This can be related to an acute traumatic injury such as a fall onto an outstretched hand with an extended and slightly flexed arm. Injury may also occur with repetitive overhead activity such as pitching. Deceleration of forearm follow-through during pitching and other overhead sports has been implicated in tension injury to the superior labrum complex (8,62,63). Overhead throwers have been shown to have an increased incidence of posterior and combined anteroposterior lesions (63). By comparison, SLAP lesions related to trauma are predominantly anterior in location. The "peel-back" mechanism has also been described in the etiology of type II SLAP lesions (21,63). This occurs when the arm is in an abducted and externally rotated position as the biceps assumes a more vertical and posterior angle. Tension on the biceps in this position causes a twisting of the biceps tendon that can result in peel-back of the anchor with repetitive overuse injury.

It is uncommon for SLAP lesions to be isolated injuries in the shoulder. Only 28% of cases with SLAP injuries were isolated in a large series (65). Associated diagnoses include rotator cuff tears, acromioclavicular joint disorders, and instability. The superior labrum functions in the stability of the shoulder in conjunction with the superior and middle glenohumeral ligaments and long head of the biceps (66). Injury to the superior labrum results in increased antero-posterior and superoinferior translation of the humeral head (14). Increased strain on the inferior glenohumeral ligament is also present following superior labrum detachment (13). An increased incidence of SLAP lesions has been shown if the shoulder is unstable (67). As noted earlier, throwers have a higher incidence of posterior SLAP lesions, which potentially leads to posterosuperior instability (63). This posterosuperior instability may predispose throwers to other shoulder injuries such as rotator cuff lesions. This may set up a vicious cycle of injury in the shoulder in which labral injury creates an environment of increased humeral head translation, which in turn predisposes for further labrum injury. It remains unclear, however, whether instability leads to labral injury or vice versa.

Treatment of SLAP Lesions

Tremendous advances have occurred over the last decade with regard to treatment of SLAP lesions. When the description of SLAP lesions first was put forth, treatment centered on debridement of degenerative and unstable lesions. Altchek reported on debridement of labral injuries

in 40 patients and found 93% of patients with continued symptoms at 2 years (68). Cordasco reported on debridement of superior labral injuries in 52 patients and found only 63% had good results at 2 years' follow-up. Treatment has shifted to fixation of unstable injuries thereafter and improved results have been seen. Segmuller and colleagues used the Suretac device to repair 17 unstable superior labral lesions with 83% reporting good results (69). However, only 53% returned to preinjury levels of activities. Field and Savoie used arthroscopic suture fixation for 20 unstable superior labral injuries and had 100% good results reported at nearly 2-year follow-up (70). Other fixation devices that have been used include arthroscopic staples and arthroscopic screws (71,72).

An algorithm for treatment of SLAP lesions is described by the Snyder four-part classification system. Type I lesions generally only require light debridement of frayed tissue at the base of the biceps anchor and superior labrum itself. The attachment site should be carefully inspected to ensure that no detachment is present. Type II lesions with a detached anchor require stabilization. Today, this is most frequently done using arthroscopic tacks, such as the Suretac, or using suture anchor fixation. The authors' preference for treatment of these lesions is using suture anchor fixation (Fig. 15-5). The standard posterior viewing portal and anterior working portal are used. An additional anterolateral portal is made using spinal needle localizaton. This portal should enter the joint through the rotator interval. The superior aspect of the glenoid is prepared using a shaver or rasp. Depending on the nature of the injury, suture anchors are placed anterior, posterior, or both in relation to the biceps tendon through the rotator interval portal. The anchor should be placed at the superior margin of the glenoid articular surface. A tissue penetrator is then placed through the superior labrum via the anterior portal. A single limb of the suture is shuttled through the labrum. Arthroscopic knots are then tied with care to place the knots superiorly on the soft tissue and not on the articular surface. Additional anchors are placed and steps repeated as needed. Type III lesions are bucket-handle tears and often are most appropriately treated with debridement. Occasionally, a type III injury involves a very large bucket-handle tear that is amenable to suture fixation. A shaver or soft tissue rasp, similar to that used for meniscal repair, can be used to prepare the bed into which the labrum will be repaired. This is achieved with the use of tissue penetrators passing suture through the intact tissue superior to the remaining intact labrum and subsequently through the torn labrum. Arthroscopic knots are tied on the tissue side of the repair. Type IV lesions involve a bucket-handle tear that extends into the biceps tendon itself. If the tear involves less than 40% to 50%, then the tear into the biceps can be debrided (66). However, when the tear involves more than 40% of the biceps, it should be repaired if possible. Repair of the tear into the biceps can be achieved using a bioabsorbable suture passed through percutaneously placed spinal needles or through the anterior cannula. This is

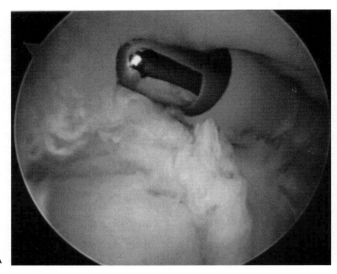
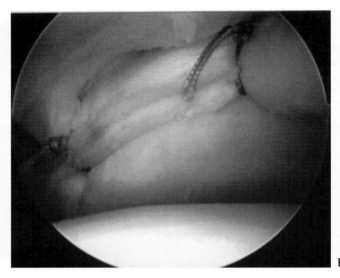

A   B

FIGURE 15-5. Type II SLAP lesion before **(A)** and after **(B)** repair using suture anchors.

similar to the repair for isolated tears in the intraarticular portion of the biceps described earlier. Arthroscopic knots are tied, affixing the tear. The bucket-handle labral tear can then be approached as mentioned for the type III lesions. If a complex or degenerative tear of the biceps involves greater than 50% of the tendon width or is not amenable to repair, then a tenodesis can be performed. Again, careful inspection of the biceps insertion should be done to ensure secure attachment as type IV lesions often have additional type II pathology present as well.

Stetson and colleagues reported an average 3.2-year clinical follow-up of 140 SLAP lesions, finding 79% good or excellent results (73). This included treatment of 19 type II lesions with glenoid abrasion only. All types I, III, and IV lesions were debrided. Results among overhead athletes and return to competition were not defined. Treatment of superior labral lesions in pitchers has been reported by Morgan and colleagues (63). Type II SLAP lesions were in 102 patients using suture anchor fixation. Fifty-three of the 102 patients were overhead athletes, including 44 baseball pitchers. This included 10 professional, 13 college, 14 high school, and seven recreational athletes. The remaining overhead athletes included four tennis players, two nonpitching baseball players, and three volleyball players. At 1-year follow-up, there were 87% excellent and 13% good results. Eight-four percent of the pitchers returned to their preinjury level of throwing subjectively.

SUMMARY

A very wide spectrum of injuries can involve the long head of the biceps tendon at the shoulder. The exact role of the biceps at the shoulder continues to be an area of controversy. The diagnosis of biceps-related pathology can be a very challenging endeavor, both clinically and radiographically. The majority of injuries to the biceps tendon occur in addition to, or as a result of, other conditions that are present in the shoulder. This is especially true for the overhead athlete who places unique demands on the biceps tendon. As a result, subtle and complex problems involving the biceps tendon and its origin at the superior labrum can occur. It is crucial to properly identify the primary cause of biceps-related symptoms early in the evaluation and treatment process to achieve optimal results in these athletes.

REFERENCES

1. Habermeyer P, Kaiser E, Knappe M, et al. (Functional anatomy and biomechanics of the long biceps tendon). *Unfallchirurg* 1987;90(7):319–329.
2. Vangsness CT Jr, Jorgenson SS, Watson T, et al. The origin of the long head of the biceps from the scapula and glenoid labrum. An anatomical study of 100 shoulders. *J Bone Joint Surg (Br)* 1994; 76 (6):951–954.
3. Cooper DE, Arnoczky SP, O'Brien SJ, et al. Anatomy, histology, and vascularity of the glenoid labrum. An anatomical study. *J Bone Joint Surg (Am)* 1992;74(1):46–52.
4. Cone RO, Danzig L, Resnick D, et al. The bicipital groove: radiographic, anatomic, and pathologic study. *AJR Am J Roentgenol* 1983;141(4):781–788.
5. Read JW, Perko M. Shoulder ultrasound: diagnostic accuracy for impingement syndrome, rotator cuff tear, and biceps tendon pathology. *J Shoulder Elbow Surg* 1998;7(3):264–271.
6. Rathbun JB, Macnab I. The microvascular pattern of the rotator cuff. *J Bone Joint Surg (Br)* 1970;52(3):540–553.
7. Neer CS 2nd. Anterior acromioplasty for the chronic impingement syndrome in the shoulder: a preliminary report. *J Bone Joint Surg (Am)* 1972;54(1):41–50.
8. Andrews JR, Carson WG Jr, McLeod WD. Glenoid labrum tears related to the long head of the biceps. *Am J Sports Med* 1985;13(5):337–341.
9. Kumar VP, Satku K, Balasubramaniam P. The role of the long

head of biceps brachii in the stabilization of the head of the humerus. *Clin Orthop* 1989;(244):172–175.

10. Warner JJ, McMahon PJ. The role of the long head of the biceps brachii in superior stability of the glenohumeral joint. *J Bone Joint Surg (Am)* 1995;77(3):366–372.

11. Yamaguchi K, Riew KD, Galatz LM, et al. Biceps activity during shoulder motion: an electromyographic analysis. *Clin Orthop* 1997;(336):122–129.

12. Levy AS, Kelly BT, Lintner SA, et al. Function of the long head of the biceps at the shoulder: electromyographic analysis. *J Shoulder Elbow Surg* 2001;10(3):250–255.

13. Rodosky MW, Harner CD, Fu FH. The role of the long head of the biceps muscle and superior glenoid labrum in anterior stability of the shoulder. *Am J Sports Med* 1994;22(1):121–130.

14. Pagnani MJ, Deng XH, Warren RF, et al. Role of the long head of the biceps brachii in glenohumeral stability: a biomechanical study in cadavera. *J Shoulder Elbow Surg* 1996;5(4):255–262.

15. Itoi E, Kuechle DK, Newman SR, et al. Stabilising function of the biceps in stable and unstable shoulders. *J Bone Joint Surg (Br)* 1993;75(4):546–550.

16. Pagnani MJ, Deng XH, Warren RF, et al. Effect of lesions of the superior portion of the glenoid labrum on glenohumeral translation. *J Bone Joint Surg (Am)* 1995;77(7):1003–1010.

17. Glousman R, Jobe F, Tibone J, et al. Dynamic electromyographic analysis of the throwing shoulder with glenohumeral instability. *J Bone Joint Surg Am* 1988;70(2):220–226.

18. Gowan ID, Jobe FW, Tibone JE, et al. A comparative electromyographic analysis of the shoulder during pitching. Professional versus amateur pitchers. *Am J Sports Med* 1987;15(6):586–590.

19. Jobe FW, Moynes DR, Tibone JE, et al. An EMG analysis of the shoulder in pitching. A second report. *Am J Sports Med* 1984;12(3):218–220.

20. Eakin CL, Faber KJ, Hawkins RJ, et al. Biceps tendon disorders in athletes. *J Am Acad Orthop Surg* 1999;7(5):300–310.

21. Burkhart SS, Morgan CD. The peel-back mechanism: its role in producing and extending posterior type II SLAP lesions and its effect on SLAP repair rehabilitation. *Arthroscopy* 1998;14(6):637–640.

22. Gerber C, Hersche O, Farron A. Isolated rupture of the subscapularis tendon. *J Bone Joint Surg (Am)* 1996;78(7):1015–1023.

23. Glousman RE. Instability versus impingement syndrome in the throwing athlete. *Orthop Clin North Am* 1993;24(1):89–99.

24. Yergason RM. Supination sign. *J Bone Joint Surg (Am)* 1931;13:160.

25. O'Brien SJ, Pagnani MJ, Fealy S, et al. The active compression test: a new and effective test for diagnosing labral tears and acromioclavicular joint abnormality. *Am J Sports Med* 1998;26(5):610–613.

26. Bell RH, Noble JS. Biceps disorders. In: Hawkins RJ, Misamore GW, eds. *Shoulder injuries in the athlete: surgical repair and rehabilitation.* New York: Churchill Livingston, 1996:267–282.

27. Ahovuo J, Paavolainen P, Slatis P. Radiographic diagnosis of biceps tendinitis. *Acta Orthop Scand* 1985;56(1):75–78.

28. Conrad MR, Nelms BA. Empty bicipital groove due to rupture and retraction of the biceps tendon. *J Ultrasound Med* 1990;9(4):231–233.

29. Middleton WD, Reinus WR, Totty WG, et al. Ultrasonographic evaluation of the rotator cuff and biceps tendon. *J Bone Joint Surg (Am)* 1986;68(3):440–450.

30. Connell DA, Potter HG, Wickiewicz TL, et al. Noncontrast magnetic resonance imaging of superior labral lesions. 102 cases confirmed at arthroscopic surgery. *Am J Sports Med* 1999;27(2):208–213.

31. Erickson SJ, Fitzgerald SW, Quinn SF, et al. Long bicipital ten-don of the shoulder: normal anatomy and pathologic findings on MR imaging. *AJR Am J Roentgenol* 1992;158(5):1091–1096.

32. Beltran J, Bencardino J, Mellado J, et al. MR arthrography of the shoulder: variants and pitfalls. *Radiographics* 1997;17(6):1403–1412; discussion 1412–1415.

33. Burns WC 2nd, Whipple TL. Anatomic relationships in the shoulder impingement syndrome. *Clin Orthop* 1993;(294):96–102.

34. Neviaser RJ. Lesions of the biceps and tendinitis of the shoulder. *Orthop Clin North Am* 1980;11(2):343–348.

35. Claessens H, Snoeck H. Tendinitis of the long head of the biceps brachii. *Acta Orthop Belg* 1972;58(1):124–128.

36. Refior HJ, Sowa D. Long tendon of the biceps brachii: sites of predilection for degenerative lesions. *J Shoulder Elbow Surg* 1995;4(6):436–440.

37. Dines D, Warren RF, Inglis AE. Surgical treatment of lesions of the long head of the biceps. *Clin Orthop* 1982;(164):165–171.

38. Neviaser TJ, Neviaser RJ, Neviaser JS. The four-in-one arthroplasty for the painful arc syndrome. *Clin Orthop* 1982;(163):107–112.

39. Petersson CJ. Spontaneous medial dislocation of the tendon of the long biceps brachii. An anatomic study of prevalence and pathomechanics. *Clin Orthop* 1986;(211):224–227.

40. Slatis P, Aalto K. Medial dislocation of the tendon of the long head of the biceps brachii. *Acta Orthop Scand* 1979;50(1):73–77.

41. Pfahler M, Branner S, Refior HJ. The role of the bicipital groove in tendinopathy of the long biceps tendon. *J Shoulder Elbow Surg* 1999;8(5):419–424.

42. Harryman DT 2nd, Sidles JA, Clark JM, et al. Translation of the humeral head on the glenoid with passive glenohumeral motion. *J Bone Joint Surg (Am)* 1990;72(9):1334–1343.

43. Fleisig GS, Escamilla RF, Andrews JR, et al. Kinematic and kinetic comparison between baseball pitching and football passing. *J Appl Biomech* 1996;12:207–224.

44. Jobe FW, Kvitne RS, Giangarra CE. Shoulder pain in the overhand or throwing athlete. The relationship of anterior instability and rotator cuff impingement. *Orthop Rev* 1989;18(9):963–975.

45. Sethi N, Wright R, Yamaguchi K. Disorders of the long head of the biceps tendon. *J Shoulder Elbow Surg* 1999;8(6):644–654.

46. Stahl S, Kaufman T. The efficacy of an injection of steroids for medial epicondylitis. A prospective study of sixty elbows. *J Bone Joint Surg (Am)* 1997;79(11):1648–1652.

47. Post M, Benca P. Primary tendinitis of the long head of the biceps. *Clin Orthop* 1989;(246):117–125.

48. Bennett WF. Specificity of the Speed's test: arthroscopic technique for evaluating the biceps tendon at the level of the bicipital groove. *Arthroscopy* 1998;14(8):789–796.

49. Crenshaw AH, Kilgore WE. Surgical treatment of bicipital tenosynovitis. *J Bone Joint Surg Am* 1966;48(8):1496–1502.

50. Becker DA, Cofield RH. Tenodesis of the long head of the biceps brachii for chronic bicipital tendinitis. Long-term results. *J Bone Joint Surg (Am)* 1989;71(3):376–381.

51. Gartsman GM, Hammerman SM. Arthroscopic biceps tenodesis: operative technique. *Arthroscopy* 2000;16(5):550–552.

52. Boileau P, Krishnan SG, Coste JS, et al. Arthroscopic biceps tenodesis: a new technique using bioabsorbable interference screw fixation. *Arthroscopy* 2002;18(9):1002–1012.

53. Klepps S, Hazrati Y, Flatow E. Arthroscopic biceps tenodesis. *Arthroscopy* 2002;18(9):1040–1045.

54. Mariani EM, Cofield RH, Askew LJ, et al. Rupture of the tendon of the long head of the biceps brachii. Surgical versus nonsurgical treatment. *Clin Orthop* 1988;(228):233–239.

55. Warren RF. Lesions of the long head of the biceps tendon. *Instr Course Lect* 1985;34:204–209.

56. Gill TJ, McIrvin E, Mair SD, et al. Results of biceps tenotomy for treatment of pathology of the long head of the biceps brachii. *J Shoulder Elbow Surg* 2001;10(3):247–249.

57. O'Donoghue DH. Subluxing biceps tendon in the athlete. *Clin Orthop* 1982;(164):26–29.

58. Curtis AS, Snyder SJ. Evaluation and treatment of biceps tendon pathology. *Orthop Clin North Am* 1993;24(1):33–43.

59. Walch G, Nove-Josserand L, Levigne C, et al. Tears of the supraspinatus tendon associated with "hidden" lesions of the rotator interval. *J Shoulder Elbow Surg* 1994;3:353–360.

60. Walch G, Nove-Josserand L, Boileau P, et al. Subluxations and dislocations of the tendon of the long head of the biceps. *J Shoulder Elbow Surg* 1998;7(2):100–108.

61. Collier SG, Wynn-Jones CH. Displacement of the biceps with subscapularis avulsion. *J Bone Joint Surg (Br)* 1990;72(1):145.

62. Snyder SJ, Karzel RP, Del Pizzo W, Ferkel RD, et al. SLAP lesions of the shoulder. *Arthroscopy* 1990;6(4):274–279.

63. Morgan CD, Burkhart SS, Palmeri M, et al. Type II SLAP lesions: three subtypes and their relationships to superior instability and rotator cuff tears. *Arthroscopy* 1998;14(6):553–565.

64. Maffet MW, Gartsman GM, Moseley B. Superior labrum-biceps tendon complex lesions of the shoulder. *Am J Sports Med* 1995; 23(1):93–98.

65. Snyder SJ, Banas MP, Karzel RP. An analysis of 140 injuries to the superior glenoid labrum. *J Shoulder Elbow Surg* 1995;4(4): 243–248.

66. Parentis MA, Mohr KJ, ElAttrache NS. Disorders of the superior labrum: review and treatment guidelines. *Clin Orthop* 2002; (400):77–87.

67. Bey MJ, Elders GJ, Huston LJ, et al. The mechanism of creation of superior labrum, anterior, and posterior lesions in a dynamic biomechanical model of the shoulder: the role of inferior subluxation. *J Shoulder Elbow Surg* 1998;7(4):397–401.

68. Altchek DW, Warren RF, Wickiewicz TL, et al. Arthroscopic labral debridement. A three-year follow-up study. *Am J Sports Med* 1992;20(6):702–706.

69. Segmuller HE, Hayes MG, Saies AD. Arthroscopic repair of glenolabral injuries with an absorbable fixation device. *J Shoulder Elbow Surg* 1997;6(4):383–392.

70. Field LD, Savoie FH 3rd. Arthroscopic suture repair of superior labral detachment lesions of the shoulder. *Am J Sports Med* 1993;21(6):783–790; discussion 790.

71. Resch H, Gosler K, Thoeni H, et al. Arthroscopic repair of superior glenoid labral detachment (the SLAP lesion). *J Shoulder Elbow Surg* 1993;2:147–155.

72. Yoneda M, Hirooka A, Saito S, et al. Arthroscopic stapling for detached superior glenoid labrum. *J Bone Joint Surg (Br)* 1991; 73(5):746–750.

73. Stetson WB, Karzel RP, Banas MP, et al. Long-term follow-up of 140 consecutive patients with injury to the superior glenoid labrum. *Arthroscopy* 1997;13(3):376–377.

16

ACROMIOCLAVICULAR JOINT DISORDERS

MARK S. SCHICKENDANTZ
RICHARD B. JONES

INTRODUCTION

Acromioclavicular (AC) joint injury is among the most common problems occurring in sports today and throughout history. This joint is not only susceptible to traumatic injury, but degenerative processes as well from prior trauma or overuse. Injuries to the AC joint are commonly confused with other problems of the shoulder complex. Hippocrates (460–377 BC) found that AC joint dislocations were often misdiagnosed as a glenohumeral injury (1). This trend continues to hold true. AC joint dislocation is more common in males (5 to 10:1) and is more often incomplete than complete (2:1) (2).

A broad spectrum of injury can occur at the AC joint and much controversy still exists in the treatment of this injury. Whether or not to treat these injuries operatively or nonoperatively has been widely debated. Furthermore, numerous techniques have been described for the operative treatment of this injury. Treatment of AC disorders in the subgroup of overhead athletes is the most debated. Disorders of the AC joint are relatively uncommon in overhead athletes. The throwing motion seems to cause little stress to the AC joint. If problems do arise, they most frequently consist of degeneration or acute or chronic instability.

ANATOMY

The AC joint is a diarthrodial joint composed of the lateral end of the clavicle and the medial margin of the acromion. Along with the sternoclavicular joint, it is the only articulation of the upper extremity with the axial skeleton. The articular surface initially consists of hyaline cartilage, which at age 17 years on the acromial side and 24 years on the clavicular side becomes fibrocartilage (3). The fibrocartilaginous intraarticular disk of the AC joint commonly undergoes degeneration throughout life; therefore, it is uncommon to find patients older than age 35 to 40 years without at least radiographic evidence of arthrosis of this joint (4,5). The AC ligaments reinforce the thin capsule. They consist of superior, inferior, anterior, and posterior capsular thickenings. The superior ligament is the strongest of the AC ligaments and blends with fibers of the deltoid and trapezius muscles, which are dynamic stabilizers of the AC joint (6). The coracoclavicular ligaments spanning from the inferior clavicle to the base of the coracoid process are the strongest static stabilizers of the AC joint. They consist of two parts, which may be separated by a bursa (Fig. 16-1). The conoid is 0.7 to 2.5 cm in length and 0.4 to 0.95 cm in width and cone shaped. Its apex attaches to the posteromedial side of the base of the coracoid process. The base of the conoid ligament attaches to the posterior inferior clavicular curve at the conoid tubercle. The trapezoid is 0.8 to 2.5 cm in length and 0.8 to 2.5 cm in width. It attaches anterolaterally to the conoid ligament on the coracoid process, extending superiorly to the undersurface of the clavicle (7,8).

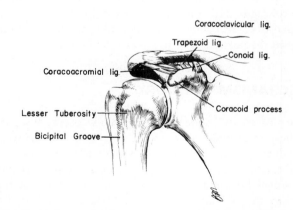

FIGURE 16-1. Anatomy of the acromioclavicular joint. (From Galatz LM, Williams GR. Acromioclavicular joint injuries. In: Bucholz RW, Heckman JD, eds. *Rockwood and Green's fractures in adults,* 5th ed., Philadelphia: Lippincott Williams & Wilkins, 2002, with permission.)

BIOMECHANICS

The primary function of the AC joint is to transmit energy to the axial skeleton from the appendicular skeleton and support the upper extremity. The rotatory motion at the AC joint has been debated. Ranges have been reported from 5 to 20 degrees of motion (9,10). Rockwood placed pins into the acromion and clavicle of volunteers and found only 5 to 8 degrees of rotation with shoulder range of motion (2). This has important implications in considering surgical fixation options for AC injuries. Rigid coracoclavicular screw fixation must be removed after healing or screw failure will eventually occur because of this normal motion. Furthermore, cerclage techniques around the distal clavicle may eventually erode the clavicle from small amount of rotatory motion.

The AC ligaments are thought to primarily control horizontal (anterior and posterior) stability. Fukuda and colleagues demonstrated that the AC ligaments are the principal restraints to axial distraction and posterior translation (11). However, Lee and co-workers found the in situ force of the trapezoid (42.9 ± 15.4 N) was significantly greater during posterior displacement than other ligaments (6).

The coracoclavicular ligaments control vertical stability of the AC joint. They help couple glenohumeral abduction and flexion to scapular rotation on the chest wall. Both the conoid and trapezoid ligaments must be disrupted to cause a complete vertical AC joint dislocation. Debski and colleagues (12) showed that, after transection of the capsule, the conoid ligament served as the primary restraint to anterosuperior loading and the trapezoid ligament was the primary restraint to posterior loading. As a result of these findings, they recommended that surgical reconstruction address both ligaments in order to restore stability in both the horizontal and vertical planes. They also concluded that injuries to the AC capsule may render the intact coracoclavicular ligaments more likely to fail with subsequent anteroposterior loading. In another similar study, Debski and colleagues (13) showed differences in the load sharing properties of the conoid and trapezoid ligaments and again stressed the possible need to reconstruct both ligaments.

MECHANISM OF INJURY

Injury of the AC joint most commonly occurs from the application of direct force. Direct force injury occurs when the athlete falls on the shoulder with arm adducted (Fig. 16-2). It can also occur with direct hits, such as those sustained in football, hockey, and karate. Most agree that the force first disrupts the AC ligaments. If the force is sufficient, this energy is transmitted to and disrupts the coracoclavicular ligaments, resulting in increased displacement of the clavicle relative to the acromion. The acromion is forced in a downward, medial, and anterior direction. During a fall, this is usually due to a combined direct impact and body roll

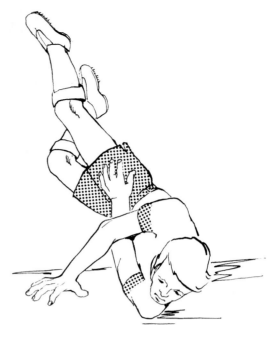

FIGURE 16-2. Illustration of typical mechanism of injury to the acromioclavicular joint. (From Galatz LM, Williams GR. Acromioclavicular joint injuries. In: Bucholz RW, Heckman JD, eds. *Rockwood and Green's fractures in adults,* 5th ed. Philadelphia: Lippincott Williams & Wilkins, 2002, with permission.)

toward the injured shoulder. Basamania (14) related that, as the body strikes the ground, the head and shoulder hit first causing rupture of the AC ligaments. With sufficient energy, the trapezoid ligament ruptures. As the force continues, the scapula and acromion are driven medially, causing the conoid to reside in a vertical position. As the force continues, the

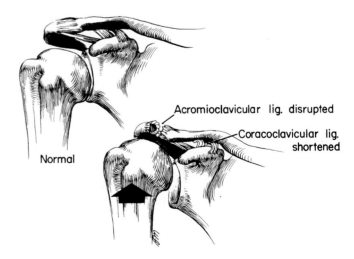

FIGURE 16-3. Illustration of injury to the acromioclavicular joint resulting from a fall on the outstretched hand. Note the decrease in the coracoclavicular space. (From Galatz LM, Williams GR. Acromioclavicular joint injuries. In: Bucholz RW, Heckman JD, eds. *Rockwood and Green's fractures in adults,* 5th ed. Philadelphia: Lippincott Williams & Wilkins, 2002, with permission.)

conoid is ruptured, allowing further medial translation of the acromion relative to the clavicle.

Indirect force injury is less common. It usually occurs when the athlete lands on an outstretched hand. The force is transmitted up the arm, through the humerus, into the humeral head, and into the acromion process. However, the energy is only directed to the AC ligaments. The coracoclavicular ligaments are not disrupted because there is a decrease in the coracoclavicular space (Fig. 16-3).

CLASSIFICATION

Like all classification systems, the classification of injuries to the AC joint should correlate to prognosis and assist with treatment. The two most popular classification systems for AC injuries are described by Allman (15) and Tossy and colleagues (16), and by Rockwood and colleagues (2). Allman (15) and Tossy (16) separated AC injuries into three distinct categories. Type I injuries involve a strain of the AC ligaments with intact coracoclavicular ligaments. Type II injuries involve ruptured AC ligaments with strained but intact coracoclavicular ligaments. Type III injuries were the worst in severity and involved ruptured AC and coracoclavicular ligaments. Rockwood, however, believed that there were varying degrees of type III injuries with different outcomes attributed to their severity. Based on his clinical findings, he proposed an expanded classification with further subdivision of Allman and Tossy's type III category (Fig. 16- 4). In Rockwood's classification system, type I injuries are essentially the same as Allman and Tossy's. Type II injuries involve disruption of the AC ligaments and strain of the coracoclavicular ligaments with up to 25% displacement of the coracoclavicular distance. A type III injury includes disruption of the AC ligaments and the coracoclavicular ligaments with a 25% to 100% displacement of the coracoclavicular interspace. Type IV injuries are similar to type III except that the clavicle is displaced posteriorly into the trapezius. This occurs with a more anteroposterior force than the typical superoinferior force. Type V injuries are a more severe form of type III, with greater than 100% displacement at the coracoclavicular interspace. The deltotrapezial fascia is usually disrupted as well. Type VI injuries are rare and associated with severe trauma. These involve inferior displacement of the clavicle beneath the coracoid. This is thought to be due to a severe hyperadduction and external rotation of the extremity (17).

PRESENTATION AND PHYSICAL EXAMINATION

The athlete should be examined in the standing or sitting position to allow downward force from the weight of the arm to intensify the deformity of the AC joint. Often a severe deformity reduces with the patient in the supine position. It is not uncommon for injuries that appear less severe initially to look worse upon later examination. Acute soft tissue swelling often hides the actual degree of deformity. As this subsides, the deformity becomes more obvious. Additionally, patients tend to initially splint their injury because of pain, and once pain subsides the weight of the arm accentuates the deformity. Grasping and gently manipulating the mid shaft of the clavicle can be done to assess the stability of the AC joint. Gross motion, particularly in the vertical plane, often indicates the presence of a high-grade injury. With an injury to the AC joint, athletes experience pain at the joint with full forward flexion of the shoulder as well as with cross-body adduction. Another examination technique involves having the athlete place the hand of the affected arm on the contralateral shoulder while the examiner applies gentle downward pressure on the affected elbow. If the athlete experiences pain at the AC joint, injury should be suspected.

With type I injuries there is usually no gross deformity. There may be mild swelling over the AC joint. There is tenderness to palpation over the AC joint but usually not in the region of the coracoclavicular ligaments. Range of motion is usually full. Overhead athletes may have pain at the extremes of motion such as the late cocking phase or follow-through phase of throwing.

Patients with type II injuries have moderate to severe tenderness at the AC joint. They usually have some mild deformity in the region as a result of swelling or slight displacement of the AC joint. These patients may have some slight motion with manipulation of the clavicle and may have palpable popping or grinding in the joint. Range of motion is usually limited by pain.

Type III injuries usually display obvious deformity (Fig. 16-5). Patients have severe pain, limited range of motion, and tenderness over the AC joint as well as the coracoclavicular region. Instability is present at the AC joint with manual manipulation. Patients usually hold the arm at their side in attempts to splint the injury, and, as mentioned earlier, this may decrease the deformity. Adducting the arm across the body usually causes severe prominence of the clavicle as a result of medial displacement of the acromion (Fig. 16-6).

Type IV injuries display posterior displacement of the clavicle into the trapezius. This may be due to the anteromedial rotation of the scapula relative to the clavicle and often reduces when the patient is in the supine position. However, the clavicle can button-hole through the trapezius fascia and be difficult to reduce. However, this is a rare injury. Patients with type V injuries have a similar presentation as type III, but usually have a more severe deformity at the AC joint. Type VI injuries are rare and are usually associated with severe trauma. Gross deformity is present often with other associated injuries. Severe neurovascular compromise may be present as well.

Patients with chronic injuries have varying degrees of deformity depending on the severity of the initial injury. They may have continued instability of the AC joint. Chronic pain at the AC joint and weakness with lack of endurance at the shoulder joint may be seen as well.

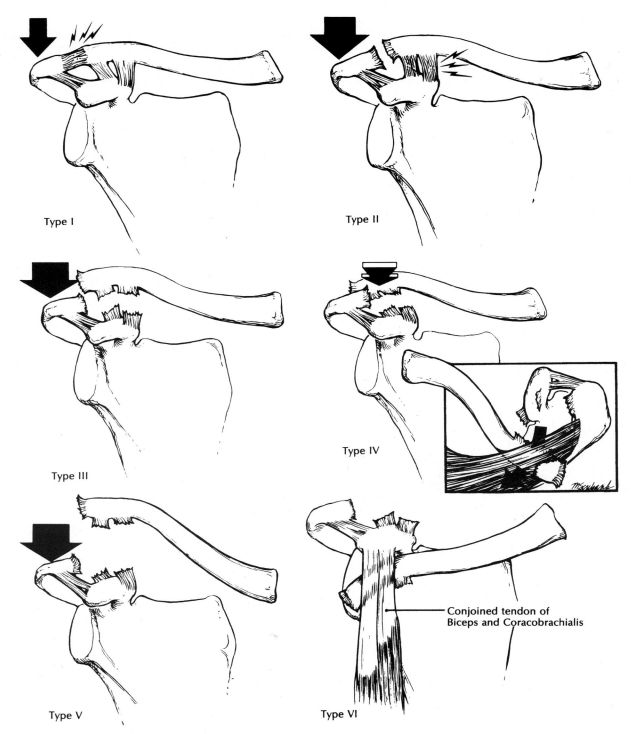

Type I

Type II

Type III

Type IV

Type V

Type VI

Conjoined tendon of
Biceps and Coracobrachialis

FIGURE 16-4. Rockwood classification of injury to the acromioclavicular joint. (From Galatz LM, Williams GR. Acromioclavicular joint injuries. In: Bucholz RW, Heckman JD, eds. *Rockwood and Green's fractures in adults,* 5th ed. Philadelphia: Lippincott Williams & Wilkins, 2002.)

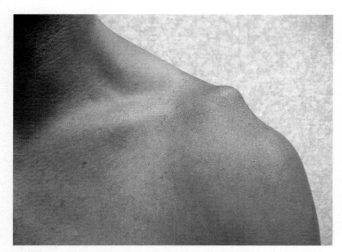

FIGURE 16-5. Clinical appearance of a grade III acromioclavicular injury.

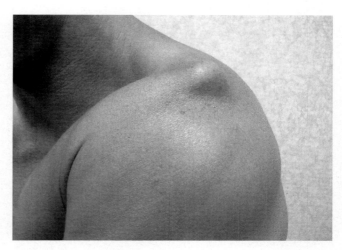

FIGURE 16-6. Accentuation of the deformity seen with a grade III acromioclavicular injury that occurs with adduction of the involved limb.

RADIOGRAPHIC AND DIAGNOSTIC EVALUATION

Radiographs are used to evaluate the extent of injury as well as exclude fractures of the acromion, clavicle, and coracoid. However, standard radiographic technique for shoulder radiographs overpenetrate and wash out the AC joint. Radiographs evaluating the AC joint should be obtained at about 50% of the intensity of those obtained for the glenohumeral joint. This helps avoid missed injuries to the area resulting from poor radiographs. It is also important to obtain a standard shoulder radiographic series in any patient with a traumatic shoulder injury to thoroughly assess the joint.

The patient should be standing or in the seated position to accentuate any deformity at the AC joint. If possible, both AC joints should be imaged on the same cassette to ensure the same technique is used in comparison. Zanca (18) showed that the optimal technique to visualize the AC joint is to angle the x-ray beam 15 degrees in the cephalad direction on an anteroposterior radiograph. This eliminates superimposition of the spine of the scapula on the AC joint.

Patients may splint the injury by supporting the injured extremity with the opposite arm or by muscular contraction, thus decreasing deformity on radiographs. Stress radiographs can be used in this situation. These are performed by suspending approximately 10 to 15 pounds from the patient's wrists while obtaining standard anteroposterior radiographs of both shoulders. Bossart and colleagues (19) believed that weighted radiographs are ineffective and offered low yield in obvious AC joint injuries, and thus should not be routinely ordered. Similarly, we have not found weighted radiographs of the AC joint to be helpful and do not recommend their routine use.

Other stress views have been described. Alexander (20) described a view in which the shoulders are pushed forward to displace the acromion inferiorly and anteriorly. A scapular lateral view is obtained in this position and compared to the opposite side. Basamania (14) described a cross-body adduction view in which the patient adducts the arm across the body and grasps it with the unaffected arm. A standard anteroposterior radiograph is then obtained. With significant injury to the AC joint, the acromion is seen displaced inferior and medial to the clavicle.

Consistent radiographic findings are present on standardized radiographs of the AC joint depending on the severity of injury. Comparison with the uninvolved side is important in all cases. With type I injuries, there is usually no joint widening or deformity. There may be mild soft tissue swelling over the AC joint. Type II injuries display a slight increase in the coracoclavicular interval, usually less than 25% greater than the opposite side (Fig. 16-7). The

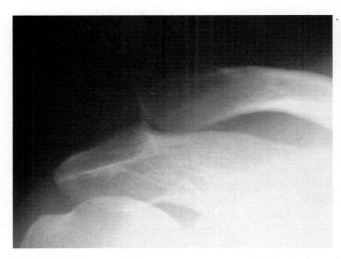

FIGURE 16-7. Radiographic appearance of a grade II acromioclavicular injury.

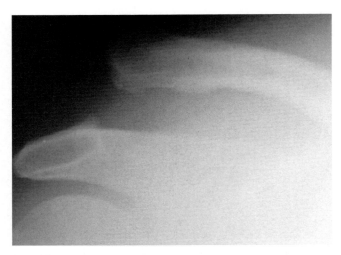

FIGURE 16-8. Radiographic appearance of a grade V acromio-clavicular joint injury.

AC joint may appear widened as a result of the slight posterior displacement by the trapezius muscle. With type III injuries, the acromion is displaced inferior to the clavicle 25% to 100% the width of the clavicle. The coracoclavicular interval is also increased 25% to 100% relative to the opposite shoulder. If the coracoclavicular distance is not increased, a fracture of the base of the coracoid should be suspected. A Stryker notch view is indicated in this case to rule out coracoid fracture.

Type IV injuries show posterior displacement of the clavicle relative to the acromion. This is best seen on an axillary view or CT scan. There are varying degrees of displacement at the AC joint and increases in the coracoclavicular interval. Type V injuries have increases in the coracoclavicular interval of greater than 100% (Fig. 16-8). There is severe displacement at the AC joint as well, reaching two to three times the width of the clavicle. Type VI injuries are rare and severe injuries that may have associated fractures or dislocations. The clavicle is displaced inferior to the coracoid process.

TREATMENT

Treatment of AC joint injuries, particularly type III, remains controversial. There have been more than 35 nonoperative treatment modalities described in the orthopedic literature and far more operative procedures described for this particular injury (2). It is well accepted that patients with AC joint injuries of type I or II should initially be treated nonoperatively. However, not all patients who experience type I or II injuries recover fully. Bergfeld and colleagues (21) looked at the long-term clinical results of type I and II AC joint injuries in Naval cadets. Symptoms were present in 39% of cadets who sustained type I injuries and in 65% of those with type II injuries.

It is also well accepted that type IV, V, and VI injuries should generally be treated operatively. However, when treating an athlete with a type III AC injury, the decision to treat the injury operatively or nonoperatively is often difficult. Historically, proponents of early operative treatment of type III injuries have cited persistent deformity, AC arthritis, and residual weakness as reasons for surgery (22–24). However, current literature suggests that most patients with type III AC injuries have comparable strength and range of motion of the shoulder with either operative or nonoperative treatment (25,26). Wojtys and Nelson (27) supported this claim, but did find increased discomfort with high activity levels in patients treated nonoperatively. Schlegel and co-workers (25) prospectively evaluated a small group of patients with type III injuries treated nonoperatively. Twenty percent believed their outcome was suboptimal. However, none experienced symptoms severe enough to warrant surgery. Objectively, no patient had significant deficits in strength or range of motion. Rockwood (2) recommends operative treatment of type III injuries in laborers and overhead, high-performance athletes. He does point out that contact athletes may be better treated nonoperatively because of the high risk of failure of surgery in this patient population.

There are relatively few peer-reviewed studies of the treatment of AC injuries in the overhead athlete in the orthopedic literature. No prospective studies compare the operative and nonoperative treatment of type III AC injuries in this group of patients. Thus, there are no absolute indications for either type of treatment of this injury in these athletes. Based on his retrospective review, Lemos (28) suggested operative treatment for high-level pitchers, open injuries, and associated brachial plexopathy. McFarland and colleagues (29) surveyed 42 orthopedic surgeons participating in the care of 28 professional baseball teams regarding their treatment for grade III AC sprains in throwing athletes: 31% recommended immediate operative treatment. This same group of physicians estimated that normal function and significant pain relief was achieved in 80% of their athletes with type III AC injuries treated nonoperatively compared with 92% of those treated operatively.

Nonoperative Treatment

Nonoperative treatment options reported for these injuries include sling (30,31), brace and harness (32–34), adhesive straps (35,36), figure-of-eight straps (37), crotch loops, stocking, garter, and strap (38,39), abduction traction and suspension (40), and casts (41,42). Historically, a common technique used to reduce the AC joint was the Kenny-Howard sling and strap. This consists of a sling combined with a strap, which wraps around the elbow. The strap is used to compress the distal clavicle in an attempt to hold it reduced. This can be problematic in that it can cause pressure necrosis of the skin over the distal clavicle.

Type I injuries are treated with ice and a sling as needed for comfort. When the athlete is pain-free and full strength and range of motion are achieved (usually 1 to 3 weeks), return to play is allowed. Type II injuries are treated similarly. Ice, analgesics, and a sling are used intermittently for the first 1 to 2 weeks. Range of motion and activities of daily living are allowed as soon as pain permits. Criteria for return to play are full strength and painless full range of motion. Unlike type I injuries, this may take up to 6 weeks to achieve. Patients must be followed up closely to ensure a more serious injury is not missed.

Nonoperative treatment of type III injuries entails the use of a sling, ice, and analgesics. The sling can be discontinued and light activities resumed when pain permits. Return to sports is allowed when there is full strength and range of motion of the injured shoulder. This may take 8 to 12 weeks.

Operative Treatment

Operative treatment of type I and II AC joint injuries is indicated when the athlete experiences symptoms referable to the AC joint after a reasonable course of nonoperative treatment. There are no indications for acute operative intervention for these injuries. As mentioned earlier, chronic pain at the AC joint may develop in a number of athletes following type I or II sprains due to injury to the fibrocartilaginous disk, synovitis, or posttraumatic arthrosis. Rarely, instability of the joint may be a cause of persistent symptoms. In these individuals, selective corticosteroid and local anesthetic injection can serve both a diagnostic and therapeutic purpose. A favorable response to injection is generally a good indication that the symptoms are referable to the AC joint. Failure of a well-placed local injection into the joint to alleviate any pain should raise the possibility of another cause for the persistent symptoms. Athletes who experience a recurrence of pain following a period of pain relief may be considered candidates for an arthroscopic evaluation of the joint. Preoperative magnetic resonance imaging (MRI) may be of value in ruling out other possible causes of pain and in planning an operative strategy. Arthroscopic distal clavicle excision has been shown to be an effective treatment for alleviating pain arising from the AC joint. However, in the face of an unstable distal clavicle, isolated excision may not be as effective as excision combined with a stabilization procedure. Instability of the distal clavicle following type I or II AC sprains is uncommon, but should be considered as a possible cause of persistent symptoms before surgical treatment is undertaken.

Arthroscopic Distal Clavicle Excision

A thorough diagnostic arthroscopy of the shoulder is performed and all associated pathology addressed appropri-

ately. The AC joint is viewed from underneath with the arthroscope in the subacromial space, viewing from the posterior portal. A clear cannula (5-mm diameter or larger) is placed through a lateral portal. To assist in locating the joint, an 18-gauge spinal needle can be placed into the AC joint from above, passing through the joint into the subacromial space. Removing the subacromial bursa aides in visualization. A clear cannula (5-mm diameter or larger) is then introduced into the subacromial space from an anterior portal, entering immediately beneath the AC joint. Generally, the same skin incision used for the anterior portal into the glenohumeral joint may be used. A radiofrequency ablation probe or mechanical shaver is used to remove the ventral capsule of the joint. Working through the anterior cannula, the fibrocartilaginous disk and other soft tissues are removed with the shaver. Attention is then directed to removing bone. Often the bone is soft enough to be removed with the shaver. At other times, a 4.5-mm diameter burr is used. Approximately 6 to 8 mm of the distal clavicle is removed (Fig. 16-9). It is safe and often advisable to remove 3 to 4 mm of the acromial side of the joint as well. Great care is taken to preserve the dorsal AC capsular ligaments.

Postoperative care involves the use of an arm sling for comfort and cryotherapy. Active assisted range-of-motion exercises are permitted as pain allows. As pain subsides and range of motion improves, progressive resistive exercises are initiated. If this procedure is performed on the dominant side of a throwing athlete, we do not allow reinstitution of a throwing program until the athlete demonstrates full, pain-free motion, balanced rotator cuff strength, and good scapular control. This typically takes at least 8 weeks to achieve.

Distal Clavicle Stabilization

Once the decision has been made to surgically stabilize the distal clavicle, the choice of which surgical approach to use must be made. A multitude of procedures have been described throughout the years for the operative treatment of AC joint injuries. These procedures can generally be placed into several different categories based on the method of fixation. These include AC fixation, coracoclavicular fixation, and dynamic muscle transfers. Various fixation devices exist within these categories including pin fixation, plates, screws, suture or tape, and autograft or allograft ligaments. Different treatment options also exist when dealing with acute versus chronic injuries.

AC fixation has been accomplished with various devices. Commonly, smooth or threaded K-wires, Steinmann pins, or screws have been used. Problems with this technique include difficulty of pin or screw placement and hardware breakage. A sloping acromion and the curve of the distal clavicle make placement of pins or screws technically demanding. Sympto-

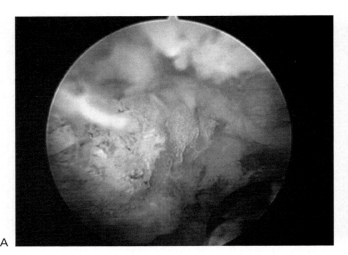
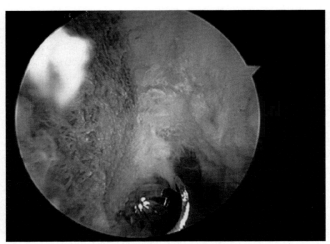

A   B

FIGURE 16-9. A: Arthroscopic appearance of acromioclavicular arthrosis viewing from the posterior portal, looking up at the ventral side of the joint. **B:** The same joint following distal clavicle resection.

matic osteolysis of the distal clavicle has been reported following this type of fixation in as many as 15% of patients (43,44). The most concerning problem with this technique is the risk of hardware migration, which has been well documented in the literature (2,45–48). A hook plate has also been described for AC fixation (49–51) but lacks popularity in the United States. This requires more extensive dissection and may cause rotator cuff symptoms. We have no experience with the hook plate technique.

Coracoclavicular fixation is probably the most commonly used type of fixation for AC joint operative stabilization. This can be accomplished with a coracoclavicular sling or more rigid fixation such as a coracoclavicular screw. Sling type fixation can be achieved with absorbable or nonabsorbable, braided or unbraided suture, or grafts, such as synthetic, autograft, or allograft tissue (2,52–55). Sutures can be placed around the clavicle or through drill holes in the clavicle. Permanent sutures and tapes, such as Mersiline, can erode through the distal clavicle over time if placed in a cerclage fashion (56–59). This type of fixation also may pull the distal clavicle anteriorly when tightened, causing posterior impingement of the AC joint. Placing sutures around the coracoid can be problematic as well. This requires extensive dissection, and it is technically demanding. Dissection around the base of the coracoid risks damage to the musculocutaneous nerve and other neurovascular structures. Breslow and co-workers (60) recently reported a technique using suture anchors in the coracoid, which was equally as strong as sutures around the coracoid. An arthroscopic technique that diminishes the dissection around the coracoid has been described as well (61). If suture is used to create a sling, size number 1 Tevdek or polydiaxone (PDS) is typically chosen, with six to nine braided strands braided into a thick bundle. This must be braided very tightly, however, or the construct will loosen.

Coracoclavicular screw fixation allows for less dissection and more rigid fixation when compared to sling-type fixation. However, a second procedure is needed to later remove the hardware. Motamedi and colleagues (62) looked at the biomechanics of coracoclavicular ligament augmentations. They looked at intact ligaments, augmentations with braided PDS, and braided polyethylene placed through or around the clavicle, and unicortical 6.5 screw fixation to the coracoid. Failure load for a unicortical screw was significantly lower than for the other fixation types. Braided PDS was significantly less stiff. The researchers recommend braided polyethylene placed around or through drill hole in clavicle to augment coracoclavicular ligament repairs. Harris and co-workers (63) looked at the structural properties of the intact and reconstructed coracoclavicular ligament complex. They concluded that coracoclavicular slings were strong but elastic and may not be suitable for severe injuries. They showed that, with bicortical placement, a coracoclavicular screw had the same stiffness as the coracoclavicular ligaments. Therefore, bicortical fixation in the coracoid should be achieved when performing this technique.

Dynamic muscle transfer, which includes transfer of the coracoid and short head of the biceps tendon to the clavicle, has been described for treating acute and chronic AC joint injuries (64,65). This is designed to hold the distal clavicle down through dynamic contraction of the biceps. Compared with other procedures, this technique offers little advantage and is not currently popular for treating these injuries.

Gurd (66) and Mumford (67) both described resection of the distal clavicle for treatment of acute and chronic AC joint injuries. Rockwood (2), however, thought that resection of the distal clavicle in the setting of ligamentous disruption was not indicated and may cause abutment of the remaining clavicle posteriorly against the acromion. Resection may further exacerbate the instability as well (67). For this reason, distal clavicle resection without concomitant stabilization of the distal clavicle is not recommended for the treatment of types III to VI AC joint sprains, either in the acute or chronic setting. Surgical treatment of chronic injuries of this severity generally entails distal clavicle excision in combination with other reconstructive procedures. Typically, no more than 10 mm of the distal clavicle needs to be resected. Taking more than this may lead to poorer results (68). Other disorders for which resection of the distal clavicle may be appropriate include degenerative disease of the AC joint or osteolysis of the distal clavicle.

Author's Preferred Operative Technique

Acute Injuries (<4 Weeks Post-injury)

The patient is placed in the beach chair position. An incision is made beginning just proximal to the clavicle approximately 1 to 2 cm medial to the AC joint extending distally over the coracoid process. Dissection is carried down to the deltotrapezial fascia. Often with severe injuries, this is torn. The distal clavicle may be buttonholed through this fascia as well. The deltotrapezial fascia should be split in line with the clavicle. A portion of the distal clavicle may be stripped of soft tissue in severe injuries. The deltoid is then split with a fine-tipped electrocautery in line with the incision. This allows exposure of the coracoid process. The coracoclavicular ligaments are then identified. They may be torn in the mid substance or avulsed from the clavicle or coracoid. Once identified, a nonabsorbable suture is placed in each end for later repair. If they are avulsed from either end, a suture anchor may be placed in the coracoid or drill hole made in the clavicle for fixation. The intraarticular disk is often torn and should be excised from the AC joint. We do not routinely resect the distal clavicle. Indications for resection of the distal clavicle include the presence of osteolysis, arthrosis of the joint, and select concomitant distal clavicle fractures that are not amenable to surgical stabilization. The AC joint is then reduced. This can be held manually or temporarily held with a K wire. Next, a ³⁄₁₆-inch or 3.5-mm drill is used to make a hole in the clavicle directly over the coracoid. This is approximately 2 to 2.5 cm medial to the AC joint. A ³⁄₆₄-inch drill is then placed through the hole and directed to the base of the coracoid. Care must be taken to ensure that it is centered in the coracoid in order to get bicortical fixation. A hole is then drilled bicortically in the base of the coracoid. A depth gauge is inserted through both holes with the AC joint reduced to determine the appropriate screw length. Next, the appropriate length coracoclavicular lag screw and washer should be chosen to allow bicortical thread purchase in the coracoid. Specially designed coracoclavicular lag screws are available; otherwise, a 6.5-mm partially

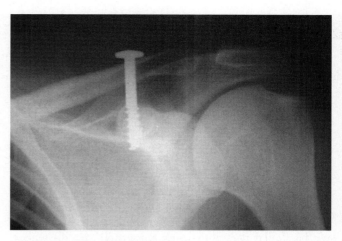

FIGURE 16-10. Coracoclavicular screw fixation of a grade III acromioclavicular joint injury.

threaded cancellous screw and washer may be used. The screw should be tightened to hold the AC joint anatomically reduced as compared to preoperative radiographs of the uninjured shoulder. This can be checked with fluoroscopy or intraoperative x-ray study (Fig. 16-10). The coracoclavicular ligaments are then repaired with the previously placed sutures. Once these are tied, the screw should be tightened one turn to take the stress off of the coracoclavicular ligament repair. During closure, the superior AC ligaments should be repaired if possible. The deltotrapezial fascia should be repaired in an imbricated fashion to assist stability. Occasionally, this needs to be repaired through drill holes in the clavicle if extensive soft tissue stripping has occurred.

Postoperative Care

Postoperatively the arm is kept in a sling and ice cuff for 1 to 2 weeks. Active and passive range of motion is then allowed, with forward flexion limited to 90 degrees. This decreases the chances of screw loosening or breakage. The patient is allowed to use the arm for light activities of daily living, lifting nothing heavier than a telephone book. The screw is removed through a small incision at approximately 8 weeks from surgery. Once the screw has been removed, full motion is allowed, but heavy lifting, pushing, or pulling is avoided for an additional 4 to 6 weeks. Return to play is allowed when the athlete has full strength and range of motion of the extremity.

CHRONIC INJURIES

When surgically treating symptomatic chronic type III, IV, and V AC joint injuries, stabilization of the joint must be achieved. As mentioned earlier, resection of the distal clavicle is routinely performed as a part of the reconstructive procedure. Thus, AC fixation techniques are not useful in this setting. Similarly, the use of rigid coracoclavicular screws is not currently recommended. Multiple techniques of ligamentous reconstruction have been described for this situation. Weaver and Dunn (69) described transfer of the coracoacromial ligament with distal clavicle resection. Their technique remains widely popular today. More recent techniques represent modifications of that described by Weaver and Dunn. Other authors have described the use of fascia lata autograft for reconstruction (70,71). Recently, Jones and colleagues (55) described a technique of AC joint reconstruction using autogenous semitendinosus tendon from the knee. The senior author (M.S.S.) has experience with a similar technique using autogenous gracilis tendon graft to reconstruct the coracoclavicular ligaments.

Authors' Operative Technique for Chronic Injuries (<4 Weeks Post-injury)

With the patient in the beach chair position, the shoulder and ipsilateral lower extremity are prepped and draped in the usual sterile fashion. Under tourniquet, the gracilis tendon is harvested for graft through a small incision centered over the pes anserinus. The tendon is generally 3 to 4 mm in diameter and does not need to be split in order to be used for a graft. The graft is prepared by carefully removing all remaining muscle and tubularizing the proximal end of the harvested tendon with number 3-0 absorbable suture on a taper needle. The final length of the graft is usually 15 to 20 cm.

Attention is then directed to the shoulder where a 6- to 8-cm incision is made along Langer's lines from a point just lateral to the posterior extent of the AC joint extending distally toward the coracoid. Skin flaps are gently mobilized. The distal end of the clavicle is readily identified and may be found button-holed though the deltotrapezial fascia. A longitudinal incision is created along the dorsal capsule of the AC joint. This incision is then carried distally along the fibers of the deltoid a distance of about 5 cm where a stay suture is placed to prevent inadvertent further splitting of the muscle. Using a needle-tipped electrocautery, the deltotrapezial fascia is then incised along the dorsum of the clavicle for a distance of 3 to 4 cm starting at the AC joint and working medially. Care is taken to stay centered along the shaft of the clavicle. Anterior and posterior muscular flaps are created and reflected from the clavicle. It is important to take great care during this dissection in order to preserve as much soft tissue as possible for later closure. Periosteal elevators are used to clear the soft tissue from the undersurface of the distal clavicle. A medium Darrach retractor is placed beneath the distal clavicle and a small Holman retractor placed behind. An oscillating saw is then used to remove the distal 1 cm of the bone. A rongeur is used to round the edges of the end of the clavicle. Staying close to the anterior edge of the lateral end of the clavicle, a 2.8-mm drill is used

to create two parallel bicortical holes in the bone directed at about a 30-degree angle posteriorly. Just posterior and between these holes, a third larger hole is created using a ¾-inch drill angled in the same direction.

Attention is then directed to the coracoid. The coracoacromial ligament is identified and followed to its origin. The base of the coracoid is carefully dissected free of enough soft tissue to pass an angled hemostat around it. The hemostat is used to pass three strands of heavy nonabsorbable suture around the base of the coracoid process. We currently use number 2 Fiberwire suture (Arthrex, Naples, FL). Two of the suture strands are to be used in the reconstruction. The third is used as a passing suture to pull the gracilis graft around the coracoid. It is recommended that the suture be passed between the coracoacromial ligament and the coracoid rather than over top of the ligament. Using the passing suture, the graft is passed around the base of the coracoid. A Hewson suture passer is brought down through the top of the large drill hole exiting the underside of the clavicle. The lateral limb of the graft is looped into the passer, which is used to pull it up through the clavicle. Next, the Hewson passer is used to pull the other two strands of suture up through the two smaller holes, resulting in a double-stranded suture in each hole. Cuff Link (Mitek/Johnson and Johnson, Westwood, MA) bone tunnel protectors are threaded onto the sutures and pushed into the holes (Fig. 16-11). The distal end of the clavicle is then held in a reduced position while the double-stranded sutures are tied. The gracilis graft is then placed under appropriate tension and sewn back onto itself using number 2 Fiberwire suture, completing the reconstruction (Fig. 16-12). Wound closure is routine.

Postoperatively, a shoulder immobilizer is used for the first 2 weeks. The arm is then placed into a simple arm sling, and passive pendulum exercises are allowed. After 4 weeks, the sling is discontinued and light daily activities are permitted. Supervised physical therapy begins 6 to 8 weeks from the time of surgery. Pushing and pulling against resistance is avoided until at least week 12. Full participation in sports is allowed once the athlete demonstrates full active shoulder motion and normal strength, usually about 6 months after surgery.

DEGENERATIVE DISEASE OF THE ACROMIOCLAVICULAR JOINT

Degenerative disease may be the most common entity affecting the AC joint in overhead athletes. The throwing motion may cause repetitive stress at the AC joint in the follow-through phase with horizontal cross arm adduction. However, weight lifting (e.g., bench press or military press) has been strongly implicated in destruction of the AC joint (72–74). Therefore, degeneration in the throwing athlete may be more related to vigorous weight training than to

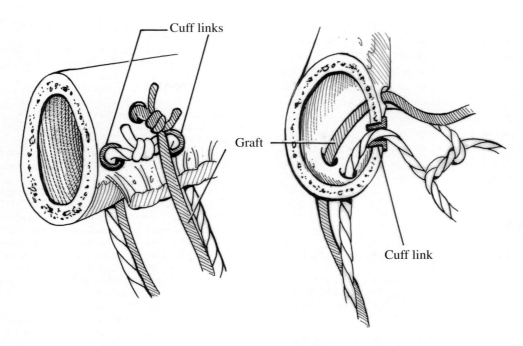

FIGURE 16-11. Illustration demonstrating the gracilis graft and reinforcing suture placement. Note the relative location of the holes and the position of the cuff links.

repetitive throwing (72). Previous injury to the AC joint may also be a source of later degeneration (21,75).

The athlete generally complains of pain in the superior aspect of the shoulder, which may radiate into the neck. The pain may be greatest during the follow-through phase of throwing and is reproduced with cross arm adduction. Instability may also be demonstrable with manual manipulation in cases of chronic injury. Radiographically, the joint often demonstrates degenerative changes such as osteophyte formation, translucency or osteolysis of the distal clavicle, and cystic changes (73). MRI may show edema in the distal clavicle, but this has been shown to be inconsistent in correlating to clinical findings at the AC joint (76).

Treatment consists initially of rest and nonsteroidal anti-inflammatory use. Failure of these modalities can be followed by corticosteroid injection of the AC joint. If this fails

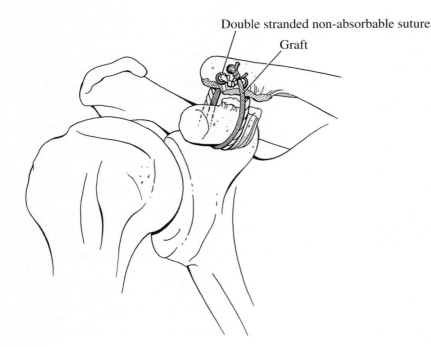

FIGURE 16-12. Final appearance of the reconstructed joint.

to relieve symptoms, resection of the distal clavicle should be considered. Distal clavicle excision has proven to be successful in overhead athletes. Cook and Tibone (72) described the procedure in an athletic population of patients. All of the baseball players were able to return to their previous level of throwing. Distal clavicle excision may be performed open or arthroscopically with success (72,74,77–80). However, care must be taken during the arthroscopic approach not to disrupt the dorsal capsular attachments, which contain the AC ligaments. This has been shown to result in postoperative AC instability (78,80,81).

REFERENCES

1. Adams FL. The genuine works of Hippocrates, vol 1 and 2. New York: William Wood, 1886.
2. Rockwood CA Jr, Williams GR, Young DC. Injuries to the acromioclavicular joint. In: Rockwood CA, Green DP, Bucholz RW, et al, eds. *Fractures in adults*, 4th ed. Philadelphia: Lippincott-Raven, 1996:1341–1413.
3. DePalma AF. *Degenerative changes in the sternoclavicular acromioclavicular joints in various decades.*. Springfield, IL: Charles C Thomas, 1957.
4. Petersson CJ. Degeneration of the acromioclavicular joint. A morphological study. *Acta Otrhop Scand* 1983;54:434–438.
5. Petersson CJ, Redlund-Jonnell I. Radiographic joint space in normal acromioclavicular joints. *Acta Otrhop Scand* 1983;54:431–433.
6. Lee K, Bebski RE, Chen C, et al. Functional evaluation of the ligaments at the acromioclavicular joint during anterioposterior and superioinferior translation. *Am J Sports Med* 1997;25(6):858–862.
7. Salter EG, Nasca RJ, Shelley BS. Anatomical observations on the acromioclavicular joint and supporting ligaments. *Am J Sports Med* 1987;15:199–206.
8. Johnston TB, Davies DV, Davies F, eds. *Gray's anatomy*, 32nd ed. London: Longmans, Green and Co, 1958.
9. Inman VT, McLaughlin HD, Nevaiser J, et al. Treatment of complete acromioclavicular dislocation. *J Bone Joint Surgery (Am)* 1962;44:1008–1011.
10. Codman EA. Rupture of the supraspinatus tendon and lesions in or about the subacromial bursa. In: Codman EA, ed. *The shoulder*. Boston: Thomas Todd, 1934.
11. Fukuda K, Craig EV, Cofield RH, et al. Biomechanical study of the ligamentous system of the acromioclavicular joint. *J Bone Joint Surg* 1986;68:434–440.
12. Debski RE, Parsons IM, Woo SL, et al. Effect of capsular injury on acromioclavicular joint mechanics. *J Bone Joint Surg (Am)* 2001;83(9):1344–1351.
13. Debski RE, Parsons IM, Fenwick J, et al. Ligament mechanics during three degree of freedom motion at the acromioclavicular joint. *Ann Biomech Eng* 2000;28(6):612–618.
14. Basamania CJ. Acromioclavicular joint injuries in athletes. In: Garrett WE, Speer KP, Kirkendall DT, eds. *Principles and practice of orthopaedic sports medicine*. Philadelphia: Lippincott Williams & Wilkins, 2000:511–534.
15. Allman FL Jr. Fractures and ligamentous injuries of the clavicle and its articulation. *J Bone Joint Surg (Am)* 1967;49:774–784.
16. Tossy JD, Mead NC, Sigmond HM. Acromioclavicular separations: useful and practical classification for treatment. *Clin Orthop* 1963;28:111–119.
17. Gerber C, Rockwood CA Jr. Subcoracoid dislocation of the lateral end of the clavicle. A report of three cases. *J Bone Joint Surg Am* 1987;69:924–927.
18. Zanca P. Shoulder pain. Involvement of the acromioclavicular joint: analysis of 1,000 cases. *Am J Roentgenol* 1971;112:493–506.
19. Bossart PJ, Joyce SM, Manaster BJ, et al. Lack of efficacy of 9weighted9 radiographs in diagnosing acute acromioclavicular separations. *Ann Emerg Med* 1988;17:20–24.
20. Alexander OM. Dislocation of the acromioclavicular joint. *Radiography* 1948;14:139.
21. Bergfeld JA, Andrish JT, Clancy WG. Evaluation of the acromioclavicular joint following first and second degree sprains. *Am J Sports Med* 1978;6(4):153–159.
22. Imatani RJ, Hanlon JJ, Cady GW. Acute, complete acromioclavicular separation. *J Bone Joint Surg Am* 1975;57:328–332.
23. Kennedy DC, Cameron J. Complete dislocations of the acromioclavicular joint. *J Bone Joint Surg Br* 1954;36:202–208.
24. Murray MP, Gore DR, Gardner GM, et al. Shoulder motion and muscle strength of normal men and women in two age groups. *Clin Orthop* 1985;192:268–273.
25. Schlegel TF, Burks RT, Marcus RL, et al. A prospective evaluation of untreated acute grade III acromioclavicular separations. *Am J Sports Med* 2001;29(6):699–703.
26. Rawes ML, Dias JJ. Long-term results of conservative treatment for acromioclavicular dislocation. *J Bone Joint Surg (Br)* 1996;78:410–412.
27. Wojtys EM, Nelson G. Conservative treatment of grade III acromioclavicular dislocations. *Clin Orthop* 1991;268:112–119.
28. Lemos MJ. The evaluation and treatment of the injured acromioclavicular joint in athletes. *Am J Sports Med* 1998;26(1):137–144.
29. McFarland EG, Blivin SJ, Doehring CB, et al. Treatment of grade III acromioclavicular separation in professional throwing athletes: Results of a survey. *Am J Orthop* 1997;26:771–774.
30. Jones R. *Injuries of joints*. London: Henry Frowde, Hodder & Stoughton, 1917:56–58.
31. Watson-Jones R. *Fractures and joint injuries*. London: Churchill Livingstone, 1982.
32. Giannestras NJ. A method of immobilization of acute acromioclavicular separation. *J Bone Joint Surg* 1944;26:597–599.
33. Warner AH. A harness for use in the treatment of acromioclavicular separation. *J Bone Joint Surg* 1937;19:1132–1133.
34. Currie DI. An apparatus for dislocation of the acromial end of the clavicle. *BMJ* 1924;1:570.
35. Rawlings G. Acromioclavicular dislocations and fractures of the clavicle: a simple method of support. *Lancet* 1939;2:789.
36. Thorndike A Jr, Quigley TB. Injuries to the acromioclavicular joint: a plea for conservative treatment. *Am J Surg* 1942;55:250–261.
37. Usadel G. Zer Behandlung der luxatio claviculae supraacromialis. *Arch Klin Chir* 1940;200:621–626.
38. Spigelman L. A harness for acromioclavicular separation. *J Bone Joint Surg (Am)* 1969;51:585–586.
39. Darrow JC, Smith JA, Lockwood RC. A new conservative method for treatment of type III acromioclavicular separations. *Orthop Clin North Am* 1980;11:727–733.
40. Caldwell GD. Treatment of complete permanent acromioclavicular dislocation by surgical arthrodesis. *J Bone Joint Surg* 1943;25:368–374.
41. Howard NJ. Acromioclavicular and sternoclavicular joint injuries. *Am J Surg* 1939;46:284–291.
42. Urist MR. Complete dislocation of the acromioclavicular joint: The nature of the traumatic lesion and effective methods of treatment with an analysis of 41 cases. *J Bone Joint Surg* 1946;28:813–837.
43. Eskola A, Vainionpaa S, Kokala O, et al. Acute complete acromioclavicular dislocation. Prospective randomized trial of

fixation with smooth or threaded Kirschner wires or cortical screw. *Ann Chir Gynaecol* 1987;76:323–326.

44. Eskola A, Vainionpaa S, Kokala O, et al. Four year outcome of operative treatment of acute acromioclavicular dislocation. *J Orthop Trauma* 1991;5:9–13.

45. Aalders GJ, Van Vroonhoven TJ, Van Der Werken C, et al. An exceptional case of pneumothorax—a new adventure of the K wire. *Injury* 1985;16:564–565.

46. Larsen E, Bjerg-Neilson A, Christensen P. Conservative or surgical treatment of acromioclavicular dislocation. A prospective, controlled, randomized study. *J Bone Joint Surg (Am)* 1986;68:552–555.

47. Lindsey RW, Gutowski WT. The migration of a broken pin following fixation of the acromioclavicular joint. A case report and review of the literature. *Orthopaedics* 1986;9:413–416.

48. Oleksiuk DI, Pelipenko VP. Migration of the fixation devices onto the mediastinum and spine after metallic osteosynthesis of the sternal and acromial ends of the clavicle. *Vestn Khir* 1979;123:121–122.

49. Albrecht F. Kohaus H, Stedtfeld HW. The Balser plate for acromioclavicular fixation. *Chirurg* 1982;53:733–734.

50. Eberle C, Fodor P, Metzger U. Hook plate (so-called Balser plate) or tension banding with the Bosworth screw in complete acromioclavicular dislocation with clavicular fracture. *Z Unfallchir Versicherungsmed* 1992;85:134–139.

51. Habernek H, Weinstabl R, Schmidt L, et al. A crook plate for treatment of acromioclavicular joint separation: indication, technique, and results after one year. *J Trauma* 1993;35:893–901.

52. Bosworth BM. Acromioclavicular separations: a new method of repair. *Surg Gynecol Obstet* 1941;73:866–871.

53. Cox JS. Current method of treatment of acromioclavicular joint dislocations. *Orthopaedics* 1992;15:1041–1044.

54. Gallay SH, Hupel TM, Beaton DE, et al. Functional outcome of acromioclavicular injuries in polytrauma patients. *J Orthop Trauma* 1998;12:159–163.

55. Jones HP, Lemos MJ, Schepsis AA. Salvage of failed acromioclavicular joint reconstruction using autogenous semitendinosus tendon from the knee. Surgical technique and case report. *Am J Sports Med* 2001;29(2):234–237.

56. Dust WN, Lenczner EM. Stress fracture of the clavicle leading to nonunion secondary to coracoclavicular reconstruction with Dacron. *Am J Sports Med* 1989;17:128–129.

57. Martell JRJ. Clavicular nonunion. Complication with the use of Mersiline tape. *Am J Sports Med* 1992;20:360–362.

58. Moneim MS, Balduini FC. Coracoid fracture as a complication of surgical treatment by coracoclavicular tape fixation. A case report. *Clin Orthop* 1982;133–135.

59. Neault MA, Nuber GW, Marymont JV. Infections after surgical repair of acromioclavicular separations with nonabsorbable tape or suture. *J Shoulder Elbow Surg* 1996;5:477–478.

60. Breslow MJ, Jazwari LM, Bernstein AD, et al. Treatment of acromioclavicular joint separation: suture or suture anchors? *J Shoulder Elbow Surg* 2002;11:225–229.

61. Wolf EM, Pennington WT. Arthroscopic reconstruction for acromioclavicular joint dislocation. *Arthroscopy* 2001;17:558–563.

62. Motamedi AR, Blevins FT, Willis MC, et al. Biomechanics of the coracoclavicular ligament complex and augmentations used in its repair and reconstruction. *Am J Sports Med* 2000;28 (3):380–384.

63. Harris RI, Wallace Al, Harper GD, et al. Structural properties of the intact and reconstructed coracoclavicular ligament complex. *Am J Sports Med* 2000;28(1):103–108.

64. Brunelli G, Brunelli F. The treatment of acromioclavicular dislocation by transfer of the short head of the biceps. *Int Orthop* 1988;12:105–108.

65. Skjeldal S, Lundblad R, Dullerud R. Coracoid process transfer for acromioclavicular dislocation. *Acta Orthop Scand* 1988;59:180–182.

66. Gurd FB. The treatment of complete dislocation of the outer end of the clavicle: a hitherto undescribed operation. *Ann Surg* 1941;63:1094–1098.

67. Mumford EB. Acromioclavicular dislocation: a new operative treatment. *J Bone Joint Surg* 1941;23:799–802.

68. Eskola A, Santavirta S, Viljakka HT, et al. The results of operative resection of the lateral end of the clavicle. *J Bone Joint Surg (Am)* 1996;78:584–587.

69. Weaver JK, Dunn HK. Treatment of acromioclavicular joint injuries, especially complete acromioclavicular separation. *J Bone Joint Surg* 1972;54:1187–1194.

70. Bunnell S. Fascial graft for dislocation of the acromioclavicular joint. *Surg Gynecol Obstet* 1928;46:563–564.

71. Lom P. Acromioclavicular disjunction. I. Diagnosis and classification. II. Surgical treatment, our modification. *Rozhl Chir* 1988;67:253–270.

72. Cook FF, Tibone JE. The Mumford procedure in athletes. An objective analysis of function. *Am J Sports Med* 1988;16:97–100.

73. Scavenius M, Iverson BF. Nontraumatic clavicular osteolysis in weight lifters. *Am J Sports Med* 1992;20:463–467.

74. Slawski DP, Cahill BR. Atraumatic osteolysis of the distal clavicle. Results of open surgical excision. *Am J Sports Med* 1994;22:267–271.

75. Cox JS. The fate of the acromioclavicular joint in athletic injuries. *Am J Sports Med* 1981;9:50–53.

76. Jordan LK, Kenter K, Griffiths HL. Relationship between MRI and clinical findings in the acromioclavicular joint. *Skeletal Radiol* 2002;31(9):516–521.

77. Auge WK, Fischer RA. Arthroscopic distal clavicle resection for isolated atraumatic osteolysis in weight lifters. *Am J Sports Med* 1998;26:189–192.

78. Flatow EL, Cordasco FA, Bigliani LU. Arthroscopic resection of the outer end of the clavicle from a superior approach: a critical, quantitative, radiographic assessment of bone removal. *Arthroscopy* 1992;8:55–64.

79. Henry MH, Liu SH, Loffredo AJ. Arthroscopic management of the acromioclavicular joint disorder. A review. *Clin Orthop* 1995;316:276–283.

80. Tolin BS, Snyder SJ. Our technique for the arthroscopic Mumford procedure. *Orthop Clin North Am* 1993;24:143–151.

81. Gartsman GM. Arthroscopic resection of the acromioclavicular joint. *Am J Sports Med* 1993;21:71–77.

17

SCAPULOTHORACIC PROBLEMS IN OVERHEAD ATHLETES

W. BEN KIBLER
JOHN MCMULLEN

INTRODUCTION

This chapter discusses injuries or pathologic processes that alter the normal articulation of the scapula and thorax. Although the observable result of the alteration is described as a scapular abnormality in relation to the thorax, the major functional result is to the glenohumeral joint. Scapular motion and arm motion are coupled in a closed chain fashion that requires the scapula to be positioned in relation to the moving arm to allow efficient force generation and force transfer with minimal joint loads (1). Altered scapular position and motion can change glenohumeral joint loads (2), and they have been frequently associated with a wide spectrum of shoulder injuries, ranging from impingement (3,4) to instability (3,5) to labral injuries (6). These alterations have been termed *scapular dyskinesis* (3,7), which collectively describes the clinically observable abnormality. This chapter evaluates scapulothoracic problems in terms of scapular dyskinesis, examines normal scapular roles, and discusses how scapular dyskinesis affects normal roles in overhead athletes.

BIOMECHANICS AND PHYSIOLOGY OF SCAPULAR MOTION AND POSITION

The scapula is inherently mobile on the thorax. Its only bony constraint is the clavicle. The clavicle acts as a strut to prevent the scapula from excessive movement forward on the thorax, and the acromioclavicular (AC) joint provides a constrained point of rotation.

Most of the constraints to excessive motion and the energy to properly position the scapula come from the periscapular muscles acting as force couples. The primary force couples for scapular control are the upper trapezius:lower trapezius/serratus anterior for upward rotation and external rotation, and the upper trapezius/lower trapezius:serratus anterior for retraction/protraction. The

levator scapulae and rhomboids are assistive muscles (8,9). These force couples are preprogrammed to interact with glenohumeral muscles to provide scapular position and stability for arm motion (1,10).

The kinematic result of the muscles acting on the pivoting scapula is scapulohumeral rhythm, which is normally a smooth coupled motion. Two-plane biomechanical analysis has shown that the average humerus:scapula ratio is approximately 2:1 with variations in the ratio within the arc of total motion (11). The instant center of rotation moves progressively from the medial spine to the AC joint. Recent three-dimensional biomechanical analysis has confirmed the 2:1 ratio but has provided much more information about scapular motion around the "ellipsoid" thorax (12,13). The scapula can move simultaneously about three axes of rotation and also translates. In arm abduction and elevation, the scapula tilts posteriorly around a horizontal axis and rotates laterally around a vertical axis (external rotation), and the lateral border and acromion upwardly rotate. This composite motion approximates what is usually called *retraction*. In arm depression, adduction, and internal rotation, the scapula tilts anteriorly and rotates medially (internal rotation), and the lateral border stays neutral. This composite motion approximates what is usually called *protraction*. The distance the medial scapular border may move on the thorax may be as high as 15 cm (14).

This integrated sequential muscle activation sequence and the resulting motion/position control allows the scapula to fulfill several specific roles in normal shoulder function.

THE ROLES OF THE SCAPULA IN SHOULDER FUNCTIONAL ACTIVITIES

The scapular roles are concerned with achieving appropriate motions and positions to facilitate shoulder function. The first role of the scapula is to be an integral part of the glenohumeral articulation. The glenoid, which is on the scapula, is the socket of the ball and socket arrangement of the glenohumeral joint. To maintain the ball and socket configuration, the scapula must move in a coordinated relationship to the moving humerus so that the instant center of rotation, the mathematical point within the humeral head that defines the axis of rotation of the glenohumeral joint, is constrained within a physiologic pattern throughout the full range of shoulder motion in throwing or serving (15). Proper alignment of the glenoid allows the optimum function of the bony constraints to glenohumeral motion and allows the most efficient position of the intrinsic muscles of the rotator cuff to allow compression into the glenoid socket, thereby enhancing the muscular constraint systems around the shoulder as well (16,17).

The second role of the scapula is three-dimensional retraction and protraction along the thoracic wall. The scapula needs to retract to facilitate the position of cocking for the baseball throw or the tennis serve. As acceleration proceeds, the scapula must protract in a smooth fashion laterally and then anteriorly around the thoracic wall to allow the scapula to maintain a normal position in relationship to the humerus and to dissipate some of the deceleration forces that occur in follow-through as the arm goes forward (11,16,18).

These first two roles confer a coupled interdependency between movements of the arm and scapula that creates dynamic stability for the glenohumeral joint in the various positions and motions encountered in athletic or work activities (1). The static relationship of the humerus and scapula has been described as a "golf ball on a tee," but in dynamic shoulder function, the more appropriate description would be a "ball on a seal's nose." The seal's nose, or scapula, must move to keep the ball, or humerus, from falling off.

The third role that the scapula plays in shoulder function is elevation of the acromion. The acromion must be elevated during the cocking and acceleration phases of throwing or arm elevation in working to clear the acromion from the moving rotator cuff to decrease impingement and coracoacromial arch compression. Although it is usually stated that rotator cuff fatigue may allow superior humeral head migration to cause subacromial impingement in this position (18), lower trapezius and serratus anterior muscle fatigue may also contribute to impingement if the acromion is not elevated (19).

The final role that the scapula plays in shoulder function is that of being a link in the proximal to distal sequencing of velocity, energy, and forces that allows the most appropriate shoulder function (18,20,21). For most shoulder activities, this sequencing starts at the ground. The individual body segments, or links, are coordinated in their movements by muscle activation and body positions to generate, summate, and transfer force through these segments to the terminal link. This sequencing is usually termed the kinetic chain. These muscle activation patterns also stabilize the scapula and increase the control of its motion and position as the arm is moved.

The scapula is pivotal in transferring the large forces and high energy from the major source for force and energy (the legs, back, and trunk) to the actual delivery mechanism of the energy and force (the arm and the hand) (20,22,23) and stabilizing the arm to absorb loads that may be generated through the long lever of the extended or elevated arm.

FACTORS CREATING SCAPULAR DYSKINESIS

Causative factors for scapular dyskinesis may be grouped as proximal (to the scapula) or distal (24). The proximal causes include postural alterations in the cervical, thoracic, or lumbar spines, hip and trunk muscle weakness or inflexibility, and neurologic lesions in the cord or peripheral nerves. They result in loss of proximal stabilization for scapular control and decreased muscle activation facilitation (10,18).

Distally based causative factors usually represent inhibition of muscle activation or muscle strength from an injury or pain-generating overload. They may include intraarticular pathology, such as labral tears or instability (5,6), rotator cuff injury or impingement (3), or soft tissue inflexibilities.

Specific factors are discussed in the following paragraphs.

Bony Posture or Injury

A resting posture of thoracic kyphosis or cervical lordosis can result in excessive scapular protraction and acromial depression in all phases of athletic activity, increasing the incidence of impingement (25). Fractures of the clavicle can shorten or angulate this important strut, which maintains proper scapular position. Third degree or AC joint separation can remove the strut and allow scapular protraction and acromial depression, leading to muscle weakness and impingement. Milder degrees of AC joint instability, due to second degree separations or arthrosis, may also alter scapular kinematics by not allowing progression of the instant center of rotation to the AC joint (11). Excessive shortening of the distal clavicle in surgery can also affect the strut function and kinematics. Bone spurs, osteochondromas, and malunions are rare causes of scapular alterations.

Muscular Alterations

Scapular dyskinesis is most frequently observed as a result of alteration of muscle activation or coordination. The rotations and translations of the scapula result from patterned muscle activation and passive positioning resulting from trunk and arm acceleration. The muscle activation patterns result in force couples for scapular control (1,8,9). The scapular stabilization pattern involves upper and lower trapezius and rhomboids coupled with serratus anterior. Scapular elevation patterns involve serratus anterior and lower trapezius coupled with upper trapezius and rhomboids. Lower trapezius activation is especially important in maintaining the normal path of the instant center of scapular motion in arm elevation, due to the mechanical advantage of its attachment at the medial aspect of the scapular spine and its straight line of pull as the arm elevates and the scapula rotates (8).

Most abnormal biomechanics and physiology that occur in scapular dyskinesis can be traced to alterations in the function of the muscles that control the scapula (4,8,11,26–28). Nerve injury either to the long thoracic nerve or the spinal accessory nerve can alter muscular function of the serratus anterior or the trapezius muscle, respectively, to give abnormal stabilization and control. This occurs in less than 5% of the problems with muscle function.

More commonly, the scapular stabilizing muscles are either directly injured from direct blow trauma, have microtrauma-induced strain in the muscles, leading to muscle weakness and force couple imbalance; become fatigued from repetitive tensile use, or are inhibited by painful conditions around the shoulder. Muscle inhibition or weakness is common in glenohumeral pathology, whether it is from instability, labral pathology, or arthrosis (16,19,26,28). The serratus anterior and the lower trapezius are the most susceptible to the effect of the inhibition, and they are more frequently involved in early phases of shoulder pathology (5,16,19). Muscle inhibition and resulting scapular dyskinesis appear to be a nonspecific response to a painful condition in the shoulder rather than a specific response to a certain glenohumeral pathologic situation. This is verified by the finding of scapular dyskinesis in as many as 68% of rotator cuff problems and 100% of glenohumeral instability problems (3,5,6). Inhibition is seen both as a decreased ability for the muscles to exert torque and stabilize the scapula and as a disorganization of the normal muscle firing patterns of the muscles around the shoulder (19,28). The exact nature of this inhibition is not clear. The nonspecific response and the disorganization of motor patterns suggest a proprioceptively based mechanism. Pain, either from direct muscle injury or indirect sources, and fatigue or uncontrolled muscle strain have been shown to alter proprioceptive input from Golgi tendon organs and muscle spindles.

Soft Tissue Inflexibility

Inflexibility or contracture of the muscles and ligaments around the shoulder can affect the position and motion of the scapula. Tightness of the pectoralis minor and short head of the biceps muscles attaching to the coracoid process creates an anterior tilt and forward pull on the scapula. Glenohumeral joint internal rotation inflexibility, due to capsular or muscular tightness, affects the smooth motion of the glenohumeral joint (6,29,30) and creates a "wind-up" effect so that the glenoid and scapula get pulled in a forward and inferior direction by the moving and rotating arm. These alterations can create an excessive amount of protraction of the scapula on the thorax as the arm continues into the horizontally adducted position in follow-through in throwing or forward arm elevation in working. Because of the ellipsoid geometry of the upper aspect of the thorax, the more the scapula is protracted in arm motions, such as arm elevation or follow-through in throwing, the farther it and its acromion move anteriorly and inferiorly around the thorax.

CLASSIFICATION OF SCAPULAR DYSKINESIS PATTERNS

Loss of control of scapular motion or position allows the scapula to exhibit dyskinetic patterns consistent with the forces applied to it through arm motion or muscle activation. These patterns can be observed by evaluation of the position of the scapula with the arms at rest down at the patient's sides, and by observation of scapular motion as the arms move in the scapular plane in ascent and descent. These dyskinetic positions have been noted to fall into three

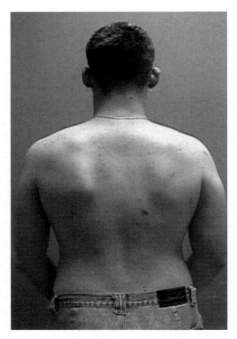

FIGURE 17-1. Type I dyskinesis with inferior medial border prominence.

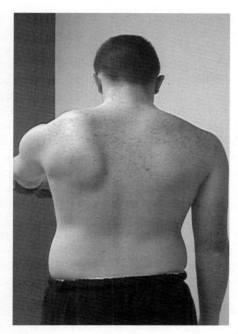

FIGURE 17-2. Type II dyskinesis with prominence of the entire medial border.

large categories, which correspond to motion in one of the three planes of possible movement on the ellipsoid thorax (31). This classification system is important to help identify how the scapula moves in abnormal relation to the arm and is involved in shoulder injury, and to understand how to address rehabilitation issues of muscle strengthening and flexibility restoration. Type I (Fig. 17-1) is characterized by prominence of the inferomedial scapular border. This motion is primarily abnormal rotation around a transverse axis. Type II (Fig. 17-2) is characterized by prominence of the entire medial scapular border and represents abnormal rotation around a vertical axis. Type III (Fig. 17-3) is char-

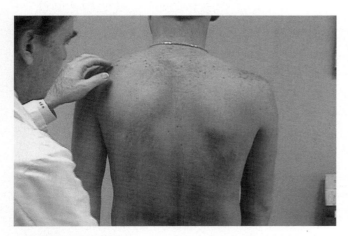

FIGURE 17-3. Type III dyskinesis with prominence of the superior medial border on the left.

acterized by superior translation of the entire scapula and prominence of the superior medial scapular border. The net effect of the scapular dyskinetic patterns is to adversely affect the normal scapular roles in shoulder function.

These patterns are more related to the position of and load on the arm and to muscle weakness than they are to specific shoulder lesions. They can change in the course of treatment as strength improves and retraction control improves.

EFFECT OF SCAPULAR DYSKINESIS ON SCAPULAR ROLES

Loss of Retraction and Protraction Control

Inability to fully retract the scapula causes inability to reach the stable cocking point in throwing or the stable base in arm elevation. Lack of full scapular protraction around the thoracic wall increases the deceleration forces on the shoulder (18) and causes alteration in the normal safe zone relationship between the glenoid and the humerus as the arm moves through the acceleration phase (1,16,18). Too much protraction caused by tightness in the glenohumeral capsule or the anterior coracoid muscles causes abnormalities of impingement as the scapula rotates down and forward (4,30). These cumulatively lead to abnormalities in concavity/compression because of the changes in the safe zone of the glenohumeral angle.

Loss of protraction control in the throwing motion also creates a relative glenoid antetilting or functional anteversion, whereby the anterior aspect of the glenohumeral joint is more open and the normal anterior bony buttress to anterior translation is deficient. This opening up and lack of bony buttress causes increased shear stresses on the rest of the anterior stabilizing structures—the labrum and glenohumeral ligaments—causing increasing risk of shear injury or strain (2). Posteriorly, glenoid antetilting increases the impingement seen between the posterosuperior glenoid and posterior rotator cuff seen in "internal impingement" (6) by moving the posterior aspect of the glenoid closer to the externally rotated and horizontally abducted arm.

Loss of Elevation Control

Lack of appropriate acromial elevation leads to impingement problems in cocking and in follow-through. This type of impingement is commonly seen not only as the sole source of impingement but also as a secondary source of impingement in other shoulder problems, such as glenohumeral instability (4,28,32,33). The serratus anterior and especially the lower trapezius appear to be the first muscles involved in inhibition-based muscle dysfunction. Lack of acromial elevation and consequent secondary impingement can be seen early in many shoulder problems such as rotator cuff tendinitis and glenohumeral instability and can play a major role in defining the clinical problems that are associated with these diagnostic entities.

Loss of the Stable Base

All of the muscles that move the arm and position the humerus in the glenoid socket have their origin on the scapula. Dyskinesis and protraction disrupt the stable base for muscle activation and shorten the effective length of the muscles (17,21,25). In severe cases of nerve palsy, the origin and insertion may be reversed. The net result is decreased apparent muscle strength on muscle activation (25), even though the muscle may test normally with scapular retraction (7).

Loss of Kinetic Chain Function

One of the most important abnormalities in abnormal scapular biomechanics is the loss of the link function in the kinetic chain. The scapula and shoulder are pivotal links in this chain, funneling the forces from the large segments, the legs and trunk, to the smaller, rapidly moving small segments of the arm (18,20). If the scapula does become deficient in motion or position, transmission of the large generated forces from the lower extremity to the upper extremity is impaired (20).

Clinical Symptoms around the Scapula

Scapular dyskinesis often has specific clinical symptoms from the alterations, in addition to the shoulder joint symptoms and signs. There is commonly point tender pain on motion to palpation over the anterior shoulder at the coracoid tip, secondary to adaptive tightness and scar in the pectoralis minor and short head of the biceps. In addition, the superomedial border or entire medial border is sore and painful to motion or palpation, because of similar tightness or scar in levator scapulae or lower trapezius insertions. Finally, there may be "trigger points," or areas of tenderness in the body of the upper trapezius. "Snapping scapula" may present as a painful bursitis, with crepitus and popping over the superior medial angle near the base of the scapular spine.

EVALUATION OF SCAPULAR DYSKINESIS IN SHOULDER PAIN

Scapular evaluation should be both inclusive and dynamic. Distant contributions to normal scapular function and dyskinesis should be evaluated, and dynamic evaluation of motion, muscular activation, and corrective maneuvers should be included.

Leg and trunk muscle activity is both large (1) and important (18) in shoulder and arm throwing, serving, and lifting activities. It is also important as a major source of facilitation of scapular muscle activation (34). Evaluation of the legs and trunk may be done by screening certain important parameters, and following with more detailed analysis on positive items. Lumbar lordosis, pelvic tilt, and hip rotational abnormalities should be checked. A good screening examination for leg and trunk strength is the "one leg stability series"—one leg stance and squat (Fig. 17-4).

Thoracic and cervical posture may be evaluated by inspection and rotation. Thoracic kyphosis or scoliosis may have a direct relationship to the motion of the scapula by creating abnormal posturing or necessitating extra motion for retraction. Excessive cervical lordosis indicates posterior cervical muscle or fascia tightness or anterior clavicular fascia tightness, which can have an effect on scapular retraction and protraction.

The evaluation of the scapula itself should be mainly done from the posterior aspect. The examination can then proceed from posterior to anterior to allow appropriate examination of all the scapular positions and motions.

Scapular position may be evaluated in several ways. Abnormalities of winging, elevation, or rotation may first be examined in the resting position. In longstanding scapular dyskinesis, resting winging may be seen. Pure serratus anterior weakness due to nerve palsy creates a prominent superomedial border and depressed acromion, whereas pure trapezius weakness due to nerve palsy creates a protracted inferior border and elevated acromion (27).

Motion and position should be examined both in the ascending phase and in the descending phase of the arm in both flexion and abduction. Muscle weakness and mild scapular dyskinesis are noted more frequently in the descending phase of the arm movement. This most commonly presents as a "hitch" or a "jump" in the otherwise smooth motion of the scapula or scapular border. It is more noticeable with several repetitions of the motions.

The dyskinetic patterns should be grouped into one of the three types based on the most predominant pattern. Some scapular dyskinesis is a mixed pattern, but there is usually one pattern that is more reproducible, that occurs for a longer time, or that is present at rest and upon motion.

A good provocative maneuver to evaluate scapular muscle strength is to do an isometric pinch of the scapulae in retraction. Scapular muscle weakness can be noted as a burning pain in less than 15 seconds. Normally, the scapula should be held in this position for 15 to 20 seconds without having the burning pain or muscle weakness. Also, wall push-ups are an effective way of evaluating serratus anterior strength. Any abnormalities of scapular winging with 5 to 10 wall push-ups may be noted.

Corrective maneuvers may be used to help assess which motion or function needs to be focused on in treatment and rehabilitation.

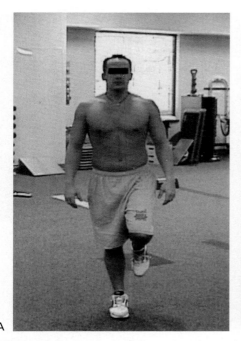
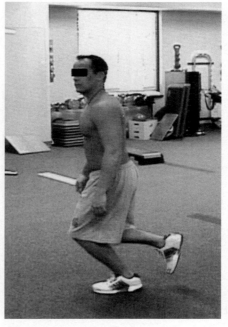

FIGURE 17-4. One-leg stability series. **A:** One-leg stance. Note balance over the stance leg. **B:** One-leg squat. The body should balance as the patient does a 45-degree squat.

The scapular assistance test (SAT) (Fig. 17-5) evaluates scapular and acromial involvement in subacromial impingement. In the patient with impingement symptoms with forward elevation or abduction, assistance for scapular elevation is provided by manually stabilizing the scapula and rotating the inferior border of the scapula as the arm moves. This procedure simulates the force couple activity of the serratus anterior and lower trapezius. Elimination or modification of the impingement symptoms indicates that these important muscles should be a major focus in the rehabilitation effort. The scapular retraction test (SRT) (Fig. 17-6)

involves manually stabilizing the scapula in a retracted position on the thorax. This position confers a stable base of origin for the rotator cuff and often improves tested rotator cuff strength. Also, this test frequently demonstrates scapular and glenoid involvement in internal impingement lesions. The positive posterior labral findings on modified Jobe relocation testing is decreased with scapular retraction and removal of the glenoid from the excessively protracted impingement position.

Quantitative measurement of scapular stabilizer strength can be achieved by the lateral slide test (Fig. 17-7). This

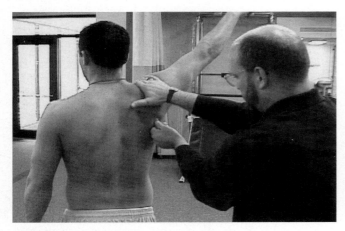

FIGURE 17-5. Scapular assistance test. The examiner assists serratus anterior and lower trapezius muscle activity as the arm is elevated. Relief of impingement symptoms is a positive test.

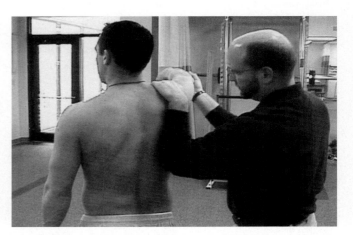

FIGURE 17-6. Scapular retraction test. The examiner stabilizes the medial scapular border as the arm is elevated or externally rotated. Relief of impingement symptoms is a positive test.

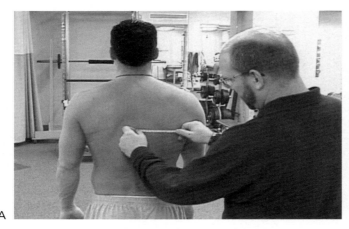

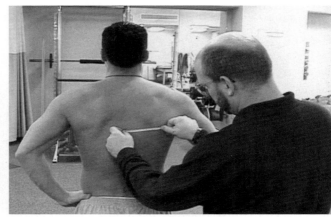

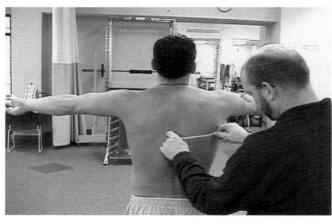

FIGURE 17-7. Lateral scapular slide. **A:** Position 1—arms at rest, at side. **B:** Position 2—arms on hips. **C:** Position 3—arms abducted below 90 degrees, maximal internal rotation.

semidynamic test evaluates the position of the scapula on the injured and noninjured sides in relationship to a fixed point on the spine as varying amounts of loads are put on the supporting musculature. The first position is with the arms relaxed at the sides. The second is with the hands on the hips with the fingers anterior and the thumb posterior with about 10 degrees of shoulder extension. The third position is with the arms at or below 90 degrees of arm elevation with maximal internal rotation at the glenohumeral joint. These positions offer a graded challenge to the functioning of the shoulder muscles to stabilize the scapula. The final position presents a challenge to the muscles in the position of most common function at 90 degrees of shoulder elevation. In position 1, the inferomedial angle of the scapula is palpated and marked on both the injured and noninjured sides. The reference point on the spine is the nearest spinous process, which is then marked with an "X." The measurements from the reference point on the spine to the medial border of the scapula are measured on both sides. In position 2, the new position of the inferomedial border of the scapula is marked, and the reference point on the spine is maintained. The distances once again are calculated on both sides. The same protocol is done for position 3. For purposes of clinical evaluation, we have established

1.5-cm asymmetry as the threshold of abnormality and accept this in any of the positions, although it is more commonly seen in position 3.

Other testing that can be done to objectify scapular position include Moire topographic analysis, which involves stroboscopic evaluation of the contours of the back. This shows the abnormalities of scapular position very well, but this is limited by the availability of these facilities.

Evaluation techniques for other structures that are pertinent to the scapular evaluation include evaluation of arthrosis or instability of the AC joint, shortening of the clavicle (from fracture or distal clavicle resection), and glenohumeral rotation and muscle strength. All of these play a role in the motion and position of the scapula.

TREATMENT CONSIDERATIONS FOR SCAPULAR DYSKINESIS

Most of the abnormalities that exist in scapular motion or position can be treated by treating the source of the problems (14,27,28). Local physical therapy treatment may relieve some of the symptoms associated with inflexibility or trigger points. Surgical treatment is usually directed at the source of the underlying problems rather than at the scapula itself.

Internal fixation of scapular or clavicular fractures may be necessary to restore normal anatomy or angulation of the glenoid or to restore the normal length to the strut of the clavicle. AC joint separations should be evaluated in terms of their contribution to scapular stability. If a third or fourth degree AC separation creates a loss of the strut function and excessive scapular protraction or dyskinesis, then functional consequences may include shoulder impingement and abnormalities in strength production. AC joints may need to be anatomically repaired in this situation. AC joint arthrosis with consequent pain or AC joint instability may need to be surgically corrected to stabilize the scapula or eliminate the pain-causing problem at the joint. Care must be taken when performing a distal clavicle resection for joint arthrosis or instability. If more than 5 to 10 mm are removed, there may be interference with clavicle strut function. Also, if the posterior AC joint capsule and ligament are resected or cut, this may cause an anteroposterior joint instability. The combination of AC joint instability and a shortened distal clavicle can have major detrimental effects on scapular kinematics. A safe operative procedure is to angle the clavicle osteotomy, removing 1 to 2 mm superiorly and 5 to 7 mm inferiorly, thereby removing the spur but maintaining clavicular length. Clinicians must always try to save and repair the posterior AC capsule and ligament.

More commonly, the underlying source of muscle inhibition or muscle imbalance needs to be addressed, whether this is the predominant glenohumeral internal derangement (e.g., instability, labral tears, rotator cuff injury, rotator cuff tendinitis with muscle weakness and inhibition) or proximal weakness leading to "disfacilitation." Superior glenoid labral tears and microtrauma-based glenohumeral instability are common pain-causing contributors to scapular dyskinesis. Once the internal derangement is corrected, scapular muscle rehabilitation may be started.

REHABILITATION CONSIDERATIONS

The ability of an athlete to return to the activity that caused the injury is often the measure of success for athletic rehabilitation. Effective rehabilitation of scapulothoracic problems considers the following: (a) Any associated glenohumeral pathology, (b) kinetic chain deficiencies that may have contributed to the pathology, (c) the role of the scapula in ultimate function, and (d) the contribution of the scapular dyskinesis and dysfunction to the pathology or decline in performance. Scapulothoracic function is rarely the final goal of rehabilitation but it is required for safe and effective upper extremity function (14). The rehabilitation should approach the scapula as a part of a kinetic chain system and exercise design should integrate the scapula within

that system whenever possible. This way the rehabilitative demands on the scapula are similar to its functional demands.

Integrating the scapula in kinetic chains for therapeutic exercise is consistent with proprioceptive neuromuscular facilitation principles. Kinetic chains, or sequential, segmental movement patterns incorporating the entire body, are fundamental to motor behavior. By incorporating multiple body segments, the stronger adjacent segments can facilitate the activation of targeted muscles through the irradiation reflex (35,36). The posture and movements of the adjacent segments complement or facilitate the scapular motion. For example, thoracic extension can stimulate scapular retraction. Adding a load to thoracic extension increases this stimulus and should increase the scapular retraction response (37). Achieving appropriate scapular motion by incorporating it into a kinetic chain is feedback sensitive. Immediate verbal, visual, and tactile feedback helps a rehabilitating athlete identify and correct errors and compensations in prescribed movement patterns (35,36).

Scapular dyskinesis patterns are often indicative of strength and flexibility problems in scapulothoracic and scapulohumeral muscles. Normalization of scapular range of motion is necessary before effective strengthening of the scapulothoracic muscles is possible. To normalize the scapular range of motion in rehabilitation, muscular, myofacial, or capsular restrictions must be eliminated through manual therapeutic techniques, modalities, appropriate rest, and stretching exercises. Common sites of these restrictions are the posterior rotator cuff and glenohumeral capsule, levator scapulae, upper trapezius, and coracoid-based musculature. The key to establishing this complete scapular motion is full scapular retraction, complete adduction, posterior tilt, lateral rotation, and upward rotation. With no soft tissue restrictions limiting retraction, exercise can then strengthen this motion (or its component scapular movements). The restoration of functional glenohumeral internal rotation increases the effectiveness of exercises to control protraction (4,6). Stretching of the posterior capsule or glenohumeral external rotators is necessary when a glenohumeral internal rotation deficit complicates the scapulothoracic problem (4,6,34).

Scapulothoracic therapeutic exercises progress from the establishment of full and appropriate motion, to strengthening within that range of motion, to complex resistive scapulohumeral movements (Table 17-1). These exercises should incorporate as many body segments as possible and begin with the scapula and shoulder girdle as the final segment in the chain. The weight of the arm is a resistive load to the scapular musculature and should be added into the kinetic chain exercises when that load does not compromise the quality of scapular motion. Scapular motion exercises begin in diagonal movement patterns such as the shoulder dump, in which the athlete simulates "dumping" a bucket backward (Fig. 17-8), and progressing into single-plane

TABLE 17–1. EXAMPLE OF INTEGRATED SCAPULOTHORACIC REHABILITATION PROGRESSION

	Weeks (Estimate)							
	1	2	3	4	5	6	7	8
Scapular motion								
Thoracic posture exercises	X	X	X					
Trunk flexion, extension, rotation	X	X	X					
Lower abdominal, hip extensor exercises	X	X	X	X	X			
Muscular flexibility								
Massage	X	X						
Modalities: e.g., ultrasound, e-stim	X	X	X					
Stretching: e.g., active-assisted, passive, PNF	X	X	X	X	X	X	X	X
Corner stretches: pectoralis minor	X	X	X					
Towel roll stretches: pectoralis minor	X	X	X					
Levator scapulae stretches	X	X	X					
"Sleeper" position stretches: shoulder external rotators	X	X	X					
Closed chain cocontraction exercise								
Weight-shifting	X	X						
Balance board	X	X						
Scapular clock	X	X						
Rhythmic ball stabilization		X						
Weight-bearing isometric extension	X	X						
Wall push-up		X						
Table push-up			X	X	X			
Modified to prone push-up					X	X	X	X
Axially loaded AROM exercise								
Scaption		X	X	X	X			
Flexion slide		X	X	X	X			
Abduction glide			X	X	X			
Diagonal slides		X	X	X	X	X		
Integrated open chain kinetic chain exercises								
Scapular motion exercises + arm elevation			X	X	X	X	X	X
Unilateral, bilateral tubing pulls with trunk motion				X	X	X	X	X
Modified shoulder dump series			X	X	X	X		
Dumbbell punches with stride: progressive height and resistance						X	X	X
Lunge series with dumbbell reaches					X	X	X	X
Plyometric sport/specific exercises								
Medicine ball toss and catch						X	X	X
Reciprocal tubing plyometrics						X	X	X

PNF, proprioceptive neuromuscular facilitation; AROM, active range of motion.

movements such as lateral tubing pulls (Fig. 17-9) and sternal lifts (Fig. 17-10). These exercises include complementary movement by the legs, hips, and trunk, which is often exaggerated, to facilitate full scapular motion and may include the arm in complementary movement. Exercises intended to improve scapular motion are reciprocal, starting from a position of scapular protraction to initiate retraction. To increase the load on active scapular motion and control, the amount of complementary motion in the proximal segments should be reduced (34).

Closed kinetic chain (CKC) exercises, with a fixed or axially loaded upper extremity, are safe and effective early in the rehabilitation process. The closed chain environment should stimulate force couple co-contractions at safe, pain-free positions (38). Exercises such as the scapular clock (Fig. 17-11) and rhythmic stabilization (Fig. 17-12) are examples of these exercises. The legs and trunk can be loaded by assuming an "athletic stance" and posture, glenohumeral elevation and scapular positioning can all be clinically controlled (34). In the "low row" exercise, performed in a similar stance, isometric shoulder extension forces thoracic extension and seems to recruit the serratus anterior/lower trapezius force couple (Fig. 17-13). This is an effective early exercise when inhibition of these muscles is contributing to the scapular dyskinesis. Rocking forward and backward in a quadriped position is an example of a CKC exercise in which scapulothoracic motion is coordinated with controlled glenohumeral motion. Moving the body over the fixed distal segments, the weight-bearing hands, produces the glenohumeral motion. The spinal posture, glenohumeral motion, and amount of weight on the hands are all clinically controlled. Similarly, the legs and hips become involved when the axially loaded hand is slid on a table or wall while standing (Fig. 17-14) (34). The axial load

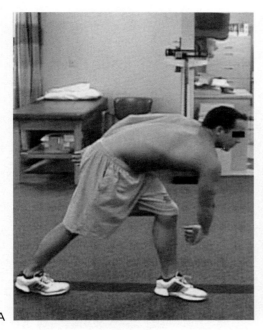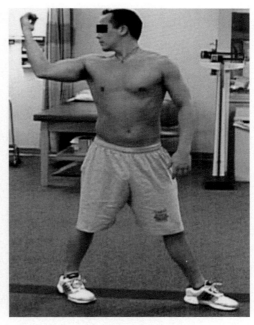

FIGURE 17-8. "Shoulder dump" exercise. **A:** Start—simulating picking up a bucket, activating contralateral hip and leg musculature. **B:** Finish— "dumping" the bucket. Extension of lower extremity, hip, and spine along with rotation to facilitate scapular retraction.

through the upper extremity effectively diminishes the weight of the arm, similar to aqua therapy, decreasing the load on the scapular musculature and rotator cuff while integrating glenohumeral elevation with appropriate scapular motion (39).

As soft tissue restrictions are relieved, scapular motion is normalized, and force couple muscle activation is reestablished, exercises progress to open kinetic chain, including the arm in the movement patterns. Integrated movement patterns progress from multiplanar diagonal patterns to

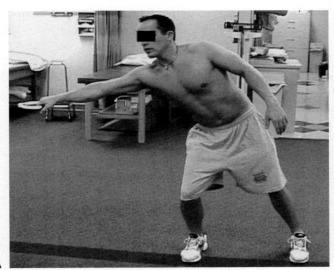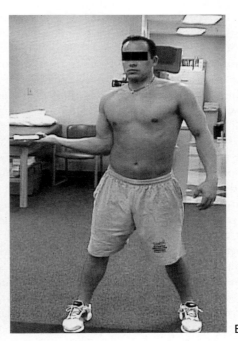

FIGURE 17-9. Lateral tubing pull. **A:** Start—body weight is lateral (activating the ipsilateral hip abductors), arm abducted to a safe, pain-free degree, and scapula abducted. **B:** Finish—ipsilateral hip abduction facilitates scapular retraction, emphasizing the frontal plane.

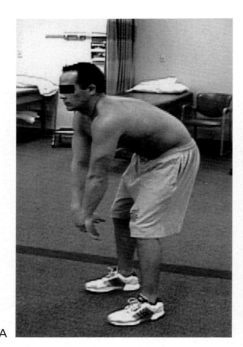
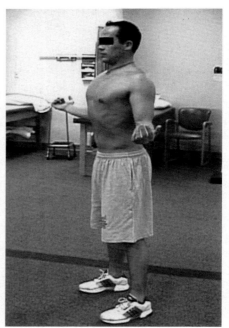

A   B

FIGURE 17-10. Sternal lift exercise. **A:** Start—kinetic chain flexion, scapular protraction. **B:** Finish—scapular retraction with hip and spine extension.

more single-plane movements. The scapular dyskinesis pattern indicates the plane of emphasis if strength deficiency is a major contributor to the dyskinesis. Type I dyskinesis suggests a sagittal plane emphasis. Type II dyskinesis is an indicator for frontal plane strengthening, as is a positive lateral slide test. In Type III dyskinesis, the lack of upward and lateral rotation of the scapula may indicate a need for strengthening in the transverse and frontal planes. Exercise movement patterns generally progress from diagonal, or transverse plane, to the plane of emphasis, continually monitoring the scapular motion for compensation. However, these are general guidelines. Multiplanar scapular stability, full range of motion, and the control of that motion is necessary for shoulder function (1–8,14).

In the final phase of scapulothoracic rehabilitation, the exercises progress to include full glenohumeral motion and integrated strengthening. The basic kinetic chain movement patterns of scapular motion exercises (e.g., the shoulder dump, sternal lift, and lateral pulls) remain the same. Elevating the arm from the body or "reaching out" during these exercises adds resistance to the scapulothoracic motion and the opportunity to add extrinsic loads such as tubing, medicine balls, or dumbbells. Horizontal dumbbell punches challenge the rotator cuff to maintain glenohumeral congruity and the scapulothoracic musculature to stabilize the scapula with an outstretched arm. These punches, overhead presses, dumbbell "cleans," and standing long pulls can all be done in various planes, with various amounts of leg and trunk contribution. There are many

possibilities when designing these types of integrated exercises, but athletes and clinicians must remain attentive to the quality of the movements and aware of muscular or movement compensations (34).

When establishing or increasing scapular motion through exaggerated integrated movements, it is acceptable for the movement of the adjacent segments to be primarily responsible for the scapular motion. Reduction of the facilitation by the adjacent segments requires greater active control of the scapula. When strengthening, compensation for weak scapular muscles by stronger scapular muscles is usu-

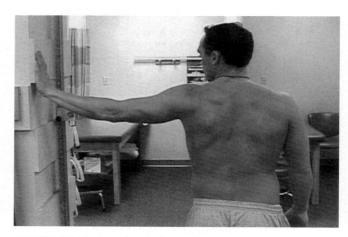

FIGURE 17-11. Scapular clock exercises. The scapula is moved to various points on the clock.

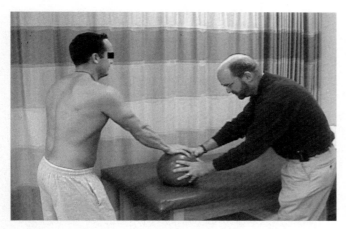

FIGURE 17-12. Rhythmic stabilization. The body may be moved in relation to the fixed arm to determine a safe and nonpainful plane of motion to start exercises.

ally unacceptable. Superior scapulothoracic muscles such as the levator scapulae and upper trapezius often compensate for more inferior muscles such as the lower trapezius and serratus anterior. Clinicians note a "shrugging" action and failure of the scapula to tilt posteriorly or rotate upwardly. Queuing the athlete to keep the "elbow pointing down" during glenohumeral elevation in abduction or scaption, or to try to "put your elbow in your hip pocket" during retraction, helps the athlete avoid this compensation. If this compensation occurs during glenohumeral flexion, the scapular center of rotation does not move laterally along its spine

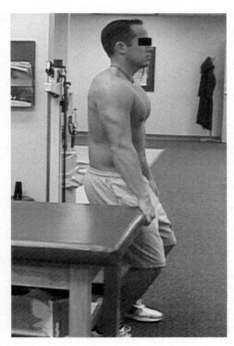

FIGURE 17-13. The "low row." Trunk extension, scapular retraction, shoulder extension to retract and depress the scapula.

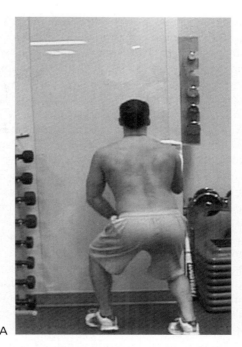

A

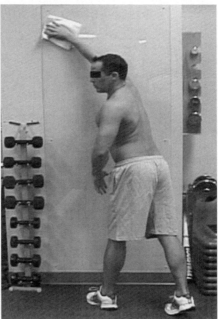

B

FIGURE 17-14. Wall slide exercise using kinetic chain with axial load through the arm. **A:** Start with arm close to body. **B:** Follow-through with hip extension/trunk rotation to facilitate scapular and rotator cuff activation.

and the scapula usually ceases rotating at approximately 60 to 90 degrees of elevation. Further elevation in the flexion plane results from scapular "shrugging" and, typically, subacromial impingement occurs. If there is sufficient activation and strength in the lower trapezius and serratus anterior to help rotate and stabilize the scapula with additional load of the flexing arm, postural corrections can aid in eliminating this compensatory tendency. Thoracic extension can facilitate the required posterior tilting of the scapula during glenohumeral flexion (10). Using the proximal-to-distal sequencing of kinetic chain motion, a concurrent ipsilateral step-up with shoulder flexion activates the ipsilateral hip extensors and can facilitate thoracic extension (1). This combination, along with some verbal queuing to correct any forward head posture ("chin back"), can significantly improve thoracoscapulohumeral rhythm during shoulder flexion (35).

For scapulothoracic rehabilitation to be effective, the scapula must be approached as a link within a kinetic chain. The scapula is dependent on the trunk and other proximal segments, just as the arm is dependent upon it for proper function (1,10,14). The therapeutic exercise component of the rehabilitation program should understand and exploit these segmental relationships. Deficits in more distant kinetic chain links may contribute to scapular dyskinesis as well, and they require evaluation and clinical attention for the rehabilitation to be complete. Thoracic spine restrictions, hip muscle tightness or weakness, low back tightness, and glenohumeral internal rotation deficit are common in overhead athletes with scapular dyskinesis (18) and are obstacles to restoring scapular motion, strength, and function. Complete scapulothoracic rehabilitation programs identify and remedy these deficiencies as well as the specific scapulothoracic motion and strength deficits (34).

REFERENCES

1. Happee R, Van Der Helm FC. Control of shoulder muscles during goal directed movements. *J Biomech* 1995;28:1179–1191.
2. Weiser WM, Lee TQ, McMaster WC. Effects of simulated scapular protraction on anterior glenohumeral stability. *Am J Sports Med* 1999;27:801–805.
3. Warner JJP, Micheli L, Arslenian L. Scapulothoracic motion in normal shoulders and shoulders with glenohumeral instability and impingement syndrome. *Clin Orthop* 1992;285:191–199.
4. Lukasiewicz AC, McClure P, Michener L. Comparison of three dimensional scapular position and orientation between subjects with and without impingement. *J Orthop Sports Phys Therapy* 1999;29:574–586.
5. Paletta GA, Warner JJP, Warren RF, et al. Shoulder kinematics with two-plane x-ray evaluation in patients with anterior instability or rotator cuff tears. *J Shoulder Elbow Surg* 1997;6:516–527.
6. Burkhart SS, Morgan CD, Kibler WB. The dead arm revisited. *Clin Sports Med* 2000;19:125–158.
7. Kibler WB, McMullen J. Scapular dyskinesis and its relation to shoulder pain. *J Am Acad Orthop Surg* 2003;11:142–151.
8. Bagg SD, Forrest WJ. EMG study of the scapular rotators during arm abduction in the scapular plane. *Am J Phys Med* 1986;65:111–124.
9. Speer KP, Garrett WE. Muscular control of motion and stability about the pectoral girdle. In: Matsen FA, Fu F, Hawkins RJ, eds. *The shoulder: a balance of mobility and stability.* Rosemont, IL: A.A.O.S., 1994:159–173.
10. Zattara M, Bouisset S. Posturo-kinetic organization during the early phase of voluntary limb alignment. *J Neurol Neurosurg Psychiatr* 1988;51:956–965.
11. Bagg SD, Forrest WJ. A biomechanical analysis of scapular rotation during arm abduction in the scapular plane. *Am J Physical Med* 1988;67:238–245.
12. McClure PW, Michener L, Sennett BJ, et al. Direct 3-dimensional measurement of scapular kinematics during dynamic movements in vivo. *J Shoulder Elbow Surg* 2001;10:269–277.
13. Ludewig PM, Cook TM, Nawoczenski DA. 3-Dimensional scapular orientation and muscle activity at selected positions of humeral elevation. *J Orthop Sports Phys Ther* 1996;24:57–65.
14. Kibler WB. The role of the scapula in athletic shoulder function. *Am J Sports Med* 1998;26:325–337.
15. Matsen FA, Harryman DT, Sidles JA. Mechanics of glenohumeral instability. *Clin Sports Med* 1991;10:783–788.
16. Pink MM, Perry J. Biomechanics of the shoulder. In: Jobe FW, ed. *Operative techniques in upper extremity sports injuries.* St. Louis: Mosby, 1996:109–123.
17. Nieminen H, Niemi J, Takala EP, et al. Load sharing patterns in the shoulder during isometric flexion tasks. *J Biomech* 1995;28:555–566.
18. Young JL, Herring SA, Press JM, et al. The influence of the spine on the shoulder in the throwing athlete. *J Back Musculoskel Rehabil* 1996;7:5–17.
19. McQuade KJ, Dawson J, Smidt GL. Scapulothoracic muscle fatigue associated with alterations in scapulohumeral rhythm kinematics during maximum resistive shoulder elevation. *J Orthop Sports Physical Therapy* 1998;5:71–87.
20. Kibler WB. Biomechanical analysis of the shoulder during tennis activities. *Clin Sports Med* 1995;14:79–85.
21. Kennedy K. Rehabilitation of the unstable shoulder. *Oper Tech Sports Med* 1993;1:311–324.
22. Elliott BC, Marshall R, Noffal G. Contributions of upper limb segment rotations during the power serve in tennis. *J Appl Biomech* 1995;11:433–442.
23. Kraemer WJ, Triplett NT, Fry AC. An in-depth sports medicine profile of women college tennis players. *J Sports Rehabil* 1995;4:79–88.
24. Rubin B, Kibler WB. Fundamental principles of shoulder rehabilitation. *Arthroscopy* 2002;18:29–39.
25. Kebatse M, McClure P, Pratt N. Thoracic position effect on shoulder range of motion, strength, and 3-dimensional scapular kinetics. *Arch Phys Med Rehabil* 1999;80:945–950.
26. Moseley JB, Jobe FW, Pink MM, et al. EMG analysis of the scapular muscles during a shoulder rehabilitation program. *Am J Sports Med* 1992;20:128–134.
27. Kuhn JE, Plancher KD, Hawkins RJ. Scapular winging. *J Am Acad Orthop Surg* 1995;3:319–325.
28. Glousman R, Jobe FW, Tibone JE. Dynamic EMG analysis of the throwing shoulder with glenohumeral instability. *J Bone Joint Surg (Am)* 1988;70:220–226.
29. Harryman DT, Sidles JA, Clark JM. Translation of the humeral head on the glenoid with passive glenohumeral motions. *J Bone Joint Surg (Am)* 1990;72:1334–1343.
30. Tyler TF, Nicholas ST, Roy T, et al. Quantification of posterior capsular tightness and motion loss in patients with shoulder impingement. *Am J Sports Med* 2000;28:668–674.
31. Kibler WB, Uhl TL. Qualitative clinical evaluation of scapular dysfunction: a reliability study. *J Shoulder Elbow Surg* 2002;11:550–556.
32. Jobe FW, Kvitne RS, Giangarra CE. Shoulder pain in the throwing athlete: the relationship of anterior instability and rotator cuff impingement. *Orthop Rev* 1989;18:963–975.
33. Bertoft ES, Thomas KA, Westerberg CE. The influence of scapular retraction and protraction on the width of the subacromial space: an MRI study. *Clin Orthop Rel Res* 1993;296:99–103.

34. Kibler WB, McMullen J, Uhl T. Shoulder rehabilitation strategies, guidelines, and practices. *Oper Tech Sports Med* 2000;8:258–267.
35. Voss DE. Proprioceptive neuromuscular facilitation. *Am J Phys Med* 1967;46:838–898.
36. Knott M, Voss DE. *Proprioceptive neuromuscular facilitation patterns and techniques,* 2nd ed. Philadelphia: Harper Row; 1968: 3–225.
37. Sherrington CS. *The interactive action of the nervous system.* New Haven, CT: Yale University Press, 1906:1–411.
38. Kibler WB. Shoulder rehabilitation: principles and practice. *Med Sci Sports Exerc* 1998;30:S40–S50.
39. Fujisawa M, Suenaga N, Minami A. Electromyographic study during isometric exercise of the shoulder in head-out water immersion. *J Shoulder Elbow Surg* 1998;7:491–494.

18

FRACTURES

SUMANT G. KRISHNAN
ROBERT J. NOWINSKI
WAYNE Z. BURKHEAD

HISTORICAL OVERVIEW

Although there is a great deal of published material on fractures of the shoulder girdle in the historical literature, these are relatively uncommon overhead sporting injuries. In the nonathletic population, fractures of the shoulder girdle are historically most common in the early adolescent patient who has open physes and in the older patient who has osteoporosis. In most active young and middle-aged overhead athletes, the bony structures of the shoulder appear to be less vulnerable to injury than the soft tissue structures (glenohumeral ligaments, labrum, and rotator cuff) about the shoulder. Shoulder instability and rotator cuff injury, therefore, are far more common than fractures in overhead athletes. However, high-energy direct or indirect trauma can cause fractures of the humerus, clavicle, or scapula.

Fractures of the shoulder girdle can lead to significant morbidity in the overhead athlete and require aggressive treatment to return to competitive sport. Precise anatomic reconstruction is often necessary to restore the shoulder to its normal biomechanical abilities. Precise diagnosis of fracture type and configuration is essential for accurate treatment. The judicious use of open reduction and internal fixation techniques has become an integral part of the treatment program to achieve anatomic restoration of the shoulder. Equally important is an early aggressive rehabilitation program designed to prevent the common problems of residual stiffness and dysfunction that can compromise the treatment of these fractures.

ANATOMY AND BIOMECHANICS

Proximal Humerus Anatomy and Biomechanics

The shoulder is the most mobile major joint in the body. The primary function is to position the hand in space to accomplish prehensile activity. The anatomic features of the proximal humerus and glenohumeral joint are well suited to provide this function. The proximal humerus consists of four well-defined parts that include the humeral head, the lesser and greater tuberosities, and the proximal humeral shaft. The proximal humerus arises from three distinct ossification centers, including one for the humeral head and one each for the lesser and greater tuberosities. The fusion of the ossification centers creates a weakened area in the construct, known as the epiphyseal scar, making these regions of the proximal humerus susceptible to fracture. The articular surface of the humeral head is two to three times larger than the surface area of the glenoid. The relatively flat glenoid produces very little constraint to humeral motion. The range of motion of the glenohumeral joint is 2:1 that of scapulothoracic motion, and their combined motion approximates to 180 degrees of abduction. The humeral neck shaft angle is approximately 45 degrees, and the head is 30 to 40 degrees retroverted relative to the epicondyles at the elbow. The anatomic configuration aligns the humeral head with the scapula as it lies along the posterolateral thorax in the anatomic plane.

The synergy between the stabilizing effect of the rotator cuff and the biceps combined with the power of the deltoid provides normal dynamic shoulder function. The deltoid is the primary motor source for the shoulder but also creates a shear stress across the joint. The rotator cuff and biceps provide stability by counterbalancing the humeral head against the deltoid shear. As internal rotation and external rotation components are added, the rotator cuff muscles provide not only humeral head depression but also stability against excessive anterior and posterior translation within the joint. Fractures of the shoulder girdle that disrupt or distort this finely tuned anatomy can alter the biomechanics of the shoulder and therefore lead to limitation of motion and function. Restoration of the anatomy along with appropriate muscle strength and coordination are necessary to return the shoulder to normal function.

Disruption of the arterial blood supply to the proximal humerus from trauma or surgical intervention can result in avascular necrosis of the humeral head. There are three main arterial contributions to the proximal humerus (1,2). The major arterial contribution to the humeral head segment is the anterior humeral circumflex artery. The terminal portion of this vessel, the arcuate artery, is interosseous in nature and perfuses the entire epiphysis. If this vessel is injured, only an anastomosis distal to the lesion can compensate for the resulting blood loss. Less significant blood supply to the proximal humerus is delivered by a branch of the posterior humeral circumflex artery, as well as the small vessels entering through the rotator cuff insertions. The posterior humeral circumflex artery, which penetrates the posteromedial cortex of the humeral head, is thought to supply only a small portion of the posteroinferior part of the articular surface of the humerus compared with the arcuate artery. The vessels that enter the epiphysis via the rotator cuff insertions are also thought to be inconsequential as well as inconsistent in their vascular supply to the humeral head.

The local nerve anatomy about the shoulder is comprised of the brachial plexus, which lies anterior to the scapula, passing below the coracoid to enter the upper arm. The axillary nerve arises from the posterior cord and courses first along the anterior surface of the subscapularis muscle belly and then below the glenohumeral joint to innervate the deltoid and teres minor. The musculocutaneous nerve arises from the lateral cord, penetrating the coracobrachialis muscle 5 to 7 cm distal to the coracoid (3). The brachial plexus therefore is tethered in its position anteromedial to the proximal humerus and is vulnerable to injury in displaced fractures. The axillary nerve is the most frequently injured portion of the plexus in proximal humerus fractures.

Clavicle Anatomy and Biomechanics

The embryologic development of the clavicle occurs through a combination of intramembranous and endochondral ossification. The central portion is the first area of ossification and is responsible for the growth of the clavicle up until the age of 5 years (4,5). Medial and lateral epiphyseal growth plates eventually develop, with only the sternal ossification center being visible radiographically (4). The medial clavicular epiphysis is the most important to longitudinal growth and contributes as much as 80% of the entire length (6). The physis fuses between the ages of 22 and 25 years.

The clavicle is the only bone that connects the trunk to the shoulder girdle. It is attached medially to the sternum and laterally to the scapula by a combination of extraarticular and capsular ligaments. The bony architecture is not only important to its function but also to providing an explanation for the pattern of fractures encountered. The clavicle has a double S-shaped curve that varies in cross-sectional area along its length. The medial portion is tubular

and resists axial loading. This portion of the clavicle protects the costoclavicular space, where the medial cord and origin of the ulnar nerve are at risk for injury with medial clavicle fractures, clavicular nonunions, and healed fractures with exuberant callus. The flat lateral portion functions to resist the muscular and ligament forces. The weakened junction of the medial tubular and flattened lateral clavicle places the middle clavicle at risk for fracture (7).

It is important to understand the relationship of the soft tissue structures to the clavicle. This knowledge lessens the risk of damage to vital structures during treatment. The clavicle is a bony framework for muscle origins and insertions. The soft tissue structures that surround the bony clavicle can be divided into the areas above, below, and behind this structure. Above the clavicle, the cervical fascia, sternocleidomastoid muscle, omohyoid, and upper third of the trapezius insert from medial to lateral onto the superior aspect of the clavicle. Below the clavicle, the clavicular head of the pectoralis major and minor attaches medially while the anterior deltoid is attached laterally. Finally, behind the clavicle, although no muscles directly insert, there is a continuous myofascial layer that lies in front of the large vessels and nerves as they pass from the root of the neck to the axilla. Behind the medial clavicle, the internal jugular and subclavian veins join to form the innominate vein. Behind the midportion are both the subclavian and axillary veins.

ETIOLOGY OF INJURY

The most common mechanism of fracture to the athletic shoulder girdle is a fall on an outstretched arm, as commonly occurs in both contact and noncontact sports. In athletic patients, significant trauma is necessary, and the resultant fracture is often more serious than those that occur in older patients with osteoporotic fractures. These younger patients commonly have displaced fractures or fracture-dislocations with substantial soft tissue disruption. Neurologic or vascular injury can occur and are related to the seriousness of the soft tissue component of the injury.

An additional mechanism of fracture of the proximal humerus occurs with excessive external rotation of the arm. The proximal humerus is wedged against the acromion in a pivotal position, and a proximal humerus fracture can occur through this area. A direct blow to the lateral arm can also cause injury to the shoulder girdle. The mechanism usually results in a fracture of the greater tuberosity, a minimally displaced fracture, or a fracture involving the articular surface. Fractures associated with primary dislocation of the shoulder, both anterior and posterior, are usually caused by the forced abducted, externally rotated position (for anterior fracture-dislocation) and forced adduction with posterior displacement (for posterior fracture-dislocation).

Clavicular fractures may result from direct or indirect trauma. Patients involved in stick sports such as lacrosse and hockey frequently sustain a direct blow to the clavicle. In addition, a fall directly onto the bone itself can result in a fracture. Clavicular injuries may also occur from a fall onto the outstretched arm, but this is probably a less common mechanism of injury. Medial clavicle fractures are most common secondary to indirect trauma from a force directed to the lateral arm.

Although the most common cause of humeral fractures is blunt trauma, a spiral fracture of the shaft of the humerus resulting from muscular violence has been reported in various overhead throwing sports, including baseball, javelin, and handball, as well as in arm wrestling. This has become a well-recognized clinical entity. Many explanations for the spiral fracture have been offered, most being variations of torsional stress injury. Powerful internal rotation is applied to the upper shaft of the humerus by the pectoralis major, subscapularis, teres major, and latissimus dorsi while a force across the forearm imparts external rotation to the distal humerus through the elbow joint.

PRESENTATION AND PHYSICAL EXAMINATION

Athletes who sustain fractures of the shoulder girdle typically describe specific trauma and can often attribute the mechanism of injury. After the fracture pain, swelling and inability to use the shoulder are seen immediately. Most patients are not able to continue to participate in the athletic activity.

A meticulous evaluation of the injured shoulder girdle begins with a visual examination by adequately exposing the shoulder girdle and upper extremity. Deformity is more common with dislocations and displaced fractures about the shoulder. Fracture-dislocations may be less apparent than true dislocations, in that the arm may hang in a more normal position at the side. In proximal humerus fractures, the deltoid and soft tissue may mask significant fracture displacement or dislocation. By 48 hours after injury, ecchymosis may extend down the chest wall or to the elbow. Posterior sternoclavicular fracture dislocations and posteriorly displaced lateral clavicle fractures can frequently be missed without a careful examination.

Other areas are evaluated in addition to obvious shoulder girdle fractures. The cervical spine is assessed for any tenderness and pain with motion. If there is any question, cervical spine radiographs are obtained before any movement of this area. Direct tenderness over a fresh or healing fracture has always been a useful clinical sign for the ribs, clavicle, acromion, and humerus and often indicates the area of concern. Pain or tenderness may be elicited indirectly with motion or with longitudinal compression or distraction.

Neurologic evaluation is carried out for all components of the upper extremity. Gentle motion and isometric contractions are generally sufficient to allow palpation of individual muscle groups as a screening test for muscle integrity and nerve supply. In the distal part of the involved limb, the color, capillary refill, and radial pulse are examined and compared with those of the uninjured upper extremity. More detailed vascular evaluation is undertaken if arterial injury is suspected.

RADIOGRAPHIC AND DIAGNOSTIC EVALUATION

The radiologic evaluation of proximal humerus fractures begins with plain radiographs. The trauma shoulder series involves three views: a true anteroposterior (AP) view of the shoulder in the plane of the scapula with the arm in internal and external rotation and an axillary lateral or a scapulolateral view (Fig. 18-1). The axillary view is a valuable view in the evaluation of the proximal humerus fracture and must not be neglected. Radiology technicians are often reluctant to position the shoulder for an axillary view due to the significant pain that the patient feels with even the slightest motion. When a supine axillary view cannot be obtained, an alternative axillary view should be obtained. These include a trauma axillary lateral view, a Velpeau axillary lateral view, or an axillary view with flexible radiographic (mammography) film (Fig. 18-2). Alternatively, a transthoracic lateral view may be helpful if the scapulolateral view (scapular Y view) or other axillary views are difficult to obtain.

When the degree of displacement of the humeral head or tuberosity fragments is uncertain, then an axial computed tomography (CT) study with 2-mm sections is indicated. CT also assists in analyzing the size of humeral head impression fractures, the extent of articular involvement in head-splitting fractures, and the displacement or extent of comminution of associated glenoid fractures. Three-dimensional reconstruction views are not routinely indicated, but may help in the preoperative planning of complex, comminuted fractures or complex malunions.

The most beneficial screening examination for clavicle fractures is the anteroposterior (AP) view. When this view is obtained, the films should include the upper third of the humerus, the shoulder girdle, and upper lung fields so that other girdle fractures or a pneumothorax can be quickly identified. When a high-energy injury occurs, a chest x-ray study should be obtained to evaluate for a pneumothorax or rib fractures. The configuration of the fracture may suggest other associated injuries. For lateral clavicle fractures, a 15-degree cephalic tilt radiograph should always be obtained to evaluate the lateral articular segment and acromioclavicular joint.

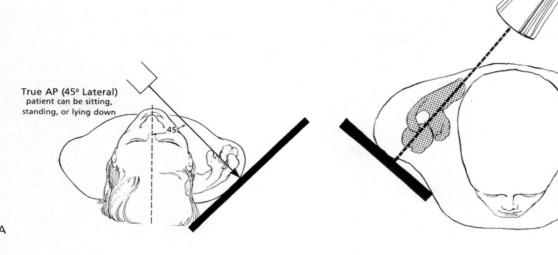

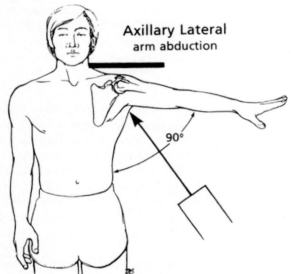

FIGURE 18-1. Trauma shoulder series. Recommended views for the evaluation of proximal humerus fractures include a true anteroposterior view in the plane of the scapula with the arm in internal and external rotation **(A)** and an axillary lateral **(B)** or scapulolateral view **(C)**. (From Rockwood CA, Jensen KL. X-ray evaluation of shoulder problems. In: Rockwood CA, Matsen FA, eds. *The shoulder,* vol. 1, 2nd ed. Philadelphia: WB Saunders, 1998:199–202, with permission.)

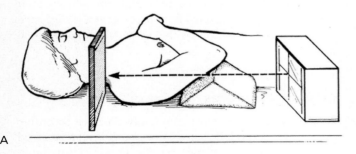

FIGURE 18-2. Modified axillary views. If the standard axillary lateral x-ray cannot be obtained, one of the modified axillary views must then be attempted. The trauma axillary lateral x-ray **(A)** positions the patient supine with the elbow elevated by a piece of foam rubber, allowing the x-ray to pass from the inferior up through the glenohumeral joint onto the x-ray cassette, which is superior to the shoulder. The Velpeau axillary lateral x-ray **(B)** positions the patient leaning the shoulder backward over a cassette with the beam directed inferiorly. A curved cassette or flexible (mammography) radiographic film can be placed in the axilla and the beam directed inferiorly through the glenohumeral joint onto the cassette. (From Rockwood CA, Jensen KL. X-ray evaluation of shoulder problems. In: Rockwood CA, Matsen FA, eds. *The shoulder,* vol 1, 2nd ed. Philadelphia: WB Saunders, 1998:202–205, with permission.)

Continued on next page

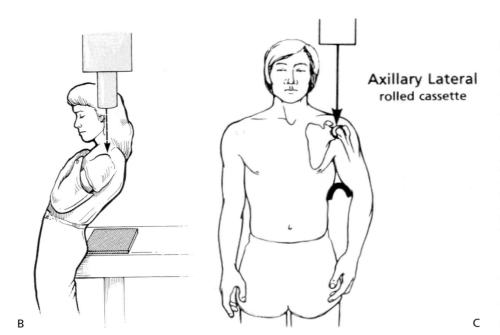

Axillary Lateral
rolled cassette

FIGURE 18-2. *Continued.* Modified axillary views. If the standard axillary lateral x-ray cannot be obtained, one of the modified axillary views must then be attempted. The trauma axillary lateral x-ray **(A)** positions the patient supine with the elbow elevated by a piece of foam rubber, allowing the x-ray to pass from the inferior up through the glenohumeral joint onto the x-ray cassette, which is superior to the shoulder. The Velpeau axillary lateral x-ray **(B)** positions the patient leaning the shoulder backward over a cassette with the beam directed inferiorly. A curved cassette or flexible (mammography) radiographic film can be placed in the axilla and the beam directed inferiorly through the glenohumeral joint onto the cassette **(C)**. (From Rockwood CA, Jensen KL. X-ray evaluation of shoulder problems. In: Rockwood CA, Matsen FA, eds. *The shoulder,* vol 1, 2nd ed. Philadelphia: WB Saunders, 1998:202–205, with permission.)

B

C

CLASSIFICATION OF INJURY

Proximal Humerus Fractures

Classification systems of proximal humerus fractures have been designed to offer a common language for discussing these fractures. The two most commonly used systems are the Neer classification and the AO/ASIF classification. The Neer classification was published in 1970 and represents a refinement of Codman's four-segment classification (i.e., articular segment, greater tuberosity, lesser tuberosity, and humeral shaft) that incorporates the concepts of displacement and vascular isolation of the articular segment (Fig. 18-3) (8,9). The system uses displacement and angulation of the segments to categorize them into one of four groups of fractures: nondisplaced fractures, fractures involving displacement of two fragments, those involving displacement of three fragments, and those involving displacement of all four fragments, with or without dislocation of the articular segment. Specific criteria for determination of a displaced fracture segment was arbitrarily defined by Neer as displacement more than 10 mm or angulation greater than 45 degrees. These values were intended merely as guidelines for differentiating nondisplaced from displaced fracture segments and remain unsubstantiated by experimental or clinical data.

The AO/ASIF group devised a proximal humerus fracture classification in 1987 that included additional subgroupings in an attempt to combine a more detailed analysis of fracture anatomy with the presumed vascular status of the articular segment (10) (Fig. 18-4). The system involves three fracture groups: type A (extraarticular fractures), type B (bifocal fractures; i.e., fracture lines at two locations), and type C (intraarticular fractures). Subgroups are divided into type 1 (nondisplaced/minimally displaced), type 2 (displaced), and type 3 (displaced with comminution/dislocated). This classification provides a more detailed method for fracture description and documentation and a more specific algorithmic approach to treatment.

Jakob and colleagues described a distinctive fracture pattern of the proximal humerus in 1991 termed the "valgus-impacted four-part fracture" (11). A valgus-impacted head fragment is the characteristic feature of this fracture pattern (Fig. 18-5). The incidence of osteonecrosis is lower with this fracture type than it is for other displaced four-part proximal humerus fractures. Either closed reduction or limited open reduction and minimal internal fixation led to a 74% satisfactory outcome in their study. The valgus-impacted four-part fracture is suggested to cause less destruction to the proximal humeral blood supply.

Clavicle Fractures

Clavicle fractures are most commonly classified according to location. Although there is not one generally accepted classification scheme, Craig's classification (12) is useful in understanding fracture anatomy, mechanism of injury,

Displaced Fractures

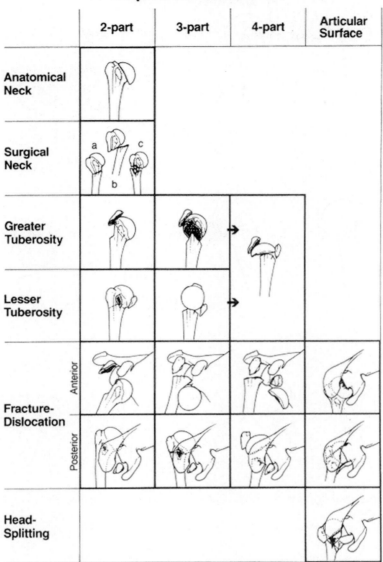

FIGURE 18-3. The anatomic (Neer) classification of proximal humerus fractures. Each of the four major segments (head, shaft, greater tuberosity, and lesser tuberosity) is considered a fracture part if it is angulated greater than 45 degrees or displaced greater than 1 cm. (From Bigliani LU, Flatow EL, Pollock RG. Fractures of the proximal humerus. In: Rockwood CA, Matsen FA, eds. *The shoulder,* vol 1, 2nd ed. Philadelphia: WB Saunders, 1998:342.)

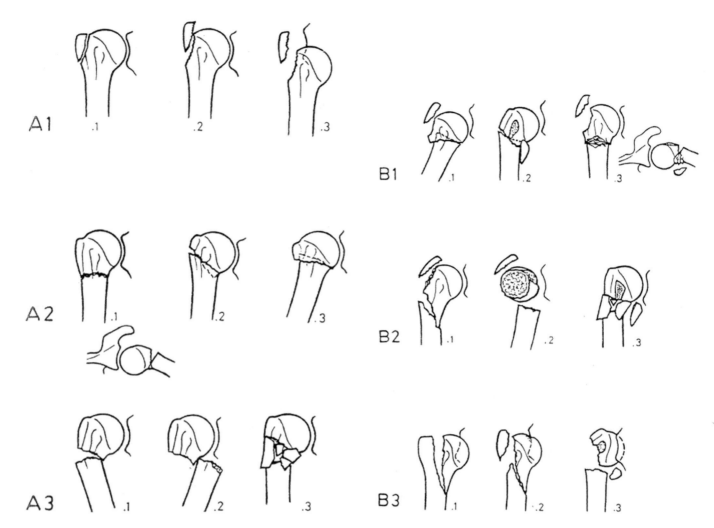

FIGURE 18-4. The AO/ASIF classification of proximal humerus fractures. **A:** Type A fractures. **B:** Type B fractures.

clinical presentation, and alternative methods of treatment. In this classification, three groups exist, depending on the anatomic location of the fracture: distal third, middle third, and inner third fractures. Middle third fractures involve the diaphyseal midshaft portion, comprise 80% of all clavicle fractures, and carry a high union rate. Inner third fractures comprise only 15% of clavicle fractures. Fractures involving the distal third make up the remaining 15% of fractures. Neer recognized the difficulties in treating distal third fractures and proposed a further subdivision into three types (13) (Fig. 18-6). Type I is a distal third fracture with minimal displacement. Type II involves a displaced fracture that occurs at the attachment of the coracoclavicular ligaments to the clavicle. This type is then further subdivided into types IIA and IIB, depending on whether the ligaments remain intact. Type IIA fractures are those in which the coronoid and trapezoid ligaments remain attached to the distal segment. In this case, because the medial fragment has no attached ligaments, it becomes unstable and displaces superiorly as a result of the pull of the sternocleidomastoid muscle. This fracture pattern results in a greater rate of nonunion. A type IIB fracture occurs within the area of the coracoclavicular ligament attachment. In these fractures, the coracoid ligament is disrupted while the trapezoid ligament remains attached to the distal segment. This pattern is more stable than the type IIA fracture. The type III fractures are intraarticular at the acromioclavicular joint.

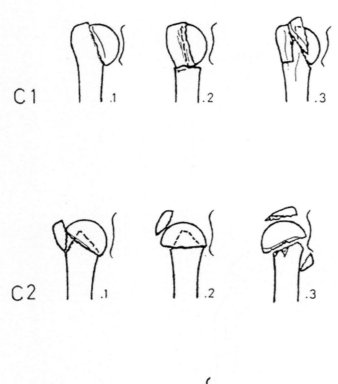

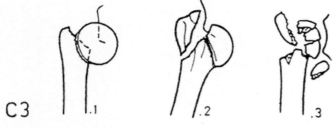

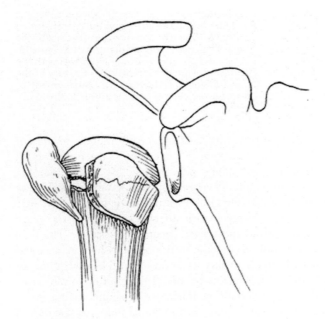

FIGURE 18-4. *Continued.* **C:** Type C fractures. (From Gerber C, Warner JJP. Alternatives to hemiarthroplasty for complex proximal-humeral fractures. In: Warner JJP, Iannotti JP, Gerber C, eds. *Complex and revision problems in shoulder surgery.* Philadelphia: Lippincott-Raven, 1997:217–218.)

FIGURE 18-5. The four-part valgus impacted fracture of the proximal humerus with an intact medial periosteal bridge. (From Naranja RJ, Iannotti JP. Displaced three- and four-part proximal humerus fractures: evaluation and management. *J Am Acad Orthop Surg* 2000;8(6):376.)

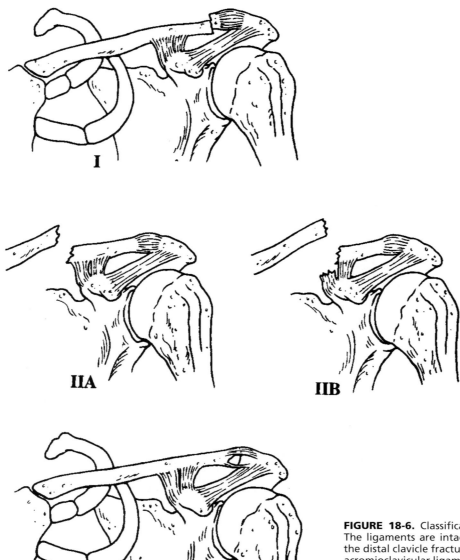

FIGURE 18-6. Classification of distal clavicle fractures. Type I: The ligaments are intact and there is minimal displacement of the distal clavicle fracture. Type **IIA**: The fracture is medial to the acromioclavicular ligaments with both ligaments intact. Type **IIB**: The fracture is between the acromioclavicular ligaments with the conoid ligament disrupted. Type **III**: Intraarticular fracture of the distal clavicle. (From Schlegel TF, Hawkins RJ. Management of distal clavicle fractures. *Oper Tech Sports Med* 1997;5(2):94.)

NONOPERATIVE TREATMENT, REHABILITATION, AND RESULTS

Nonoperative care is typically reserved for minimally displaced or nondisplaced fractures of the shoulder girdle. Most shoulder girdle fractures (80% to 85%) belong to this category. Fractures with minimal degrees of displacement and angulation are typically well tolerated functionally even in the throwing athlete. A short period of initial immobilization followed by early motion has been consistently described by most authors as having a high degree of success in treating these fractures.

Most treatment programs stress early motion to prevent the formation of scarring in the capsule, subacromial space, and other surrounding soft tissues that often leads to decreased function. Therapy programs for the nonoperative treatment of shoulder girdle fractures are typically divided into three phases: (a) the passive stretching phase, (b) the active stretching phase, and (c) the strengthening phase. The time frame for individual phases varies between fracture area and configuration (i.e., stable versus unstable). The time frame for each phase can therefore be modified according to the extent of the injury. Specific nonoperative programs for the treatment of clavicle fractures and proximal humerus fractures in the overhead athlete are outlined in Tables 18-1 and 18-2.

TABLE 18–1. NONOPERATIVE SHOULDER CONDITIONING THERAPY FOR CLAVICLE FRACTURES

Phase I: 0–2 weeks
1. ICE
   a. 7 days per week
   b. 2–3 times per day after exercising or as necessary
   c. 15–20 min "ON" maximum, 60 min "OFF" minimum
2. STRETCHING: PASSIVE MOTION
   a. 7 days per week, 3 times per day
   b. Pendulum exercise: short arc, 1–2 sets, 20–30 repetitions (reps)
   c. Standing internal rotation to belt line (thumb behind back): 1–2 sets, 5–10 reps
   d. Supine-seated forward elevation to 90°, 1–2 sets, 5–10 reps
3. STATIONARY CYCLING
   a. 5 days per week, 1 time per day
   b. Spin or light resistance and increase as tolerated: 10–15–20–30 minutes

Phase II: 2–6 weeks
1. ICE as per phase I
2. STRETCHING: ACTIVE MOTION (WITH TERMINAL STRETCH)
   a. 7 days per week, 3 times per day
   b. Pendulum exercise: short arc, 1–2 sets, 20–30 reps
   c. Standing internal rotation to belt line (thumb behind back): 1–2 sets, 5–10 reps
   d. Seated forward elevation (overhead elbow lift): 1–2 sets, 5–10 reps
3. CORD STRENGTHENING
   a. 7 days per week, 1–2 times per day
   b. Internal rotation: 1–2 sets, 10–15 reps
   c. Standing forward punch: 1–2 sets, 10–15 reps
4. STATIONARY CYCLING
   a. 5 days per week, 1 time per day
   b. Spin or light resistance and increase as tolerated: 15–30–45 minutes
5. STAIR STEPPER (e.g., Stair Master)
   a. 1–2 times per week, 1 time per day
   b. Progressive resistance, increase as tolerated: 20–30 min

Phase III: 3–6 weeks and after
1. ICE as per phase I
2. STRETCHING: ACTIVE MOTION (WITH TERMINAL STRETCH)
   a. 7 days per week, 3 times per day
   b. Pendulum exercises: 1–2 sets, 20–30 reps
   c. Seated external rotation: 1–2 sets, 10–15 reps
   d. Seated forward elevation (overhead elbow lift): 1–2 sets, 5–10 reps
   e. Standing internal rotation (thumb behind back): 1–2 sets, 5–10 reps
   f. Cross-arm push (adduction): 1–2 sets, 5–10 reps
3. CORD STRENGTHENING
   a. 7 days per week, 1–2 times per day
   b. External rotation: 1–2 sets, 10–15 reps
   c. Internal rotation: 1–2 sets, 10–15 reps
   d. Shoulder shrug: 1–2 sets, 10–20–30 reps
   e. Seated row (narrow-middle-wide grip): 1–2 sets, 10–15 reps
   f. Standing forward punch: 1–2 sets, 10–15 reps
   g. Biceps curls: 1–2 sets, 10–15 reps
   h. Latissimus pulls: 1–2 sets, 5–10 reps
   i. Overhead punch press: 1–2 sets, 10–15 reps
4. CYCLING
   a. 3 times per week, 1 time per day
   b. 30–45 minutes, progressive resistance
   c. Stationary or outdoor
   d. Mountain or road bikes
   e. Few hills and remain on seat
5. WATER WORKOUT
   a. 2 times per week, 1 time per day
   b. Aqua jogger exercise, 20–30 minutes
6. STAIR STEPPER (e.g., Stair Master)
   a. 1–2 times per week, 1 time per day
   b. Progressive resistance

TABLE 18–2. NONOPERATIVE SHOULDER CONDITIONING THERAPY FOR STABLE, NONDISPLACED SHOULDER FRACTURES

Phase I: 0–1 week

1. ICE
   a. 7 days per week
   b. 2–3 times per day after exercising or as necessary
   c. 15–20 min "ON" maximum, 60 min "OFF" minimum
2. STRETCHING: PASSIVE MOTION
   a. 7 days per week, 3 times per day
   b. For dislocations, avoid provocative positions for 6 weeks
   c. Pendulum exercise-short arc: 1–2 sets, 20–30 reps
   d. Standing internal rotation to belt line (thumb behind back): 1–2 sets, 5–10 reps
   e. Supine-seated forward elevation: 1–2 sets, 5–10 reps
   f. Supine-seated external rotation: 1–2 sets, 10–15 reps
3. STATIONARY CYCLING
   a. 5 days per week, 1 time per day
   b. Spin or light resistance and increase as tolerated
   c. 10–15–20–30 minutes

Phase II: 1–2 weeks

1. ICE as per phase I
2. STRETCHING: ACTIVE MOTION (WITH TERMINAL STRETCH)
   a. 7 days per week, 3 times per day
   b. For dislocations, avoid provocative positions for 6 weeks
   c. Pendulum exercise-short arc: 1–2 sets, 20–30 reps
   d. Standing internal rotation (thumb behind back): 1–2 sets, 5–10 reps
   e. Seated forward elevation (overhead elbow lift): 1–2 sets, 5–10 reps
   f. Seated external rotation: 1–2 sets, 10–15 reps
3. STATIONARY CYCLING
   a. As per phase I
   b. Increase resistance and time
4. STAIR STEPPER (e.g., Stair Master)
   a. 1–2 times per week, 1 time per day
   b. Progressive resistance increase as tolerated
   c. 20–30 minutes

Phase III: 2 weeks and after

1. ICE as necessary
2. STRETCHING
   a. As per phase II
   b. Progress according to range of motion and pain
3. CORD STRENGTHENING
   a. 7 days per week, 1–2 times per day
   b. External rotation: 1–2 sets, 10–15 reps
   c. Internal rotation: 1–2 sets, 10–15 reps
   d. Shoulder shrug: 1–2 sets, 10–20–30 reps
   e. Seated row: 1–2 sets, 10–15 reps
   f. Standing forward punch: 1–2 sets, 10–15 reps
   g. Biceps curls: 1–2 sets, 10–15 reps
4. CYCLING
   a. 3 times per week, 1 time per day
   b. 30–45 minutes, progressive resistance
   c. Stationary or outdoor
   d. Mountain or road bikes
   e. Few hills and remain on seat
5. WATER WORKOUT
   a. 2 times per week, 1 time per day
   b. Aqua jogger exercise, 20–30 minutes
6. STAIR STEPPER (e.g., Stair Master)
   a. 1–2 times per week, 1 time per day
   b. Progressive resistance, 20–30 minutes

Proximal Humerus Fractures

Most proximal humerus fractures are nondisplaced and can be managed with conservative care. The periosteum, capsule, and rotator cuff limit fracture displacement so the reduction is unnecessary. The constrained design of the glenohumeral joint and the global range of motion of the shoulder motion provide the advantage that it can compensate for even moderate amounts of residual fracture displacement.

Assisted motion exercises may begin when the fragments move in union. This can be determined by the examiner grasping the humeral head between the thumb and index finger of one hand and rotating the elbow with the opposite hand. The absence of pain, crepitus, and movement between the shaft and the proximal humerus suggests clinical continuity. Once this has been documented, passive range of motion may begin as early as 2 but more often after 3 weeks after the fracture. Overly aggressive activity before this stage may distract the minimally displaced fracture, resulting in either malunion or nonunion of the fracture. Intermittent radiographs are necessary to confirm that there is no displacement of the fracture during healing and physical therapy exercises.

As the fracture becomes more stable, it is then possible to progress therapy to include active exercises with terminal stretch and eventually resisted strengthening exercises. This program should be well designed and carefully monitored and continued until union. Satisfactory functional outcome often takes place between 6 and 12 months.

Clavicle Fractures

Nonoperative treatment is typically recommended for most clavicle fractures. Type I and type III distal clavicle fractures usually require no special treatment and have a favorable outcome with rapid healing after symptomatic care. A sling or figure-of-eight splint is provided for comfort until the pain subsides. Early motion is initiated as tolerated and can begin within days of the injury. Resistive strengthening can begin when the fracture is healed. Recovery is usually rapid and outcome expected to be good. Persistent symptoms occur in a very small percentage of patients. Neer (14) reported that only 2 of 75 patients treated nonoperatively with type I fractures had difficulties. Similarly, Nordquist (15) documented that only 11% of his patients treated nonoperatively went on to have residual problems. There are conflicting results on the long-term complications of type III fractures. Neer found that these often led to AC arthrosis or osteolysis. Nordquist, on the other hand, found no evidence of AC arthritis or distal clavicle osteolysis in his study. If late symptoms develop in either type I or III fractures, then a distal clavicle resection can be performed with good results.

Most fractures of the clavicular shaft can be managed with a well-padded commercial figure-of-eight splint or sling for comfort only. Occasionally, a closed reduction is necessary. A postreduction radiograph is used to evaluate the reduction. Rehabilitation is started as soon as the patient can participate comfortably. It is rare that a fracture of the shaft of the clavicle requires an open reduction and internal fixation. If a completely displaced fracture of the midshaft of the clavicle cannot be reduced with closed manipulation, the patient is observed for 2 to 3 weeks in the figure-of-eight splint. If after observation the complete displacement persists, open reduction and internal fixation can be recommended.

Recent studies have evaluated the sequelae and deficits following conservative treatment of displaced clavicle fractures. Nowak and associates (16) reported that 46% of patients with clavicle fractures demonstrated sequelae (pain during activity, pain at rest, or cosmetic defects) at a 9- to 10-year follow-up. Nonunion occurred in 6% of these patients. No bony contact was the strongest radiographic predictor for sequelae. Comminuted fractures with transversely placed fragments had a significantly increased risk for remaining symptoms, as had older patients. Fracture location and shortening did not predict outcome, except for cosmetic defects. McKee and associates (17) reported on previously unrecognized deficits following conservative treatment of displaced midshaft clavicle fractures and detected residual deficits in shoulder strength, especially endurance. They concluded that the significant level of dissatisfaction following conservative care should encourage more active treatment options in selected patients.

Spiral Humerus Shaft Fractures

The nonsurgical treatment of spiral diaphyseal humeral fractures has long been known to render satisfactory results in most instances. Plate fixation and intramedullary nailing can be associated with a relatively high incidence of complications, such as nonunion, infection, and nerve palsy. Functional bracing of these fractures can offer effective nonoperative management of the majority of these fractures. Indications for functional bracing of humeral shaft fractures include closed diaphyseal fractures without marked distraction between the fragments and closed fractures associated with initial radial nerve palsy. Open fractures without significant soft tissue damage can also be treated with functional bracing following surgical irrigation and debridement and closure of the open wound. Contraindications include bilateral humeral fractures on fractures in polytraumatized patients unless they are able to stand erect early and ambulate with external support on the opposite side.

Functional bracing of humeral shaft fractures begins with stabilization in an above-the-elbow cast or a coaptation splint that holds the elbow in 90 degrees of flexion. A cuff and collar are added for support. On occasion, when the fracture is the result of a low-energy injury and there is minimal swelling of the extremity, the functional brace can be applied at the first encounter. Otherwise, it is best to use a cast or splint until the acute symptoms and swelling subside. In most instances, the brace is applied approximately 12 days after the injury (18–20).

Pendulum exercises are begun the first postinjury day and are continued after the application of the brace to prevent contracture of the shoulder joint. Active elevation and abduction are avoided. The cuff and collar are discontinued when the elbow reaches full extension but should be used during recumbency for an additional 2 weeks. During ambulation, the arm hangs at the side of the body and swings normally. The brace must be adjusted and fastened with Velcro straps to maintain constant compression of the soft tissues and to prevent displacement of the brace, which is likely to occur as swelling subsides and atrophy develops.

Radiographic evaluation of the fracture should follow the application of the brace and be repeated 1 week later and then at 3- to 4-week intervals. Failure to obtain acceptable alignment of the fragments calls for abandoning the closed treatment and beginning of a different treatment modality. Once the brace is discontinued, there is frequently limitation of motion of the shoulder. However, it improves after return to normal activities. The limitation of shoulder motion ranges from 0 to 15 degrees (18–20). Limitation of motion at the elbow is less, ranging from 0 to 10 degrees.

OPERATIVE TREATMENT, REHABILITATION, AND RESULTS

In the competitive athlete who requires the arm for throwing or overhead motion (as in playing baseball, playing football, throwing javelin, or swimming), a more rigorous effort should be made to restore anatomy and obtain rigid fixation. Subtle unrecognized deficits after nonoperative management of certain shoulder girdle fractures may not be readily apparent to the layperson; however, these potential functional deficits may have a career-altering effect on the overhead athlete. Therefore, every attempt should be made to regain anatomic alignment of shoulder fractures to minimize postinjury sequelae. Subtle weakness and loss of motion due to fracture incongruity may well be tolerated in most cases by the sedentary patient, but these must be addressed in the athletic patient.

Proximal Humerus Fractures

The operative management of proximal humerus fractures relies on several factors, including the patient's preinjury activity level, the classification type of the fracture, and the experience of the surgeon. Appropriate and realistic goals for the eventual function of the shoulder must be discussed with the patient. The patient's general medical health, physiologic age, ability to cooperate with postoperative rehabilitation, and functional expectations should all be considered. Based on these features, some patients should be treated operatively. Bone quality, fracture pattern, and associated injuries influence the treatment program and rehabilitation. Finally, the operating surgeon must make a self-appraisal with regard to his or her knowledge and expertise. Fixation options for the treatment of proximal humerus fractures include closed reduction techniques with percutaneous fixation and open reduction internal fixation. Hemiarthroplasty, although an excellent option for the elderly patient with osteoporotic bone, is not a viable initial treatment option for the overhead athlete.

Percutaneous Fixation Techniques

Closed reduction and percutaneous fixation techniques have been advocated to avoid several problems unique to proximal humerus fractures. Open techniques can require a large dissection with soft tissue stripping, thereby potentially disrupting some of the blood supply to the proximal humerus. Avascular necrosis of the humeral head can occur in 3% to 14% of patients with displaced fractures with open treatment (21). Percutaneous techniques that can avoid these problems include the use of pin fixation and screw fixation.

Closed reduction and percutaneous pin fixation of proximal humerus fractures has been described using a variety of devices, including terminally threaded pins, dynamic hip screw guide pins, Schantz pins, and Kirschner wires (21). Terminally threaded pins, however, are recommended due to the increased risk of pin loosening and migration and potential loss of fracture fixation with smooth wires. K-wires have been shown to have a failure rate of up to 100%, attributable to the small diameter of the pin and the smooth tip.

A thorough knowledge of proximal humeral anatomy is crucial for proper pin placement. Percutaneous pin placement options for surgical neck fractures include retrograde lateral, retrograde anterior, retrograde anterolateral, and antegrade superolateral through the greater tuberosity (22) (Fig. 18-7). Retrograde pins are angled approximately 45 degrees to the shaft in the coronal plane and 30 degrees to the shaft in the sagittal plane, so that it is aimed at the central portion of the humeral head (22). Pins should begin above the insertion of the deltoid to avoid injury to the radial nerve as it courses in the spiral groove. The starting point of the pins, however, allows best purchase of the shaft when they are started at least 2 cm distal to the fracture. This provides a more rigid construct, thereby preventing motion and failure of the pin. Stability of the construct is also increased with a wide pin spread. This must be assessed on multiple fluoroscopic planes to prevent triangulation of the pins. Retrograde pins should be placed with a soft tissue protector to avoid injuring the axillary nerve. Finally, the

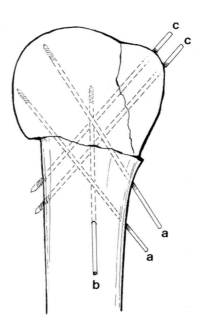

FIGURE 18-7. Placement options for percutaneous fixation using terminally threaded AO pins, 2.5 mm in diameter. Two retrograde lateral pins are inserted just above the deltoid insertion (a), and a third is inserted retrograde through the anterior cortex (b). If the greater or lesser tuberosities are displaced, two or more pins are inserted in an antegrade direction for reduction and fixation (c). (From Gerber C, Warner JJP. Alternatives to hemiarthroplasty for complex proximal-humeral fractures. In: Warner JJP, Iannotti JP, Gerber C, eds. *Complex and revision problems in shoulder surgery.* Philadelphia: Lippincott-Raven, 1997:224, with permission.)

threaded tip of the pins should be placed into but not through the subchondral region of the humeral head. Penetration of the pins through the head increases the potential for loosening as the mechanical advantage is lost.

The shoulder is then brought through a range of motion under fluoroscopy to assess stability of the construct. If there is any question about fixation, another pin should be placed. Pins are cut as short as possible below the skin, and the wounds are closed. Pendulum exercises are started early in the postoperative period.

Temporary pins may be used to aid closed reduction, or they may be left in situ for 4 to 6 weeks to hold the reduction. The usual sites of insertion are two wires from above the deltoid insertion into the humeral head, one wire from the greater tuberosity to the medial humeral shaft, and an optional forth wire from the anterior humeral shaft into the humeral head. Additional pins are inserted as needed for added stability.

Percutaneous pin fixation of proximal humerus fractures has a few limitations. First, antegrade superolateral pins can interfere with early pendulum exercises by impinging on the lateral border of the acromion. Second, subcutaneous pins can cause local skin irritation and breakdown and can irritate or scar the penetrated deltoid muscle. Third, pin fixation can require a second operation for pin removal if the patient cannot tolerate removal in the office. For these reasons, percutaneous screw fixation with cannulated screws may provide a better option for some fractures.

Three- and four-part proximal humerus fractures can be managed with percutaneous screws when a few criteria are met. Satisfactory reduction must first be achieved with percutaneous guidewire fixation. The shoulder is brought through a range of motion under fluoroscopy and must be stable. There must be adequate bone stock on the lateral surface of the proximal humerus to accept the screw head. Extensive metaphyseal comminution and severely osteoporotic bone are contraindications for this technique.

Partially threaded 6.5-mm cancellous screws (cannulated) are typically used, although smaller screws can be substituted (Fig. 18-8). Percutaneous guide pins are first inserted in proper configuration. Typically, the same configuration for percutaneous pin fixation is used (Fig. 18-9). Screws are then placed over the guidewires and advanced until they engage the subchondral bone of the humeral head. Washers may be used with the screw heads to assist with either lateral wall fixation or fixation of the tuberosity fragments. Percutaneous screws can also be used in conjunction with percutaneous pin fixation in selected cases.

Stable constructs using percutaneous screw fixation allow early pendulum and range-of-motion exercises without irritating subcutaneous pins. Screw fixation also avoids the need for secondary surgery for pin removal. Cases in which a stable screw construct can be obtained therefore allow early motion and avoid the complications associated with pin fixation.

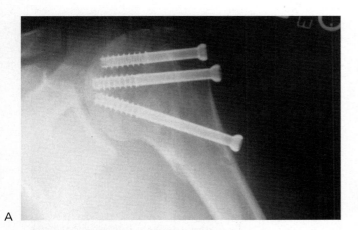

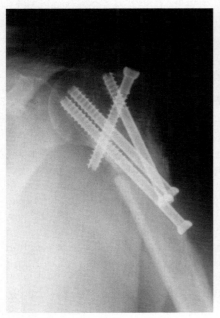

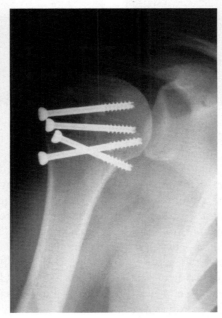

FIGURE 18-8. Partially threaded 6.5 mm **(A)**, 4.0 mm **(B)**, or 3.5 mm **(C)** cannulated screws can be used as an alternative to percutaneous pin fixation for proximal humerus fractures.

A

B

C

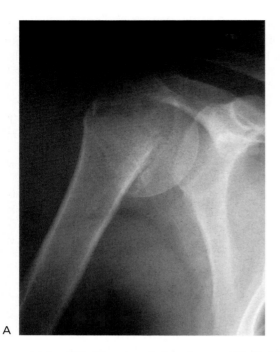

A

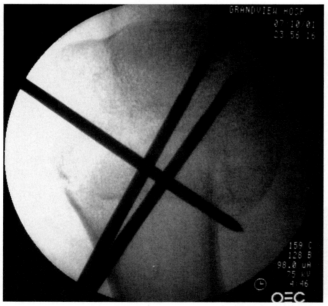

B

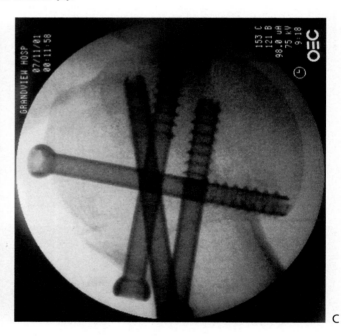

C

FIGURE 18-9. The technique of percutaneous screw fixation begins with fracture reduction **(A)**, followed by percutaneous pin fixation **(B)**, and finally cannulated screw fixation **(C)**.

Open Reduction and Internal Fixation Techniques

Open reduction and internal fixation of proximal humerus fractures are typically managed through a deltopectoral approach. The tendon of the long head of the biceps is identified and used as a reference for proximal humeral anatomy. Minimal dissection of the soft tissues is performed to identify and mobilize the tuberosity fragments. Extensive stripping is to be avoided to preserve the vascularity of the articular segment. Nonabsorbable suture can be placed through the rotator cuff insertion on the tuberosity for mobilization and reduction of the fractures. Once reduction has been achieved, the surgeon has the option of several fixation techniques. These include tension band fixation techniques with sutures or wires (with or without intramedullary support) and various plating techniques with screws. Alternatively, an open reduction may be performed followed by percutaneous pin or screw fixation techniques as previously described. This is a viable option for patients with little metaphyseal comminution and good bone quality. Additional security can be achieved with wires, cables, or suture tension bands to augment the pin fixation.

Valgus-impacted four-part fractures without lateral displacement of the humeral shaft, as described by Jakob (11), can be managed with open reduction and minimal internal fixation (Fig. 18-10). In four-part fractures without lateral displacement of the humeral shaft, the periosteum along the medial humeral neck should be intact, thereby protecting the articular segment from osteonecrosis. Resch and associates (23) described a technique of lifting the head segment into an anatomic position, bone grafting under the head, and buttressing the head segment in a reduced position using the tuberosity fragments. Fixation was achieved with interosseous sutures and interfragmentary screws and percutaneously placed Kirschner wires. Overall, the clinical results were excellent, particularly when anatomic reduction was achieved and maintained. Twenty of the 22 patients showed no evidence of osteonecrosis at the mean follow-up of 36 months. Ultimately, however, decisions regarding method of treatment should be based on the degree of bone quality and the patient's activity level.

Hawkins and associates first described their results using the tension band technique for fixation of three-part proximal humerus fractures in 1986 (24). Since that time, several variations of the technique have evolved. These include the use of the tension band technique in combination with Enders nails, lag screws, Kirschner wires, or an AO T-plate.

The technique for tension band fixation first requires reduction of tuberosity fragments to the humeral head piece (Fig. 18-11). Two 14-gauge colpotomy needles with stylets are passed through the subscapularis and lesser tuberosity, through the head, and out through the greater tuberosity and supraspinatus tendon. The malrotation of the head on the shaft is reduced. Two holes are drilled through the anterior humeral shaft below the greater tuberosity and lesser tuberosity and deep to the biceps tendon. Two 20-gauge wires or number 5 nonabsorbable braided sutures are used. The first is passed through the shaft, crossing the fracture in a figure-of-eight centered on the surgical neck fracture with one end through the colpotomy needle. This needle is then removed, and the suture is tied securely. The process is repeated with a second figure-of-eight through the second colpotomy needle, thereby converting this to a stable one-part fracture. The rotator interval is repaired. Stability is checked as the shoulder is brought through a full range of motion.

In order to achieve a more stable construct, variations of the tension band technique have been described using both intramedullary and extramedullary devices. The placement of intramedullary rods and accompanying tension band is technically demanding but provides intramedullary fixation, tension band compression over the fracture site, and sutures to keep the rods from migrating proximally. Ender nail intramedullary fixation combined with a tension band has been used for two-part surgical neck fractures and three-part proximal humerus fractures. Alternatively, Rush rods can be used with a suture hole through the top hook.

The technique of intramedullary rod and tension band fixation uses a deltopectoral approach and protected mobilization of the fracture fragments (Fig. 18-12). Two preliminary drill holes are made at the articular margin of the greater tuberosity for the two intramedullary rods that will be passed. A number 5 nonabsorbable suture is then passed into one of the drill holes and exits through the other. This

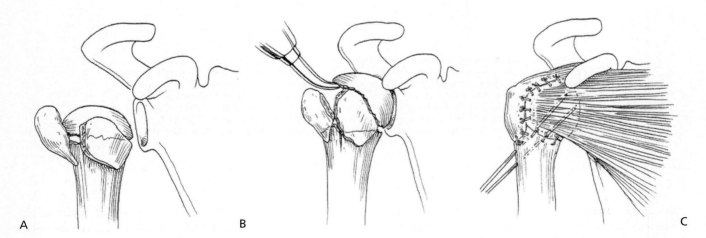

A   B   C

FIGURE 18-10. Technique for open reduction and internal fixation of a valgus-impacted four-part fracture. **A:** Four-part valgus-impacted fracture with an intact medial periosteal bridge. **B:** Periosteal elevator is used to elevate the impacted humeral head fragment. The greater and lesser tuberosities are placed under the humeral head as a buttress. **C:** Two or three percutaneously placed, terminally threaded Kirschner wires secure the humeral shaft to the humeral head fragment. Intraosseous and rotator cuff sutures secure the tuberosity fragment to each other and the humeral shaft. (From Naranja RJ, Iannotti JP. Displaced three- and four-part proximal humerus fractures: evaluation and management. *J Am Acad Orthop Surg* 2000;8(6):376.)

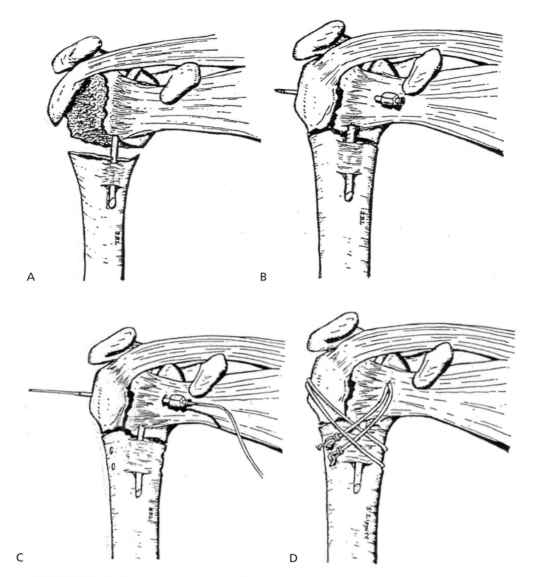

FIGURE 18-11. Tension band technique. **A:** A three-part fracture with a displaced greater tuberosity and an unimpacted, displaced segment of the head. **B:** The fracture is reduced and a colpotomy needle is passed from the lesser to the greater tuberosity, incorporating the tendons of the rotator cuff. **C:** With the needle in place, a free wire is passed and the drill holes are made along the anterior aspect of the humeral shaft. **D:** The fracture is reduced and the first wire is crossed, passed through the humeral shaft, and tightened. With the fracture stabilized, a second wire is applied in a similar fashion. (From Hawkins RJ, Bell RH, Gurr K. The three-part fracture of the proximal humerus: operative treatment. *J Bone Joint Surg (Am)* 1986;68(9): 1411–1412.)

serves as the top portion of the figure-of-eight construct of the tension band repair. The two free ends are then passed through the top hole of the intramedullary rod. Ender nails can be modified by placing a drill hole through the tip of the rod just above the standard slot in the rod (25) (Fig. 18-13). When sutures are passed through the more proximal hole in the tip of the rod, less of the rod protrudes from the greater tuberosity, thereby making it less prominent. A second set of drill holes is made in the shaft at a distance from

the fracture site equal to that of the entrance point of the intramedullary rods. The figure-of-eight suture then crosses the fracture site and one end is passed through the distal drill holes in the shaft. Additional sutures through the rods and secured through the drill holes distal to the fracture site preclude the rods from migrating into the subacromial space. The intramedullary rods are then passed through the entrance holes, past the fracture site, and into the medullary canal. The fracture is anatomically reduced and the rods are

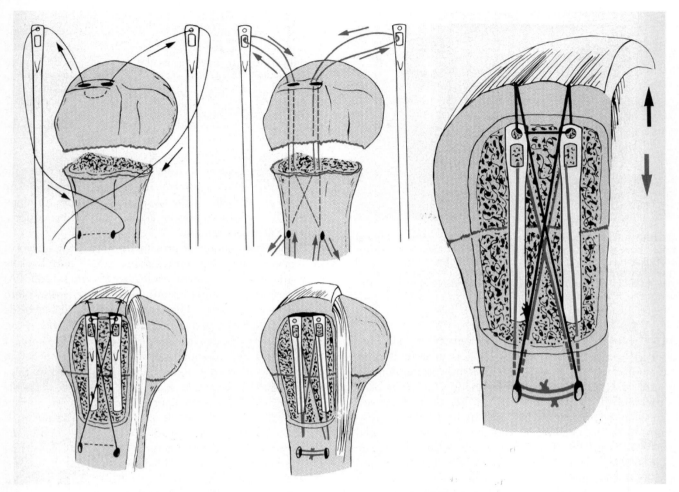

FIGURE 18-12. Technique of open reduction and internal fixation with modified Ender rods. The superior hole is used for a figure-of-eight tension band. Additional sutures through the rods and secured through drill holes beyond the fracture site preclude the rods from migrating into the subacromial space. (From Norris TR, Green A. Proximal humerus fractures and glenohumeral dislocations. In: Browner BD, Jupiter JB, Levine AM, et al, eds. *Skeletal trauma,* vol 2, 2nd ed. Philadelphia: WB Saunders, 1998:1594, with permission.)

inserted just beneath the cortical entrance point proximally. The sutures are through each rod and are tied distally to prevent the rods from migrating proximally with the tension band. The tension band is then tightened to provide secure fixation and compress the fracture site. Finally, the shoulder is brought through a range of motion to test fracture stability and closure is made.

Various types of plate fixation for proximal humerus fractures have been described, including AO plates (modified cloverleaf small fragment and large fragment T or L plates) (26–28) and blade plate devices (AO proximal humerus blade plate and bent semitubular plates) (22,29). Regardless of the type of fixation used, it must be able to secure the displaced tuberosity to both the head and shaft.

Plate fixation of displaced proximal humerus fractures relies on the buttress plating principles described by the AO/ASIF group. Plate fixation can restore the anatomy of

the proximal humerus and result in restoration of function with a useful range of motion and good strength. The use of screws and a plate, however, requires that adequate bone be present for stable fixation to be achieved. Youth, greater activity, and good bone quality may be the best indications for this technique. These patients typically respond poorly to closed treatment for three- and four-part fractures and often are not candidates for arthroplasty because of their age and activity level.

Plate fixation of the proximal humerus is achieved through a deltopectoral approach. Kirschner wires are used for temporary reduction of the fragments. An AO T- or L-plate is then buttressed against the lateral surface of the humerus adjacent to the bicipital groove (26). Alternatively, a modified AO cloverleaf plate may be used (27,28). Both superior and anterior arms are cut to avoid impingement between the greater tuberosity and the acromion (Fig. 18-

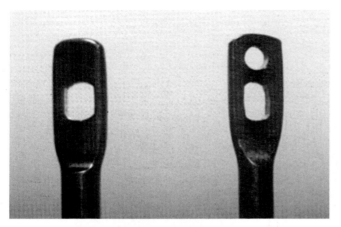

FIGURE 18-13. Modified 3.5-mm Enders nail with additional hole above eyelet to allow deeper insertion below the rotator cuff. (From Norris TR, Green A. Proximal humerus fractures and glenohumeral dislocations. In: Browner BD, Jupiter JB, Levine AM, et al, eds. *Skeletal trauma,* vol 2, 2nd ed. Philadelphia: WB Saunders, 1998:1593.)

14). The role of a prophylactic acromioplasty after plate fixation of the proximal humerus remains unclear. Patients treated in one study, however, had a slightly greater range of motion and, consequently, better function (26). The plate is premolded to exactly fit the lateral side of the humerus. Cancellous screws are used in the proximal holes for fixation into the humeral head, while cortical screws are used distally to secure the plate to the proximal shaft. Inadequate fixation that does not allow early motion, loss of fixation and reduction, and technical errors are the most common causes of unsatisfactory results with plate fixation.

The AO T-plate has been a popular technique for fixation of three- and four-part fractures; however, some authors have reported poor results with the plate. Reported complications included avascular necrosis secondary to extensive soft tissue stripping, superior placement of the plate leading to impingement, and loss of plate fixation with screw loosening, malunion, and infection. The AO T-plate is relatively stiff and therefore cannot be bent to fit the exact anatomy of the proximal lateral humerus or the tuberosities. Only two holes are available proximally for large cancellous screw fixation into the head. In order for these screws to obtain purchase in the tuberosities, the plate must be placed high on the bone and may cause impingement. The anterior arm of the T-plate can also rest undesirably on the biceps tendon.

Blade plate fixation of proximal humerus fractures can be achieved by using a premanufactured, commercially available 90-degree humeral blade plate (Synthes, Paoli, PA) or by custom fashioning a semitubular plate (Synthes) into a blade plate (22,29). The commercially available blade plate is constructed with a cannulated blade so that it can be passed over a guidewire. The plate portion of the implant consists of a limited-contact dynamic compression design that allows for compression of the head or tuberosity fragment to the shaft fragment. Blade plate fixation is preferable if the proximal fragment contains enough of the greater tuberosity to allow placement of the blade. The bone quality of the shaft must also be adequate to allow good bicortical fixation. Three-part fractures can be managed using this technique; however, the blade portion typically cannot achieve adequate fixation of both tuberosities in displaced four-part fractures (Fig. 18-15).

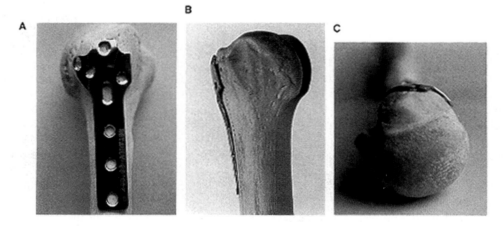

FIGURE 18-14. The modified cloverleaf plate. **A:** Both superior and anterior arms of the plate are cut, and 4.0-mm cancellous screws are used to fix the humeral head and the tuberosities. **B** and **C:** The plate is precontoured to exactly fit the lateral side of the humerus and greater tuberosity. It rests lateral to the biceps tendon and its low profile allows a superior placement on the humerus without impingement. (From Esser RD. Treatment of three- and four-part fractures of the proximal humerus with a modified cloverleaf plate. *J Orthop Trauma* 1994;8(1):18.)

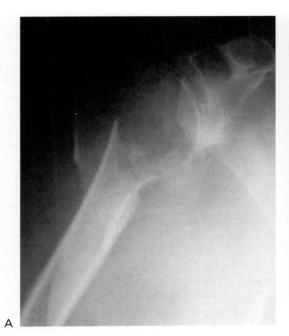
A

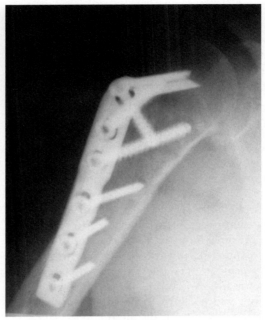
B

FIGURE 18-15. A,B: The commercially available AO blade plate can be used for two- and three-part fractures of the proximal humerus provided that bicortical fixation can be achieved with the distal screws. The blade plate cannot typically maintain reduction for displaced four-part fractures and other fixation methods must be utilized.

Blade plate fixation is approached through an extended deltopectoral incision. The long head of the biceps is identified distally at the level of the pectoralis major insertion. Typically, the biceps tendon is entrapped proximally between the tuberosity fragment and the head in three-part fractures and must be removed. The tendon is retracted and reduction of the fracture is performed. Provisional fixation can be achieved with pins. The guide pin for the cannulated blade is then inserted perpendicular to the long axis of the humeral shaft through the greater tuberosity fragment and into the subchondral bone of the humeral head. The recommended entry point for the guidewire is 1 to 2 cm distal to the tip of the greater tuberosity and 0.5 to 1 cm posterior to the lateral lip of the bicipital groove. Blade length is then measured from the inserted guidewire. If the measured blade length is between sizes, a second pin is inserted distal and parallel to the first pin in order to transverse more of the humeral head and achieve an available blade length.

A long enough plate should be selected to allow three to four bicortical screws in the distal humeral shaft. The plate portion may also require contouring before insertion to allow an anatomic fit against the lateral cortex of the proximal humerus. The lateral cortex at the blade insertion site may be predrilled before blade insertion if the bone is thick. Typically, the thin, metaphyseal bone can easily be penetrated with the blade portion. The blade is inserted directly over the guidewire and impacted until flush with the lateral cortex. The blade is fixed to the shaft with 4.5-mm cortical screws. The proximal most screw hole at the junction of the

blade portion can be used to direct a 4.5- or 6.5-mm cancellous screw into the humeral head for additional fixation. A partially threaded screw can be substituted in this hole to obtain additional compression across fracture fragments. Alternatively, the proximal hole can be used to secure suture fixation of the rotator cuff to the plate, thereby achieving some degree of rotational control of the proximal fragments.

Intramedullary Nailing Techniques

Several intramedullary devices and techniques have been designed for the treatment of three- and four-part proximal humerus fractures. Designs were created as an alternative to rigid plate fixation to avoid excessive soft tissue dissection. Intramedullary devices that were unlocked have been associated with proximal migration of the rod, leading to subacromial impingement and necessitating their early removal. Intramedullary devices with a facility for locking have been designed to allow control of rotation and prevent proximal migration.

In 1986, Mouradian reported his 7-year experience with a modified Zickel supracondylar device for the treatment of displaced proximal humerus fractures (30). The device offers screw fixation in cancellous bone and a flexible intramedullary portion for diaphyseal fixation. Fracture fixation is not rigid and allows for some telescoping of the fracture site. Mouradian's technique employed two screws for fixation into the humeral head directed 15 degrees cephalad. In addition to fixation of displaced three- and four-part fractures and dislocations, the device was also used for two-part fractures, pathologic fractures, and selected fractures of the proximal humeral shaft. There was a slight correlation between increasing age and decreasing clinical result. There were no nonunions, vascular injuries, or infection. Avascular necrosis occurred in three patients with four-part fractures; however, there was no collapse of the articular surface, no significant pain, and no decrease in functional score with time.

The Polarus Nail (Accumed, Inc., Beaverton, OR) was designed to provide a more rigid internal fixation system for proximal humerus fractures while preserving soft tissue attachments (Fig. 18-16). Unfavorable surgical results seen with other systems are commonly attributed to poor bone quality of the proximal humerus and the extensive soft tissue stripping required to visualize the fracture fragments. Intramedullary nailing attempts to solve the dilemma between the extensive exposure required to achieve rigid internal fixation, which allows early active motion, and fracture ischemia and soft tissue disruption.

Intramedullary nailing offers the advantages of creating a strong stable fixation that is effective in protecting the fracture from bending and axial loading. With the addition of interlocking screws, the construct is also stable in torsion. Wheeler and Colville showed in a biomechanical comparison that the intramedullary nailing provided a stronger,

more stable, and durable fixation option than did percutaneous pin fixation for large-fragment multipart proximal humerus fractures with minimal comminution (31). The intramedullary device was shown to have a greater stiffness and less angular displacement of fragments during cyclic loading when compared with percutaneous pin fixation. When loading the constructs to failure, the nail proved to have greater failure torques, stiffness, energy absorbed, and angular displacement before failure. In another biomechanical study, Ruch and colleagues compared the stability of tension band wires with supplemental Enders nails, modified the cloverleaf plate and screws, and the intramedullary nail (32). Plate and screw fixation and intramedullary nailing was shown to provide greater torsional and bending stiffness compared with tension band wires with Enders nails. There was no statistically significant difference in torsional or bending stiffness between intramedullary nailing with interlocks and plate and screw fixation.

The technique of intramedullary nail insertion uses a deltoid splitting approach. The patient is placed on a radiolucent table in the beach chair position. A longitudinal incision is made in line with the greater tuberosity and the deltoid muscle is bluntly divided in the line of its fibers. A 1-cm longitudinal incision is created in the supraspinatus tendon. A bone awl is then used to create an entry hole immediately medial to the greater tuberosity and approximately 1.5 cm posterior to the bicipital groove. Fracture

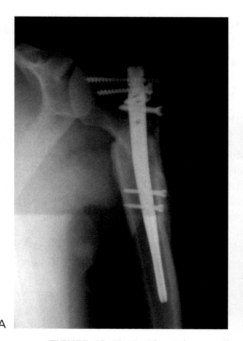

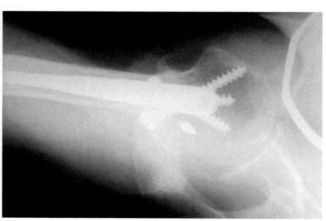

A

B

FIGURE 18-16. A: The Polarus nail was designed to offer rigid fixation of multipart proximal humerus fractures with minimal soft tissue disruption. The angled positioning of proximal holes allows screws to be placed in multiple planes to capture the tuberosity fragments and secure them to the head piece. **B:** Axillary radiographs are mandatory during nailing for proximal humerus fractures to ensure that no screws penetrate through the articular surface of the humeral head.

reduction is achieved by closed methods whenever possible. Open reduction is necessary if reduction is impeded by soft tissue interposition or adhesions, as in delayed cases. A 2-mm guidewire is then passed across the fracture site, followed by an optional cannulated broach. The nail is then inserted over the guidewire and locked proximally and distally under fluoroscopic guidance in both anteroposterior and axillary planes. The supraspinatus incision is closed with nonabsorbable suture, followed by closure of the deltoid muscle and skin. Postoperatively, mobilization is achieved through active assisted exercises until tuberosity union is achieved radiographically, then progressing to active exercises.

Early clinical reports using the Polarus nail have demonstrated good functional results in the treatment of displaced proximal humerus fractures in both the young and the elderly patient with osteopenic bone. Rajasekhar and co-workers reported on 30 patients treated with the Polarus nail, 14 of whom were older than 60 years of age (33). By Constant score, 20 of 25 patients (80%) showed satisfactory to excellent functional outcomes. Complications included one nonunion, one patient with shoulder stiffness, one case of avascular necrosis, and one case of a screw backing out. Adedapo and Ikpeme reported on 23 patients with acute displaced three- and four-part proximal humerus fractures, including seven patients with associated shaft involvement, treated with the Polarus nail (34). At 1-year follow-up, the median Neer scores were 89 and 60 for the three- and four-part fractures, respectively. Three patients (13%), all in the four-part group, continued to have significant pain at final review. In three patients, complications included proximal screw loosening and extrusion, which required removal, and one patient had avascular necrosis with head collapse and nail protrusion, which necessitated removal of the entire device.

Intramedullary nail fixation should be used with caution in the overhead athletic population, because the rotator cuff is violated during nail insertion. Although nonathletes may not suffer postoperative functional difficulties, the competitive overhead athlete may not be as fortunate because of the repetitive function of the rotator cuff needed during any overhead sporting activity.

Distal Clavicle Fractures

Although the majority of type I and III distal clavicle fractures are recommended to be treated nonoperatively, there still remains considerable debate regarding the ideal method of treatment for type II fractures (Fig. 18-17). These fractures have been reported to have an increased incidence of nonunion and prolonged convalescence when treated nonoperatively. Displacement of the fracture fragments (the weight of the arm pulls the distal fragment inferiorly and the trapezius pulls the proximal fragment superiorly) makes this type of fracture difficult to manage.

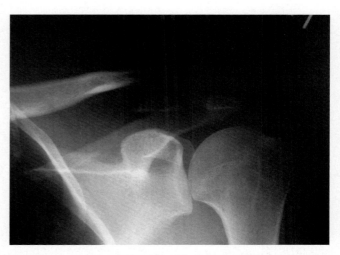

FIGURE 18-17. Type II distal clavicle fracture. This fracture was treated with excision of the distal fragments and modified Weaver Dunn reconstruction of the remaining clavicle segment.

It may be possible to achieve a closed reduction; however, the difficulty comes in maintaining the reduction. The standard figure-of-eight bandage is almost always inadequate. The Kenny-Howard sling may be used to hold the distal clavicle reduced in a manner similar to its use with a grade III acromioclavicular joint separation. This device, however, requires continual wear and adjustment for optimal results. For this reason, compliance is often poor.

Nonoperative management may not be the most conservative method of management for these displaced fractures, especially in the overhead athlete. The incidence of nonunion with the closed treatment has been reported to be as high as 30% (13). Pain and functional limitations develop in many of the individuals whose injury goes on to a nonunion. The incidence of symptomatic nonunions has been reported to be as high as 80% (35). In addition to this increased risk of nonunion, a prolonged convalescence period is almost inevitable with nonoperative treatment. Neer (35) reported on 17 patients treated with closed reduction and some form of external support. None of these fractures were united with callus before 16 weeks after injury. Of those fractures that went on to heal, all were considered delayed in union.

Because of the high rate of nonunion and delayed convalescence, many investigators have advocated surgery for these injuries. Many techniques have been described, ranging from primary excision of the distal clavicle fragment with repair of the disrupted coracoclavicular ligaments to open reduction and internal fixation of the fracture. Neer (35) was the first to document that early internal fixation of these fractures without ligament repair resulted in improved outcome when compared with nonoperative management. He recommended that when this lesion is encountered, open reduction and internal fixation is indicated unless precluded by the general condition of the patient.

Many methods of surgical stabilization exist for treatment of type II fractures. When the outer clavicle segment is small and comminuted, the distal fragment can be excised and the clavicle can be fixed to the coracoid in a similar fashion to the Weaver-Dunn procedure. When the distal segment is larger, a plate may be considered. With this method, caution must be taken to ensure that at least four cortices can be achieved in the lateral fragment. If this is not possible, failure of the fixation almost always occurs. Proper surgical intervention does not always ensure a satisfactory outcome. Complication and failure rates have ranged in the literature from 17% to 30%. For this reason, the type II distal clavicle fractures remain the most challenging clavicle fracture to treat.

Midshaft Clavicle Fractures

The indications for surgery for midshaft clavicle fractures include open fractures, displaced fractures with potential compromise of the overlying skin, and fracture associated with neurovascular injury. In cases of severe fracture displacement, without an open wound or neurovascular compromise, an attempt at closed reduction may be warranted. When there is greater than 100% overlap of the fracture fragments, a higher incidence of nonunion exists. In the athlete, this may represent an indication for surgery to prevent a prolonged convalescence. Typically, a 3.5-mm AO reconstruction or dynamic compression plate, or some form of intramedullary fixation, is the most appropriate form of surgical stabilization.

AO plates are malleable, allowing them to be contoured to the curved shape of the clavicle. By contrast, intramedullary devices, by their nature, avoid the irregular exterior of the clavicle, achieving their stability internally by three-point fixation. Smooth pins should be avoided because of risk of migration. In general, if surgery is required, a plate is the preferred method of fixation. Exceptions include thin individuals in whom the plate may lead to skin erosion or when there is extensive fracture comminution that precludes food screws purchase. The hardware should be removed in athletes before returning to collision sports.

Displaced midshaft fractures are exposed using a curvilinear incision 1 cm anterior, and therefore inferior, to the clavicle. This is taken down through subcutaneous tissue to the platysma and trapezius fascia. The fracture is subperiosteally exposed and reduced. Standard AO technique is used to achieve fixation. A 3.5-mm reconstruction or dynamic compression plate is used, allowing contouring to the clavicular shape. Extreme care is necessary to avoid the neurovascular structures inferior and posterior to the clavicle, especially during the drilling and determination of screw length. The plate is ideally placed superior on the clavicle, which represents the tension side of this fracture. The plate can alternatively be placed on the anteroinferior aspect of the clavicle. This has the advantages of less skin compromise and potentially decreasing the risk of injury to the neurovascular structures. If fracture orientation allows, the plate in this position allows the direction of the drill, tap, and screw to be from anteroinferior to posterosuperior, providing the least opportunity for neurovascular compromise.

A similar but shorter incision is made when using intramedullary fixation and the fracture is exposed. The lateral or distal fragment is elevated, exposing its medullary canal. Several forms of intramedullary fixation devices have been historically described. The Rockwood Clavicular Screw (DePuy, Warsaw, IN) is a current popular intramedullary device. With the medullary canal exposed, the screw is advanced though the distal fragment medullary canal, exiting the posterior clavicle just before the acromioclavicular joint. The fracture is then reduced and the screw is advanced into the medullary canal of the medial fragment, thereby engaging the threaded shaft and resisting migration. Once the fracture has been stabilized, the screw is left just within the subcutaneous tissue so that it may later be removed once union has been achieved. If not needed for additional compression across the fracture site, the nut should not be used because it may cause significant irritation just under the skin.

Spiral Humeral Shaft Fractures

Most spiral humeral shaft fractures can be treated successfully with closed management, usually with a coaptation splint followed by functional bracing as previously described. Generally, these fractures heal within 6 to 10 weeks. Open treatment has been reported in 16 cases in the literature, usually for failure to obtain closed reduction (36). Muscle interposition at the fracture site was noted in a number of these cases. Heilbronner and associates have stated that open reduction and internal fixation should be reserved for markedly displaced segmental fractures, fractures associated with elbow articular injuries requiring early mobilization, fractures associated with vascular injuries, radial nerve palsy present after a manipulation of the fracture, and inability to obtain reduction due to soft tissue interposition (36).

There is no series in the literature that demonstrates superiority of open reduction and internal fixation over closed management of these fractures. These fractures are the result of low-energy trauma, which in most cases preserves the periosteal and muscular envelope of the humerus. With uneventful healing of the humeral fracture at 3 months, a full range of motion should be present, and strengthening exercises from 3 to 6 months are then required. When strength returns, sports are resumed. Contact sports require a functional humeral brace or a protective pad during the first year of competition.

POSTOPERATIVE REHABILITATION

The postoperative program for shoulder conditioning therapy (Table 18-3) following surgery is divided into three

TABLE 18–3. THREE-PHASE SHOULDER CONDITIONING THERAPY FOR THE POSTOPERATIVE MANAGEMENT OF SHOULDER GIRDLE FRACTURES

Phase 1
1. ICE
   Or as necessary

Days per week: 7   Times per day: 4–5
15–20 minutes "ON" maximum
60 minutes "OFF" maximum

2. STRETCHING: PASSIVE MOTION
   Days per week: 7 — Times per day: 4–5

Exercise	Sets	Reps
Pendulum exercise	1–2 sets	20–30 reps
Supine external rotation	1–2 sets	10–15 reps
Supine forward elevation (overhead elbow lift)	1–2 sets	5–10 reps
Standing internal rotation (thumb behind back)	1–2 sets	5–10 reps

Phase 2
1. ICE — See phase 1
2. STRETCHING: ACTIVE MOTION (WITH TERMINAL STRETCH)
   Days per week: 7 — Times per day: 3–4

Exercise	Sets	Reps
Pendulum exercise	1–2 sets	20–30 reps
Supine-seated external rotation	1–2 sets	10–15 reps
Supine-seated forward elevation (overhead elbow lift)	1–2 sets	5–10 reps
Standing internal rotation (thumb behind back)	1–2 sets	5–10 reps

Phase 3
1. ICE: — See phase 1
2. STRETCHING: ACTIVE MOTION (WITH TERMINAL STRETCH). See phase 2
   ADD LATE TERMINAL STRETCHING: Days per week: 7 Times per day: 3–4

Exercise	Sets	Reps
Side door stretch	1–2 sets	5–10 reps
Overhead door stretch	1–2 sets	5–10 reps
Double-arm door stretch	1–2 sets	5–10 reps

3. CORD STRENGTHENING
   Days per week: 7 — Times per day: 1–2

Exercise	Sets	Reps
External rotation	1–2 sets	10–15 reps
Internal rotation	1–2 sets	10–15 reps
Standing forward punch	1–2 sets	10–15 reps
Shoulder shrug	1–2 sets	10–15 reps
Seated row	1–2 sets	10–15 reps

phases: (a) the passive stretching phase, (b) the active stretching phase, and (c) the cord strengthening phase. Individual postoperative therapy programs are outlined for clavicle open reduction-internal fixation (ORIF) (Table 18-4), proximal humerus percutaneous pinning (Table 18-5), and proximal humerus ORIF (Table 18-6).

Icing is recommended during the first two phases to reduce pain, swelling, and discomfort. Icing is performed for 15 to 20 minutes with at least a 60-minute break in between. Ice is placed in a towel or in zipper lock bag and a towel and applied to the injured area. Ice is never placed directly on the skin.

Shoulder stretching is divided into two phases. Phase 1, or passive range of motion, is always performed with the uninjured arm assisting or helping the operated arm. Phase 2, or active range of motion with a terminal stretch, is only performed with the operated arm. In most instances, passive range of motion is weaned by using the uninjured arm in isolated incidents to assist the operated arm. The other major difference between passive and active stretching involves the "terminal stretch." During active stretching and upon reaching the endpoint of pain or movement, the operated arm is pushed with the uninjured hand another 5

TABLE 18–4. POSTOPERATIVE SHOULDER CONDITIONING THERAPY FOLLOWING ORIF OF DISTAL AND MIDSHAFT CLAVICLE FRACTURES

Weeks Postoperative	Treatment
0–4 weeks	Sling immobilization
4–5 weeks	Phase I
5–6 weeks	Phase II
6 weeks	Phase III
Return to Activities	
Weight training	3 months
	No long lever-arm exercises
	No abducted positions
	No impingement positions
Computer	5 weeks
Golf	3–3.5 months
Tennis	4 months
Contact sports	4–5 months

ORIF, open reduction-internal fixation.

TABLE 18–5. POSTOPERATIVE SHOULDER CONDITIONING THERAPY FOLLOWING PERCUTANEOUS PINNING OF PROXIMAL HUMERUS FRACTURES

Weeks Postoperative	Treatment
0–6 weeks	Sling immobilization
3 weeks	Pins removed in office
3–6 weeks	Phase I (continue to use sling)
6–10 weeks	Phase II (discontinue sling)
10 weeks	Phase III
16 weeks	Late terminal stretching
Return to Activities	
Computer	2 months
Golf	4 months
Tennis	5 months
Contact sports	5–6 months

to 10 degrees for additional movement. This final movement is called *terminal stretch*. Maximum motion for each patient remains the goal and terminal stretching assists in achieving this goal.

All stretching exercises should be done slowly to maximize muscle and soft connective tissue involvement. When stretching, the goal is to reach the maximum range of motion for the individual patient. The reason for multiple sets and repetitions stems from "warming up" the shoulder so it can actually stretch further in the last few repetitions. The first few repetitions prepare the stiffened or swollen shoulder for initial movement. Because there is more than one repetition per set, the first one or two repetitions are warm-up repetitions, with very little pain, and range of motion is gradually increased during following repetitions.

It is important to let pain be a guide during passive stretching. The arm is moved to the endpoint (which is dictated by pain). The goal is to increase the endpoint as often as possible until full range of motion is achieved. Excruciating pain is to be avoided, but uncomfortable pain is toler-

ated, as long as the pain does not remain for a prolonged period of time. A basic rule to follow when stretching is that if the pain does not linger, then stretching was not performed far enough.

Specific passive stretching exercises in the first phase of rehabilitation include pendulum exercises, supine external rotation, supine forward elevation (overhead elbow lift), and standing internal rotation (thumb behind back). Pendulum exercises, although not considered a "true" stretch, acts as a warm-up exercise. The program should always begin with pendulum exercises. In addition to supine stretching exercises, pulley exercises can be added during this phase to assist with forward flexion, abduction, external rotation, and internal rotation.

Phase two exercises include icing and pendulum exercises, as well as advances to active motion stretching with terminal stretch. These exercises include supine-seated external rotation, supine-seated forward elevation (overhead elbow lift), and standing internal rotation (thumb behind back). Additionally, the towel modification can be added to assist with internal rotation up the back.

Phase three exercises also include icing, pendulum exercises for warm-up, and active motion stretching with terminal stretch, but adds more aggressive stretching exercises and cord strengthening. Additional stretching exercises during this phase include side-arm door stretching, overhead door stretching, and double-arm door stretching. Cord strengthening exercises are resistance exercises that should be done very slowly in *both* directions. The goal is to achieve a maximum amount of strengthening while listening to the endpoint of pain. Strengthening is achieved throughout the full range of motion. It is important for this exercise to be done slowly, not only when the exercise is completed (concentric), but also when coming back to the starting position (eccentric). A slower motion achieves the maximal contraction throughout the full range of motion. Specific cord strengthening exercises include external rotation, internal rotation, standing forward punch, shoulder shrug, and seated rows (narrow-middle-wide grip).

TABLE 18–6. POSTOPERATIVE SHOULDER CONDITIONING THERAPY FOLLOWING ORIF OF PROXIMAL HUMERUS FRACTURES

Weeks Postoperative	Treatment
0–6 weeks	Sling immobilization
0–6 weeks	Phase I
6–10 weeks	Phase II
10 weeks	Phase III
16 weeks	Late terminal stretching
Return to Activities	
Computer	2 months
Golf	4 months
Tennis	5 months
Contact sports	5–6 months

ORIF, open reduction-internal fixation.

COMPLICATIONS

Proximal Humerus Fractures

In the past 25 years, open reduction and internal fixation has been widely advocated for the treatment of displaced three- and four-part proximal humerus fractures. In many cases, the deformity cannot be maintained by closed reduction techniques and immobilization. The blood supply to the humeral head is at significant risk not only from the injury, but also from the dissection of soft tissues during open reduction and fixation. Avascular necrosis of the humeral head following fracture is considered particularly deleterious and can potentially be associated with a painful and functionally poor outcome. An incidence between 3% and 14% has been reported for three-part fractures, whereas the incidence in four-part fractures has been reported to be between 13% and 34% (37). A proximal humerus fracture that is at risk for avascular necrosis has to be reduced anatomically if joint-preserving treatment is selected.

Malunion of a proximal humerus fracture is a potential complication that can result from inadequate operative reduction, loss of operative reduction, or nonoperative treatment of a displaced fracture. Most patients with malunions of the proximal humerus present with pain and stiffness of the shoulder, which often cause severe functional impairment. Disruption of the normal anatomic relationships can result in a loss of motion and strength of the shoulder. Osseous abnormalities can involve malposition of the greater or lesser tuberosities, incongruity of the articular surface, or malalignment of the articular segment (38). In addition to the osseous involvement of the malunion, soft tissue scarring and tears of the tendons of the rotator cuff can also contribute to stiffness and loss of strength. Successful operative management is achieved only if all osseous and soft tissue abnormalities are corrected at the time of operation.

Nonunion of a fracture of the proximal humerus is uncommon and associated with pain, stiffness, and disability of the affected shoulder. Nonunions are most frequent after displaced two-part surgical neck fractures, but can less commonly occur with three- and four-part fractures. Factors identified with the development of nonunion include inadequate immobilization or premature motion, failed internal fixation, soft tissue interposition, osteopenia, wide separation or distraction of the fracture, and systemic medical disease. Although satisfactory reconstruction of these nonunions can be obtained, the overall outcome in most studies is only fair.

Complications of percutaneous pin fixation include pin loosening and migration. Young patients with adequate bone stock rarely experience this complication, whereas patients with poor bone quality or lack of compliance during aftercare are more likely. Insufficient reduction of the fracture leading to an unstable construct is a common factor that can lead to pin loosening and migration. Other factors have also been identified including unstable reduction, too few pins, lack of a proximal to distal pin counterbalancing the varus force of the cuff, and the use of pins that lie too close together and fail to provide rotational stability. Poor bone quality and metaphyseal comminution can likely lead to loss of fixation and failure of union.

Pin migration is a potential problem that can occur with percutaneous pinning. Terminally threaded pins should always be used and smooth wires avoided. Serial radiographs in the postoperative period should be obtained to identify and remove any loose pins. Pin tract infections are a possible complication if the pins are not cut well below the surface of the skin. Permanent loss of motion due to

scarring is a potential problem after transcutaneous fixation, although it is uncommon. Another uncommon complication that has been reported is a fracture through the pin holes after pin removal.

Complications of tension band techniques include a poor rotator cuff that requires mobilization and repair and less than adequate holding power in the soft bone. Wire can be tied with greater compression compared to suture, but can also cut through osteoporotic bone. Wires have a propensity to break and migration of their pieces poses a significant problem. Although tension band technique paired with Ender rods has the additional advantage of intramedullary fixation, complications are similar to those reported for tension band alone.

Plate fixation of proximal humerus fractures also has unique complications. The use of a plate increases the possibility of postoperative impingement between the greater tuberosity and the acromion. This complication is common when the plate is placed too high on the greater tuberosity. The additional surgical exposure potentially increases the risk for avascular necrosis of the humeral head.

Intramedullary nailing offers the potential for stable fixation of proximal humerus fractures with minimal soft tissue disruption. Early published studies reported few complications with device, including fracture nonunion, shoulder stiffness, avascular necrosis, and proximal screw loosening. There is concern with antegrade humeral nailing techniques that involve violation of the rotator cuff with an opening incision. Meticulous closure with nonabsorbable suture must be achieved to optimize soft tissue healing in these cases. Another potential complication of humeral nailing is leaving the proximal portion of the nail proud, thereby irritating the overlying supraspinatus tendon and causing mechanical impingement under the acromion. Finally, with early motion of the shoulder with intramedullary nail fixation, the proximal locking screws can have a tendency to loosen and back out, thereby potentially loosing fixation of the proximal fragments. Loose screws cause mechanical irritation and must be removed or replaced to prevent further complications.

Clavicle Fractures

The most common complication with distal clavicle fractures is nonunion. In adults, most fractures heal in 6 weeks. Nonunion is generally determined when the fracture has failed to show clinical or radiographic progression of healing at 4 to 6 months (39). Distal clavicle fractures have a higher incidence in nonunion and account for more than half of the ununited fractures after closed treatment (14). Increasing severity of trauma has been reported to be responsible for up to 50% of the nonunions (39). Healed fractures are thought to have an altered blood supply, making them susceptible to nonunion. If a fracture occurs through a previously healed area, it is thought that further alteration of the vascularity occurs (40). With increasing degrees of displacement, there is a higher likelihood of soft tissue interposition, which alters healing (39). Finally, poor internal fixation may play a primary role in nonunion. If a nonunion occurs, the patient is often asymptomatic and requires no further treatment. Nordquist (15) reported a nonunion rate of 22% in his series of distal clavicle fractures treated nonoperatively. Of those with a nonunion, 80% were asymptomatic. The remaining 20% were asymptomatic, but not enough to require surgery. Malunion is common, but rarely symptomatic. These usually represent a cosmetic problem. If nonunion develops and is painful or a malunion is symptomatic, a salvage procedure such as a Mumford or a Weaver-Dunn reconstruction can be performed.

Neurovascular compromise often is the result of abundant callus, malunion, or fracture displacement. The vascular structures that have been reported to be involved in compression syndromes include the carotid artery, subclavian vein, and subclavian artery. The brachial plexus can be injured as a result of neuropraxia or a progressive compres-

sion effect on the medial cord. This usually presents clinically as ulnar nerve symptoms. Finally, posttraumatic symptoms of the joint may follow intraarticular injuries of the acromioclavicular joint. This is often the result of an unrecognized type III distal clavicle fracture.

AUTHORS' PREFERRED TREATMENT ALGORITHMS AND TECHNIQUES

Proximal Humerus Fractures

Eighty percent to 85% of proximal humerus fracture can be treated nonoperatively as previously outlined. For those fractures with displacement of greater than 1 cm and angulation greater than 45 degrees, surgery to restore normal anatomy of the proximal humerus is required. Greater tuberosity fractures that are displaced as little as 5 mm are also surgical candidates, especially in the overhead athlete. Irreducible fracture-dislocations and those reducible fracture-dislocations with residual displacement require surgical reconstruction.

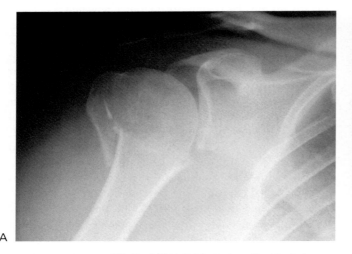
A

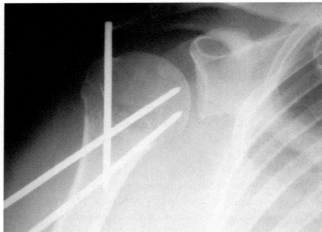
B

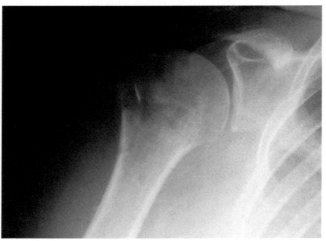
C

FIGURE 18-18. A,B: Closed reduction of this proximal humerus fracture allowed percutaneous pin fixation with three terminally threaded guide wires. Pin were removed at 3 weeks in the office and led to successful healing of the fracture **(C).**

Our surgical protocol for displaced proximal humerus fractures begins with an attempt at a closed reduction under general anesthesia. If an anatomic reduction is achieved, the fracture is then checked for stability under live fluoroscopy. If a stable reduction is obvious, then the fracture is treated closed according to the conservative treatment outline. If a guarded or unstable reduction is achieved, then a percutaneous pinning technique is used (Fig. 18-18). Two terminally threaded pins are used in a retrograde fashion to secure the humeral shaft to the humeral head fragment. If a greater tuberosity fragment exists, then a third pin is advanced through the tuberosity in an antegrade fashion, engaging the inferomedial cortex, just below the surgical neck fracture line. Finally, if a lesser tuberosity fragment exists, a single pin is inserted anterosuperior to inferoposterior to capture and secure this fragment. The shoulder is then brought through a range of motion under live fluoroscopy to assess stability of the repair. Additional pins are inserted for added stability if required. If a stable repair cannot be achieved, the percutaneous technique is abandoned for a open reduction and internal fixation method. Final radiographs in the AP and axillary planes are checked to confirm that no pin penetrates the humeral head. The pins are then removed at 3 weeks. Postoperative therapy program is followed as previously outlined.

When an open reduction and internal fixation technique is required, our current protocol uses the Synthes AO 3.5-mm LCP Proximal Humerus Plate (Fig. 18-19). The locking compression plate (LCP) for the proximal humerus was designed to address complex fractures of the proximal humerus including fractures and fracture-dislocations, osteotomies, and nonunions of the proximal humerus, particularly for patients with osteopenic bone. This plate has distinct characteristics over previous plates used for proximal humerus fractures because it is anatomically shaped for the proximal humerus anatomy. Multiple proximal locking holes accept 3.5-mm locking screws, which function as individual fixed angled devices in both divergent and convergent patterns for added stability. Ten suture holes are located around the perimeter of the proximal end of the plate to assist with additional suture repair of the tuberosities or the rotator cuff.

The LCP Proximal Humerus Plate is applied through the standard deltopectoral approach as previously described. A temporary reduction of the fragments can be held with K-wires to assist with plate application. This particular plate is an excellent choice for two-part surgical neck fractures and three-part neck and greater tuberosity fractures (Fig. 18-20). Four-part fractures of the proximal humerus, as with all other plating techniques for the proximal humerus, require supplemental suture or screw fixation of the lesser tuberosity fragment. This plating technique allows rigid anatomic fixation of proximal humerus fractures so that early passive motion can be instituted to prevent postoperative stiffness.

Distal Clavicle Fractures

Type I and III fractures of the distal clavicle are typically treated nonoperatively with a graduated therapy program as previously outlined. Type II distal clavicle fractures are usually managed surgically because of their high potential for complications with conservative care. The size of the distal fragment dictates which surgical technique will be used. In situations with a small or comminuted distal fragment, our first choice is to excise the distal fragment and then perform a modified Weaver-Dunn type procedure with concomitant coracoclavicular fixation. This secures the distal end of the medial fragment to the coracoid using a transferred coracoacromial ligament as an autograft. The repair is further augmented with a braided nine-strand number 0 PDS (polydioxanone) suture, which is passed around the coracoid and through a drill hole in the clavicle in a figure-of-eight technique. If necessary, this is further supplemented with an autogenous hamstring tendon for coracoclavicular reconstruction as well as acromioclavicular joint superior capsular reconstruction (to resist anteroposterior plane clavicular instability).

If the distal fragment is large, then we prefer rigid fixation with a plate and screw construct. This technique requires a minimum of four cortices in the distal fragment. Bone grafting is recommended to increase the rate of healing. The distal clavicle plate fixation is further supplemented with a braided nine-strand number 0 PDS (polydioxanone) suture and autogenous palmaris or hamstring tendon passed around the coracoid and over the clavicle.

Midshaft Clavicle Fractures

We manage most midshaft fractures with a well-padded commercial figure-of-eight splint or sling for comfort. Occasionally a closed reduction is necessary. A postreduction radiograph is used to evaluate the reduction. Rehabilitation as outlined previously is started as soon as the patient can participate comfortably.

It is rare that a fracture of the shaft of the clavicle requires an open reduction and internal fixation. If a completely displaced fracture of the midshaft of the clavicle cannot be reduced with closed manipulation, we observe the patient for 2 weeks in the figure-of-eight splint. If after observation the complete displacement persists, we recommend open reduction and internal fixation with a 3.5-mm reconstruction or dynamic compression plate as previously described.

Humeral Shaft Fractures

Humeral shaft fractures are treated with a coaptation splint for 2 weeks and then converted to a functional fracture brace for a total of 6 weeks. By 6 weeks, these fractures are usually nontender and demonstrate radiographic callus. A

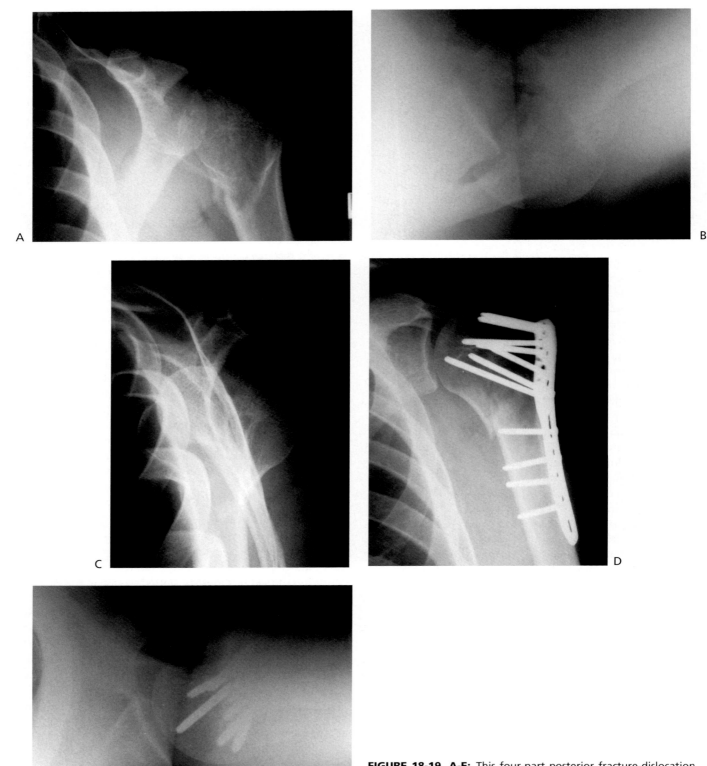

FIGURE 18-19. A-E: This four-part posterior fracture-dislocation was treated with the AO locking compression plate (LCP) for the proximal humerus. The lesser tuberosity fragment was stabilized with transosseous suture fixation. Stable fixation allowed for early passive motion and eventual healing.

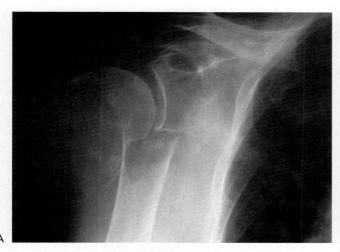

A

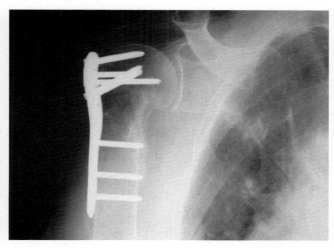

B

FIGURE 18-20. A,B: The AO-LCP plate is also an excellent option for displaced two-part proximal humerus fractures that require open reduction.

graduated range-of-motion and strengthening program is resumed at this time. Particular emphasis is placed on regaining external rotation, which is important for the overhead athlete (Fig. 18–21).

Open reduction and internal fixation with plate fixation is reserved only for severely displaced fractures that cannot be reduced, combined vascular injuries that require repair, loss of radial nerve function after manipulation, and ipsilateral elbow or forearm fractures. We do not use intramedullary nail fixation for the treatment of displaced humeral shaft fractures in the overhead athlete because of the previously mentioned potential for postoperative rotator cuff dysfunction or subacromial impingement and pain from the nail insertion.

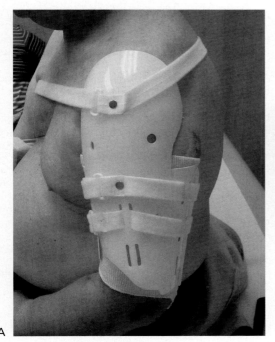

A

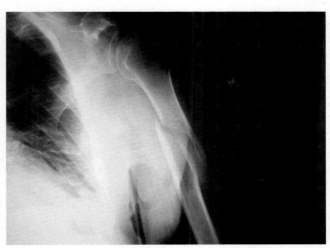

B

FIGURE 18-21. A: Preferred treatment for spiral humeral shaft fractures is functional fracture bracing. B: A radiograph with the brace applied is obtained to confirm appropriate alignment of the fracture fragments.

REFERENCES

1. Hagg O, Lundberg G. Apsects of prognostic factors of comminuted and dislocated proximal humerus fractures. In: Bateman JE, Welsh RP, eds: *Surgery of the shoulder.* Philadelphia: BC Decker, 1984.
2. Landin LA. Fracture patterns in children. *Acta Orthop Scand* 1983;202[Suppl]:1–109.
3. Flatow EL, Bigliani LU, April EW. An anatomic study of the musculocutaneous nerve and its relationship to the coracoid process. *Clin Orthop* 1989;244:166–171.
4. Dameron TB, Rockwood CA. Fractures of the shaft of the clavicle. In Rockwood CA, Wilkins KE, King RE, eds. *Fractures in children.* Philadelphia: JB Lippincott, 1984:608.
5. Fawcett J. The development and ossification of the human clavicle. *J Anat* 1913;47:225–234.
6. Ogden JA, Conologue GJ, Bronson NL. Radiology of postnatal skeletal development. Vol 3. The clavicle. *Skeletal Radiol* 1979;4:196–203.
7. Ljunggren AE. Clavicular function. *Acta Orthop Scand* 1979;50:261–268.
8. Neer CS II. Displaced proximal humeral fractures. Part I. Classification and evaluation. *J Bone Joint Surg (Am)* 1970;52(6):1077–1089.
9. Neer CS II. Displaced proximal humeral fractures. Part II. Treatment of three-part and four-part displacement. *J Bone Joint Surg (Am)* 1970;52(6):1090–1103.
10. Muller ME, Nazarian S, Koch P, et al. The comprehensive classification of fractures of long bones. Berlin: Springer-Verlag, 1990:54.
11. Jakob RP, Miniaci A, Anson PS, et al. Four-part valgus impacted fractures of the proximal humerus. *J Bone Joint Surg (Br)* 1991;73:295–298.
12. Craig EV. Fractures of the clavicle. In Rockwood CA, Matsen FA, eds. *The shoulder.* Philadelphia: WB Saunders, 1990.
13. Neer CS II: Fractures of the distal third of the clavicle. *Clin Orthop* 1968;58:43–50..
14. Neer CS II. Nonunion of the clavicle. *JAMA* 1960;172:1006–1011.
15. Nordquist A, Petersson C, Redlund-Johnell I. The natural course of lateral clavicle fracture. *Acta Orthop Scand* 1993;64:87–91.
16. Nowak J, Holgersson M, Larsson S. Can we predict sequelae following fractures of clavicle based on initial findings? A prospective study with 9-10 years follow up. Presented at the American Shoulder and Elbows Surgeons 18th Open Meeting, Dallas, Texas, February 16, 2002.
17. McKee MD, Pederson B, Jones C, et al. Previously unrecognized deficits following conservative treatment of displaced, mid-shaft fracture of the clavicle detected by patient-based outcome measures and objective muscle strength testing. Presented at the American Shoulder and Elbows Surgeons 19th Open Meeting, New Orleans, Louisiana, February 8, 2003.
18. Sarmiento A, Kinman PB, Galvin EG, et al. Functional bracing of fractures of the shaft of the humerus. *J Bone Joint Surg Am* 1977;59:596–601.
19. Wallny T, Westerman K, Sagebiel C, et al. Functional treatment of humeral shaft fractures: indications and results. *J Orthop Trauma* 1991;11:283–287.
20. Balfour GW, Mooney V, Ashby ME. Diaphyseal fractures of the humerus treated with a ready-made fracture brace. *J Bone Joint Surg (Am)* 1982;64:1–15.
21. Herscovici D, Saunders DT, Johnson MP, et al. Percutaneous fixation of proximal humeral fractures. *Clin Orthop* 2000;375:97–104.
22. Williams GR, Wong KL. Two-part and three-part fractures: open reduction and internal fixation versus closed reduction and percutaneous pinning. *Orthop Clin North Am* 2000;31(1):1–21.
23. Resch H, Beck E, Bayley I. Reconstruction of the valgus-impacted humeral head fracture. *J Shoulder Elbow Surg* 1995;4:73–80.
24. Hawkins RJ, Bell RH, Gurr K. The three-part fracture of the proximal humerus: operative treatment. *J Bone Joint Surg (Am)* 1986;68(9):1410–1414.
25. Cuomo F, Zuckerman JD. Open reduction and internal fixation of two- and three-part proximal humerus fractures. *Tech Orthop* 1994;9(2):141–153.
26. Savoie FH, Geissler WB, Vander Griend RA. Open reduction and internal fixation of three-part fractures of the proximal humerus. *Orthopedics* 1989;12(1):65–70.
27. Esser RD. Treatment of three- and four-part fractures of the proximal humerus with a modified cloverleaf plate. *J Orthop Trauma* 1994;8(1):15–22.
28. Esser RD. Open reduction and internal fixation of three- and four-part fractures of the proximal humerus. *Clin Orthop* 1994;299:244–251.
29. Hintermann B, Trouillier HH, Schäfer D. Rigid internal fixation of fractures of the proximal humerus in older patients. *J Bone Joint Surg (Br)* 2000;82(8):1107–1112.
30. Mouradian WH. Displaced proximal humerus fractures. Seven years' experience with a modified Zickel supracondylar device. *Clin Orthop* 1986;212:209–218.
31. Wheeler DL, Colville MR. Biomechanical comparison of intramedullary and percutaneous pin fixation for proximal humeral fracture fixation. *J Orthop Trauma* 1997;11(5):363–367.
32. Ruch DS, Glisson RR, Marr AW, et al. Fixation of three-part proximal humeral fractures: a biomechanical evaluation. *J Orthop Trauma* 2000;14(1):36–40.
33. Rajasekhar C, Ray PS, Bhamra MS. Fixation of proximal humeral fractures with the Polarus nail. *J Shoulder Elbow Surg* 2001;10(1):7–10.
34. Adedapo AO, Ikpeme JO. The results of internal fixation of three- and four-part proximal humeral fractures with the Polarus nail. *Injury* 2001;32:115–121.
35. Neer CS II. Fractures of the distal clavicle with detachment of the coracoclavicular ligaments in adults. *J Trauma* 1963;3:99–110.
36. Heilbronner DM, Manoli A, Morawa LG. Fractures of the humerus in arm wrestlers. *Clin Orthop* 1980;149:169–171.
37. Gerber C, Hersche O, Berberat C. The clinical relevance of post-traumatic avascular necrosis of the humeral head. *J Shoulder Elbow Surg* 1998;7(6):586–590.
38. Beredjiklian PK, Iannotti JP, Norris TR, et al. Operative treatment of malunion of a fracture of the proximal humerus. *J Bone Joint Surg (Am)* 1998;80(10):1484–1497.
39. Jupiter JB, Leffert RD. Nonunion of the clavicle. *J Bone Joint Surg (Am)* 1987;69:753–760.
40. Watson-Jones R. *Fractures and joint injuries,* 5th ed. Baltimore: Williams & Wilkins, 1955.

19

NEUROLOGIC AND VASCULAR LESIONS

LOUIS U. BIGLIANI
WALTER G. STANWOOD
WILLIAM N. LEVINE

Neurologic and vascular lesions around the shoulder in an athlete can present with signs and symptoms that may overlap with other causes and can be a diagnostic challenge. Often the patient's complaints are vague and inconsistent. It is therefore imperative that the treating physician have a high index of suspicion when treating this patient population. This chapter outlines the diagnostic workup of the many neurologic and vascular lesions around the shoulder and presents both nonoperative and operative management of these challenging cases.

SUPRASCAPULAR NEUROPATHY

Historical Overview

Neuropathies of the shoulder are rare injuries and comprise less than 2% of all patients with pain and weakness in this region, which may lead to overlooking this diagnosis (1). In addition other diagnoses such as internal impingement, instability, and rotator cuff pathology may cloud the clinical picture in the overhead athlete.

Suprascapular neuropathy was first described by Andre Thomas in 1936 and was subsequently described as occurring at the suprascapular notch in the American literature by Kopell and Thompson (2,3). Initially repetitive motion was believed to be a primary etiologic factor. Since then numerous other causes of nerve injury have been described including tumors, ganglion cysts, traction injuries, and direct trauma (4–6).

Suprascapular neuropathy at the spinoglenoid notch was initially described by Ganzhorn and colleagues in 1981 and subsequently by Aiello and co-workers in 1982 (4,7). Volleyball players have been the subjects of the majority of spinoglenoid notch pathology (8–12), although suprascapular neuropathy has been described in baseball pitchers, archers, swimmers, weightlifters, football players, and tennis players (7,8,12–16).

Anatomy

The suprascapular nerve originates from the upper trunk of the brachial plexus, which is formed by the C5 and C6 roots. The nerve traverses the posterior cervical triangle, paralleling the omohyoid, and then going under the trapezius muscle. It then passes through the suprascapular notch below the transverse scapular ligament. The suprascapular artery and vein parallel the nerve passing cephalad to the ligament. The variable anatomy of the suprascapular notch has been elucidated by Hrdlicka and others, which has theoretical implications in the development of symptoms at this site (5,17,18). Hypertrophy and calcification of the transverse scapular ligament has also been identified as sources of nerve injury (17,19,20).

After passing through the notch, the nerve begins to arborize, with a variable number of motor branches to the supraspinatus and sensory innervation to the glenohumeral joint, acromioclavicular joint, coracohumeral ligament, and coracoacromial ligament (21–23). Two thirds of the shoulder joint has sensory and sympathetic innervation from the suprascapular nerve (16). Additionally, a cadaveric study identified a cutaneous innervation of the nerve in the proximal-lateral one third of the arm in approximately 15% of the specimens (24).

An anatomic study by Bigliani and colleagues further defined the course of the suprascapular nerve, identifying two or more branches to the infraspinatus as it travels around the spinoglenoid notch (21). The presence of an inferior transverse scapular ligament at the level of the spinoglenoid notch has been reported with variable incidence of 3% to 80% in the literature (17,25,26).

Etiology of Injury

Overhead athletes continually put their arms in the extremes of motion that can create large torques about the shoulder. This can establish a cycle of repetitive microtrauma to the nerve that can manifest itself in many ways. Injury can also be seen in the form of direct trauma to the nerve in the form of a fracture, dislocation, blunt trauma, or traction injury (4,5,27).

Injury at the level of the suprascapular notch has been described by Rengachary and co-workers as well as others (5,28–30) as the sling effect, occurring with hyperabduction of the shoulder. A recent study demonstrated a correlation between increased shoulder range of motion and suprascapular nerve entrapment in symptomatic volleyball players (31). A vascular etiology for injury to this nerve has been discussed by Ringel and colleagues (14). They described an intimal injury to the axillary or suprascapular artery during the pitching motion that could cause microemboli to lodge in the vasa nervorum and cause an ischemic injury.

Feretti and associates have proposed a mechanism of injury by which an eccentric contraction of the infraspinatus during the overhead smash in volleyball creates tension on the nerve as it passes around the spinoglenoid notch (10). Alternatively, Sandow and others theorize that the supraspinatus in its confluence with the infraspinatus tendon compresses the nerve at the spinoglenoid notch in the position of maximal abduction and external rotation (9). This compressive effect is primarily produced by contraction of the supraspinatus muscle in this model.

Compression of the nerve by a ganglion cyst has been described with an incidence of 1% to 4.2% (17,32,33). Compression can occur at either the suprascapular notch or the spinoglenoid notch. Cadaveric and MRI studies have shown that the cyst commonly originates from labral pathology within the glenohumeral joint (17,32,33).

History and Physical Examination

Injury to the nerve along its course may produce varied symptoms. Patients may present after an acute event, but often they present after repetitive trauma that is subtler in onset. Most commonly, pain is the primary presenting symptom. It is usually localized to the posterior shoulder and can be characterized as a deep, dull ache that is exacerbated by their sports overhead shoulder motion. Ringel and associates revealed reproducible pain during the cocking and release phase of the pitching motion (14). A lesion at the level of the suprascapular notch is more likely to produce pain than a more distally based lesion (34,35). Accordingly, many patients may present with painless weakness of the affected shoulder (11,36). Numbness in the region of the posterolateral shoulder should also be considered as a presenting symptom (24,37).

Other important causes of shoulder dysfunction must be assessed. A complete physical examination rules out cervical spine disease, brachial plexopathy, glenohumeral pathology, and rotator cuff tears. Observation of atrophy within the supraspinatus or infraspinatus fossa can be helpful (Fig. 19-1). Diminution in abduction and external rotation strength

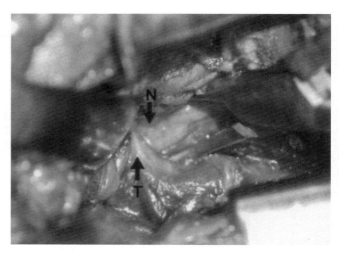

FIGURE 19-1. Intraoperative photo of quadrilateral space demonstrating long head of triceps (T) impinging on axillary nerve (N).

may be demonstrated. Palpation at the apex of the clavicle and scapular spine may reproduce pain at the suprascapular notch. More distally based pathology may elicit symptoms at the spinoglenoid notch. A positive cross-body adduction test has been reported to be a useful diagnostic aid (29,35). With this test, the nerve is stretched at the level of the suprascapular notch, exacerbating the patient's symptoms. Rose and Kelly have described a more invasive diagnostic test consisting of injection of local anesthetic into the notch. Resolution of symptoms can be helpful in confirming the diagnosis, but proper needle placement is imperative to prevent false-negative results (38).

Diagnostic Studies

All patients being evaluated for shoulder pathology should receive the standard shoulder series: anteroposterior (AP) in the scapular plane, scapular Y, and axillary radiographic views. To better assess the suprascapular notch, a Stryker notch view can be obtained. When osseous malformations or fractures have been excluded and the history and physical examination point to a nerve lesion, electrodiagnostic studies are a valuable adjunct in confirming the diagnosis. These studies are generally able to demonstrate neuropathy and its severity. Nerve conduction velocities show prolonged motor latencies from Erb's point to the supraspinatus or infraspinatus, depending on the level of the pathology (34,35,39). Electromyography (EMG) shows fibrillations, positive sharp waves, decreased amplitudes, and polyphasics (16,34,40).

Magnetic resonance imaging (MRI) is a useful tool in imaging the soft tissues of the shoulder. It has been shown to be reproducible in identifying space-occupying lesions of the suprascapular nerve (6,33,41,42). Most commonly these manifest as ganglion cysts. The course of the nerve is best seen on the T2-weighted sagittal oblique images (35). The supraspinatus and infraspinatus muscle bellies have been shown to demonstrate changes in their signal intensity with damage to the nerve (34). These include decreased muscle bulk, fatty degeneration, and altered signal intensity (6,9). However, these findings are nonspecific to denervation and can be seen independently in the face of rotator cuff tears (43,44).

Nonoperative Management

Nonoperative management of suprascapular nerve entrapment is indicated as the initial treatment modality. This has been successful in several studies, especially if the symptoms are not from a space-occupying lesion (36,40,45–48). The true success of treatment is unknown because many of these studies were retrospective or case reports with a heterogeneous group of patients. It has been suggested that 6 to 12 months of nonoperative management is indicated before surgery should be considered. In a competitive overhead athlete, the compliance or tolerance for prolonged restricted involvement of activities is limited. Furthermore, these patients can have symptoms for 10 months to 2.8 years before presentation for surgery (8,40,49). In patients with advanced entrapment, there may be significant muscle wasting, which is often irreversible (16). This underscores the importance of a quick and accurate diagnosis to facilitate appropriate intervention.

Physical therapy is directed at preserving glenohumeral motion while strengthening the rotator cuff and deltoid, as well as providing scapular stabilization. Exercises directed toward scapular retraction and toward maintaining posture and strengthening of the trapezius, rhomboids, and serratus anterior are instituted (35). Local injections of steroids have also been described with limited success (50).

Operative Intervention

Decompression of the nerve at the level of the suprascapular notch has traditionally been performed through a posterior approach (51). The patient is typically in the semiprone or lateral position, although the beach chair position can be used (35). The incision is 10 to 12 cm and is parallel and cephalad to the scapular spine. The trapezius is elevated of the scapular spine superiorly. The supraspinatus is reflected posteriorly, exposing the notch. Once the suprascapular artery and vein have been retracted, the transverse scapular ligament is transected, while protecting the nerve beneath. Osseous malformations of the notch causing impingement of the nerve are also addressed at this time.

The posterior approach may also be used when addressing isolated pathology at the spinoglenoid notch. The incision is placed directly overlying the spine or just caudad to it. The deltoid is split in line with its fibers or may be taken down off of the spine. The infraspinatus belly is dissected off of the spine and retracted inferiorly. Judicious dissection through the vascular fibrous tissue overlying the notch reveals the nerve as it delivers branches to the infraspinatus (22). Hama and colleagues and Sandow and associates have illustrated a technique of deepening the spinoglenoid notch to address the suprascapular nerve at this level (9,52). Caution should be exercised with this technique, because removal of more than 1 cm may predispose to fracture at the acromial base. Both of these series deal with high-level volleyball players. All patients in both series had resolution of pain and return to their previous level of competition (9,52). Ringel and colleagues reported on a series of two professional pitchers who underwent decompression of the nerve (14). One patient had no visible area of compression at the suprascapular notch or the spinoglenoid notch. The second patient had an anomalous motor branch to the supraspinatus that traveled over the transverse scapular ligament. Both returned to pitching for their respective teams. Vastamaki and Goransson reported on a mixed population of laborers and those with athletic injuries (12). Overall, 72% had complete relief or minimal pain; 81% rated their result as excellent or good at a minimum of 5.6 years of follow-up. A recent study compared the outcomes of nonoperative versus operative treatment (40). Overall, there was improvement noted in both groups, but significantly more in the operative group. Patients with traumatic lesions improved with either nonoperative or operative management, but there was no significant difference between the two groups. Compressive lesions did significantly better with surgery than with nonoperative treatment.

Successful decompression of the nerve secondary to compression from a ganglion cyst has been reported with both open and arthroscopic means (4,53–61). However, an open approach to the nerve does not allow surgical repair of the labral pathology that is invariably present. This may account for the recurrences that have been documented (58,62). An open or arthroscopic approach to decompression of the cyst with concomitant arthroscopic management of the labrum has shown reproducible results (35,58,59,61). The one recurrence noted with this approach was thought to be secondary to unrecognized labral pathology at the index procedure (58).

Authors' Preferred Method

The approach to open management of suprascapular nerve entrapment at our institution is similar to that of Post and Mayer (51). A posterior approach with an incision parallel to the spine of the scapula is used. It is placed just cephalad or caudad to the spine, depending on whether the pathology is at the suprascapular or spinoglenoid notch, respectively. The trapezius muscle is not split; rather, elevation of the entire trapezius off the spine is performed to prevent injury to the spinal accessory nerve during retraction. Judicious dissection of the fatty layer underlying the trapezius exposes the supraspinatus. Access to the suprascapular notch is facilitated with minimal retraction of the supraspinatus inferiorly. The transverse scapular ligament is defined with the use of a small sponge stick, while the overlying artery and vein are retracted. The nerve is protected below and the ligament is transected.

If the nerve is involved at the level of the spinoglenoid notch, the supraspinatus is retracted superiorly and the infraspinatus inferiorly. The inferior transverse scapular ligament, if present, is transected and the notch is deepened with a high-speed burr. The osseous resection is limited to 1 cm to minimize potential iatrogenic fracture of the acromion base (9).

AXILLARY NERVE INJURY

Historical Overview

Axillary nerve injuries account for less than 1% of all nerve lesions, but are the most common peripheral nerve injury to the shoulder (63,64). It has been described as an injury in contact sports, with direct blunt injury, traction, and dislocation being the most common mechanisms (65–67). The quadrilateral space syndrome also involves the axillary nerve, in addition to the posterior humeral circumflex artery. This entity was originally described by Cahill and Palmer and is seen primarily as a noncontact injury and therefore is a more plausible etiology for dysfunction in the overhead athlete (68).

Anatomy

The axillary nerve is a terminal branch of the posterior cord of the brachial plexus arising from the C5 and C6 nerve roots. It courses along the subscapularis obliquely from superomedial to inferolateral, crossing 3 to 5 mm from the musculotendinous junction (69). It then passes through the quadrilateral space with the posterior humeral circumflex artery. This space is bound by the teres minor superiorly, the teres major inferiorly, the long head of the triceps medially, and the shaft of the humerus laterally. After exiting the space, the nerve forms two major trunks. The anterior trunk continues around the humeral shaft to give branches to the middle and anterior deltoid on the undersurface of the muscle. The posterior trunk supplies the posterior deltoid and the teres minor. The branch to the teres minor arborizes while in the quadrilateral space or just after exiting. Ultimately, the posterior trunk becomes the superior lateral brachial cutaneous nerve.

Etiology

The overhead athlete who sustains an anterior shoulder dislocation is at risk for an axillary nerve injury, although this is relatively uncommon in persons younger than age 50 years (70,71). Direct blows to the lateral shoulder have been noted to cause axillary nerve injury in contact athletes (65,72). This mechanism of injury is less common in the overhead athlete. A more likely etiology in this subset of patients is the quadrilateral space syndrome. As the axillary nerve and posterior humeral circumflex artery traverse the space, it is possible that they can become compressed. Overuse of the extremity may cause the formation of fibrotic bands or hypertrophy of the long head of the triceps tendon causing compression (1,68,73). This triceps pathoanatomy has been demonstrated at our institution (see Fig. 19-1). Most of the recent cases of quadrilateral space syndrome have involved overhead athletes, providing additional support that repetitive motion is integral to the pathology (74–77). This theory is further supported by the fact that the syndrome is rarely seen in the inactive elderly population (68,76,78).

History and Physical Examination

The overhead athlete, in the absence of acute trauma, may present to the clinician with vague complaints of easy fatigability of the arm while playing their sport, poorly localized pain in the posterior shoulder, and numbness to the lateral shoulder. Often, these patients are able to compensate for the loss of deltoid function for activities of daily living. In the overuse patient, symptoms can be insidious in onset and may have been undiagnosed or misdiagnosed.

Sensation over the deltoid should be assessed, noting any paresthesias. However, complete deltoid motor loss can occur in the face of minimal sensation loss. Atrophy of the deltoid and teres minor should be assessed. Squaring of the shoulder is observed with significant denervation of the deltoid. Muscle wasting can be more difficult to assess in incomplete lesions of the deltoid. These patients may retain full range of motion, but when the extremity is exercised they demonstrate abduction weakness (67). Delineating the function of the deltoid from the rotator cuff through extension of the shoulder has recently been proposed by two independent authors. Nishijima and colleagues have described the swallow-tail sign, wherein the injured shoulder is unable to extend fully with respect to the contralateral side (79). The deltoid extension lag sign has been described by Hertel and co-workers (80). When the arm is passively brought into full extension, the patient is unable to maintain this position when support is withdrawn and the arm drops.

In an athlete suspected of having quadrilateral space syndrome, palpation over the space reliably reproduces their pain (68,76,78). Placement of the arm in an abducted and externally rotated position for 1 minute may reproduce symptoms (68). Paresthesias were originally described as occurring in a nondermatomal pattern in the arm and forearm, although subsequent reports are variable in accounting for their presence.

Diagnostic Studies

Plain radiographs should be obtained to rule out any osseous pathology. Electrodiagnostic studies are an important part of the workup in a patient with a suspected nerve lesion. In the face of known blunt injury or dislocation, EMG is especially useful. These studies should not be performed before 3 weeks from the injury because fibrillation potentials are not evident until that time. Repeat studies should be performed 3 months after injury if no clinical improvement is noted, because electrical improvement in the nerve may be present despite the clinical picture.

In the case of the overhead athlete, acute trauma is less likely and the diagnosis of quadrilateral space syndrome should be considered. The use of EMG in this setting has been reported with variable success, but it may aid in confirmation (68,76–78,81).

Although quadrilateral space syndrome has been described as primarily a lesion of the axillary nerve, arteriography is essential to its diagnosis. With the arm at the side, the posterior humeral circumflex artery is patent; when the arm is brought into abduction and external rotation, the artery occludes (Fig. 19-2). This finding has been described as pathognomonic for this syndrome (68,74,76, 82–84).

Atrophy and fatty degeneration have been described in the radiologic literature as useful findings on MRI (85,86). A case report of a paralabral cyst extending into the quadrilateral space has been documented on MRI (86). Despite these reports, support for its widespread use in this setting has not been subsequently substantiated.

Nonoperative Management

The body of literature that exists for nonoperative management of axillary nerve pathology in athletes is largely from a traumatic etiology. Perlmutter and co-workers reported on axillary nerve injury following a direct blow to the shoulder in 11 football players (72). Nonoperative treatment consisted of rotator cuff, deltoid, and periscapular muscle strengthening. Four of the 11 patients eventually required surgical exploration for persistent clinical and electromyographic deficiencies. Ten of the 11 ultimately returned to their prior level of participation. All patients had good to excellent manual muscle testing results, although cutaneous sensory abnormalities persisted in all of the patients.

In another series addressing peripheral nerve injuries in sports, there were six axillary nerve injuries. Five of six resolved with physical therapy alone. Redler and colleagues presented successful nonoperative management of a pitcher with quadrilateral space syndrome (75). Retraining from an overhead motion to three quarters was instituted. Additionally, internal rotation stretching of the shoulder joint, horizontal stretching in adduction, and rotator cuff strengthening have been advocated with quadrilateral space syndrome (82).

Operative Management

Given the length of the axillary nerve and the known rate of nerve recovery, 3 to 6 months of nonoperative management should show significant improvement. When this fails, operative intervention should be considered. Studies have shown inferior results of operative intervention when performed more than 1 year after injury (87).

As previously stated, direct trauma to the overhead athlete's shoulder is rare. In most cases, patients with axillary nerve pathology and antecedent trauma require an anterior and posterior approach to the nerve. All approaches are briefly discussed here. The patient is positioned in the lateral decubitus position, allowing access to the front and back of the shoulder as well as sural nerve for grafting if needed. The anterior deltopectoral approach allows assessment of the nerve from its origin off the posterior cord to

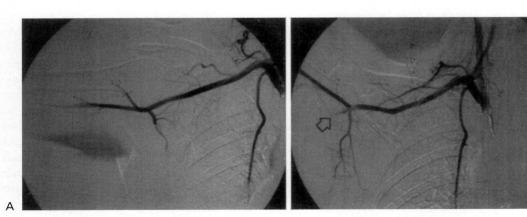

FIGURE 19-2. A: (Image on left), Arteriogram of upper extremity in abduction showing patent branches of axillary artery. **B:** (Image on right) Arm in abduction and external rotation demonstrating obliteration of flow of posterior humeral circumflex artery (*arrow*).

its entrance into the quadrilateral space. Once dissection to the clavipectoral fascia is completed, the muscles originating from the coracoid are removed and tagged or a coracoid osteotomy is performed (69). This facilitates proximal visualization of the nerve.

If no pathology is identified at this point or if a nerve graft must be used, a posterior approach is also necessary (88). This approach has been described in conjunction with the quadrilateral space syndrome (68). The skin incision is an inverted "L" with the horizontal limb parallel and just inferior to the spine of the scapula. The vertical limb trails inferiorly overlying the humerus. A full thickness flap is then developed down to the deltoid fascia. The inferior border of the deltoid fascia is then identified. This is facilitated by beginning development of this plane inferolaterally and proceeding superomedially, separating the deltoid from the teres muscle bellies. The deltoid origin is then removed from the spine of the scapula, leaving a cuff of tissue behind for later reattachment. The teres minor insertion is detached and retracted medially. A combination of blunt and sharp dissection of the quadrilateral space follows, with excision of any fibrous bands. When decompression is complete, a finger is placed on the posterior humeral circumflex artery and the arm is put into abduction and external rotation. A persistent pulse verifies an adequate decompression. The teres minor is not reattached. The deltoid is sutured to the spine.

In the original description, 89% of patients (16 of 18) showed improvement in symptoms following decompression (68). Similarly, Francel and associates reported on five patients with improvement in symptoms in all patients (78). Several other case reports give similar results (76,83).

Authors' Preferred Method

Surgical management of quadrilateral space syndrome at this institution involves a posterior approach similar to that described by Francel and associates (78). The patient is positioned in the prone position. A longitudinal incision approximately 6 to 8 cm in length is placed within the posterior axillary fold and extends proximally toward the lateral edge of the acromion. Full thickness skin flaps are developed down to the deltoid fascia. The deltoid is not taken off the scapula; therefore the plane between the deltoid and the posterior cuff muscles must be exploited to maximize visualization. The adipose at the inferior edge of the deltoid can create difficulties in developing this plane. To facilitate this aspect of the case, dissection should begin at the inferolateral aspect of the deltoid, where the long head of the triceps crosses, and proceed proximally and medially. The muscle bellies of the teres are isolated and decompression of the space follows. The teres minor is not released from its insertion, but if there are pathologic elements contributing to the compression, they are released locally at the level of the neurovascular bundle. Any fibrotic bands tethering the

bundle are transected. Additionally, we have found that the long head of the triceps may have hypertrophic bands, which play a role in the pathology and are resected accordingly (see Fig. 19-1). Confirmation of decompression is made with insertion of a finger into the space without constriction. Visualization of axillary fat can also be used as a guide. Closure of the wound only involves approximation of the skin flaps; no muscles are taken down. Patients may begin range-of-motion exercises as soon as 1 week postoperatively and advance to full sports involvement as soon as the wound is healed.

An axillary approach is also described to address axillary nerve pathology (see later discussion), but this approach places the intercostal brachial nerve at risk, which can have significant morbidity in some patients. Additionally, the vessels cover the nerve and require meticulous dissection for proper exposure. It is for these reasons that the anterior and posterior approaches are primarily used.

VASCULAR INJURIES

History

Thoracic outlet syndrome was originally described by Hunald in 1743 with compression from a cervical rib causing the pathology (89). Since that time, the first thoracic rib, fibrous bands, and anomalous or hypertrophied scalene muscles have been described as well (90–93). The repetitive use of the extremity in an abducted and externally rotated position puts the overhead athlete at risk for this vascular insult. Additional reports have discussed humeral hypertrophy, pectoralis minor hypertrophy, and subtle glenohumeral instability as causative factors (94–96). In addition, the rotational torques at the shoulder during the pitching motion create a mechanism for repetitive stretching of the axillary artery in that the circumflex scapular vessels can create a tethering effect (97).

Anatomy

The thoracic outlet is defined by three anatomic passages by which the neurovascular supply to the upper extremity must traverse. The superior thoracic outlet is bound anteriorly by the manubrium, posteriorly by the spine, and laterally by the first thoracic rib (98). Continuing laterally, the bundle passes through a triangle bound by the anterior scalene, middle scalene, and the first rib that forms the floor of the triangle. Finally, the costoclavicular passage, which is bound by the clavicle and subclavius muscles anteriorly, the subscapularis posteriorly, and the first rib medially. As the plexus and vessels continue, they pass beneath the coracoid with the pectoralis minor anteriorly and the humerus posteriorly. The neurovascular bundle is at risk anywhere along this course.

Etiology

The first thoracic rib is present at all levels of the thoracic outlet and therefore is central to the discussion of the vascular pathology in thoracic outlet syndrome. It has been noted to be the etiology of symptoms in several series that have included overhead athletes (98–100). It has been proposed that the relationship between the first rib and the clavicle can cause ischemia (101). In addition, it has been demonstrated that weakness or injury to the shoulder girdle can cause compression of the neurovascular bundle as it passes between the clavicle and the first rib (98). The presence of a cervical rib has been implicated as the pathologic structure in many series (98–100,102). The vessels around the shoulder are subjected to very high rotational torques in the overhead athlete. The subclavian and axillary arteries are most commonly involved. This repetitive stretching may predispose them to intimal injury, which can ultimately lead to aneurysm formation. The relationship of the circumflex vessels to the axillary artery can create a leash effect as the arm is brought into the extremes of motion (95,97,103). This puts the axillary artery and the circumflex vessels at risk. Branch artery aneurysms have also been reported by several other authors in high-level overhead athletes (95,103,104).

The pectoralis minor has been shown to cause compression of the axillary artery when the arm is placed in the abducted and externally rotated position (94,95,103–105). The ultimate manifestation of the vascular insult is aneurysm formation with subsequent thrombus propagation. The clot causes local ischemic effects at the shoulder, as well as distally in the hand from the showering of emboli.

Glenohumeral instability has also been implicated as a factor in producing vascular compromise in this patient population (94). Paralleling this aspect of inciting factors is hypertrophy of the humeral head, which has been discussed by Nuber and colleagues as well as others (94,100). Roher and associates evaluated the incidence of axillary artery compression in the abducted and externally rotated position (96). They demonstrated that the artery was compressed 83% of the time at the level of the humeral head. In only 7.6% of cases was the compression greater than 50% of the lumen. There was no difference in the rate of compression in professional pitchers and control subjects. This mechanism of compression has been demonstrated in symptomatic athletes by other authors (94,95,100,102).

Although less common, venous thrombosis of the axillary or subclavian vein, or effort thrombosis, has also been described (82,106). The vein can become compressed within the thoracic outlet and cause thrombosis. Several case reports are documented in overhead athletes (107–110).

History and Physical Examination

The typical athlete who presents with ischemia of the upper extremity is a pitcher, but it has also been described in volleyball players, weightlifters, kayakers, golfers, and tennis players (94,96,97,102–104,111). It usually involves the dominant extremity. They may present with only symptoms of a heaviness of the arm or easy fatigability when playing their sport. Pain is also described in the arm that is exacerbated by use of the arm.

Typically these patients have some manifestation of distal ischemia, which can take the form of cyanosis of the digits, new-onset cold intolerance, numbness, focal ulceration, and even gangrene. In addition, unilateral Raynaud's phenomenon may be present. If this is found during the workup, the diagnosis of thoracic outlet should be entertained (99,102).

On examination, these patients may have completely normal pulses with the extremity at the side. Bruits should be assessed from the supraclavicular region distally to the hand. A complete motor and neurologic examination should be performed to exclude other causes. A complete examination also notes the condition of the skin, whether or not there is pallor, ulcerations, or frank necrosis. Patients with a suspected venous thrombosis may have a normal neuromuscular examination. These patients may have swelling of the entire extremity, mottled and cold skin, and, variably, a cordlike band can be palpated in the axilla (82).

The Adson test should be performed when thoracic outlet obstruction is suspected (112). The patient is seated with arms resting on knees. The patient is then asked to take a deep breath, elevate the chin and turn the chin to the affected side. A diminution or obliteration of the radial pulse or a change in blood pressure is highly suggestive of compression of the subclavian artery by the anterior scalene muscle. The hyperabduction test has the seated patient abduct and externally rotate the arm above the plane of the shoulder. Reproduction of the symptoms and a loss of a distal pulse should raise the clinician's suspicions for compression of neurovascular structures underneath the pectoralis minor as well as between the clavicle and first rib (113).

Diagnostic Tests

Initial radiographs should be obtained of any patient presenting with shoulder complaints. It is possible to detect cervical ribs, clavicular nonunions, and other anomalous osseous formations. When this does not lead to a definitive diagnosis and a vascular etiology is suspected, there are several options. The use of arterial photoplethysmographic techniques in neutral and provocative positions can assess the effect of distal flow from proximal compression. Doppler ultrasound can be used as a noninvasive means of primarily assessing the subclavian and axillary arteries (100,102). Arteriography is used as the confirmatory test, which is performed with the arm in neutral and in provocative positions. Additionally this study can be used as a preoperative planning device.

Venography has been described by several authors to confirm the diagnosis of effort thrombosis in athletes

(82,107,108,110). Duplex ultrasound has also been used as an adjunct, but it has limited use in the axilla and shoulder (107, 114). This technique also remains highly technician-dependent and, therefore, venography remains the study of choice for confirmation of the diagnosis.

Nonoperative Management

Patients with vascular pathology usually benefit from cessation of play with the involved extremity. However, the improvement in symptoms is short-lived because invariably the symptoms return when they resume play. For this reason, nonoperative management in the competitive athlete who wants to return to competition may be difficult. More importantly, reports of gangrene of the fingers, aneurysm rupture, and stroke have been reported in delayed or untreated cases (115–117).

Operative Management

Initial acute invasive management of patients with axillary, subclavian, or branch arterial ischemic lesions has involved the use of thrombolytics for dissolution of digital emboli (102). This has not been found to be effective in addressing the proximal thrombus in the shoulder (97,101). However, those patients with effort thrombosis have shown a favorable response to thrombolytics followed by excision of the source of compression (107,108, 110,118,119).

When there is evidence of aneurysm formation, there are several surgical options available. Excision and direct repair is ideal, providing an end-to-end repair. This approach is limited by two factors. If the lesion is too large, a primary repair creates tension. In addition, given the high torques created in the shoulder by overhead athletes, shortening the length of the vulnerable vessel segment is ill advised. Lateral patching of the artery is an option if the pathoanatomy allows. When the humeral head is responsible for compression of the axillary artery without vessel damage, lateral patch grafting has been described to increase the diameter of the vessel so that flow is not compromised (100,102). Synthetic grafts in this setting are not considered because there is no healing of artery to the graft and the strength of the repair relies solely on the sutures. Interposition vein grafting is a viable option and has demonstrated success in multiple studies (94,95,97,99,100,111,120).

The surgical approach depends on the location of the pathology. Traditionally, a supraclavicular approach has been used for release of the anterior scalene, resection of a cervical rib, and fibrous band excision. The proximal subclavian artery can be assessed from this approach. Yao and colleagues have described a two-incision supraclavicular and infraclavicular approach to address the aforementioned pathology as well as the first part of the axillary artery (102).

The supraclavicular approach involves a transverse incision just cephalad and parallel to the clavicle. The platysma is incised off the clavicle followed by retraction of the scalene fat pad. The phrenic nerve is dissected free of the anterior scalene. Subsequent to this, the scalene muscles, cervical ribs, and anomalous fibrous bands can be addressed. A second infraclavicular incision can then be used. After the transverse incision is made caudad to the clavicle, the pectoralis major is split in line with its fibers. If the pectoralis minor is involved in the compression it can be incised, facilitating assessment of the axillary artery. Additionally, the first rib is transected if needed.

Pathology of the second and third parts of the axillary artery can be addressed with a transaxillary approach (97,98,100,102). The transverse incision is placed immediately caudad to the axillary hairline, between the pectoralis major and latissimus dorsi. All attempts are made to preserve the intercostal brachial nerve within the field. The pectoralis major and minor are retracted superiorly. The axillary artery is observed in intimate contact with the brachial plexus. The anterior and posterior circumflex humeral arteries are assessed because they often arise from a common trunk and represent a well-documented site of pathology (95,97,103,104,111). Direct repair of the artery as well as ligation have been described. McCarthy and colleagues also described branch artery occlusion involving the suprascapular artery and subscapular artery; corresponding compression arises from the anterior scalene and pectoralis minor respectively.

The results of surgical intervention in athletes have generally been successful. McCarthy and colleagues reported on six high-level baseball pitchers who had either a pectoralis minor or anterior scalene release. All of them returned to their previous level of play. A larger follow-up study showed 12 of 13 patients returned to their previous level of competition. Follow-up noninvasive testing revealed no compression of the vessel in any patient. A collection of four studies treating injury to the anterior and posterior circumflex scapular arteries revealed eight of eight patients returning to competition (97,103,104,111).

More recently, Arko and associates in a larger study of vascular pathology in athletes presented a subset of seven overhead athletes with either axillary or subclavian artery involvement (120). Six of the seven patients returned to their premorbid level of competition. In the same study, 12 patients with effort thrombosis of the axillary or subclavian vein were followed up. All of these patients underwent thrombolysis. Eight patients exhibited persistent symptoms of venous occlusion requiring subsequent excision of the first rib. At a mean of 13.9 months, all 12 patients had returned to their previous level of play. In the absence of any compressive structure and a preserved intima, thrombolytics alone can work. This was shown in a case report of a wrestler who had the onset of venous engorgement, arm swelling, and pain 3 days after a match. Thrombolytics followed by 6 weeks of warfarin resolved his symptoms and he returned to athletics.

When there is venographic evidence of compression of the vein, thrombolytics followed by surgical resection has been successful. Vogel and co-workers reported a case of a competitive swimmer who presented with a subclavian vein thrombosis secondary to thoracic outlet syndrome. The vein was successfully recanalized with streptokinase. The first rib was subsequently removed and the patient returned to the previous level of swimming (107). More recently, DiFelice and colleagues reported on a series of four professional baseball players with effort thrombosis (108). All were treated with urokinase followed by first rib resection and 3 months of anticoagulation. All have since returned to playing professional baseball.

Authors' Preferred Method

Nonoperative measures including the use of thrombolytics are used initially. When surgery is necessary, however, we use a transaxillary approach to branch artery aneurysm formation at the common origin of the anterior and posterior circumflex arteries. Operative management includes ligation of the circumflex arteries and excision of the aneurysm with reverse saphenous vein interposition.

Active range-of-motion exercises begin 6 weeks postoperatively. "Soft tossing" exercises start at 8 weeks and throwing from the mound at 12 weeks. Four months after surgery, patients are allowed to return to their previous level of performance, including the professional level.

SERRATUS ANTERIOR PALSY

History

Winging of the scapula was first described by Winslow in 1723 (121). In 1837, Velpeau was the first to specifically describe serratus anterior palsy as an etiology. The management of this entity has been successful with both operative and nonoperative approaches. In 1904, Tubby was the first to describe surgical management (122). This consisted of transfer of the sternal portion of the pectoralis major into the substance of the serratus anterior. Since then, several methods have been described for surgical correction of scapular winging secondary to serratus palsy. Management of the overhead athlete presents a challenge because return to play and restoration or maintenance of function is essential to the athlete's success. Operative intervention involves an extended time out from athletic involvement, but nonoperative methods can often take up to a year to be successful. Discussion as to the ultimate goals of the athlete and realistic expectations facilitate successful outcomes.

Anatomy

The long thoracic nerve is solely a motor nerve and innervates the serratus anterior muscle. It originates from the cervical roots of C5, C6, and C7. The C5 and C6 roots emerge through the scalenus medius muscle. They are joined by the C7 root at this point to form the long thoracic nerve. The nerve continues distally and laterally, remaining posterior to the brachial plexus and axillary vessels. It follows the axillary border of the latissimus dorsi on the chest wall and terminates 30 cm from the spine within the distal mass of the serratus at the level of the ninth and tenth rib (123).

The serratus anterior originates from the upper nine ribs and inserts on the anteromedial border of the scapula. The distal digitations of the muscle insert on the inferior angle of the scapula, which serves the important function of scapular stability during arm elevation. The serratus provides cephalad rotation and protraction of the scapula. It acts to stabilize the scapula against the chest wall during elevation of the arm. This motion aids in moving the coracoacromial arch out of the path of the greater tuberosity during elevation, preventing impingement (124).

Etiology

Multiple etiologies of serratus anterior palsy have been described. Both traumatic and nontraumatic events may precipitate its occurrence (125–127). In the largest series to date, Vastamaki and colleagues reported on 197 patients with serratus palsy and found that 26% were secondary to trauma (127). Exertion was the cause in 35% of cases, which included work-related activity as well as sports activities. Iatrogenic injury occurred in 11% and infection accounted for 7% of the diagnosis.

In the overhead athlete, direct trauma to the nerve is less likely. Chronic repetitive motion more commonly elicits the injury. It has been shown to occur in players of the following sports: tennis, basketball, bowling, archery, weightlifting, marksmanship, football, cross country skiing, and rowing (123,127–131). Case reports document acute palsy after rigorous stretching in ballet and following specific weightlifting maneuvers (129,132). An avulsion of the serratus anterior off the chest wall while rowing has been reported as well (133). Holden and colleagues reported on seven cases of rib fractures in female athletes associated with an acute increase in their training regimens (130). Less commonly, brachial neuritis or Parsonage-Turner syndrome can be the cause and should be included as part of the differential diagnosis.

A recent cadaveric study demonstrated tethering of the long thoracic nerve within a fascial sling formed between the first rib and proximal serratus anterior medially and the brachial plexus laterally (134). This tethering effect was most dramatic with the arm in an abducted and externally rotated position with the head rotated to the contralateral side. Additionally, Bora and colleagues found that the length of the long thoracic nerve doubled with elevation of the arm in conjunction with contralateral head rotation (135). The clinical correlate to this anatomic finding may be important in the overhead athlete who puts his or her arm in this position of risk.

History and Physical Examination

Patients with serratus anterior palsy, as with many of the lesions described previously, may be incorrectly diagnosed because of its indolent course and often overlapping symptoms. With incomplete paralysis of the serratus anterior, the patient may not perceive scapular winging and may present with shoulder pain secondary to impingement as the primary complaint. A painful clicking or popping that increases with activity may be described. In cases associated with rib fractures, pain is often referred to the posterior thorax along the spine of the scapula. Patients may report shoulder weakness or easy fatigability and limited shoulder motion specific to their sport.

Weakness or paralysis of the serratus anterior causes medial and cephalad winging of the scapula. The degree of displacement correlates with the amount of dysfunction of the muscle. Subtle differences in the position of the scapulae can be noted while observing patients with their arms at their sides and then with their hands resting on their waist. Gregg and colleagues noted that, in cases of complete serratus, palsy patients were unable to elevate their arm beyond 110 degrees (123). Performing a wall push-up demonstrates scapular winging. Raising the arm against resistance also reveals the characteristic displacement. Pure abduction of the arm may not produce winging and is important in delineating serratus palsy from trapezius dysfunction.

Diagnostic Studies

Standard x-ray examination is usually not indicated in cases of suspected serratus anterior palsy unless the dysfunction is secondary to rib fractures. EMG analysis can aid in the diagnosis and is helpful to give a baseline assessment. It is often necessary to communicate with the neurodiagnostician before the test because it can be difficult to document serratus anterior palsy. Subsequent examinations at 3- to 4-month intervals can follow the nerve's electrical recovery and potential for clinical improvement.

Nonoperative Management

Functional recovery from serratus anterior injury can usually be expected. Most cases spontaneously resolve, usually within 6 to 9 months (131). Several case reports in athletes have shown a high return to competition after 6 weeks to several months of therapy (123,128–131), although it can take up to 2 years to regain function in cases of Parsonage-Turner syndrome. Acutely, treatment is aimed at pain reduction and preservation of motion. Physical therapy focuses on reestablishing smooth scapulothoracic and glenohumeral motion in conjunction with strengthening the periscapular musculature. Once strength and premorbid range of motion are restored, patients may return to play. The use of a scapular orthosis has had variable success in stabilizing the shoulder girdle (126,136). Its application in an athlete should be limited to the acute rehabilitation phase, because long-term use likely limits competitive competition because of their cumbersome nature and variable compliance with use.

Operative Management

When nonoperative measures fail to regain effective shoulder girdle motion by 12 months, operative management should be considered. Early attempts at operative correction included transferring the pectoralis major directly into the dysfunctional serratus anterior and transfer of the pectoralis minor directly into the scapula via fascia lata grafts (122,137). Others attempted to sew a fascia lata graft from the vertebral border of the scapula into the adjacent spinous processes (138). These procedures tended to fail because they were not durable and the grafts stretched over time.

Dickson used the pectoralis major with a fascia lata graft placed through the scapula (139). More recently, efforts have focused on using the pectoralis major tendon in conjunction with a fascia lata graft rolled into a tube (140,141). An extension of this technique has been described by Post in an effort to further decrease the amount of stretching of the graft (142). The fascia lata graft is tightly coiled or spiraled with nonabsorbable suture holding it in place. One end of the graft is subsequently woven through the myotendinous junction of the pectoralis major and secured with suture, and then the pectoralis is sutured back on itself. The other end is passed through the vertebral border of the scapula. All patients in that series had excellent results.

Authors' Preferred Method

We have used a similar approach to these patients (143). Ten of 11 patients in this series had a satisfactory result at an average follow-up of 41 months (143).

However, we have modified this method to a two-incision technique. The modifications include elimination of the fascia lata graft and use of a much smaller incision anteriorly and a small accessory incision posteriorly. A small axillary incision is made in the axillary skin crease. The insertion of the pectoralis major is identified on the humerus and the interval between the sternal and clavicular head is exploited by abduction and external rotation of the arm. The sternal head of the tendon is then sharply dissected off the humerus and mobilized of any fascial restraints medial to allow maximum excursion. Dissection continues within the axilla, taking care to remain medial against the chest wall to avoid the laterally oriented neurovascular structures within the axilla.

The inferior angle of the scapula is then palpated and a small incision is made directly overlying it. Subperiosteal dissection of the subscapularis, infraspinatus, and serratus anterior is then performed to expose the entire inferomedial scapula. Multiple sutures are then placed in the scapula and the sutures from the pectoralis major are then retrieved from the anterior incision. An assistant then reduces the scapula to the chest wall and the sternal head of the pectoralis major tendon is secured directly to the scapula.

The patient is placed in a sling for 6 weeks. Gentle pendulum and isometric exercises are performed during this time. Following removal of the sling, progressive strengthening exercises are initiated. No heavy lifting or full activity is allowed for 6 months.

There is a paucity of data in the competitive athlete to make any strong recommendations. However, a study by Perlmutter and Leffert, showed good and excellent results in 13 of 16 patients following a pectoralis major transfer with fascia lata autograft, but only 9 of 16 patients were able to return to sports activities (144). Additionally, Post has recommended that patients avoid repetitive lifting of objects weighing more than 20 pounds after this surgery (142). Finally, in the case of penetrating trauma or iatrogenic injury, direct repair or nerve grafting should be considered (145). There are limited reports of successful nerve grafting with idiopathic serratus anterior weakness (146). More favorable results have been shown when the nerve is addressed within a year of the injury (147)

TRAPEZIUS DYSFUNCTION

History

The trapezius plays an integral role in smooth scapulothoracic motion. Both Codman and Inmann and associates made early contributions to the understanding of the complexities of linked scapulothoracic motion (148,149). The term *scapulohumeral rhythm* was first introduced by Codman, whereas Inmann and associates helped identify the three separate functional components of the trapezius muscle (148,149). Dickson attempted stabilization of the scapula using fascia lata grafts secured to the cervical muscles and the spinous process of the first thoracic vertebra (139). Similar procedures were described by Henry and Whitman (138,150). All of these procedures tended to fail, however, because of stretching of the graft. The combination of a static fascial stabilization with a dynamic muscle transfer was described by Dewar and Harris (151). This also failed because the transfer of the levator scapulae alone was

not sufficient to overcome the trapezius dysfunction. Eden and Lange were the first to describe the dynamic transfer of the levator scapulae, rhomboid major, and rhomboid minor to substitute for the loss of trapezius function (152, 153). This transfer functionally reproduces the three aspects of the trapezius and has been shown to have reproducible, durable results at our institution (147,154).

Direct repair, grafting, and neurolysis in cases of iatrogenic injury or penetrating trauma to the spinal accessory nerve have had variable success. Favorable results are seen when the nerve is addressed within 6 months of the injury; outcomes deteriorate when more than a year elapses since injury (155,156).

Anatomy

The trapezius takes its origin from the spinous processes of the seventh cervical vertebra to the twelfth thoracic vertebra. There are cephalad attachments of its origin on the ligamentum nuchae and the external occipital protuberance. The upper portion of the trapezius inserts onto the lateral third of the clavicle, the middle portion onto the medial acromion and superior spine of the scapula, and the inferior portion onto the inferior aspect of the spine of the scapula.

The trapezius muscle acts in synchrony to elevate, retract, and rotate the scapula. Together with the levator scapulae, the rhomboids, and the serratus anterior, they provide smooth scapulothoracic stabilization and linked scapulohumeral motion. The upper portion of the trapezius elevates the scapula and provides cephalad rotation of the lateral angle. The middle portion adducts the scapula, while the inferior portion depresses and caudally rotates the scapula. In its resting state, the trapezius supports the entire upper extremity at the end of the clavicular lever arm.

The spinal accessory nerve (cranial nerve XI) provides the sole motor innervation to the trapezius. Proprioceptive fibers from the second, third, or fourth cervical nerve may also join the accessory nerve (157). Before the nerve innervates the trapezius, it must first pass through the posterior cervical triangle. This triangle is bordered by the sternocleidomastoid anteriorly, the trapezius posteriorly, and the clavicle inferiorly. The roof is formed by the superficial layer of the deep cervical fascia. The nerve is very superficial within the triangle and vulnerable to injury. The spinal accessory nerve emerges from the triangle to course along the superficial lateral surface of the levator scapulae. It then passes along the medial half of the trapezius, innervating the muscle as it descends medial to the vertebral border of the scapula (158).

Etiology

Injury to the spinal accessory nerve from surgical dissection in the neck occurred in up to 50% of cases in the 1950s (159). Alterations in neck dissections have led to a decrease in its incidence (160,161). Penetrating trauma is also a reported cause of injury, although rare (162,163). The incidence in athletes is also infrequent, although there have been reports in players of hockey, lacrosse, football, skiing, and wrestling (67,147,164–166). The mechanism of injury typically involves either a direct blow from a stick or a traction injury.

Diagnostic Studies

Dedicated shoulder radiographs should be obtained to rule out any osseous pathology. Additional imaging studies can be obtained based on the history and physical examination. A baseline EMG study and nerve conduction study can be obtained at 3 months. Serial examinations can then be performed at 6-week intervals to assess the potential for recovery and aid in following a treatment algorithm of either nerve exploration or muscle transfer. All potential muscles for transfer should be assessed in addition to the serratus anterior. Results can be negatively affected if serratus dysfunction coexists with trapezial palsy (159). A negative or inconclusive EMG does not, however, exclude the diagnosis of trapezius palsy. In a study from our institution, 12 of 35 electromyographic studies performed for presumed trapezial dysfunction were incorrect, incomplete, or inconclusive (154).

History and Physical Examination

This diagnosis can be elusive. In a study by Bigliani and colleagues, 14 of 22 patients initially had an incorrect diagnosis (154). A meticulous history and physical examination is essential to the expeditious diagnosis and treatment of these patients. A history of overt trauma to the neck or shoulder can be helpful, but more occult trauma or traction injuries should be drawn out in the history. Subtle dysfunction in an overhead athlete may present with signs and symptoms of impingement because they are unable to clear the acromion from the greater tuberosity (145). Additionally, they may have secondary symptoms of adhesive capsulitis, thoracic outlet syndrome, instability, and radiculitis from tension on the brachial plexus (147,154,155,167). This shoulder dysfunction usually precludes them from participating in their sport. Pain that is proportional to the use of the extremity is a common complaint. They often describe a dull ache and heaviness of the extremity. Not surprisingly, there is difficulty with overhead activities and heavy lifting.

In the presence of trapezial palsy, the entire shoulder is depressed with lateral and caudal migration of the scapula. They have an asymmetric neckline and women often describe difficulty with maintaining their bra strap. The winging of the scapula can create a "scapular hump" as the superior angle migrates in a cephalad direction. It is usually located equidistant between the neck and acromion. Weakness in elevation and abduction is a ubiquitous finding.

Winging is exacerbated by these movements; especially in abduction. Although not uniform in its presence, most patients exhibit difficulty in raising the extremity above the horizontal. In the presence of a rested levator scapulae, the shrug test may be negative (168). In addition, the weight duration test can aid in documenting fatigue and pain by having the patient hold a chair or weighted object at arm's length (169).

Nonoperative Management

A trial of physical therapy is indicated in these patients to maximize the function of the remaining scapular stabilizers while the trapezius recovers. Injury secondary to blunt trauma or a stretching injury can take up to 1 year to recover. This can be a frustrating proposition for a competitive athlete. It has been suggested that the potential for functional recovery in younger patients is guarded (170). Therefore, in a patient compliant with physical therapy who has functionally plateaued at a suboptimal level, operative intervention is reasonable to consider at an earlier date. However, when trapezial dysfunction is secondary to an infectious etiology, nonoperative management can provide improvement in up to 18 to 24 months.

Operative Management

Operative management of trapezius palsy historically has included scapular stabilization with fascia lata graft and transfer of the levator scapulae alone or in combination with a fascia lata. These techniques failed as a result of graft stretching or because the levator alone was unable to substitute for the trapezius. Scapulothoracic fasciodesis has also been described and involves static fixation of the scapula to the rib cage (171). This represents a salvage procedure suited for individuals with fascioscapulohumeral dystrophy.

The dynamic muscle transfer described by Eden and Lange represent the current standard for operative intervention of trapezial palsy. The rhomboid major and minor as well as the levator scapulae are removed from their anatomic insertions and lateralized on the scapulae to substitute for the trapezius. The rhomboid major, in part, reproduces the lower trapezius. The rhomboid major and minor function as the middle portion and the levator substitutes for the upper portion. A modification of the Eden-Lange procedure has been published at our institution and its description follows (147,154).

Authors' Preferred Method

The patient is placed in the lateral decubitus position with the table elevated 15 degrees. A longitudinal incision is made midway between the spinous process and the medial border of the scapula. It extends from the superior angle to the base of the scapula. The atrophied trapezius is dissected out and transected at the scapular border. The levator scapulae, rhomboid minor, and rhomboid major are then individually identified (Fig. 19-3). The three muscles for transfer are then removed from their native insertion on the scapula.

Attention is then directed to separating the muscles and dissecting proximally and medially. Separation of the two rhomboids represents one of the modifications of the Eden-Lange that allows for a more anatomic reproduction of trapezial function. Care must be exercised during mobilization of the muscles as the dorsal scapular nerve and transverse scapular artery run superficial to the levator and then terminate deep to the rhomboids near the scapula. Maximizing the mobilization of the levator to its attachment on the cervical vertebrae facilitates its new lateral insertion.

The supraspinatus and infraspinatus are then elevated off of their respective fossae for a distance of 5 to 6 cm (Fig. 19-4). This represents another modification that allows transfer of the rhomboid minor into the supraspinatus fossa to function as the middle trapezius. Two drill holes are made in the supraspinatus fossa and four or five are made into the infraspinatus fossa approximately 4 cm lateral to the medial border of the scapula. This allows for transfer of the rhomboid minor and major, respectively. Two nonabsorbable sutures are used for the rhomboid minor and four for the rhomboid major. This is done with the scapula in a reduced position with the arm abducted 90 degrees.

Next, a second incision 4 cm in length is made over the spine of the scapula starting 3 cm medial to the posterior tip of the acromion and extends medially. The atrophied trapezius, the deltoid, and supraspinatus are elevated to facilitate placement of three drill holes in the spine of the scapula. A tunnel through the soft tissue in line with the trapezial fibers is made to facilitate passage of the levator scapulae. The optimum position of the transferred levator is

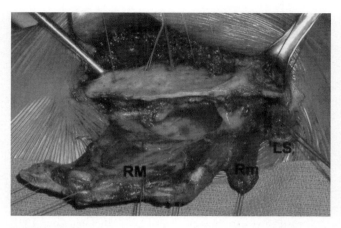

FIGURE 19-4. Intraoperative photo demonstrating mobilization of rhomboid major (RM), rhomboid minor (Rm), and levator scapulae (LS) muscles. Supraspinatus and infraspinatus have been dissected off of their respective fossae and anchoring stitches have been placed.

5 to 7 cm from the posterior lateral corner of the scapular spine. This prevents the occurrence of webbing, which can occur if the muscle is transferred too far laterally.

The incisions are then closed in layers followed by application of an abduction foam wedge. It has been our experience that the wedge is better tolerated than an abduction brace. The wedge is used for 4 weeks postoperatively, keeping the arm in 60 to 70 degrees of abduction. Passive range-of-motion exercises are begun the first day after surgery, with the arm being elevated to 140 degrees and externally rotated to 40 degrees. At 4 weeks, the wedge is discarded and a progressive strengthening program is started. A combination of free weights, rubber sheeting, and medicine ball throwing is used to improve dynamic scapular stability.

In our follow-up study of 22 patients, 13 had excellent results with normal function and shoulder symmetry and six had satisfactory outcomes, noting mild neck asymmetry and functional deficits (154). Adequate pain relief was attained in 19 of 22 patients. Extrapolation of these results to a competitive overhead athlete should be done with caution. Twelve of these patients were involved with strenuous athletic activity postoperatively, including volleyball, tennis, golf, swimming, skiing, racquetball, karate, and bowling. However, they needed to adhere to a specific exercise regimen to maintain their function.

COMPLICATIONS

Patients undergoing these elective procedures have a very low complication rate. There has been a report of a phrenic nerve palsy following a thoracic outlet decompression. It was manifested by shortness of breath during wind-sprints but did ultimately resolve. (95). A postoperative hematoma following a pectoralis major transfer for serratus anterior

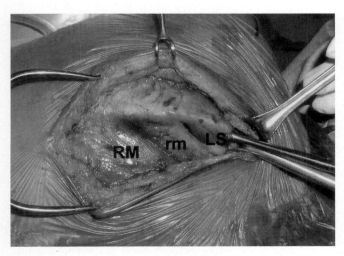

FIGURE 19-3. Intraoperative photo of rhomboid major (RM), rhomboid minor (rm), and levator scapulae (LS) before dissection off of the scapula.

palsy has also been reported (142). This too resolved without additional operative intervention. Most of the reported complications are related to failure of a repair or transfer secondary to patient compliance issues. This underscores the importance of patient selection. An aggressive athlete, who wants a return to play as soon as possible, may require extensive counseling on the consequences of advancing postoperative therapy beyond the stated limits.

REFERENCES

1. Narakas A. Compression and traction neuropathies about the shoulder and arm. In: Gelberman RH, ed. *Operative nerve repair and reconstruction.* Philadelphia: JB Lippincott, 1991: 1147–1175.
2. Thomas A. La paralysie du muscle sous-epineux *Presse Med* 1936;64:1283–1284.
3. Kopell H, Thompson W. Pain and the frozen shoulder. *Surg Gynecol Obstet* 1959;109:92–96.
4. Ganzhorn RW, et al. Suprascapular-nerve entrapment. *J Bone Joint Surg (Am)* 1981;63(3):492–494.
5. Rengachary SS, et al. Suprascapular entrapment neuropathy: a clinical, anatomical, and comparative study. Part 3: Comparative study. *Neurosurgery* 1979;5(4):452–455.
6. Inokuchi W, Ogawa K, Horiuchi Y. Magnetic resonance imaging of suprascapular nerve palsy. *J Shoulder Elbow Surg* 1998;7 (3):223–227.
7. Aiello I, et al. Entrapment of the suprascapular nerve at the spinoglenoid notch. *Ann Neurol* 1982;12(3):314–316.
8. Fabre T, et al. Entrapment of the suprascapular nerve. *J Bone Joint Surg (Br)* 1999;81(3):414–419.
9. Sandow MJ, Ilic J. Suprascapular nerve rotator cuff compression syndrome in volleyball players. *J Shoulder Elbow Surg* 1998; 7(5):516–521.
10. Ferretti A, Cerullo G, Russo G. Suprascapular neuropathy in volleyball players. *J Bone Joint Surg (Am)* 1987;69(2):260–263.
11. Ferretti A, De Carli A, Fontana M. Injury of the suprascapular nerve at the spinoglenoid notch. The natural history of infraspinatus atrophy in volleyball players. *Am J Sports Med* 1998;26 (6):759–763.
12. Vastamaki M, Goransson H. Suprascapular nerve entrapment. *Clin Orthop* 1993;(297):135–143.
13. Zuckerman JD, Polonsky L, Edelson G. Suprascapular nerve palsy in a young athlete. *Bull Hosp Jt Dis* 1993;53(2):11–12.
14. Ringel SP, et al. Suprascapular neuropathy in pitchers. *Am J Sports Med* 1990;18(1):80–86.
15. Cummins CA, et al. Suprascapular nerve entrapment at the spinoglenoid notch in a professional baseball pitcher. *Am J Sports Med* 1999;27(6):810–812.
16. Post M. Diagnosis and treatment of suprascapular nerve entrapment. *Clin Orthop* 1999(368):92–100.
17. Ticker JB, et al. The incidence of ganglion cysts and other variations in anatomy along the course of the suprascapular nerve. *J Shoulder Elbow Surg* 1998;7(5):472–478.
18. Hrdlicka A. The scapula: visual observations. *Am J Phys Anthropol* 1942;29:73–94.
19. Cohen SB, Dines DM, Moorman CT. Familial calcification of the superior transverse scapular ligament causing neuropathy. *Clin Orthop* 1997;(334):131–135.
20. Alon M, et al. Bilateral suprascapular nerve entrapment syndrome due to an anomalous transverse scapular ligament. *Clin Orthop* 1988;(234):31–33.
21. Bigliani LU, et al. An anatomical study of the suprascapular nerve. *Arthroscopy* 1990;6(4):301–305.
22. Warner JP, et al. Anatomy and relationships of the suprascapular nerve: anatomical constraints to mobilization of the supraspinatus and infraspinatus muscles in the management of massive rotator-cuff tears. *J Bone Joint Surg (Am)* 1992;74(1): 36–45.
23. Ozer Y, Grossman JA, Gilbert A. Anatomic observations on the suprascapular nerve. *Hand Clin* 1995;11(4):539–544.
24. Ajmani ML. The cutaneous branch of the human suprascapular nerve. *J Anat* 1994;185(Pt 2):439–4442.
25. Demirhan M, et al. The spinoglenoid ligament and its relationship to the suprascapular nerve. *J Shoulder Elbow Surg* 1998;7 (3):238–243.
26. Cummins CA, et al. Anatomy and histological characteristics of the spinoglenoid ligament. *J Bone Joint Surg (Am)* 1998;80(11): 1622–1625.
27. Gelberman RH, Verdeck WN, Brodhead WT. Supraclavicular nerve-entrapment syndrome. *J Bone Joint Surg (Am)* 1975;57 (1):119.
28. Agre JC, et al. Suprascapular neuropathy after intensive progressive resistive exercise: case report. *Arch Phys Med Rehabil* 1987;68(4):236–238.
29. Callahan JD, et al. Suprascapular nerve entrapment. A series of 27 cases. *J Neurosurg* 1991;74(6):893–896.
30. Mizuno K, et al. Compression neuropathy of the suprascapular nerve as a cause of pain in palsy of the accessory nerve. A case report. *J Bone Joint Surg (Am)* 1990;72(6):938–939.
31. Witvrouw E, et al. Suprascapular neuropathy in volleyball players. *Br J Sports Med* 2000;34(3):174–180.
32. Fritz RC, et al. Suprascapular nerve entrapment: evaluation with MR imaging. *Radiology* 1992;182(2):437–444.
33. Tirman PF, et al. Association of glenoid labral cysts with labral tears and glenohumeral instability: radiologic findings and clinical significance. *Radiology* 1994;190(3):653–658.
34. Cummins CA, Messer TM, Nuber GW. Suprascapular nerve entrapment. *J Bone Joint Surg (Am)* 2000;82(3):415–424.
35. Romeo AA, Rotenberg DD, Bach BR Jr. Suprascapular neuropathy. *J Am Acad Orthop Surg* 1999;7(6):358–367.
36. Steiman, I. Painless infraspinatus atrophy due to suprascapular nerve entrapment. *Arch Phys Med Rehabil* 1988;69(8):641–643.
37. Harbaugh KS, Swenson R, Saunders RL. Shoulder numbness in a patient with suprascapular nerve entrapment syndrome: cutaneous branch of the suprascapular nerve: case report. *Neurosurgery* 2000;47(6):1452–1455; discussion 1455–1456.
38. Rose DL, Kelly CR. Shoulder pain. Suprascapular nerve block in shoulder pain. *J Kans Med Soc* 1969;70(3):135–136.
39. Khalili A. Neuromuscular electrodiagnostic studies in entrapment neuropathy of the suprascapular nerve. *Orhop Rev* 1974; 3:27–28.
40. Antoniou J, et al. Suprascapular neuropathy. Variability in the diagnosis, treatment, and outcome. *Clin Orthop* 2001;(386): 131–138.
41. Herzog R. Magnetic resonance imaging of the shoulder. *J Bone Joint Surg (Am)* 1997;79:934–953.
42. Goss TP, Aronow MS, Coumas JM. The use of MRI to diagnose suprascapular nerve entrapment caused by a ganglion. *Orthopedics* 1994;17(4):359–362.
43. Fuchs B, et al. Fatty degeneration of the muscles of the rotator cuff: assessment by computed tomography versus magnetic resonance imaging. *J Shoulder Elbow Surg* 1999;8(6):599–605.
44. Zanetti M, Gerber C, Hodler J. Quantitative assessment of the muscles of the rotator cuff with magnetic resonance imaging. *Invest Radiol* 1998;33(3):163–170.
45. Martin SD, et al. Suprascapular neuropathy. Results of non-

operative treatment. *J Bone Joint Surg (Am)* 1997;79(8): 1159–1165.

46. Jackson DL, et al. Suprascapular neuropathy in athletes: case reports. *Clin J Sport Med* 1995;5(2):134–136; discussion 136–137.

47. Black KP, Lombardo JA. Suprascapular nerve injuries with isolated paralysis of the infraspinatus. *Am J Sports Med* 1990;18(3): 225–228.

48. Bryan WJ, Wild JJ Jr. Isolated infraspinatus atrophy. A common cause of posterior shoulder pain and weakness in throwing athletes? *Am J Sports Med* 1989;17(1):130–131.

49. Vastamaki M. (Suprascapular nerve entrapment). *Duodecim* 1986;102(6):369–375.

50. Hadley MN, Sonntag VK, Pittman HW. Suprascapular nerve entrapment. A summary of seven cases. *J Neurosurg* 1986;64 (6):843–848.

51. Post M, Mayer J. Suprascapular nerve entrapment. Diagnosis and treatment. *Clin Orthop* 1987;(223):126–136.

52. Hama H, et al. A new strategy for treatment of suprascapular entrapment neuropathy in athletes: shaving of the base of the scapular spine. *J Shoulder Elbow Surg* 1992;1(5):253–260.

53. Hirayama T, Takemitsu Y. Compression of the suprascapular nerve by a ganglion at the suprascapular notch. *Clin Orthop* 1981;(155):95–96.

54. Neviaser TJ, Ain BR, Neviaser RJ. Suprascapular nerve denervation secondary to attenuation by a ganglionic cyst. *J Bone Joint Surg (Am)* 1986;68(4):627–628.

55. Ogino T, et al. Entrapment neuropathy of the suprascapular nerve by a ganglion. A report of three cases. *J Bone Joint Surg (Am)* 1991;73(1):141–147.

56. Rachbauer F, Sterzinger W, Frischhut B. Suprascapular nerve entrapment at the spinoglenoid notch caused by a ganglion cyst. *J Shoulder Elbow Surg* 1996;5(2 Pt 1): 150–152.

57. Thompson RC Jr, Schneider W, Kennedy T. Entrapment neuropathy of the inferior branch of the suprascapular nerve by ganglia. *Clin Orthop* 1982;(166):185–187.

58. Moore TP, et al. Suprascapular nerve entrapment caused by supraglenoid cyst compression. *J Shoulder Elbow Surg* 1997;6 (5):455–462.

59. Iannotti JP, Ramsey ML. Arthroscopic decompression of a ganglion cyst causing suprascapular nerve compression. *Arthroscopy* 1996;12(6):739–745.

60. Chochole MH, et al. Glenoid-labral cyst entrapping the suprascapular nerve: dissolution after arthroscopic debridement of an extended SLAP lesion. *Arthroscopy* 1997;13(6):753–755.

61. Fehrman DA, Orwin JF, Jennings RM. Suprascapular nerve entrapment by ganglion cysts: a report of six cases with arthroscopic findings and review of the literature. *Arthroscopy* 1995; 11(6):727–734.

62. Skirving AP, Kozak TK, Davis SJ. Infraspinatus paralysis due to spinoglenoid notch ganglion. *J Bone Joint Surg (Br)* 1994;76(4): 588–591.

63. McIlveen SJ, et al. Isolated nerve injuries about the shoulder. *Clin Orthop* 1994;(306):54–63.

64. Perlmutter GS. Axillary nerve injury. *Clin Orthop* 1999;(368): 28–36.

65. Hirasawa Y, Sakakida K. Sports and peripheral nerve injury. *Am J Sports Med* 1983;11(6):420–426.

66. Perlmutter GS, Apruzzese W. Axillary nerve injuries in contact sports: recommendations for treatment and rehabilitation. *Sports Med* 1998;26(5):351–361.

67. Bateman J. Nerve injuries about the shoulder in sports. *J Bone Joint Surg* 1967.

68. Cahill BR, Palmer RE. Quadrilateral space syndrome. *J Hand Surg (Am)* 1983;8(1):65–69.

69. Steinmann S, Moran E. Axillary nerve injury: diagnosis and treatment. *J Am Acad Orthop Surg* 2001;9(5):328–335.

70. Gumina S, Postacchini F. Anterior dislocation of the shoulder in elderly patients. *J Bone Joint Surg (Br)* 1997;79(4):540–543.

71. Pasila M, et al. Early complications of primary shoulder dislocations. *Acta Orthop Scand* 1978;49(3):260–263.

72. Perlmutter GS, Leffert RD, Zarins B. Direct injury to the axillary nerve in athletes playing contact sports. *Am J Sports Med* 1997;25(1):65–68.

73. Iannotti J, Williams GR. Biomechanics and pathologic lesions in the overhead athlete. In: Iannotti JP, Williams GR, eds. *Disorders of the shoulder: diagnosis and management. Philadelphia: Lippincott Williams & Wilkins: 1999:248.*

74. Cormier PJ, Matalon TA, Wolin PM. Quadrilateral space syndrome: a rare cause of shoulder pain. *Radiology* 1988;167(3): 797–798.

75. Redler MR, Ruland LJ 3rd, McCue FC 3rd. Quadrilateral space syndrome in a throwing athlete. *Am J Sports Med* 1986;14(6): 511–513.

76. Lester B, et al. Quadrilateral space syndrome: diagnosis, pathology, and treatment. *Am J Orthop* 1999;28(12):718–722, 725.

77. Paladini D, et al. Axillary neuropathy in volleyball players: report of two cases and literature review. *J Neurol Neurosurg Psychiatry* 1996;60(3):345–347.

78. Francel TJ, Dellon AL, Campbell JN. Quadrilateral space syndrome: diagnosis and operative decompression technique. *Plast Reconstr Surg* 1991;87(5):911–916.

79. Nishijima N, et al. The swallow-tail sign: a test of deltoid function. *J Bone Joint Surg (Br)* 1994;77:152–153.

80. Hertel R, Lambert SM, Ballmer FT. The deltoid extension lag sign for diagnosis and grading of axillary nerve palsy. *J Shoulder Elbow Surg* 1998;7(2):97–99.

81. Lubahn JD, Cermak MB. Uncommon nerve compression syndromes of the upper extremity. *J Am Acad Orthop Surg* 1998;6 (6):378–386.

82. Baker CL Jr, Liu SH. Neurovascular injuries to the shoulder. *J Orthop Sports Phys Ther* 1993;18(1):360–364.

83. McKowen HC, Voorhies RM. Axillary nerve entrapment in the quadrilateral space. Case report. *J Neurosurg* 1987;66(6): 932–934.

84. Okino S, Miyaji H, Matoba M. The quadrilateral space syndrome. *Neuroradiology* 1995;37(4):311–312.

85. Linker CS, Helms CA, Fritz RC. Quadrilateral space syndrome: findings at MR imaging. *Radiology* 1993;188(3):675–676.

86. Sanders TG, Tirman PF. Paralabral cyst: an unusual cause of quadrilateral space syndrome. *Arthroscopy* 1999;15(6):632–637.

87. Coene LN, Narakas AO. Operative management of lesions of the axillary nerve, isolated or combined with other nerve lesions. *Clin Neurol Neurosurg* 1992;94[Suppl]:S64–S66.

88. Petrucci FS, Morelli A, Raimondi PL. Axillary nerve injuries— 21 cases treated by nerve graft and neurolysis. *J Hand Surg (Am)* 1982;7(3):271–278.

89. Tyson RR, Kaplan GF. Modern concepts of diagnosis and treatment of the thoracic outlet syndrome. *Orthop Clin North Am* 1975;6:507—518.

90. Thomas G, et al. The middle scalene muscle and its contribution to the thoracic outlet syndrome. *Am J Surg* 1983;145: 589–592.

91. Bonney G. The scalenus medius band. *J Bone Joint Surg (Br)* 1965;47:381–384.

92. Lusskin R, Weiss C, Winer J. The role of the subclavius muscle in the subclavian vein syndrome (costoclavicular syndrome) following fracture of the clavicle. *Clin Orthop* 1967;54:75–83.

93. Roos D. The place for scalenectomy and first rib resection in thoracic outlet syndrome. *Surgery* 1982;92:1077–1084.

94. Nuber GW, et al. Arterial abnormalities of the shoulder in athletes. *Am J Sports Med* 1990;18(5):514–519.

95. McCarthy WJ, et al. Upper extremity arterial injury in athletes. *J Vasc Surg* 1989;9(2):317–327.

96. Rohrer MJ, et al. Axillary artery compression and thrombosis in throwing athletes. *J Vasc Surg* 1990;11(6):761–768; discussion 768–769.

97. Todd GJ, et al. Aneurysms of the mid axillary artery in major league baseball pitchers—a report of two cases. *J Vasc Surg* 1998;28(4):702–707.

98. Leffert R. Thoracic outlet syndrome. In: Gelberman RH, ed. *Operative nerve repair and reconstruction.* Philadelphia: JB Lippincott, 1991:1177–1195.

99. Nehler MR, et al. Upper extremity ischemia from subclavian artery aneurysm caused by bony abnormalities of the thoracic outlet. *Arch Surg* 1997;132(5):527–532.

100. Durham JR, et al. Arterial injuries in the thoracic outlet syndrome. *J Vasc Surg* 1995;21(1):57–69; discussion 70.

101. Todd T. The descent of the shoulder after birth. *Anatomisher Anzeiger Centralblatt fur die gesamte wissenschaftliche Anatomie* 1912;14:358–397.

102. Yao JS. Upper extremity ischemia in athletes. Semin Vasc Surg 1998;11(2):96–105.

103. Reekers JA, et al. Traumatic aneurysm of the posterior circumflex humeral artery: a volleyball player's disease? *J Vasc Interv Radiol* 1993;4(3):405–408.

104. Kee ST, et al. Ischemia of the throwing hand in major league baseball pitchers: embolic occlusion from aneurysms of axillary artery branches. *J Vasc Interv Radiol* 1995;6(6):979–982.

105. Tullos HS, et al. Unusual lesions of the pitching arm. *Clin Orthop* 1972;88:169–182.

106. Kleinsasser L. Effort thrombosis of the axillary and subclavian vein. *Arch Surg* 1949;59:258–274.

107. Vogel CM, Jensen JE. 9Effort9 thrombosis of the subclavian vein in a competitive swimmer. *Am J Sports Med* 1985;13 (4):269–272.

108. DiFelice GS, et al. Effort thrombosis in the elite throwing athlete. *Am J Sports Med* 2002;30(5):708–712.

109. McMaster WC. Swimming injuries. An overview. *Sports Med* 1996;22(5):332–336.

110. Medler RG, McQueen DA. Effort thrombosis in a young wrestler. A case report. *J Bone Joint Surg (Am)* 1993;75(7):1071–1073.

111. Schneider K, et al. An aneurysm involving the axillary artery and its branch vessels in a major league baseball pitcher. A case report and review of the literature. *Am J Sports Med* 1999;27 (3):370–375.

112. Adson A, Coffey J. Cervical rib: method of anterior approach for relief of symptoms by division of scalenus anticus. *Ann Surg* 1927;85:839–857.

113. Wright I. The neurovascular syndrome produced by hyperabduction of the arms. *Am Heart J* 1945;29(1):1–19.

114. Dugas JR, Weiland AJ. Vascular pathology in the throwing athlete. *Hand Clin* 2000;16(3):477–485.

115. McCready RA, et al. Recurrence and rupture of an axillary artery aneurysm. *Am Surg* 1982;48(5):241–242.

116. Brooks A, Fowler B. Axillary artery thrombosis after prolonged use of crutches. *J Bone Joint Surg (Am)* 1964;46:863–864.

117. Fields WS, Lemak NA, Ben-Menachem Y. Thoracic outlet syndrome: review and reference to stroke in a major league pitcher. *AJR Am J Roentgenol* 1986;146(4):809–814.

118. Urschel HC Jr, Razzuk MA. Improved management of the Paget-Schroetter syndrome secondary to thoracic outlet compression. *Ann Thorac Surg* 1991;52(6):1217–1221.

119. Taylor LM Jr, et al. Thrombolytic therapy followed by first rib resection for spontaneous (9effort9) subclavian vein thrombosis. *Am J Surg* 1985;149(5):644–647.

120. Arko FR, et al. Vascular complications in high-performance athletes. *J Vasc Surg* 2001;33(5):935–942.

121. Winslow M. Sur quelques mouvements extraordinaires des omoplates et des bras, et sur une nouvelle espece de muscles. *Mem Acad Royale Sci* 1723:98–112.

122. Tubby A. A case illustrating the operative treatment of paralysis of the serratus magnus muscle by muscle grafting. *Br Med J* 1904:1159–1160.

123. Gregg JR, et al. Serratus anterior paralysis in the young athlete. *J Bone Joint Surg (Am)* 1979;61(6):825–832.

124. Schulte KR, Warner JJ. Uncommon causes of shoulder pain in the athlete. *Orthop Clin North Am* 1995;26(3):505–528.

125. Wiater JM, Flatow EL. Long thoracic nerve injury. *Clin Orthop* 1999;(368):17–27.

126. Warner JJ, Navarro RA. Serratus anterior dysfunction. Recognition and treatment. *Clin Orthop* 1998;(349):139–148.

127. Vastamaki M, Kauppila LI. Etiologic factors in isolated paralysis of the serratus anterior muscle: A report of 197 cases. *J Shoulder Elbow Surg* 1993;2(5):240–243.

128. Woodhead AB 3rd. Paralysis of the serratus anterior in a world class marksman. A case study. *Am J Sports Med* 1985;13(5): 359–362.

129. Stanish WD, Lamb H. Isolated paralysis of the serratus anterior muscle: a weight training injury. Case report. *Am J Sports Med* 1978;6(6):385–386.

130. Holden DL, Jackson DW. Stress fracture of the ribs in female rowers. *Am J Sports Med* 1985;13(5):342–348.

131. Foo CL, Swann M. Isolated paralysis of the serratus anterior. A report of 20 cases. *J Bone Joint Surg (Br)* 1983;65(5): 552–556.

132. White SM, Witten CM. Long thoracic nerve palsy in a professional ballet dancer. *Am J Sports Med* 1993;21(4):626–628.

133. Gaffney KM. Avulsion injury of the serratus anterior: a case history. *Clin J Sport Med* 1997;7(2):134–136.

134. Hester P, Caborn DN, Nyland J. Cause of long thoracic nerve palsy: a possible dynamic fascial sling cause. *J Shoulder Elbow Surg* 2000;9(1):31–35.

135. Bora F, Pleasure D, Didzian N. A study of nerve regeneration and neuroma formation after nerve suture by various techniques. *J Hand Surg* 1976;1:138–143.

136. Marin R. Scapula winger's brace: a case series on the management of long thoracic nerve palsy. *Arch Phys Med Rehabil* 1998;79(10):1226–130.

137. Chaves J. Pectoralis minor transplant for paralysis of the serratus anterior. *J Bone Joint Surg (Br)* 1951;33:228–230.

138. Whitman A. Congenital elevation of the scapula and paralysis of serratus magnus muscle. *JAMA* 1932;99:1332–1334.

139. Dickson F. Fascial transplants in paralytic and other conditions. *J Bone Joint Surg* 1937;19:405–412.

140. Durman D. An operation for paralysis of the serratus anterior. *J Bone Joint Surg* 1945;27:380–382.

141. Gozna ER, Harris WR. Traumatic winging of the scapula. *J Bone Joint Surg (Am)* 1979;61(8):1230–1233.

142. Post M. Pectoralis major transfer for winging of the scapula. *J Shoulder Elbow Surg* 1995;4(1 Pt 1):1–9.

143. Connor PM, et al. Split pectoralis major transfer for serratus anterior palsy. *Clin Orthop* 1997;(341):134–142.

144. Perlmutter GS, Leffert RD. Results of transfer of the pectoralis major tendon to treat paralysis of the serratus anterior muscle. *J Bone Joint Surg (Am)* 1999;81(3):377–384.

145. Wiater JM, Bigliani LU. Spinal accessory nerve injury. *Clin Orthop* 1999;(368):5–16.

146. Novak CB, Mackinnon SE. Surgical treatment of a long thoracic nerve palsy. *Ann Thorac Surg* 2002;73(5):1643–1645.

147. Bigliani LU, Perez-Sanz JR, Wolfe IN. Treatment of trapezius paralysis. *J Bone Joint Surg (Am)* 1985;67(6):871–877.

148. Inman V, Saunders J, Dec M. Observations on the function of the shoulder joint. *J Bone Joint Surg* 1944;26:1–30.

149. Codman E. Rupture of the supraspinatus tendon and other lesions in or about the subacromial bursa. In: *The shoulder.* Boston: Thomas Todd, 1934.

150. Henry A. An operation for slinging a dropped shoulder. *Br J Surg* 1927;15:95–98.

151. Dewar F, Harris R. Restoration of function of the shoulder following paralysis of the trapezius by fascial sling fixation and transplantation of the levator scapulae. *Ann Surg* 1950;132: 1111–1115.

152. Lange M. Die behandlung der irreparablem trapeziusmahlung. *Langenbecks Arch Klin Chir* 1951;270:437–439.

153. Eden R. Zur behandlung der trapeziuslahmung mittelst muskelplastik. *Deustche Zeitschr Chir* 1924;184:387–397.

154. Bigliani LU, et al. Transfer of the levator scapulae, rhomboid major, and rhomboid minor for paralysis of the trapezius. *J Bone Joint Surg (Am)* 1996;78(10):1534–1540.

155. Dunn AW. Trapezius paralysis after minor surgical procedures in the posterior cervical triangle. *South Med J* 1974;67(3): 312–315.

156. Dellon AL, Campbell JN, Cornblath D. Stretch palsy of the spinal accessory nerve. Case report. *J Neurosurg* 1990;72(3): 500–502.

157. Hollinshead W. Pectoral region, axilla, shoulder and arm. In: *Textbook of anatomy.* Hagerstown, MD: Harper and Row, 1974: 193.

158. Jobe CM, Kropp WE, Wood VE. Spinal accessory nerve in a trapezius-splitting surgical approach. *J Shoulder Elbow Surg* 1996;5(3):206–208.

159. Barron O, Levine WN, Bigliani LU. Surgical management of chronic trapezius dysfunction. In: Warner JJ, Iannotti JP, Ger- ber C, eds. *Complex and revision problems in shoulder surgery.* Philadelphia: Lippincott-Raven, 1997:377–384.

160. Remmler D, et al. A prospective study of shoulder disability resulting from radical and modified neck dissections. *Head Neck Surg* 1986;8(4):280–286.

161. Brandenburg JH, Lee CY. The eleventh nerve in radical neck surgery. *Laryngoscope* 1981;91(11):1851–1859.

162. Vandeweyer E, Goldschmidt D, de Fontaine S. Traumatic spinal accessory nerve palsy. *J Reconstr Microsurg* 1998;14(4): 259–261.

163. Vastamaki M, Solonen KA. Accessory nerve injury. *Acta Orthop Scand* 1984;55(3):296–299.

164. Kocher MS, Dupre MM, Feagin JA Jr. Shoulder injuries from alpine skiing and snowboarding. Aetiology, treatment and pre- vention. *Sports Med* 1998;25(3):201–211.

165. Cohn B, Brahms M, Cohn M. Injury to the eleventh cranial nerve in a high school wrestler. *Orthop Rev* 1986;15:59–64.

166. Lorei MP, Hershman EB. Peripheral nerve injuries in athletes. Treatment and prevention. *Sports Med* 1993;16(2):130–147.

167. Wright TA. Accessory spinal nerve injury. *Clin Orthop* 1975; (108):15–18.

168. Gabel G, Nuley N. Spinal accessory nerve. In: Gelberaman R, ed. Operative nerve repair and reconstruction. Philadelphia: JB Lippincott, 1991:445.

169. Neer C. Less frequent procedures. In: *Shoulder reconstruction.* Philadelphia: WB Saunders, 1990:451.

170. Post M. Orthopaedic management of neuromuscular disorders. In: Post M, et al, eds. *The shoulder: operative technique.* Balti- more: Lippincott Williams & Wilkins, 1998:201–233.

171. Ketenjian AY. Scapulocostal stabilization for scapular winging in facioscapulohumeral muscular dystrophy. *J Bone Joint Surg (Am)* 1978;60(4):476–480.

20

DISORDERS IN PEDIATRIC ATHLETES

MININDER S. KOCHER
JAMES O'HOLLERAN

INTRODUCTION

Injuries to the shoulder in pediatric and adolescent athletes are increasingly being seen with expanded participation and higher competitive levels of youth sports. Injury patterns are unique to the growing musculoskeletal system and specific to the demands of the involved sport (1–4). Recognition of injury patterns with early activity modification and the initiation of efficacious treatment can prevent disability and return the youth athlete to sport. This chapter reviews the diagnosis and management of common shoulder injuries in the pediatric athlete.

DEVELOPMENTAL ANATOMY AND GROWTH

The shoulder complex involves four articulations and multiple ossification centers. Growth occurs through the cartilaginous physis. Bony development occurs through the primary and secondary centers of ossification and through periosteal bone formation. The cartilaginous physis is particularly vulnerable to acute macrotraumatic and repetitive microtraumatic injury (5).

Prenatally, the limb buds develop during the fourth gestational week (1–4). The central core of the humerus appears as a cartilaginous anlage and the clavicle begins to ossify through intramembranous ossification by the fifth week. The scapula also appears around this time and is positioned proximally at the level of C4-5. The precursor to the shoulder joint, the interzone, also appears between the humerus and scapula. During the sixth gestational week, the hand begins to develop, bone formation occurs in the primary center of ossification of the humerus, and the interzone develops a layered configuration with a chondrified layer on either side of a loose layer of central cells. In the seventh week, the upper limbs rotate laterally, the shoulder joint is formed, and the scapula descends to its position between the first and fifth ribs. The muscular, tendinous, and ligamentous structures of the shoulder become distinct by the 13th gestational week and continue to mature throughout the gestational period.

The secondary center of ossification of the proximal humeral epiphysis is usually seen after 6 months of age. Additional ossification centers appear at the greater tuberosity between 7 months and 3 years of age and at the lesser tuberosity is seen 2 years later. By age 5 to 7 years, these centers coalesce to form the proximal humeral epiphysis. The proximal humeral physis is extraarticular, except medially where the capsule extends beyond the anatomic neck, inserting on the medial metaphysis (Fig. 20-1). The proximal humeral physis contributes approximately 80% of the longitudinal growth of the humerus and usually fuses between 19 and 22 years of age. Fractures of the proximal humeral physis often occur through the zone of hypertrophy (Fig. 20-2).

The clavicle forms by intramembranous ossification. The medial secondary ossification center appears between 12 and 19 years of age and does not fuse to the shaft until age 22 to 25 years. The lateral epiphysis is inconstant, appearing, ossifying, and fusing over a period of a few months at about age 19 years.

The scapula appears as a cartilaginous anlage in the first gestational week at the C4-5 level and gradually descends to its adult-like position overlying the first to fifth ribs. Failure to descend results in persistent elevation of the scapula and limited glenohumeral motion (Sprengel's deformity). The scapula ossifies via intramembranous ossification with multiple remaining secondary ossification centers (Fig. 20-3). The ossification center of the coracoid process appears at approximately 1 year of age, coalescing with the ossification center of the upper glenoid by age 10 years. The acromion ossifies by multiple (two to five) ossification centers which usually appear about puberty and fuse by age 22 years. Failure of fusion of one of these ossification centers may result in an os acromiale. Various other scapular malformations may occur, including bipartite coracoid, acromion duplication, glenoid dysplasia, and scapular clefts. In the first 2 years of life, the glenoid is retroverted approximately 6 degrees, but reaches adult retroversion of 2 to 6 degrees by the end of the first decade of life.

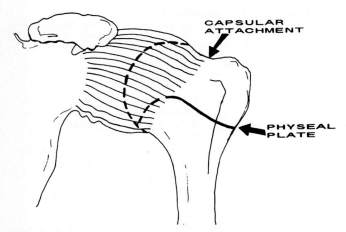

FIGURE 20-1. Proximal humeral physis and glenohumeral joint capsule. The physis is mostly extraarticular except medially. (From Curtis RJ. Anatomy, biomechanics, and kinesiology of the child's shoulder. In: DeLee JC, Drez D, Miller MD, eds. *Orthopaedic sports medicine: principles and practice,* 2nd ed. Philadelphia: WB Saunders, 2003, with permission.)

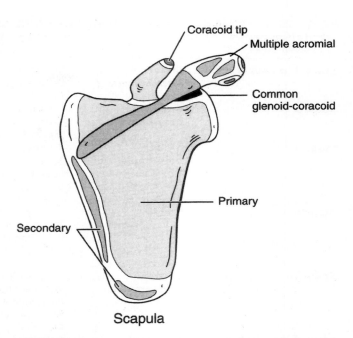

FIGURE 20-3. Ossification centers of the scapula. (From Curtis RJ. Anatomy, biomechanics, and kinesiology of the child's shoulder. In: DeLee JC, Drez D, Miller MD, eds. *Orthopaedic sports medicine: principles and practice,* 2nd ed. Philadelphia: WB Saunders, 2003, with permission.)

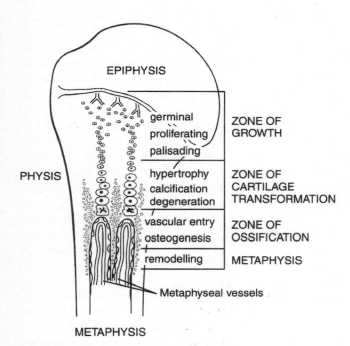

FIGURE 20-2. Proximal humeral physis. Fractures often occur through the zone of hypertrophy. (From Curtis RJ. Anatomy, biomechanics, and kinesiology of the child's shoulder. In: DeLee JC, Drez D, Miller MD, eds. *Orthopaedic sports medicine: principles and practice,* 2nd ed. Philadelphia: WB Saunders, 2003, with permission.)

Maturation and Laxity

In addition to longitudinal growth of the upper and lower extremities, the pediatric athlete is developing in terms of maturation (1–4). The child's stage of maturation is often an important factor in injury patterns. In addition, girls mature at an earlier age than boys. Less mature children often have less muscular development and may be in a period of rapid longitudinal growth, predisposing to repetitive overuse injuries. More mature children may have increased muscular development and less longitudinal growth remaining, leading to acute, macrotraumatic injuries. The Tanner staging system is usually used to classify children with respect to secondary sexual development and maturation (Table 20-1).

During childhood and adolescence, changes in laxity also occur. Laxity is common in younger children and less common through adolescence. In newborns, type III collagen is synthesized, and the fibers formed from type III collagen are supple and elastic. With each passing decade, collagen-producing cells make less type III collagen and progressively convert to making type I collagen, which is more nonelastic. This changing ratio of type I and III collagen is so reliable that the chronologic age of an individual can be determined by analyzing the type III collagen of a skin sample (6). Some patients, particularly girls, may exhibit generalized ligamentous laxity of multiple joints (7–9). Because of the importance of capsuloligamentous

TABLE 20–1. TANNER STAGING CLASSIFICATION OF SECONDARY SEXUAL CHARACTERISTICS

Tanner Stage		Male	Female
Stage 1 (prepubertal)	**Growth**	5–6 cm/yr	5–6 cm/yr
	Development	Testes <4 mL or <2.5 cm	No breast development
		No pubic hair	No pubic hair
Stage 2	**Growth**	5–6 cm/yr	7–8 cm/yr
	Development	Testes 4 mL or 2.5–3.2 cm	Breast buds
		Minimal pubic hair at base of penis	Minimal pubic hair on labia
Stage 3	**Growth**	7–8 cm/yr	8 cm/yr
	Development	Testes 12 mL or 3.6 cm	Elevation of breast; areolae enlarge
		Pubic hair over pubis	Pubic hair of mons pubis
		Voice changes	Axillary hair
		Muscle mass increases	Acne
Stage 4	**Growth**	10 cm/yr	7 cm/yr
	Development	Testes 4.1–4.5 cm	Areolae enlarge
		Pubic hair as adult	Pubic hair as adult
		Axillary hair	
		Acne	
Stage 5	**Growth**	No growth	No growth
	Development	Testes as adult	Adult breast contour
		Pubic hair as adult	Pubic hair as adult
		Facial hair as adult	
		Mature physique	
Other		Peak height velocity: 13.5 years	Adrenarche: 6–8 years
			Menarche: 12.7 years
			Peak height velocity: 11.5 years

restraints for shoulder stability, patients with laxity may experience difficulty with glenohumeral instability.

EPIDEMIOLOGY AND INJURY PATTERNS

Injuries to the pediatric athlete's shoulder are being seen with increased frequency. There has been increased participation in youth sports (10). In addition, children are participating in organized athletics at higher competitive levels with increased intensity. It is not uncommon to see a youth pitcher with a sore shoulder who plays in two concurrent leagues, throws a large number of pitches during games and practices, and who has been taught split finger pitches. Less than 10% of the 2.5 million volunteer coaches and less than one third of the interscholastic coaches in the United States have had any type of coaching education. The sequelae of these injuries are of importance. Sports injuries to youth ages 0 to 14 years for 29 sports in 1997 cost the U.S. public nearly $50 billion according to the U.S. Consumer Product Safety Commission (11). In addition, injuries to youth athletes can result in permanent disability and deformity.

Injury patterns to the pediatric athlete's shoulder tend to be sport specific. In football, the shoulder ranks second only to the knee in number of overall injuries (12–14). These injuries tend to result from macrotrauma, such as glenohumeral dislocation, acromioclavicular separation, and clavicle fractures. Bicycling is a popular recreational and

sporting activity among children and adolescents. Sixty percent of all bicycle injuries occur in children between the ages of 5 and 14 years and 85% of injuries involve the upper extremity (10,15). A common injury pattern during bicycling involves lateral clavicle fracture or acromioclavicular separation from landing on the point of the shoulder when thrown from the bicycle. Shoulder injuries during alpine skiing and snowboarding are being seen with increased frequency and account for approximately 40% of upper extremity injuries and 10% of all injuries (16,17). Thirty percent of wrestling injuries occur in the upper extremity, with the shoulder being the most commonly involved location. Injury to the acromioclavicular joint is frequent, resulting from a direct blow of the shoulder against the mat (18).

The pediatric shoulder is particularly vulnerable in overhead athletes. In baseball, injury to the pediatric shoulder from throwing is a result of microtrauma from repetitive motions of large rotational forces (19–35). The proximal humeral physis is particularly vulnerable to these large, repetitive forces, resulting in a chronic physeal stress fracture (Little League shoulder) (36–45). The shoulder in tennis is similarly subjected to repetitive overhead motions involving large torques. Impingement and depression of the shoulder (tennis shoulder) may result (46). Repetitive microtrauma also frequently leads to shoulder dysfunction in swimmers (47). The risk of injury is related to competitive level and event type. Injuries include impingement syndrome and glenohumeral instability. Multidirectional instability is often seen and is related to the underlying ligamentous laxity often seen in swimmers. Similarly, multidirectional instability can be seen in gymnasts who also frequently demonstrate generalized ligamentous laxity. Additional shoulder injuries unique to gymnasts include cortical hypertrophy at the pectoralis major insertion (ringman's shoulder) and supraspinatus tendinitis (48–54).

SPECIFIC INJURIES

Sternoclavicular Joint Injury

True sternoclavicular joint dislocations are rare in the skeletally immature. The characteristic injury involves a physeal fracture of the medial clavicle, commonly a Salter-Harris I or II injury, in that the medial clavicular physis does not fuse until the early 20s (55–60). The epiphysis stays attached to the sternum via the stout sternoclavicular ligaments and the medial clavicular shaft displaces posteriorly or anteriorly. Medial clavicular injury often results from an indirect force transmitted along the clavicle from a direct blow during contact sports to the lateral shoulder. If the shoulder is driven forward, posterior displacement of the medial clavicle occurs. Conversely, if the shoulder is driven posteriorly, anterior displacement of the medial clavicle occurs.

The patient often describes a pop in the region of the sternoclavicular joint and there is tenderness to palpation of the medial clavicle. The direction of displacement may be obscured by marked swelling. Posterior displacement can be a medical emergency because the medial clavicle can impinge on vital mediastinal structures including the innominate great vessels, trachea, and esophagus (Fig. 20-4). Venous congestion, diminished pulses, dysphagia, or dyspnea should alert the clinician to the possibility of such injury. Standard anteroposterior (AP) radiographs of the

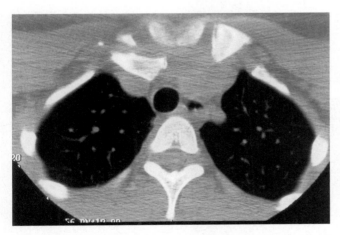

FIGURE 20-4. Sternoclavicular joint injury. Axial computed tomography scan demonstrating physeal fracture/separation of the medial clavicle with compression of the innominate vein in a 16-year-old female.

chest or sternoclavicular joint are often hard to interpret given the overlapping spinal, thoracic, and mediastinal structures. A tangential radiograph obtained in a 40-degree cephalad-directed manner (the serendipity view) may aid in visualization of the medial clavicle displacement. Definitive delineation of the fracture pattern and direction of displacement is provided by computed tomography scan.

Minimally displaced fractures heal readily. Attempted reduction of anteriorly displaced fractures can be accomplished under local anesthesia or sedation by placing the patient supine with a bolster between the scapulae. The arm is abducted 90 degrees and then extended with gentle posterior pressure directly over the medial clavicle followed by protraction of the shoulder. After reduction, the shoulder is immobilized in a figure-of-eight dressing or shoulder immobilizer and gentle range of motion exercises are started as pain allows. Most fractures heal in 3 to 4 weeks and return to sport requires full painless range of motion and strength. Unstable fractures usually heal and remodel rapidly. Posteriorly displaced medial clavicular fractures with impingement of mediastinal structures require emergent reduction with thoracic surgery standby for the rare but potential injury of the major thoracic vessels. Under general anesthesia with the patient supine, traction is applied to the arm with the shoulder extended, and a towel clip can be used to reduce the medial clavicle. There is little indication for open reduction and internal fixation of medial clavicular physeal fractures, and catastrophic complications of pin migration from hardware about the sternoclavicular joint has been reported. On rare occasion, open reduction with stabilization may be indicated for patients with recurrent, symptomatic instability. In younger children, repair of the torn periosteum is usually sufficient for stability, whereas older children and adolescents require reconstruction of the medial sternoclavicular ligamentous structures using palmaris tendon or semitendinosus tendon graft.

Clavicle Fracture

The clavicular shaft is vulnerable to injury from direct blows during contact sports. In addition, indirect forces on the outstretched arm may lead to clavicular fracture. The clavicular shaft is mechanically vulnerable as a strut given its S-shaped configuration and the strong ligamentous bindings at either end. With fracture, there is limited shoulder motion and tenderness over the fracture site, and the skin overlying the fracture may be tented and compromised. The proximal fragment may be elevated superiorly due to spasm of the sternocleidomastoid or trapezius muscles. Significant neurovascular injury is rare but should be assessed clinically given the proximity of the subclavian vessels and the brachial plexus. Radiographs are usually sufficient for diagnosis and management. Younger children may exhibit a greenstick fracture or plastic deformation.

The prognosis of most clavicular shaft fractures in children is excellent (61–63). Immobilization is accomplished by a figure-of-eight bandage or shoulder immobilizer. Slings that exert significant pressure to effect a reduction should be avoided. Even displaced fractures usually heal readily with a bump of healing callus that remodels over a period of 6 to 12 months. Return to sport is allowed when the clavicle is nontender, there is radiographic union, and motion and strength are full. This usually occurs by 4 to 6 weeks in younger children and by 6 to 10 weeks in the ado-

lescent. Significant malunion that does not remodel and nonunion of clavicular shaft fractures in the skeletally immature are rare. Malunion with a symptomatic bump can be treated after healing with osteoplasty. Open reduction and internal fixation is indicated for open fractures, fractures with significant neurovascular compromise, threatened skin from fracture displacement (Fig. 20-5), and floating shoulder injuries.

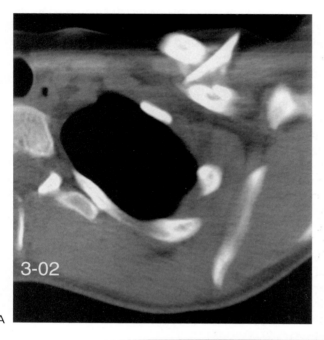

A

FIGURE 20-5. Clavicle fracture. A comminuted clavicle fracture in a 14-year-old female athlete. **A:** Computed tomography scan demonstrates the comminuted fragment tenting the skin. Preoperative **(B)** and postoperative **(C)** radiographs obtained after open reduction and internal fixation.

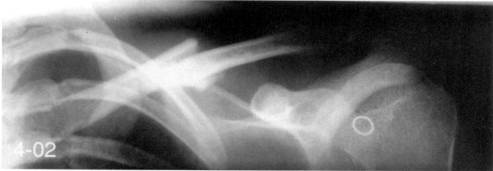

B

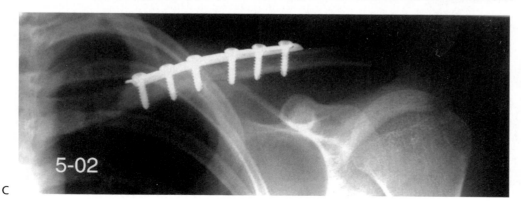

C

Acromioclavicular Joint Injury

A fall on the point of the shoulder usually results in acromioclavicular separation in the adult and older adolescent, but results in physeal fracture of the lateral clavicle in children (63–71). With lateral clavicle fracture and true acromioclavicular separation in the pediatric patient, displacement of the lateral clavicle occurs superiorly through a tear in the thick periosteal tube surrounding the distal clavicle (Fig. 20-6). The lateral clavicular epiphysis along with the acromioclavicular and coracoclavicular ligaments usually remain intact to the periosteal tube.

The pediatric athlete with lateral clavicle physeal fracture or acromioclavicular injury usually presents after a fall or contact to the point of the shoulder. Pain and deformity are localized to the acromioclavicular joint. Plane radiographs are usually sufficient to evaluate the injury and stress radiographs with 5 to 10 pounds of traction may aid in delineating the degree of instability. An axillary lateral view demonstrates AP displacement. Like for adult acromioclavicular injuries, Rockwood has classified pediatric acromioclavicular injuries based on the position of the lateral clavicle and the accompanying injury to the periosteal tube (71). Type I injuries involve mild sprain of the acromioclavicular ligaments without disruption of the periosteal tube. Type II injuries involve partial disruption of the dorsal periosteal tube with slight widening of the acromioclavicular joint.

Type III injuries involve a large dorsal disruption of the periosteal tube with gross instability of the distal clavicle. Type IV injuries involve disruption of the periosteal tube with posterior displacement of the lateral clavicle (Fig. 20-7). Type V injuries involve periosteal tube disruption with greater than 100% superior subcutaneous displacement of the lateral clavicle. Type VI injuries involve an inferior subcoracoid dislocation of the lateral clavicle.

Nonoperative management of acromioclavicular injuries in children younger than 13 years old is the mainstay of treatment because these injuries usually represent a physeal fracture rather than a true acromioclavicular joint dislocation (63–71). Thus, these injuries exhibit a great potential for healing and remodeling because the periosteal tube usually remains in continuity with the epiphyseal fragment and acromioclavicular and coracoclavicular ligaments. For type IV, V, and VI injuries with very large displacement, operative stabilization may be indicated. Repair of the periosteal tube with or without internal fixation is usually performed. For late adolescent and adult-type true acromioclavicular joint separations, nonoperative management results in good outcomes for type I and II injuries, whereas operative management is indicated for type IV, V, and VI injuries. The management of type III injuries in the older adolescent athlete remains controversial, as with adults, with many clinicians recommending initial nonoperative management (64,68,69).

Osteolysis of the Distal Clavicle

Osteolysis of the distal clavicle is an overuse injury resulting from repetitive microtrauma (72). It has also been described as a sequela following traumatic injury to the distal clavicle or acromioclavicular joint; however it is seen most commonly in adult weightlifters. In addition, this entity is being identified in other sports since cross-training has become more popular and in younger athletes who are weight training year-round for higher level sports. Patients complain of an aching discomfort about the acromioclavicular joint after workouts, with the pain progressing to interfere with training and eventually with activities of daily living. There is tenderness to palpation of the distal clavicle and pain with cross-chest adduction. Treatment consists of rest, particularly from weight training, and antiinflammatory medications. For those who fail conservative treatment or who are unable to refrain from weight training, distal clavicle resection usually results in resolution of pain and return to sport.

Little League Shoulder

As a result of repetitive microtrauma from the large rotational torques involved in throwing, chronic stress fracture of the proximal humeral physis can occur (19–35). This entity has been termed *Little League shoulder* and is most commonly seen in high-performance male pitchers between

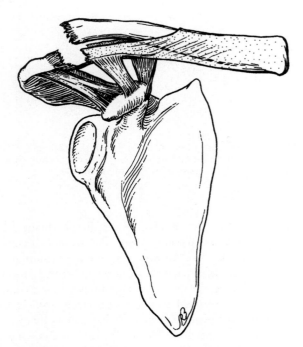

FIGURE 20-6. Acromioclavicular injury. Displacement of the distal clavicle occurs through a tear in the periosteal tube of the clavicle. The acromioclavicular and sternoclavicular ligaments remain intact to the periosteal tube. (From Beim GM, Warner JP. Clinical and radiographic evaluation of the acromioclavicular joint. *Oper Tech Sports Med* 1997;5:68, with permission.)

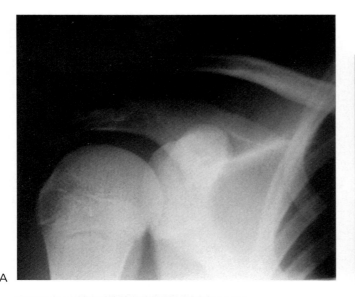

A

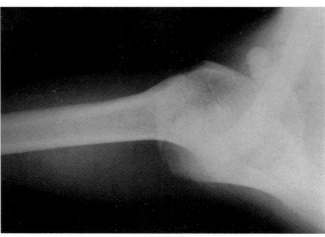

B

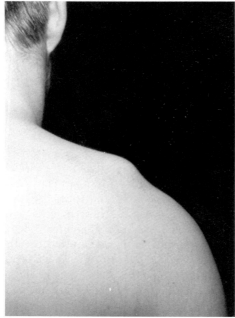

C

FIGURE 20-7. Type IV acromioclavicular injury. **A:** Anteroposterior radiograph. **B:** Axillary lateral view demonstrating posterior displacement. **C:** Photograph showing posterior prominence of lateral clavicle in a 16-year-old male.

12 and 14 years old (36–45). The rotator cuff muscles attach proximal to the proximal humeral physis, whereas the pectoralis major, deltoid, and triceps muscles attach distally. In addition to age and the large rotational forces of pitching, poor throwing mechanics and frequent pitching may predispose to injury. In an extensive study of Little League pitchers, Albright found that those who had poor pitching skills were more likely to be symptomatic (20).

Patients complain of shoulder pain and there is typically widening of the proximal humeral physis with lateral fragmentation (Fig. 20-8) on x-ray study. Bilateral AP radiographs in internal and external rotation are useful to compare the extent of physeal widening with that on the noninvolved side. Good results can usually be obtained by enforcing rest from pitching until the patient becomes asymptomatic (36–45). Growth disturbances resulting in arm length discrepancy are rare. However, repetitive stress to the proximal humeral physis in young throwers may account, in part, for the increased humeral retroversion seen in the throwing shoulder of adult throwers, which allows for greater external rotation and ball velocity. Return to throwing is through an interval program that emphasizes a vigorous preseason conditioning program and limits the frequency of pitching during the subsequent year with attention paid to shoulder pain. Proper throwing mechanics should be stressed, with control rather than speed being emphasized.

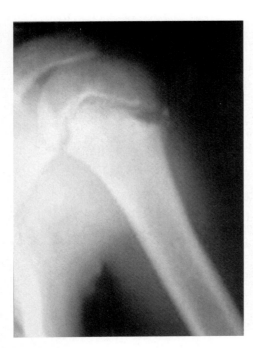

FIGURE 20-8. Little League shoulder. Anteroposterior radiograph demonstrating widening and lateral sclerosis of the proximal humeral physis in a 14-year-old adolescent male.

Proximal Humerus Fracture

Approximately 20% of proximal humeral fractures in the skeletally immature occur in sporting events (73–79). The peak age is 10 to 14 years. Two thirds of cases involve the proximal humeral metaphysis and one third involve the proximal humeral physis. Approximately one fourth of fractures in this region occur through unicameral bone cysts. Proximal metaphyseal fractures are characteristically more likely in children younger than 10 years old. Most physeal fractures in this region are Salter-Harris type I or II lesions, with type II fractures being more common in children older than 10 years of age. With physeal fractures, the distal fragment usually displaces anteriorly and laterally through a relatively weaker area of periosteum. Patients present with shoulder pain, limited motion, and tenderness to palpation. Routine roentgenograms are usually sufficient to demonstrate the fracture pattern, amount of displacement, or presence of a unicameral bone cyst.

Nondisplaced or minimally angulated metaphyseal or physeal fractures can usually be treated adequately with a shoulder immobilizer. Because most of these fractures are intrinsically stable, shoulder motion can be initiated early. There is tremendous potential for remodeling of proximal humerus fractures because the physis is so active. Thus, many moderately displaced, angulated, or bayoneted fractures can be accepted in less than anatomic alignment with good functional outcomes in younger children (73–79). For severely angulated or displaced fractures in adolescents, closed reduction should be performed. Reduction is usually achieved by bringing the distal shaft fragment into flexion,

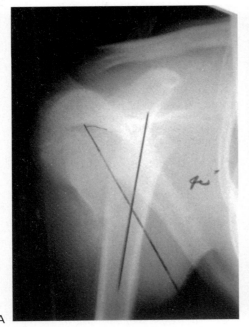
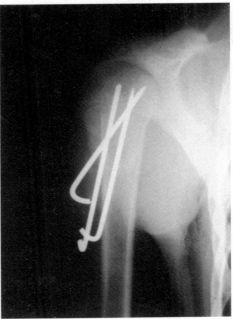

FIGURE 20-9. Proximal humerus fracture. Preoperative oblique view **(A)** and oblique view **(B)** after reduction and percutaneous pinning in a 16-year-old male.

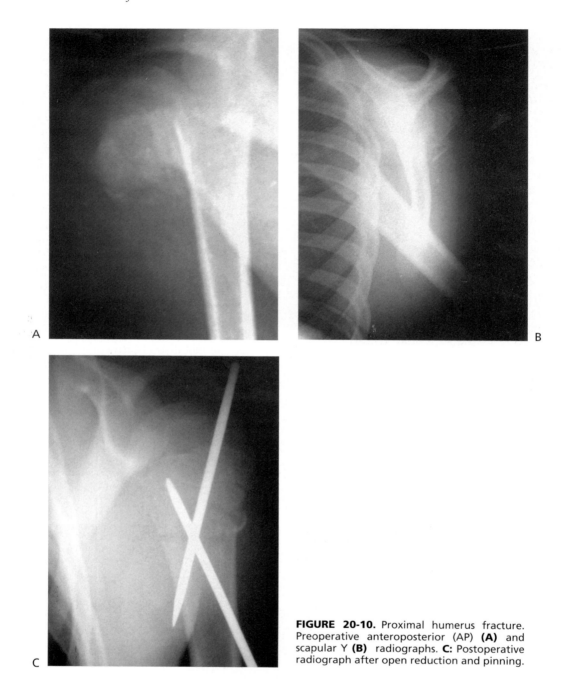

FIGURE 20-10. Proximal humerus fracture. Preoperative anteroposterior (AP) **(A)** and scapular Y **(B)** radiographs. **C:** Postoperative radiograph after open reduction and pinning.

abduction, and external rotation to align it with the proximal fragment. If stable after reduction, the fracture can be immobilized next to the chest. If unstable, the reduction must be held immobilized by a shoulder spica cast or shoulder spica brace. These are usually poorly tolerated by patients and parents, and thus percutaneous pinning is advantageous because it allows immobilization in an immobilizer (Fig. 20-9). In older adolescents, closed reduction of displaced fractures is often unsuccessful with periosteum, deltoid muscle, or long head of biceps tendon preventing

reduction. In these cases, open reduction with internal fixation is required (Fig. 20-10).

Glenohumeral Instability

The glenohumeral joint is the most commonly dislocated large joint in adolescents and adults, but is less commonly involved in children before skeletal maturity. In large series of patients with glenohumeral instability, the proportion of skeletally immature patients ranges from 1% to 5%

(80–143). Traumatic anterior dislocation is by far the most common type of instability seen in adolescent athletes, although multidirectional instability, posterior subluxation, and recurrent subluxation are being recognized with increased frequency, particularly in gymnasts, swimmers, and throwers.

The patient with a traumatic anterior dislocation presents with pain, limited motion, and deformity. The humeral head may be palpated anteriorly or in the axilla and the arm is typically held in a slightly abducted, externally rotated position. Careful examination, particularly of the axillary nerve, is essential to rule out neurovascular injury. With posterior dislocation, the coracoid process may be prominent anteriorly and the arm is often held in internal rotation and adduction. AP and lateral views of the glenohumeral joint demonstrate the dislocation and identify associated fractures or Hill-Sachs lesions (Fig. 20-11). Posterior dislocations may be missed because of inadequate lateral images. Gentle reduction of an anterior dislocation is performed by one of several techniques including traction-countertraction, Stimson maneuver, or abduction maneuvers. After a brief period of immobilization, a rehabilitation program focused on rotator cuff strengthening and avoiding the apprehension position is initiated.

Rates of recurrent instability in adolescents and young adults vary between 25% and 90% in various series (80–143). Rowe reported 100% recurrence in children younger than 10 years old and 94% recurrence in patients between 11 and 20 years old (132–134). Rockwood reported a recurrence rate of 50% in adolescent patients

between 14 and 16 years old and Marans and colleagues reported a 100% recurrence rate in children between 4 and 15 years old with open physes at the time of dislocation (71,116). Higher recurrence rates in younger patients may be related to an increased percentage of elastic type III collagen, greater ligamentous laxity in general, and greater demands. Management of the adolescent patient with significant recurrent instability is usually surgical, involving capsulorrhaphy or a Bankart type repair for capsuloligamentous disruption. Both arthroscopic and open techniques have been used with, in general, higher recurrence rates with arthroscopic repair. Surgical results have been reported in pediatric shoulder instability, with overall improvement of stability and function (80–143).

Atraumatic instability is seen in the pediatric athlete without a clear history of trauma and may occur with throwing, hitting, swimming, or overhead serving. Initially, there is a lack of pain with these episodes of subluxation with spontaneous reduction. Clinical examination often reveals signs of generalized ligamentous laxity including hyperextensibility of the of the elbows, knees, and metacarpophalangeal joints. Examination may also show signs of multidirectional instability including the sulcus sign and excessive translation with anterior and posterior drawer tests or the load and shift test. A vigorous rehabilitation program stressing rotator cuff strengthening is successful in most patients. For patients who fail nonoperative management, a capsular shift reconstruction is recommended (122). This can be performed open or arthroscopically, with, in general, higher recurrence rates with arthroscopic capsulorraphy.

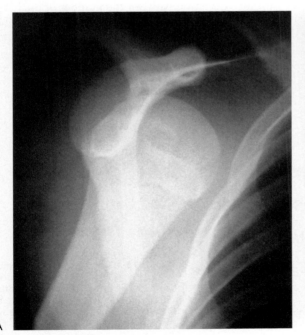
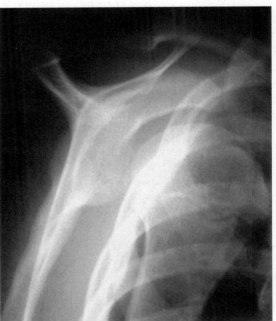

FIGURE 20-11. Anterior glenohumeral dislocation. Anteroposterior **(A)** and scapular Y **(B)** radiographs.

Rotator Cuff Injury

Much less common than in adults, rotator cuff tendinitis and subacromial impingement can occur in the pediatric overhead athlete (144–148). Repetitive microtrauma in high-level overhead sports such as swimming, baseball, and tennis can lead to tendinitis, secondary muscle weakness, mechanical imbalance, and secondary instability. In the pediatric athlete with joint laxity, true impingement with compromise of the subacromial space is uncommon (144–148). Rather, impingement secondary to muscle imbalance and instability is seen. The usual presenting symptom is pain with overhead activities progressing to constant pain or night pain. As the process continues, range of motion and strength may be diminished. Impingement may be elicited with forward elevation or secondary to provocative instability tests. Magnetic resonance imaging may be useful to assess the integrity of the rotator cuff; however, full-thickness tears in the pediatric or adolescent shoulder are uncommon. Internal impingement, with fraying of the undersurface rotator cuff at the posterior superior glenoid margin, can be seen in the overhead athlete (146). A symptomatic os acromiale can mimic impingement symptoms (Fig. 20-12). Because many of the scapular apophyses do not fuse until the early 20s, care should be taken when interpreting radiographs.

Treatment of rotator cuff tendinitis consists of rest, nonsteroidal antiinflammatory medications, and a rehabilitation program emphasizing range of motion, parascapular stabilization, and rotator cuff strengthening to restore dynamic stability. Rehabilitation of secondary impingement should focus on improving dynamic joint stability instead of the subacromial space. For cases refractory to nonoperative management, shoulder arthroscopy may be of benefit for debridement or repair of partial tears and assessing intraarticular lesions such as superior labral tears (144–148). Subacromial decompression is rarely indicated in the pediatric athlete.

Scapulothoracic Dysfunction

Scapulothoracic bursitis and crepitus can be seen in the adolescent overhead athlete (1). Symptoms typically involve pain or crepitus with scapulothoracic and coordinated upper extremity motion. Scapular winging should be ruled out on physical examination and an osteochondroma of the ventral scapula should be ruled out on imaging.

Treatment consists of activity restriction and periscapular muscle strengthening. Crepitus without pain or dysfunction should be observed. Symptomatic crepitus that is refractory to nonoperative treatment, nonsteroidal antiinflammatory drugs, and time can be treated surgically with scapulothoracic bursoscopy or open excision of the superomedial scapular angle.

PREVENTION

Most repetitive, overuse injuries to the pediatric overhead athlete's shoulder can be prevented by attention to symptoms of pain, emphasis on proper mechanics, and limiting the potential for overuse.

In a prospective cohort study of 476 youth pitchers over one season, Lyman and colleagues found that half of the subjects experienced elbow or shoulder pain during the season (31). The curve ball was associated with a 52% increased risk of shoulder pain and the slider was associated with an 86% increased risk of elbow pain. There was a significant association between the number of pitches thrown in a game and during the season to the rate of elbow and shoulder pain. Also, fatigue and satisfaction were associated with pain.

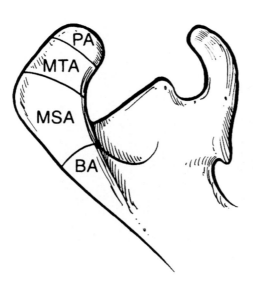

PA = Pre-acromion

MSA = Meso-acromion

MTA = Meta-acromion

BA = Basi-acromion

FIGURE 20-12. Os acromiale. The most common site of failure of ossification occurs at the junction of the mesoacromion and metaacromion. (From Deutsch A, Williams GR. Glenoid and scapula fractures in adults and children. In: DeLee JC, Drez D, Miller MD, eds. *Orthopaedic sports medicine: principles and practice,* 2nd ed. Philadelphia: WB Saunders, 2003, with permission.)

Recommendations for the prevention of shoulder injuries in youth pitchers include avoidance of the curve ball and the slider. The change-up and fastball are considered "safe" pitches. High pitch counts should be avoided. Limits on the number of pitches instead of the number of innings pitched appears more reasonable because an inning can have large variability in terms of the number of pitches. In the aforementioned study, there was a substantially increased risk of shoulder pain with greater than 75 pitches per game and greater than 800 pitches per season (31). A USA Baseball survey has recommended limits of 52 pitches for 8- to 10-year-old pitchers, 68 for 11- to 12-year-old pitchers, and 76 for 13- to 14-year-old pitchers (31). In addition, proper mechanics must be emphasized and taught, with an emphasis on control and not speed (19–35).

REFERENCES

1. Kocher MS, Waters PM, Micheli LJ. Upper extremity injuries in the paediatric athlete. *Sports Med* 2000;30:117–135.
2. Ireland ML, Hutchinson MR. Upper extremity injuries in young athletes. *Clin Sports Med* 1995;14:533.
3. Patel PR, Warner JJP. Shoulder injuries in the skeletally immature athlete. *Sports Med Arthrosc Rev* 1996;4:99–113.
4. Tibone JE. Shoulder problems of adolescents: how they differ from those of adults. *Clin Sports Med* 1983;2:423–427.
5. Bright RW, Burstein AH, Elmore SM. Epiphyseal-plate cartilage: a biomechanical and histological analysis of failure modes. *J Bone Joint Surg (Am)* 1974;56:688–703.
6. Bakerman S. Quantitative extraction of acid-soluble human skin collagen with age. *Nature* 1962;196:375–376.
7. Carter C, Sweetnam R. Recurrent dislocation of the patella and the shoulder: their association with familial joint laxity. *J Bone Joint Surg (Br)* 1960;42:721–727.
8. Finsterbush A, Pogrund H. The hypermobility syndrome: musculoskeletal complaints in 100 consecutive cases of generalized joint hypermobility. *Clin Orthop* 1982;168:124.
9. Jesse E, Owen D, Sagar K. The benign hypermobile syndrome. *Arthritis Rheum* 1980;23:1053.
10. Zaricznyj B, Shattuck LJ, Mast TA, et al. Sports-related injuries in school-aged children. *Am J Sports Med* 1980;8:318–324.
11. Consumer Product Safety Commission. Bicycle related injuries: data from the National Electronic Injury Surveillance System. *JAMA* 1987;257:3334–3337.
12. Culpepper MI, Niemann KMW. High school football injuries in Birmingham, Alabama. *South Med J* 1983;76:873–878.
13. Olson OC. The Spokane study: high school football injuries. *Phys Sportsmed* 1979;7:75–82.
14. Goldberg B, Rosenthal PP, Nicholas JA. Injuries in youth football. *Phys Sportsmed* 1984;12:122–132.
15. Kirburz D, Jacobs R, Reckling F, et al. Bicycle accidents and injuries among adult cyclists. *Am J Sports Med* 1986;14:416–419.
16. Blitzer CM, Johnson RJ, Ettlinger CF, et al. Downhill skiing injuries in children. *Am J Sports Med* 1984;12:142–147.
17. Kocher MS, Feagin JA Jr. Shoulder injuries during alpine skiing. *Am J Sports Med* 1996;24:665–669.
18. Requa R, Garrick JG. Injuries in interscholastic wrestling. *Phys Sportsmed* 1981;9:44–51.
19. Abrams JS. Special shoulder problems in the throwing athlete:

pathology, diagnosis, and nonoperative management. *Clin Sports Med* 1991;10:839–861.
20. Albright JA, Jokl P, Shaw R, et al. Clinical study of baseball pitchers: correlation of injury to the throwing arm with method of delivery. *Am J Sports Med* 1978;6:15–21.
21. American Academy of Pediatrics Committee on Sports Medicine. Risk of injury from baseball and softball in children 5 to 14 years of age. *Pediatrics* 1994;93:690–692.
22. Andrews JR, Fleisig GS. Preventing throwing injuries. *J Orthop Sports Phys Ther* 1998;27:187–188.
23. Axe MJ, Snyder-Mackler L, Konin JG, et al. Development of a distance-based interval throwing program for Little League-aged athletes. *Am J Sports Med* 1996;24:594–602.
24. Crockett HC, Gross LB, Wilk KE, et al. Osseous adaptation and range of motion at the glenohumeral joint in professional baseball pitchers. *Am J Sports Med* 2002;30:20–26.
25. Dillman CJ, Fleisig GS, Andrews JR. Biomechanics of pitching with emphasis upon shoulder kinematics. *J Orthop Sports Phys Ther* 1993;18:402–408.
26. Escamilla RF, Fleisig GS, Alexander E, et al. A kinematic and kinetic comparison while throwing different types of baseball pitches. *Med Sci Sports Exerc* 1994;26:S175.
27. Escamilla RF, Fleisig GS, Barrentine SW, et al. Kinematic comparisons of throwing different types of baseball pitches. *J Appl Biomech* 1998;14:1–23.
28. Fleisig GS, Barrentine SW, Zheng N, et al. Kinematic and kinetic comparison of baseball pitching among various levels of development. *J Biomech* 1999;32:1371–1375.
29. Gainor BM, Piotrowski G, et al. The throw: biomechanics and acute injury. *Am J Sports Med* 1980;8:114–118.
30. Lipscomb AB. Baseball injuries in growing athletes. *J Sports Med* 1975;3:25–34.
31. Lyman S, Fleisig GS, Waterbor JW, et al. Longitudinal study of elbow and shoulder pain in youth baseball pitchers. *Med Sci Sports Exerc* 2001;33:1803–1810.
32. Oberlander MA, Chisar MA, Campbell B. Epidemiology of shoulder injuries in throwing and overhead athletes. *Sports Med Arthrosc Rev* 2000;8:115–123.
33. Pasternack JS, Veenema KR, Callahan CM. Baseball injuries: a Little League survey. *Pediatrics* 1996;98:445–448.
34. Slager RF. From Little League to the big league, the weak spot is the arm. *Am J Sports Med* 1977;5:37–48.
35. Torg JS, Pollack H, Sweterlitsch P. The effect of competitive pitching on the shoulders and elbows of preadolescent baseball players. *Pediatrics* 1972;49:267–272.
36. Adams JE. Little League shoulder: osteochondrosis of the proximal humeral epiphysis in boy baseball pitchers. *Calif Med* 1966;105:22–25.
37. Albert MJ, Drvaric DM. Little League shoulder: case report. *Orthopedics* 1990;13:779–781.
38. Barnett LS. Little league shoulder syndrome: proximal humeral epiphysis in adolescent baseball pitchers. *J Bone Joint Surg (Am)* 1985;67:495–496.
39. Cahill BR, Tullos HS, Fain RH. Little League shoulder: lesions of the proximal humeral epiphyseal plate. *Sports Med* 1974;2:150–151.
40. Carson WG Jr, Gasser SI. Little Leaguer's shoulder: a report of 23 cases. *Am J Sports Med* 1998;26:575–580.
41. Dotter WE. Little leaguer's shoulder: a fracture of the proximal epiphyseal cartilage of the humerus due to baseball pitching. *Guthrie Clinic Bull* 1953;23:68–72.
42. Gugenheim JJ, Stanley RF, Wood GW, et al. Little League survey: the Houston study. *Am J Sports Med* 1976;4:189–200.
43. Larson RL, Singer KM, Bergstrom R, et al. Little League survey: the Eugene study. *Am J Sports Med* 1976;4:201–209.
44. Tullos HS, Fain RH. Little league shoulder: rotational stress

fracture of proximal humeral epiphysis. *J Sports Med* 1974;2: 152–153.

45. Tullos HS, King JW. Lesions of the pitching arm in adolescents. *JAMA* 1972;220:264–271.

46. Priest JD, Nagel DA. Tennis shoulder. *Am J Sports Med* 1976;4: 28–42.

47. Richardson AB, Jobe FW, Collins HR. The shoulder in competitive swimming. *Am J Sports Med* 1980;8:159–163.

48. Aronem JG. Problems of the upper extremity in gymnastics. *Clin Sports Med* 1985;4:61–71.

49. Fulton NN, Albright JP, El-Khoury GY. Cortical desmoid-like lesion of the proximal humerus and its occurrence in gymnasts. *Am J Sports Med* 1979;7:57–61.

50. Garrick JF, Regua RK. Epidemiology of women's gymnastic injuries. *Am J Sports Med* 1980;8:261–264.

51. Goldberg MJ. Gymnastic injuries. *Orthop Clin North Am* 1980; 11:717–732.

52. Snook GA. Injuries in women's gymnastics: a 5 year study. *Am J Sports Med* 1979;7:242–244.

53. Snook GA. Injuries in intercollegiate wrestling: a 5 year study. *Am J Sports Med* 1982;10:142–144.

54. Chambers RB. Orthopedic injuries in athletes (ages 6 to 17). *Am J Sports Med* 1979;7:195–197.

55. Clark RL, Milgram JW, Yawn DH. Fatal aortic perforation and cardiac tamponade due to Kirschner wire migrating from the right sternoclavicular joint. *South Med J* 1974;67:316–318.

56. Denham RH, Dingley AF. Epiphyseal separation of the medial clavicle. *J Bone Joint Surg (Am)* 1967;49:1179–1183.

57. Destouet JM, Gilula LA, Murphy WA, et al. Computed tomography of the sternoclavicular joint and sternum. *Radiology* 1981;138:123–128.

58. Lewonowski K, Bassett GS. Complete posterior retrosternal epiphyseal separation: a case report and review of the literature. *Clin Orthop* 1992;281,84–88.

59. Selesnick FH, Jablon M, Frank C, et al. Retrosternal dislocation of the clavicle. *J Bone Joint Surg (Am)* 1984;66:297.

60. Winter J, Sterner S, Maurer D, et al. Retrosternal epiphyseal disruption of medial clavicle: case and review in children. *J Emerg Med* 1989;7:9–13.

61. Zenni EJ, Krieg JK, Rosen MJ. Open reduction and internal fixation of clavicular fractures. *J Bone Joint Surg (Am)* 1981;63: 147–151.

62. Brooks AL, Henning GD. Injury to the proximal clavicular epiphysis. *J Bone Joint Surg (Am)* 1972;54:1347–1351.

63. Havranek P. Injuries of the distal clavicular physis in children. *J Pediatr Orthop* 1989;9:213–215.

64. Bjerneld H, Hovelius L, Thorling J. Acromioclavicular separations treated conservatively. *Acta Orthop Scand* 1983;54: 743–745.

65. Black GB, McPherson JA, Reed MH. Traumatic pseudodislocation of the acromioclavicular joint in children. *Am J Sports Med* 1991;19:644–646.

66. Eidman DK, Siff SJ, Tullos HS. Acromioclavicular lesions in children. *Am J Sports Med* 1981;9:150–154.

67. Falstie-Jensen S, Mikkelsen P. Pseudodislocation of the acromioclavicular joint. *J Bone Joint Surg (Br)* 1982;64:368–369.

68. Galpin RD, Hawkins RJ, Grainger RW. A comparative analysis of operative versus nonoperative management of grade III acromioclavicular separations. *Clin Orthop* 1985;193:150–155.

69. Larsen E, Bjerg-Nielsen A, Christensen P. Conservative or surgical treatment of acromioclavicular dislocation. *J Bone Joint Surg (Am)* 1986;68:552–555.

70. Ogden JA. Distal clavicular physeal injury. *Clin Orthop* 1984; 188:68–73.

71. Rockwood CA. Fractures of outer clavicle in children and adults. *J Bone Joint Surg (Br)* 1982;64:642–649.

72. Cahill BR. Atraumatic osteolysis of the distal clavicle: a review. *Sports Med* 1992;13:214–222.

73. Baxter MP, Wiley J. Fractures of the proximal humeral epiphysis: their influence on humeral growth. *J Bone Joint Surg (Br)* 1986;68:570–573.

74. Dameron TB, Reibel DB. Fractures involving the proximal humeral epiphyseal plate. *J Bone Joint Surg (Am)* 1969;51: 289–297.

75. Mann DC, Rajmaira S. Distribution of physeal and non-physeal fractures in 2650 long bone fractures in children aged 0-16 years. *J Pediatr Orthop* 1990;10:713–716.

76. Neer CS, Horowitz BS. Fractures of the proximal humeral epiphyseal plate. *Clin Orthop* 1965;41:24–31.

77. Nilsson S, Svartholm F. Fracture of the upper end of the humerus in children. *Acta Chir Scand* 1965;130:433–439.

78. Sherk H, Probst C. Fractures of the proximal humeral epiphysis. *Orthop Clin North Am* 1975;6:401–413.

79. Williams DJ. The mechanisms producing fracture separation of the proximal humeral epiphysis. *J Bone Joint Surg (Br)* 1981;63: 102–107.

80. Allen AA, Warner JJP. Shoulder instability in the athlete. *Orthop Clin North Am* 1995;26:487–504.

81. Altchek DW, Warren RF, Skyhar MJ, et al. T-plasty modification of the Bankart procedure for multidirectional instability of the anterior and inferior types. *J Bone Joint Surg (Am)* 1991;73: 105–112.

82. Arnoczky SP, Aksan A. Thermal modification of connective tissues: basic science considerations and clinical implications. *J Am Acad Orthop Surg* 2000;8:305–313.

83. Aronen JG, Regan K. Decreasing the incidence of recurrence of first time anterior shoulder dislocation with rehabilitation. *Am J Sports Med* 1984;12:283–291.

84. Asher MA. Dislocations of the upper extremity in children. *Orthop Clin North Am* 1976;7:583–591.

85. Bankart ASB. The pathology and treatment of recurrent dislocation of the shoulder joint. *Br J Surg* 1938;26:23–28.

86. Bigliani LU, Kelkar R, Flatow EL, et al. Glenohumeral stability. Biomechanical properties of passive and active stabilizers. *Clin Orthop* 1996;330:13–30.

87. Bigliani LU, Pollock RG, Soslowsky LJ, et al. Tensile properties of the inferior glenohumeral ligament. *J Orthop Res* 1992;10: 187–197.

88. Blasier RB, Soslowsky LJ, Malicky DM, et al. Posterior glenohumeral subluxation: active and passive stabilization in a biomechanical model. *J Bone Joint Surg (Am)* 1997;79:433–440.

89. Bowen MK, Warren RF. Ligamentous control of shoulder stability based on selective cutting and static translation experiments. *Clin Sports Med* 1991;10:757–782.

90. Bradley JP, Tibone JE. Electromyographic analysis of muscle action about the shoulder. *Clin Sports Med* 1991;10:789–805.

91. Burkhead WZ, Rockwood CA. Treatment of instability of the shoulder with an exercise program. *J Bone Joint Surg (Am)* 1992; 74:890–896.

92. Cain PR, Mutschler TA, Fu FH, et al. Anterior stability of the glenohumeral joint. A dynamic model. *Am J Sports Med* 1987; 15:144–148.

93. Callanan M, Tzannes A, Hayes K, et al. Shoulder instability. Diagnosis and management. *Aust Fam Physician* 2001;30 :655–661.

94. Cole BJ, L'Insalata J, Irrgang J, et al. Comparison of arthroscopic and open anterior shoulder stabilization. A two to six-year follow-up study. *J Bone Joint Surg (Am)* 2000;82: 1108–1114.

95. Curl LA, Warren RF. Glenohumeral joint stability. Selective cutting studies on the static capsular restraints. *Clin Orthop* 1996;330:54–65.

96. DeBerardino TM, Arciero RA, Taylor DC. Arthroscopic stabilization of acute initial anterior shoulder dislocation: The West Point experience. *J South Orthop Assoc* 1996;5:263–271.

97. Dines DM, Levinson M. The conservative management of the unstable shoulder including rehabilitation. *Clin Sports Med* 1995;14:797–816.

98. Dora C, Gerber C. Shoulder function after arthroscopic anterior stabilization of the glenohumeral joint using an absorbable tac. *J Shoulder Elbow Surg* 2000;9:294–298.

99. Emery R, Mullaji A. Glenohumeral joint instability in normal adolescents: incidence and significance. *J Bone Joint Surg (Br)* 1991;73:406.

100. Field LD, Warren RF, O'Brien SJ, et al. Isolated closure of rotator interval defects for shoulder instability. *Am J Sports Med* 1995;23:557–563.

101. Gartsman GM, Roddey TS, Hammerman SM. Arthroscopic treatment of anterior-inferior glenohumeral instability. Two to five-year follow-up. *J Bone Joint Surg (Am)* 2000;82:991–1003.

102. Gill TJ, Micheli LJ, Gebhard F, et al. Bankart repair for anterior instability of the shoulder. Long-term outcome. *J Bone Joint Surg (Am)* 1997;79:850–857.

103. Guanche CA, Quick DC, Sodergren KM, et al. Arthroscopic versus open reconstruction of the shoulder in patients with isolated Bankart lesions. *Am J Sports Med* 1996;24:144–148.

104. Harryman DT II, Sidles JA, Clark JM, et al. Translation of the humeral head on the glenoid with passive glenohumeral motion. *J Bone Joint Surg (Am)* 1990;72:1334–1343.

105. Harryman DT II, Sidles JA, Harris SL, et al. The role of the rotator interval capsule in passive motion and stability of the shoulder. *J Bone Joint Surg (Am)* 1992;74:53–66.

106. Hoffmann F, Reif G. Arthroscopic shoulder stabilization using Mitek anchors. *Knee Surg Sports Traumatol Arthrosc* 1995;3:50–54.

107. Hovelius L. Anterior dislocation of the shoulder in teenagers and young adults. *J Bone Joint Surg* 1987;69:393–399.

108. Hovelius L, Augustini BG, Fredin H, et al. Primary anterior dislocation of the shoulder in young patients. A ten-year prospective study. *J Bone Joint Surg (Am)* 1996;78:1677–1684.

109. Hovelius L, Eriksson K, Fredin H, et al. Recurrences after initial dislocation of the shoulder. Results of a prospective study of treatment. *J Bone Joint Surg (Am)* 1983;65:343–349.

110. Itoi E, Newman SR, Kuechle DK, et al. Dynamic anterior stabilisers of the shoulder with the arm in abduction. *J Bone Joint Surg (Br)* 1994;76:834–836.

111. Itoi E, Sashi R, Minagawa H, et al. Position of immobilization after dislocation of the glenohumeral joint. A study with use of magnetic resonance imaging. *J Bone Joint Surg (Am)* 2001;83:661–667.

112. Kirkley A, Griffin S, Richards C, et al. Prospective randomized clinical trial comparing the effectiveness of immediate arthroscopic stabilization versus immobilization and rehabilitation in first traumatic anterior dislocations of the shoulder. *Arthroscopy* 1999;15:507–514.

113. Kvitne RS, Jobe FW. The diagnosis and treatment of anterior instability in the throwing athlete. *Clin Orthop* 1993;291:107–123.

114. Levy O, Wilson M, Williams H, et al. Thermal capsular shrinkage for shoulder instability: mid-term longitudinal outcome study. *J Bone Joint Surg (Br)* 2001;83:640–645.

115. Mallon WJ, Speer KP. Multidirectional instability: current concepts. *J Shoulder Elbow Surg* 1995;4:54–64.

116. Marans HJ, Angel KR, Schemitsch EH, et al. The fate of traumatic anterior dislocation of the shoulder in children. *J Bone Joint Surg. (Am)* 1992;74:1242–1244.

117. Marcacci M, Zaffagnini S, Petitto A, et al. Arthroscopic management of recurrent anterior dislocation of the shoulder: analysis of technical modifications on the Caspari procedure. *Arthroscopy* 1996;12:144–149.

118. Matsen FA III, Harryman DT II, Sidles JA. Mechanics of glenohumeral instability. *Clin Sports Med* 1991;10:783–788.

119. McLaughlin HL, Cavallaro WU. Primary anterior dislocation of the shoulder. *Am J Surg* 1950;80:615–621.

120. Moseley JB Jr, Jobe FW, Pink M, et al. EMG analysis of the scapular muscles during a shoulder rehabilitation program. *Am J Sports Med* 1992;20:128–134.

121. Murrell GAC, Warren RF. The surgical treatment of posterior shoulder instability. *Clin Sports Med* 1995;14:903–915.

122. Neer CS, Foster DR. Inferior capsular shift for involuntary inferior and multidirectional instability of the shoulder. *J Bone Joint Surg (Am)* 1980;62:897–908.

123. O'Brien SJ, Neves MC, Arnoczky SP, et al. The anatomy and histology of the inferior glenohumeral ligament complex of the shoulder. *Am J Sports Med* 1990;18:449–456.

124. O'Brien SJ, Warren RF, Schwartz E. Anterior shoulder instability. *Orthop Clin North Am* 1987;18:395–408.

125. O'Neill DB. Arthroscopic Bankart repair of anterior detachments of the glenoid labrum: a prospective study. *J Bone Joint Surg (Am)* 1999;81:1357–1366.

126. Pagnani MJ, Deng X-H, Warren RF, et al. Role of the long head of the biceps brachii in glenohumeral stability: a biomechanical study in cadavera. *J Shoulder Elbow Surg* 1996;5:255–262.

127. Pagnani MJ, Warren RF. Stabilizers of the glenohumeral joint. *J Shoulder Elbow Surg* 1994;3:173–190.

128. Pagnani MJ, Warren RF. Multidirectional instability: medial T-plasty and selective capsular repairs. *Sports Med Arthrosc Rev* 1993;1:249–258.

129. Pagnani MJ, Warren RF, Altchek DW, et al. Arthroscopic shoulder stabilization using transglenoid sutures: a four-year minimum followup. *Am J Sports Med* 1996;24:459–467.

130. Paxinos A, Walton J, Tzannes A, et al. Advances in the management of traumatic anterior and atraumatic multidirectional shoulder instability. *Sports Med* 2001;31:819–828.

131. Pollock RG, Owens JM, Flatow EL, et al. Operative results of the inferior capsular shift procedure for multidirectional instability of the shoulder. *J Bone Joint Surg (Am)* 2000;82:919–928.

132. Rowe CR. Prognosis in dislocations of the shoulder. *J Bone Joint Surg (Am)* 1956;38:957–977.

133. Rowe CR, Zarins B. Recurrent transient subluxation of the shoulder. *J Bone Joint Surg (Am)* 1981;63:863–872.

134. Rowe CR, Zarins B, Cuillo JV. Recurrent anterior dislocation of the shoulder after surgical repair: apparent causes of failure and treatment. *J Bone Joint Surg (Am)* 1984;66:159–168.

135. Simonet WT, Cofield RH. Prognosis in anterior shoulder dislocation. *Am J Sports Med* 1984;12:19–24.

136. Speer KP, Deng X, Borrero S, et al. Biomechanical evaluation of a simulated Bankart lesion. *J Bone Joint Surg (Am)* 1994;76:1819–1826.

137. Wagner KT, Lyne ED. Adolescent traumatic dislocations of the shoulder with open epiphysis. *J Pediatr Orthop* 1983;3:61–62.

138. Wall MS, Deng X-H, Torzilli PA, et al. Thermal modification of collagen. *J Shoulder Elbow Surg* 1999;8:339–344.

139. Warner JJ, Beim GM. Combined Bankart and HAGL lesion associated with anterior shoulder instability. *Arthroscopy* 1997;13:749–752.

140. Warner JJ, Deng XH, Warren RF, et al. Static capsuloligamentous restraints to superior-inferior translation of the glenohumeral joint. *Am J Sports Med* 1992;20:675–685.

141. Wickiewicz TL, Pagnani MJ, Kennedy K. Rehabilitation of the unstable shoulder. *Sports Med Arthrosc Rev* 1993;1:227–235.

142. Wilk KE, Arrigo CA, Andrews JR. Current concepts: the stabilizing structures of the glenohumeral joint. *J Orthop Sports Phys Ther* 1997;25:364–379.

143. Wolf EM, Cheng JC, Dickson K. Humeral avulsion of gleno-humeral ligaments as a cause of anterior shoulder instability. *Arthroscopy* 1995;11:600–607.

144. Bigliani LU, D'Alessandro DF, Duralde XA, et al. Anterior acromioplasty for subacromial impingement in patients younger than 40 years of age. *Clin Orthop* 1989;246:111–116.

145. Hawkins RJ, Kennedy JC. Impingement syndrome in athletes. *Am J Sports Med* 1980;8:151–157.

146. Jobe CM. Superior glenoid impingement. *Orthop Clin North Am* 1997;28:137–143.

147. Levitz CL, Dugas J, Andrews JR. The use of arthroscopic thermal capsulorrhaphy to treat internal impingement in baseball players. *Arthroscopy* 2001;17:573–577.

148. Tibone JE, Elrod B, Jobe FW, et al. Surgical treatment of tears of the rotator cuff in athletes. *J Bone Joint Surg (Am)* 1986; 68:887–891.

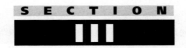

SPORT-SPECIFIC SHOULDER INJURIES AND MANAGEMENT IN OVERHEAD ATHLETES

21

BASEBALL

JAMES R. ANDREWS
CHRISTOPHER G. MAZOUÉ

INTRODUCTION

Baseball pitching is one of the most demanding motions on the shoulder in sports. Each pitch requires the generation of tremendous forces and torques on the shoulder to create the acceleration necessary to propel a baseball at high velocities, then decelerate the upper extremity after the ball has been released. Each baseball pitch can result in humeral angular velocities of 7,000 to 8,000 degrees per second making it one of the fastest movements in sports (1,2). For this energy to be produced during a pitch, the shoulder must allow for extremes in range of motion and flexibility, yet must provide a certain level of stability in a joint that has little inherent stability. Thus, the shoulder must maintain a delicate balance of mobility and stability while generating levels of energy via muscular contractions that are believed to be near physiologic limits for each of the hundreds or thousands of pitches that may be thrown over the course of each year. The dynamic and static tissues of the shoulder that provide this balance and energy generation are highly susceptible to overuse injuries in the context of the demands that are placed upon them.

With the large numbers of individuals of all ages participating in baseball, injuries to the shoulder are commonplace. An extensive amount of both biomechanical and clinical research has been focused on the baseball player in order to greater understand the kinetics and kinematics of the baseball pitch and the pathophysiology of the shoulder in the baseball player. This chapter concentrates on our experience with the throwing shoulder in the baseball player and our approaches to the diagnosis, nonoperative treatment, surgical techniques, and rehabilitation protocols for baseball players.

PITCHING MECHANICS

To understand the pathophysiology of the throwing shoulder in the baseball player, it is helpful to have a basic knowledge of the mechanics of the baseball pitch. Based on analyses of hundreds of baseball pitchers using high-speed video and computerized motion analysis at the American Sports Medicine Institute (ASMI), we have divided the baseball pitch into six phases (Fig. 21-1): wind-up, stride, arm cocking, arm acceleration, arm deceleration, and follow-through (1).

The *wind-up phase* starts from a two-legged stance. The pitcher brings the front leg to a tucked position, preparing the body for the remainder of the pitch sequence. This phase ends when the ball is removed from the glove. There is no excessive strain placed upon the pitcher's shoulder and electromyographic (EMG) analysis has revealed little muscular activity across the shoulder during this phase (3–10).

Stride is defined as the sequence of activities from the end of the wind-up phase until the front foot strikes the ground. During this maneuver, the body is advanced forward; however, the hand and ball remain positioned behind the body. This places an eccentric load on the humeral adductors and internal rotators, effectively creating a preload on these muscles as they prepare to accelerate the shoulder.

The sequence from foot contact until achievement of maximal external rotation of the throwing shoulder is defined as the *arm cocking phase*. During this phase, shoulder external rotation can reach 165 to 180 degrees and an anterior translation force of approximately 50% body weight is generated (1,11,12). Significant stresses are placed on the anterior capsule and soft tissues of the shoulder during this phase, especially at the anterior band of the inferior glenohumeral ligament. As the shoulder is repetitively placed in this position of maximal external rotation, attenuation of these anterior static restraints may occur through repetitive microtrauma (13). This, in turn, may lead to pathologic laxity of the anterior ligaments and capsule, producing occult instability or microinstability of the shoulder (13). The rotator cuff muscles, as dynamic stabilizers of the shoulder, must therefore work to prevent abnormal anterior translation of the shoulder in this position. This predisposes these muscles to overuse injuries.

From the position of maximal external rotation of the throwing shoulder until ball release is the *arm acceleration*

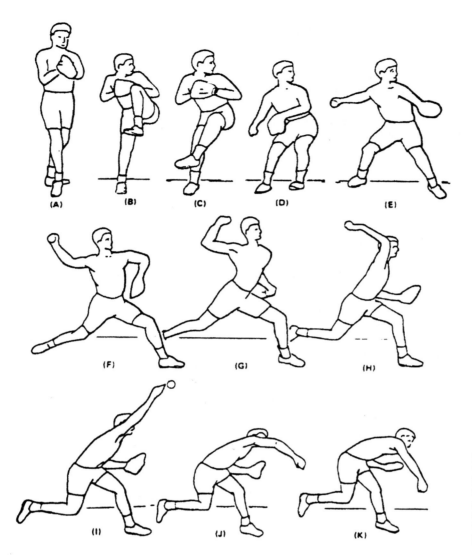

FIGURE 21-1. The six phases of pitching: wind-up (A-C), stride (C-F), arm cocking (F-H), arm deceleration (I-J) and follow-through (J-K). (From Dillman CJ, Fleisig GS, Andrews JR. Biomechanics of pitching with emphasis upon shoulder kinematics. *J Orthop Sports Phys Ther* 1993;18:402, with permission.)

phase. Within approximately 0.05 to 0.08 second, the baseball is accelerated forward from a stationary position to speeds in excess of 80 mph in high-level athletes (12). The rotator cuff and scapular stabilizing muscles all demonstrate high levels of activity during this phase (3–10).

The *arm deceleration phase* progresses from ball release until maximal shoulder internal rotation. Large shoulder forces and torques are required to decelerate the upper extremity and counteract the anterior distraction forces on the shoulder joint, which may approach body weight (12). This phase is the most violent phase on the shoulder. The rotator cuff must both decelerate the shoulder via large eccentric contractions and stabilize the shoulder against anterior translation. Any underlying anterior instability of the shoulder requires even greater activity of these dynamic stabilizers. These large, repetitive loads on the rotator cuff during deceleration may result in tension injuries. In addition, large tensile loads are applied to the posterior capsule

during deceleration, which may lead to chronic attenuation of the posterior capsule and posterior laxity.

The final phase is the *follow-through*. Posterior shoulder muscles continue to eccentrically contract during this phase. This phase is important for final dissipation of the energy generated during the throwing motion.

PATHOPHYSIOLOGY OF PITCHING

The activity of the scapula and its stabilizing muscles and the coordination of scapular function during the pitch cannot be overemphasized. The scapula functions as a mobile base for the shoulder. The movement of the scapula allows maintenance of proper length-tension relationships for the deltoid and rotator cuff muscles (14). Failure of coordinated scapular movements can increase both tensile and compressive stresses on the rotator cuff, increasing the possibility of failure of these structures. Diminished EMG activities of the scapular stabilizing muscles during the pitch in patients with glenohumeral instability supports the role that these muscles play in creating a stable base for overhead activities (4).

Although we have concentrated on the shoulder, we cannot forget that the baseball pitch requires a coordinated transfer of energy from the legs and pelvis, trunk, shoulder, upper arm, forearm, and finally the hand as the ball is delivered. The sequential transfer of energy from the legs and pelvis to the hand is defined as the kinetic chain (14). Any loss of energy or coordination from this chain can lead to failure or fatigue of the remainder of the chain, leading to injury.

The severe stresses placed upon the shoulder during the throwing motion can lead to developmental changes in the function and anatomy of the shoulder. In most mature baseball pitchers, there is an increased external rotation and decreased internal rotation of the throwing shoulder in abduction as compared with those of the nonthrowing shoulder (1,15,16). The total arc of motion of the throwing shoulder is, therefore, not increased, but simply moved posteriorly. It has been postulated that this shift in rotation of the shoulder is secondary to increases in anterior capsular laxity and posterior capsular tightness in the overhead athlete (17). More recent literature proposes an alternative theory behind this rotational shift in the arc of motion in baseball players. This theory suggests that the dominant humeral head in the young overhead athlete undergoes an osseous adaptation secondary to the stresses placed on the immature proximal humerus during the throwing motion. This osseous adaptation produces increased retroversion of the dominant shoulder, which, in turn, results in decreased internal rotation and increased external rotation (18–20). In a recent study looking at professional baseball pitchers, the dominant shoulder was found to have 17 degrees more humeral head retroversion and 3 degrees more glenoid retroversion than the nondominant shoulder (18). This same study compared range of motions of the dominant shoulder compared with those of the nondominant shoulder, with the dominant shoulder exhibiting 9 degrees more external rotation and 9 degrees less internal rotation than the nondominant shoulder. Therefore, as previously discussed, the total arc of motion (189 degrees) was the same for both shoulders in the throwing athlete with the arc of motion rotated posteriorly in the dominant shoulder. These findings again illustrate how significant the stresses are to the shoulder in throwing athletes and how the body adapts to offset these stresses.

HISTORY AND PHYSICAL EXAMINATION

A thorough history is invaluable in the diagnosis of throwing injuries in baseball players. Because most injuries in

overhead athletes are secondary to overuse and fatigue, it is crucial to gain an understanding of the onset of symptoms and a detailed history of the throwing activities since the onset of symptoms. Table 21-1 (21) provides a baseline for establishing a thorough history in baseball players with shoulder pain. Table 21-2 (21) provides a guideline for the physical examination. The physical examination is used to further localize the possible site of injury that is suspected based on the history. It is imperative for an examiner to become familiar with a consistent routine to evaluate the thrower's shoulder. Although the examination is used to correlate a patient's symptoms with anatomic pathology, all possible sources of injury should be evaluated in each shoulder. Of particular importance in throwing athletes, espe-

TABLE 21–1. HISTORY IN THE THROWING SHOULDER

I. **General information**
   Age
   Gender
   Dominant handedness
   Position
   Years throwing
   Level of competition
II. **Injury pattern**
   Onset of symptoms—acute or chronic
   History of trauma or sudden injury
III. **Symptom characteristics**
   Location of symptoms—anterior, lateral, posterior
   Quality of symptoms—sharp, dull, burning
   Presence of mechanical symptoms
   Presence of weakness or instability
   Severity of symptoms
   Duration of symptoms
   Activities that worsen symptoms
   Activities that relieve symptoms
   Duration of symptoms
   Presence of neurosensory changes
   Phase of throwing-producing symptoms
   Type of pitch-producing symptoms
   Innings pitched in season/year
   Frequency of starts/relief appearances
   Change in velocity of pitches
   Loss of control/location of pitches
IV. **Treatment/rehabilitation**
   Amount of rest from throwing
   Type and duration of rehabilitation
   Type, location, frequency of injections
V. **Related symptoms**
   Neck pain
   Radicular symptoms
   Brachial plexus injury
   Peripheral nerve entrapment
VI. **Medical information**
   Past medical/surgical history
   Medications
   Allergies
   Family/social history
   Review of symptoms

TABLE 21–2. PHYSICAL EXAM IN THE THROWING SHOULDER

SITTING POSITION
I. **Inspection**
II. **Palpation**
Sternoclavicular joint
Acromioclavicular joint
Clavicle, acromion, coracoid
Bicipital groove
Scapula
Musculature
III. **Range of motion**
Crepitus
Glenohumeral motion
Scapulothoracic motion
IV. **Motor strength**
Rotator cuff
Scapular winging
V. **Impingement signs**
Neer/Hawkins signs
Cross chest adduction test
VI. **Stability tests**
Anterior, posterior, inferior stability
VII. **Special tests—biceps**
Speed's test
Yergason's test
VIII. **Special tests—SLAP**
O'Brien's test
Crank test
Lemak test
Mimori test
IX. **Neurologic examination**
X. **Cervical examination**

SUPINE POSITION
I. **Range of motion**
II. **Anterior instability tests**
Anterior drawer
Apprehension test
Relocation test
III. **Posterior instability test**
Posterior drawer
Apprehension test
IV. **SLAP test**
Clunk test
V. **Internal impingement test**

PRONE POSITION
I. **Palpation posterior shoulder**
II. **Stability test**
Anterior apprehension

cially with regard to range of motion and stability, is examination of both the dominant and nondominant shoulders.

For every overhead athlete, we obtain a standard "thrower's series" of radiographs, which includes true anteroposterior views with the arm in maximum internal rotation and external rotation, a modified Stryker's notch view, and an axillary lateral view. A scapular outlet view may be obtained when external impingement is suspected. When magnetic resonance imaging (MRI) is required, we prefer MR arthrography following intraarticular saline injections. This technique greatly enhances visualization of the glenoid labrum and subtle rotator cuff tears.

The ultimate diagnosis of shoulder injuries in baseball players can be difficult. The soft tissues of the shoulder are subjected to tremendous stresses from throwing a baseball that result in overuse injuries. Partial thickness rotator cuff tears and labral tears are common findings on MRI in baseball players. Yet, not all of these rotator cuff and labral tears are symptomatic. It is the job of the examiner to determine whether radiographic findings correlate with the patient's symptoms and physical examination. This can be challenging.

REHABILITATION

Because most shoulder injuries in baseball players are secondary to overuse and fatigue, most of these injuries can be treated with initial active rest, followed by a strict supervised physical therapy program. Active rest involves the athlete participating in activities that do not require throwing a baseball or engaging in other overhead activities. Based on the patient's symptoms and suspected diagnosis, we often rest a player for 6 to 12 weeks. During this time, we start a supervised physical therapy program. This program must focus on strengthening the rotator cuff muscles as the dynamic stabilizers of the glenohumeral joint and improving coordination of the rotator cuff and scapular stabilizing muscles. We teach our overhead athletes a program called the "thrower's 10" (Chapter 7), which consists of 10 exercises for the muscles of the shoulder and scapula that were developed on the basis of the contribution of these various muscles during the throwing motion as determined by EMG (22–24). These exercises can be used as a rehabilitation tool or as a group of core exercises to be used for maintenance throughout the year. Following progression through the thrower's 10 program, we encourage use of plyometric exercises. These are movements that focus on eccentric muscular contractions before concentric contractions. These exercises enhance strength and dynamic stability of the shoulder and are excellent transitional exercise before throwing activities are resumed. When the athlete is ready to resume throwing, following the appropriate period of active rest and initial physical therapy, an interval throwing program is begun. The baseball player must be monitored throughout this interval throwing program and must be patient with its progression. If an individual progresses through the entire throwing program without symptoms, then the athlete is cleared for competitive activities.

For hitters, we have developed an interval hitting program to ease the baseball player back into full swings (Table 21-3). We often initiate this program before beginning the interval throwing program following a surgical procedure to the shoulder.

In most cases of shoulder injuries in baseball players, we do not consider surgical intervention until the athlete has

TABLE 21–3. INTERVAL HITTING PROGRAM

Off a tee stand
  Step 1: 50% effort (15–20 swings)
  Step 2: 50% effort (2 sets of 15 swings)
  Step 3: 65%–70% effort (2 sets of 15 swings)
  Step 4: 70%–75% effort (2 sets of 20–25 swings)
  Step 5: 80%–90% effort (2 sets of 25 swings)
Soft toss swings: Warm-up using a tee stand
  Step 6: 50%–60% effort (15–20 swings)
  Step 7: 65%–70% effort (2 sets of 20–25 swings)
  Step 8: 80%–90% effort (2 sets of 25 swings)
Batting practice swings: Warm-up with soft toss swings
  Step 9: 50%–65% effort (2 sets of 25 swings)
  Step 10: 70%–75% effort (2 sets of 30 swings)
  Step 11: 80%–90% effort (2 sets of 30–35 swings)
  Hit 3 times per week with a day off in between.
  Perform each step for 2 days before progressing to next step.

failed a prescribed, supervised shoulder rehabilitation program after 3 months. Most baseball players do well with nonoperative treatment.

GLENOHUMERAL INSTABILITY

Glenohumeral laxity is defined by the amount of translation of the humeral head upon the glenoid (25). Individuals often exhibit considerable variations in laxity of the glenohumeral joint. Glenohumeral instability is a clinical condition in which excessive translation of the humeral head on the glenoid results in symptoms (25). Instability may arise in an atraumatic nature in those individuals born with loose connective tissues; however, in athletes, most cases of shoulder instability are acquired through trauma to the soft tissues of the glenohumeral joint. Acquired instability may develop secondary to a high-energy trauma to the shoulder, leading to significant injury to the anterior labrum, ligaments, and capsule of the glenohumeral joint, or it may develop from repetitive stress to the anterior soft tissues of the shoulder joint. Jobe and colleagues described this latter pattern of injury to the shoulder with overhead activities as microtrauma (13).

The most common instability pattern found in baseball players is recurrent, involuntary, microtraumatic, chronic anterior subluxation. The extreme ranges of motion achieved during each baseball pitch and the large forces and torques applied to the shoulder during each baseball pitch produce large stresses on the static restraints of the glenohumeral joint, that is, the labrum, capsule, and glenohumeral ligaments. As a consequence, these restraints become attenuated over time, leading to laxity of the glenohumeral joint. As these static restraints become lax, the dynamic stabilizers of the glenohumeral joint (i.e., the rotator cuff muscles) must compensate for this increased laxity to prevent subluxation of the humeral head on the glenoid.

Any fatigue of these dynamic restraints or any loss of coordination of the rotator cuff and scapular stabilizing muscles can lead to further increased stresses on the static restraints, resulting in even greater laxity of these structures. Thus, a pattern of recurrent, microtraumatic, chronic subluxation of the glenohumeral joint develops. Instability is diagnosed when symptoms develop secondary to the excessive laxity of the glenohumeral joint. We believe that many shoulder injuries in baseball players are directly related to this instability.

The most common direction of glenohumeral instability found in baseball players is anterior. As the shoulder reaches the cocked position, the anterior forces on the glenohumeral joint reach one half times body weight (12). The anterior band of the inferior glenohumeral ligament is the primary restraint to anterior translation of the glenohumeral joint with the shoulder in the position of abduction and external rotation (26). As this ligament is chronically stressed, it becomes attenuated. Because this ligament is able to undergo substantial plastic deformation before failure (27), a significant amount of anterior laxity may develop in the glenohumeral joint, leading to anterior subluxation. The posterior rotator cuff must, therefore, prevent this anterior subluxation. This is especially important in the deceleration phase of throwing during which the glenohumeral joint is exposed to a tremendous anterior force. For this reason, the posterior supraspinatus and the infraspinatus are common sites of injury in baseball players with pathologic anterior laxity, because these muscles must stabilize the joint. This large anterior translation force during the deceleration phase also results in large stresses applied to the posterior capsule of the glenohumeral joint. This may lead to posterior capsulitis and posterior capsular laxity. This, in turn, may worsen the anterior laxity through the circle concept of shoulder instability as described by Warren and colleagues (28). In this theory, capsular laxity is required both anteriorly and posteriorly to produce excessive translation of the glenohumeral joint. Many baseball players, in fact, have posterior laxity on examination. Although posterior instability is not a common cause of disability in overhead athletes, posterior laxity may contribute to the development of anterior laxity and instability.

Besides rotator cuff injury, anterior subluxation has also been implicated in labral injuries, SLAP (superior labrum anterior-to-posterior) lesions, and internal impingement. Therefore, we make every attempt to identify pathologic laxity in injured baseball players and address this laxity appropriately to prevent recurrence of injury.

The history in baseball players with recurrent occult or microtraumatic instability is often vague. It is rare for the overhead athlete to describe a feeling of instability with this injury pattern. Rowe described the "dead-arm syndrome" in patients with anterior subluxation (29). Pitchers may complain of loss of velocity or control. Often, the complaints associated with occult instability are those resulting from the associated injuries such as rotator cuff tears or SLAP lesions.

Most cases of baseball players with occult instability can be treated with active rest and a strict supervised physical therapy program. This program must focus on strengthening the rotator cuff muscles as the dynamic stabilizers of the glenohumeral joint and aid in improving coordination of the rotator cuff and scapular stabilizing muscles.

If operative treatment is indicated in the baseball player, we make every effort via our history, physical examination, radiographic studies, examination under anesthesia, and diagnostic arthroscopy to determine the instability pattern of the involved shoulder. Once we have treated any underlying pathology of the shoulder (e.g., a partial thickness rotator cuff tear or labral injury), we address the capsular laxity with thermal-assisted capsular shrinkage (TACS) using a temperature-controlled monopolar radiofrequency probe. The thermal energy is directed at specific sites based on our appreciation of the patient's pattern of laxity. When we first began using TACS in 1997, we were more liberal in the amount of capsule being treated. Our improved understanding of the effects of TACS on the soft tissues of the shoulder, the rehabilitation of athletes following TACS, and the patterns of instability seen in baseball players have led us to become more conservative in our indications for TACS and the amount of capsule and ligamentous tissue treated. The amount of TACS performed is tailored to each individual based on the history, physical examination, and intraoperative findings. At this time, it is common for us to only treat the anterior band of the inferior glenohumeral ligament; however, based on the physical examination and our appreciation of the degree of anterior laxity, we may be more aggressive in our use of TACS. We occasionally treat the posterior band of the inferior glenohumeral ligament, if a player complains of posterior shoulder pain in the deceleration phase.

Perhaps more important than the amount of tissue treated with thermal energy is the rehabilitation following TACS. The physical therapist plays a crucial role in determining the outcome following TACS. There are several keys to successful rehabilitation following TACS. The physical therapist must adjust the rehabilitation program based on the type of instability pattern and the patient's response to the surgery. Each patient responds differently to the effects of TACS. It is imperative that the therapist understand the patient's response to the surgery and adjust the rehabilitation program accordingly. It is also helpful to have benchmarks for progression of range of motion following TACS. In our program, we like to see 75 degrees of external rotation of the affected shoulder with the shoulder at 90 degrees of abduction by 6 weeks. Having such standards for range of motion following TACS allows for an adjustment of the rehabilitation program based on the patient's response to the surgery.

Although microtraumatic instability is the most common pattern of instability found in baseball players, we do see players who have sustained macrotrauma to the shoulder that has produced anterior shoulder dislocations. The question arises as to what is the appropriate treatment for these shoulder dislocations in the throwing athlete. In the dominant shoulder of baseball players, especially pitchers, we often consider an arthroscopic Bankart repair following the initial dislocation. This provides for an acceptable repair with limited dissection of the anterior soft tissues of the shoulder, thereby avoiding possible crucial loss of external rotation of the glenohumeral joint. In the nondominant shoulder, we usually recommend nonoperative treatment following the initial dislocation. If this treatment fails (i.e., recurrent dislocations develop), we usually proceed with an open anterior Bankart repair. Our indications for treatment of anterior glenohumeral instability are continuing to evolve as our experience with arthroscopic techniques evolves. Our goals for arthroscopic stabilization are to perform the same procedure arthroscopically as is done with open technique with the same or better results as with an open procedure and with a low complication rate. Currently, our relative contraindications to arthroscopic anterior stabilization procedures for anterior shoulder dislocations include loss of continuity of the labral-glenohumeral ligament complex, multidirectional instability, severe instability with a large Hill-Sachs lesion, and intention of returning to high-risk collision sports.

In throwers requiring an open anterior Bankart repair or an open capsular shift for multidirectional instability in their dominant shoulders, we perform an "anatomic capsular shift" (30). This technique uses a subscapularis split with the option of taking down the upper lateral corner of the subscapularis. The anterior capsule of the glenohumeral joint is incised at its humeral insertion, beginning at its most superior insertion at the anatomic humeral neck. The length of this capsular incision is based on the severity of the instability and the presence of a multidirectional component (Fig. 21-2). With the anterior capsule reflected medially, the Bankart lesion can be repaired via suture anchors. The medial capsule is then anchored to the glenoid with suture anchors. Then, with the shoulder positioned at 30 to 45 degrees of abduction and 15 to 45 degrees of external rotation, the lateral portion of the incised anterior capsule is translated superiorly and stabilized to the humerus via suture anchors. Careful attention is paid to limiting the amount of lateral advancement of the capsule to avoid loss of external rotation. Approximating the superior edge of the middle glenohumeral ligament to the inferior edge of the superior glenohumeral ligament closes the rotator interval (Fig. 21-3). Finally, the subscapularis split is repaired anatomically. The rehabilitation following this procedure, as with most surgical procedures in the throwing athlete, is critical in achieving appropriate range of motion postoperatively while protecting the repair.

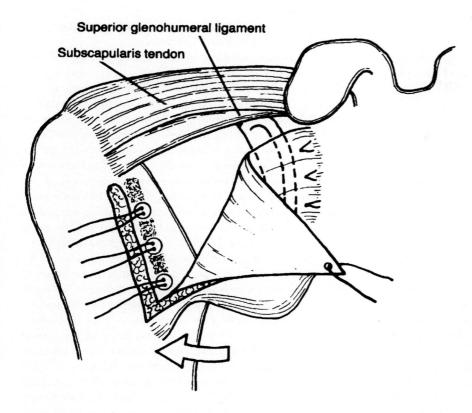

Superior glenohumeral ligament

Subscapularis tendon

FIGURE 21-2. Anatomic capsular shift—the anterior capsule is incised at its humeral insertion from superior to inferior. (From Andrews JR, Satterwhite YE. Anatomic capsular shift. *J Orthop Tech* 1993;1:151–160, with permission.)

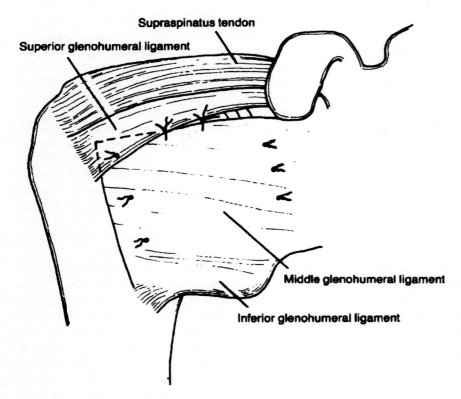

Supraspinatus tendon

Superior glenohumeral ligament

Middle glenohumeral ligament

Inferior glenohumeral ligament

FIGURE 21-3. Anatomic capsular shift—the medial capsule is anchored to the glenoid with suture anchors. The lateral edge of the anterior capsule is translated superiorly and stabilized to the humerus with suture anchors. The rotator interval is then closed. (From Andrews JR, Satterwhite YE. Anatomic capsular shift. *J Orthop Tech* 1993;1:151–160, with permission.)

tial thickness tear and convert it to a full thickness tear in hopes of achieving a more stable insertion. Our first choice on most partial thickness tears requiring surgical treatment is to limit our procedure to an arthroscopic debridement, with or without thermal capsulorrhaphy. For tears that affect greater than 75% of the thickness of the tendon, especially when associated with significant shoulder instability, we consider converting these tears into full thickness tears and repairing them with an arthroscopic versus miniopen technique.

Full thickness rotator cuff tears are uncommon in baseball players. When they do occur, surgical intervention is warranted to prevent propagation of the tear. Currently, we treat most full thickness tears with an arthroscopic subacromial decompression followed by a mini-open repair of the cuff. This repair consists of a two-level anatomic repair using suture anchors placed just lateral to the articular surface and bony tunnels at the lateral aspect of the insertion of the rotator cuff into the greater tuberosity (Fig. 21-4). Our indications for arthroscopic rotator cuff repairs in overhead athletes continue to evolve. For simple, unretracted tears, we consider an arthroscopic repair using suture anchors; however, we are currently looking at methods to recreate our two-layer anatomic repair via an all-arthroscopic technique.

LABRUM INJURIES

SLAP Lesions

The advent and advances in arthroscopy over the past 3 decades has introduced the glenoid labrum as a common site of injury in the throwing shoulder. In 1985, Andrews and colleagues first described superior labrum tears related to the long head of the biceps in a population of throwing athletes (35). The authors postulated that the strong eccentric contraction of the biceps tendon during the deceleration phase of throwing produced a significant traction force at the superior labrum, producing tears of the anterosuperior glenoid labrum over a period of time. In 1990, Snyder and co-workers introduced the term *SLAP lesion* to describe an injury to the *s*uperior *l*abrum *a*nterior-to-*p*osterior and provided a useful classification for these injuries (36) (Fig. 21-5). Unlike the repetitive traction mechanism postulated by Andrews and colleagues in their population of throwing athletes (35), the injuries in this study by Snyder and co-workers were thought to be secondary to acute trauma, either due to a fall onto the outstretched arm producing a compressive force to the shoulder or due to a sudden traction force on the arm. More recently, Burkhart and Morgan described a new mechanism for injury to the superior

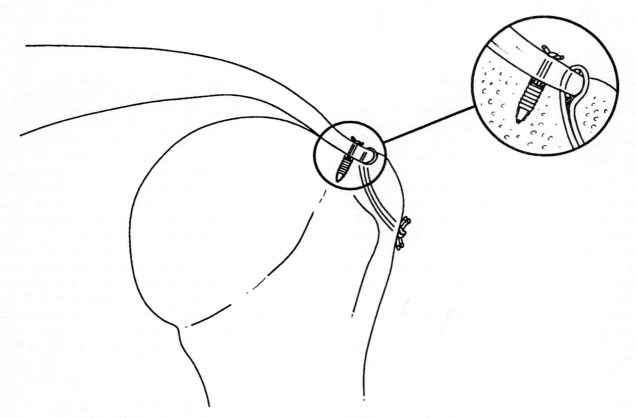

FIGURE 21-4. Anteroposterior (AP) view of completed two-level anatomic repair of a full-thickness rotator cuff tear using suture anchors and bony tunnels.

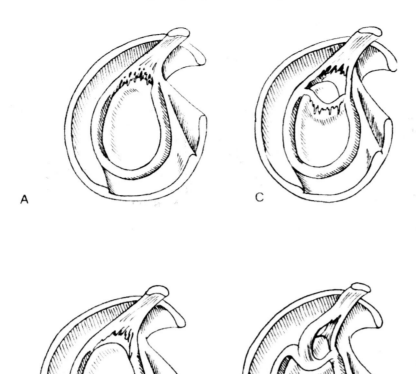

FIGURE 21-5. Classification of SLAP (superior *l*abrum *a*nterior-to-*p*osterior) lesions. **A:** Type I—Degeneration of superior glenoid labrum. **B:** Type II—Detachment of superior glenoid labrum and biceps tendon from the glenoid rim. **C:** Type III—Bucket-handle type tear of the superior labrum with intact biceps anchor. **D:** Detachment of the superior glenoid labrum with tear extending lengthwise through the biceps tendon anchor such that a portion of the biceps anchor attached to the superior labrum is detached from glenoid.

labrum (37). As opposed to the traction theory, in which the labrum fails secondary to a tensile force, these authors observed a "peel-back" phenomenon on the superior labrum. This theory is based on the torsional load applied to the labrum through the biceps. As the shoulder rotates into extreme abduction and external rotation during the cocking phase, the biceps tendon force vector shifts from an anterior-horizontal direction to a more vertical, posterior direction. This produces a torsional force at the base of the biceps that is transmitted to the posterosuperior labrum. As the superior labrum is subjected to these torsional forces over time, failure occurs and produces tears. These lesions tend to be located more posterior on the superior labrum secondary to the vectors of force applied to the labrum.

The diagnosis of SLAP lesions can be difficult. As with most injuries in the throwing shoulder, most SLAP lesions develop over time through repetitive loads placed on the biceps and superior labrum complex. Patients with these lesions often have nonspecific symptoms. Some patients may complain of mechanical symptoms in the shoulder such as catching or slipping as fragments of the labral tear become interposed between the humeral head and glenoid. The various special tests to aid in the diagnosis of SLAP lesions including O'Brien's test, the crank test, the clunk

test, Mimori's test, the Lemak test, and the biceps active test are all included in our physical examination; however, none of these tests has been shown to have a high sensitivity or specificity for diagnosing SLAP lesions. MRI, especially with intraarticular contrast, is helpful in the diagnosis of SLAP lesions, yet, in our experience, MRI tends to overdiagnose SLAP lesions. Ultimately, the true evaluation of a SLAP lesion is made at the time of arthroscopy. Only upon direct visualization and manipulation of the superior labrum can a truly accurate assessment be made with regard to the presence and severity of a SLAP lesion.

Our surgical treatment of SLAP lesions consists of repair of the unstable superior labrum and, in most cases, thermal capsulorrhaphy. Our initial step in surgical management of these lesions is understanding the exact nature of the injury to the superior labrum. Type I and III SLAP lesions are usually treated adequately with arthroscopic debridement of the unstable tissue. For type II and IV SLAP lesions, we reattach the unstable biceps-labrum complex to the glenoid. This technique involves the arthroscopic placement of suture anchors at the superior glenoid rim following debridement of the cortical bone to a bleeding bed just off of the articular surface of the superior glenoid. A single limb of the suture anchor is placed under the labrum using a suture passer and the suture is tied in a lasso fashion over the superior labrum. We then perform a thermal capsulorrhaphy if we feel the patient has excessive laxity of the glenohumeral joint.

Anteroposterior Labrum Injuries

Anterior and posterior glenoid labral tears and fraying are common in baseball players due to the repetitive stresses placed upon these structures in the act of throwing. In individuals with occult instability, the labrum is subjected to even greater compression and shear forces as the humeral head subluxes over the labrum. Most of these labral tears are asymptomatic in baseball players and can be treated nonoperatively. On occasion, a labral tear causes mechanical symptoms within the glenohumeral joint. In most of these cases, arthroscopic debridement of the tear is sufficient to relieve symptoms and allow for a stable joint. Some tears, based on their location, the extent of the tear, and other associated injuries, would benefit from arthroscopic repair with suture anchors.

POSTERIOR GLENOID EXOSTOSIS

The posterior glenoid exostosis (Bennett's lesion) is an abnormal extraarticular ossification located at the posteroinferior glenoid. Although a relatively uncommon finding, this lesion should be suspected in any baseball player with posterior shoulder pain.

Bennett, in his 1941 review of shoulder and elbow lesions in professional baseball players, believed that these lesions were a primary source of posterior shoulder pain secondary to local irritation of the posterior shoulder capsule and circumflex nerve (38). However, more recent literature suggests that these lesions may not be the primary source of pain in these athletes, but rather may be an asymptomatic finding in shoulders with other sources of posterior shoulder pain such as labral tears or undersurface rotator cuff tears (39–41). At this time, the exact contribution of the posterior glenoid exostosis to an overhead athlete's symptoms is uncertain. What is certain is that the presence of these exostoses correlates highly with other pathology of the glenohumeral joint such as labral tears and undersurface rotator cuff tears (39–41).

Clinically, most baseball players with symptomatic posterior glenoid exostoses give a history of posterior shoulder pain present only during the act of throwing, usually in the late cocking and early acceleration phases. A consistent finding on physical examination is tenderness to palpation at the posterior rotator cuff, capsule, and glenoid. The ultimate diagnosis of this lesion is made on Stryker's notch radiographs in which an ossification is seen at the posteroinferior border of the glenoid (Fig. 21-6).

The treatment of athletes with posterior glenoid exostoses is controversial. Some authors have concluded that

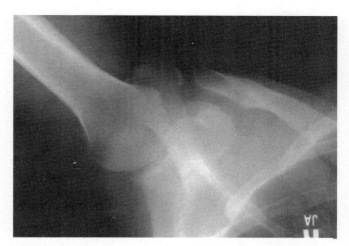

FIGURE 21-6. Radiograph showing of a high-level baseball pitcher with a posterior glenoid exostosis (Bennett's lesion).

excision of these exostoses is not warranted (41,42), whereas others believe that selected lesions should be excised (39,40). Meister and co-workers suggested that large exostoses, especially those greater than 100 mm^2, in baseball players with posterior shoulder pain and tenderness at the posterior shoulder, should be excised via arthroscopic techniques (40). For Yoneda and colleagues, arthroscopic excision of a Bennett's lesion is warranted when the following four criteria are met: (a) the presence of a posterior glenoid exostosis on radiographs, (b) posterior shoulder pain, especially in the follow-through phase, (c) tenderness at the posteroinferior shoulder, and (d) relief of symptoms following injection of the lesion with local anesthetics.

We believe that the presence of a posterior glenoid exostosis is highly predictive of an undersurface rotator cuff tear caused by internal impingement and injury to the posterior labrum. We initially treat our baseball players with these lesions with a period of active rest and supervised rehabilitation. If nonoperative treatment fails, and the patient presents with posterior shoulder pain and tenderness over the posterior glenoid with a large exostosis, we strongly consider arthroscopic excision of the lesion. During the procedure, we initially treat any underlying intraarticular pathology. We then place a 70-degree arthroscope through the anterior portal to improve visualization beyond the posterior glenoid rim. The posterior glenoid exostosis is uncovered through a small incision at the medial edge of the posteroinferior capsule. A small round burr is then employed to debride the exostosis back to the normal contour of the posterior glenoid rim. Patients postoperatively are placed in a supervised physical therapy program. As part of the surgical procedure, it is important to address any underlying instability in these patients because any pathologic laxity may predispose the soft tissues of the glenohumeral joint to further injury and possible recurrence of the exostosis.

NEUROVASCULAR PATHOLOGY ABOUT THE SHOULDER

Neurovascular disorders about the shoulder seen in baseball players include thoracic outlet syndrome, suprascapular nerve entrapment, quadrilateral space syndrome, and long thoracic nerve palsy. These injuries are often a function of the extreme ranges of motion about the shoulder girdle and muscular forces generated about the shoulder girdle that place the neurovascular structures around the shoulder at risk of tensile or compressive forces. In evaluating possible neurologic injuries around the shoulder, it is important to consider cervical spine disease and brachial neuritis as part of the differential diagnosis.

Thoracic Outlet Syndrome

Thoracic outlet syndrome is a condition characterized by abnormal compression of the major neurovascular structures around the neck and shoulder, including the brachial plexus, the subclavian and axillary arteries, and the subclavian vein. The compression may be caused by any number of bony and myofascial structures that surround these neurovascular structures including a cervical rib, the anterior or middle scalene muscles, or the pectoralis minor (Fig. 21-7). Wilburn and Porter have classified thoracic outlet syndromes based on the compressed neurovascular structure to include arterial, venous, neurogenic, and nonspecific thoracic outlet syndromes (43).

Patients with thoracic outlet syndrome often have vague symptoms that are only elicited with exertion. Symptoms include fatigue, claudication, paresthesias, and motor deficits. Several tests have been developed to help with the clinical assessment of thoracic outlet syndrome such as the Adson test, the Wright test, and the Roos maneuver; however, most of these tests have a low specificity.

For suspected vascular thoracic outlet syndrome, Doppler examinations, arteriograms, and venograms can help with the diagnosis. For neurogenic thoracic outlet syndrome, EMG with nerve conduction velocity testing may be helpful. The findings with these tests are usually restricted to the ulnar nerve distribution because the neural compression is often located at the lower trunk of the brachial plexus via a cervical rib, enlarged transverse process of C7, or fibrous bands extending from the cervical rib to the first rib (44). Nonspecific thoracic outlet syndrome is usually associated with poor posture and extensive myofascial restrictions about the thoracic outlet. The postural attitude responsible for this syndrome commonly results from relative hyperflexion of the lower cervical and upper thoracic spine, leading to adaptive shortening of the neck and anterior chest myofascial structures and elevation of the first rib.

Treatment of nonspecific thoracic outlet syndrome is nonsurgical with an emphasis on stretching of the anterior

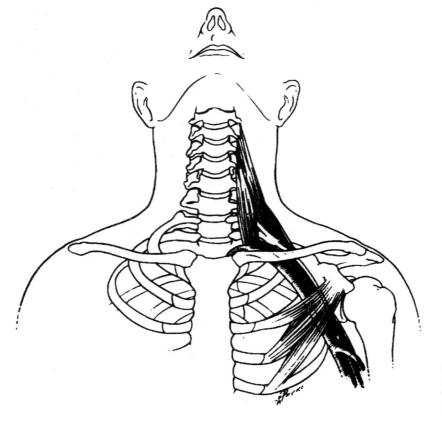

FIGURE 21-7. Anatomy of the thoracic outlet. (From Wilburn AJ, Porter JM. Thoracic outlet syndrome. *Spine: State Art Rev* 1988;2:598, with permission.)

chest and neck muscles and strengthening of the postural muscles of the shoulder girdle and thoracic spine.

Vascular and neurogenic thoracic outlet syndrome can also be successfully treated with physical therapy to open up the thoracic outlet. If nonoperative treatment fails, surgical intervention may be warranted. For arterial thoracic outlet syndrome, surgical procedures include transaxillary first rib resection, supraclavicular anterior scalenectomy, or pectoralis minor resection. Venous thoracic outlet syndrome is characterized by venous thrombosis; therefore, treatment is early anticoagulation, possible thrombolysis, and possible first rib resection.

DiFelice and co-workers recently presented the cases of four baseball players diagnosed with effort thrombosis in their dominant arms (45). *Effort thrombosis* has been used to describe venous thrombosis of the upper extremity because of its common association with repetitive upper extremity activities. These four players complained of upper extremity fatigue and swelling over a period of 2 to 7 days. Diagnosis was confirmed by contrast venography and all patients were treated with urokinase thrombolysis, oral anticoagulation for 3 months, and delayed resection of the first rib. All four players were able to resume playing at or above their previous levels.

Treatment of neurogenic thoracic outlet syndrome following failed nonoperative treatment is usually resection of the first rib and fibrous bands.

Suprascapular Nerve Entrapment

The suprascapular nerve may sustain a traction injury from the large forces around the shoulder during pitching or may be compressed at the spinoglenoid or suprascapular notches by their respective ligaments (46) or by a ganglion cyst (47,48). Cysts at the spinoglenoid notch may develop secondary to glenoid labral pathology, such as a SLAP lesion (49). Athletes with suprascapular neuropathy present with a dead arm, loss of velocity, or impingement secondary to loss of the stabilizing effects of the supraspinatus and infraspinatus. Symptoms of suprascapular nerve entrapment may progress during the season because the nerve is continuously subjected to traction or compression forces. Diagnostic studies for suspected suprascapular nerve entrapment include an MRI study, which may identify a labral cyst, and electrodiagnostic tests, which may reveal denervation of the supraspinatus or infraspinatus. Because most of these injuries in baseball players are secondary to traction from the force of throwing, we treat most patients with active rest and a supervised physical therapy program. Any decompression of a ganglion cyst is done arthroscopically.

Quadrilateral Space Syndrome

Quadrilateral space syndrome is characterized by compression of the posterior humeral circumflex artery and axillary nerve, or branches of the axillary nerve, within the quadrilateral space. This space is located in the back of the shoulder and is bordered by the teres minor superiorly, teres major inferiorly, humerus laterally, and long head of the triceps medially (50) (Fig. 21-8). The compression of these neurovascular structures is maximized with the shoulder in abduction and external rotation; therefore, baseball players, as they achieve the cocking position, may repetitively over-

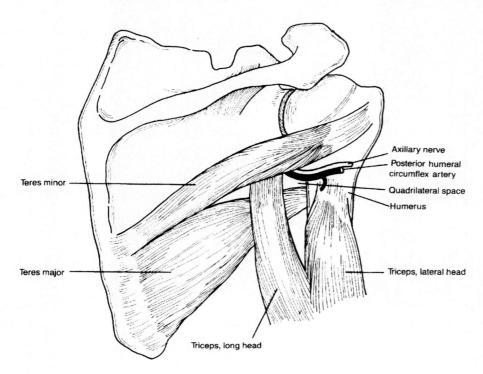

FIGURE 21-8. Anatomy of the quadrilateral space. (From Gardner E, Gray DJ, O'Rahilly R. *Anatomy: a regional study of human structure,* 5th ed. Philadelphia: WB Saunders, 1986, with permission.)

load the axillary nerve and posterior humeral circumflex artery. This may eventually lead to the formation of fibrous bands at the quadrilateral space, resulting in worsening compression of these neurovascular structures (51). Clinical findings include vague anterolateral shoulder pain, paresthesias around the shoulder, and pinpoint tenderness posteriorly at the quadrilateral space. These findings are amplified with the shoulder in a position of abduction and external rotation, compromising the quadrilateral space. Most patients with quadrilateral space syndrome can be treated nonoperatively with aggressive stretching of the posterior shoulder. If nonoperative treatment fails, a subclavian arteriogram may show occlusion of the posterior humeral circumflex artery as the shoulder is maneuvered from neutral to the cocked position. Surgical treatment involves release of the teres minor at its humeral insertion and release of the fibrous bands at the quadrilateral space.

Long Thoracic Nerve Palsy

The long thoracic nerve is also subject to traction and compression injury in baseball players. Loss of this nerve results in weakness of the serratus anterior, a scapular stabilizing muscle; therefore, players may present with a loss of throwing velocity and subacromial impingement signs, in addition to the finding of scapular winging. Treatment of long thoracic nerve palsy is nonoperative. Recovery of this nerve may take months to years.

ADOLESCENT INJURIES

The adolescent shoulder is different than that of an adult, primarily because of the presence of the physis in the skeletally immature athlete. Unlike the adult shoulder in which the soft tissues are most susceptible to injury, in the young baseball player, the physis is the "weak link" in the shoulder. If the shoulder is subjected to large, repetitive stresses, the physis is a potential site for injury.

Little Leaguer's shoulder is a result of excessive stress to the physis of the proximal humerus in a skeletally immature overhead athlete (52). It is believed that this injury is secondary to repetitive tension and torsional loads to the proximal humeral physis producing a fatigue fracture of the physis (53). Young baseball players with this injury usually have a several month history of mild shoulder pain that may escalate with throwing activities. On examination, the proximal humerus is tender to palpation and shoulder range of motion is painful and decreased on the affected extremity. Radiographs demonstrate widening of the proximal humeral physis. Views of the contralateral shoulder are often helpful to provide comparison of the physes (Fig. 21-9). Treatment consists of active rest, daily gentle range-of-motion exercises, and a mild rotator cuff strengthening program as symptoms subside. No throwing is permitted for 6 weeks. Once clinical and radiographic evidence of healing is present, a more aggressive rotator cuff strengthening program is initiated, followed by an interval throwing program.

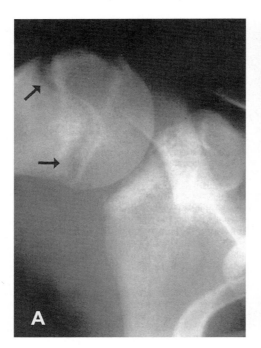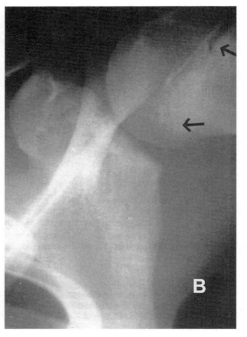

FIGURE 21-9. Radiographs of young right-hand dominant baseball player with 2-month history of right shoulder pain. **A:** Radiographs of painful right shoulder showing increased radiolucency and widening across proximal humerus physis consistent with Little Leaguer's shoulder. **B:** Radiograph of normal left shoulder.

Another injury seen in skeletally immature overhead athletes is proximal humeral epiphysiolysis. This is a separate entity from classic Little Leaguer's shoulder. This diagnosis is given when the proximal humeral epiphysis demonstrates avascular necrosis and has a much more guarded prognosis with regard to returning to overhead athletics than does a proximal humeral epiphyseal plate fatigue fracture (54).

Glenohumeral instability and rotator cuff injuries do occur in adolescent baseball players, as they do in adults. The treatment algorithms are similar; however, nonoperative treatment is pursued for a much longer period of time in younger athletes. Often, a prolonged period of active rest and supervised physical therapy, in conjunction with maturation of the young athlete, leads to successful outcomes in most adolescent baseball players with shoulder injuries.

To prevent injury in young baseball players, it is often helpful to have a young pitcher's throwing motion evaluated by a coach or instructor familiar with normal biomechanics. Incorrect form when pitching may predispose the shoulder to excessive forces, resulting in a greater potential for injury. Probably the greatest measure that a coach, parent, or league official can take to prevent shoulder injuries in young baseball players is to avoid overuse by limiting the number of pitches a young athlete can make in a game and season. Our recommendations are set forth in the following section.

Other potential shoulder injuries in the skeletally immature baseball player include spiral oblique fractures of the proximal humerus, epiphyseal avulsion fractures of the coracoid process with resultant acromioclavicular joint separation, true acromioclavicular joint separations, and os acromiale (42,55–57).

PITCH LIMITS IN YOUNG BASEBALL PLAYERS

Shoulder injuries are common in baseball pitchers, and the risk of shoulder injury increases with age and level of competition. It is likely that this increased risk is due to the cumulative microtrauma that the shoulder has been subjected to from the athlete's days of youth baseball. It is reasonable to assume that the amount of stress placed on a young pitcher's shoulder from repetitive pitching appearances increases the risk of injury both in the present and the future. With the advent of year-round baseball, young baseball players are subjecting themselves to injury now more than ever. In addition, they are subjecting their shoulders to stresses that may lead to more serious injuries in the future.

With the support of the USA Baseball Medical and Safety Committee and the U.S. Olympic Committee, we conducted a study through ASMI and the American Baseball Foundation (ABF) to understand why youth baseball pitchers develop arm problems and to provide information for establishing safety recommendations (58). A prospective

study of 476 youth baseball players ages 9 to 14 was conducted over the 1999 spring baseball season examining the relationship between number and types of pitches and presence of shoulder and elbow pain. The study divided the subjects into three age groups: 9 to 10 year olds, 11 to 12 year olds, and 13 to 14 year olds. A total of 3,789 pitching appearances were analyzed. More than 9% of all pitching appearances resulted in shoulder pain, with 35% of all subjects reporting shoulder pain at least once during the season. With regard to types of pitches thrown, use of a curve ball produced a 52% increased risk of shoulder pain, without variation in age groups. With regard to pitch counts, a significant direct relationship between an increased number of game pitches and presence of shoulder pain was found. In addition, a significant direct relationship between number of pitches thrown during the season and risk of shoulder pain was also found.

These findings provide statistical support to the long held conventions that the greater numbers of pitches thrown in both a game and season and the types of pitches thrown can result in shoulder pain in a youth pitcher. It is our opinion that this pain is evidence of overuse in these youth pitchers that may eventually lead to more significant injuries as these youths continue to stress their shoulders over the courses of their careers.

Based on our results from this study, we established a set of recommendations for youth pitching. Pitchers between 9 and 14 years of age should not throw curve balls or sliders. In support of this recommendation, USA Baseball concluded that pitchers should first learn the fastball (recommended age 8 ± 2 years), then the change-up (10 ± 3 years), followed by the curve ball (14 ± 2 years), and, finally, the slider (16 ± 2 years) (59). We recommend that youth baseball pitchers be limited to 75 pitches in a game and 600 pitches in a season. An alternative method to limit pitch counts is to limit the number of batters faced in a game and season to 15 and 120, respectively. These pitch limits should be inclusive of all leagues in which a player participates and should not be circumvented by participation in more than one league at a time. These recommendations apply to competitive game pitches only. They do not apply to warm-up pitches, practice pitches, throwing from other positions, or throwing drills.

CONCLUSION

The act of throwing a baseball requires a complex sequence of muscle activation to place the shoulder in extremes of motion and generate tremendous forces to accelerate the baseball. This places tremendous stresses on the soft tissues of the shoulder, often leading to injury. Most shoulder injuries in baseball players can be treated nonoperatively with a period of active rest followed by a supervised rehabilitation program. If a prolonged period of nonoperative treatment fails, arthroscopic intervention is a useful tool to evaluate and treat the injured shoulder. It should be the goal of the clinician to be aware of the causes of injuries in baseball players and to make every attempt to educate these players with the hope of preventing injury.

REFERENCES

1. Dillman CJ, Fleisig GS, Andrews JR. Biomechanics of pitching with emphasis upon shoulder kinematics. *J Orthop Sports Phys Ther* 1993;18:402–408.
2. Fleisig GS, Dillman CJ, Andrews JR. A biomechanical description of the shoulder joint during pitching. *Sports Med Update* 1991;6:10.
3. Jobe FW, Moynes DR, Tibone JE, et al. An EMG analysis of the shoulder in pitching. A second report. *Am J Sports Med* 1984; 12:218–220.
4. Glousman R, Jobe F, Tibone J, et al. Dynamic electromyographic analysis of the throwing shoulder with glenohumeral instability. *J Bone Joint Surg (Am)* 1988;70:220–226.
5. Moynes DR, Perry J, Antonelli DJ, et al. Electromyography and motion analysis of the upper extremity in sports. *Phys Ther* 1986;66:1905–1911.
6. DiGiovine NM, Jobe FW, Pink M, Perry J. An electromyographic analysis of the upper extremity in pitching. *J Shoulder Elbow Surg* 2002;1:15–25.
7. Gowan ID, Jobe FW, Tibone JE, et al. A comparative electromyographic analysis of the shoulder during pitching. Professional versus amateur pitchers. *Am J Sports Med* 1987;15:586–590.
8. Bradley JP, Tibone JE. Electromyographic analysis of muscle action about the shoulder. *Clin Sports Med* 1991;10:789–805.
9. Sisto DJ, Jobe FW, Moynes DR, et al. An electromyographic analysis of the elbow in pitching. *Am J Sports Med* 1987;15:260–263.
10. Jobe FW, Tibone JE, Perry J, et al. An EMG analysis of the shoulder in throwing and pitching. A preliminary report. *Am J Sports Med* 1983;11:3–5.
11. Feltner M, Dapena J. Dynamics of the shoulder and elbow joints of the throwing arm during the baseball pitch. *Int J Sport Biomech* 1986;2:235–259.
12. Fleisig GS, Dillman CJ, Andrews JR. Proper mechanics for baseball pitching. *Clin Sports Med* 1989;1:151–170.
13. Jobe FW, Jobe CM. Painful athletic injuries of the shoulder. *Clin Orthop* 1983;173:117–124.
14. Bisson LJ, Andrews JR. Classification and mechanism of shoulder injuries in throwers. In: Andrews JR, Zarins B, Wilk KE, eds. *Injuries in baseball.* Philadelphia: Lippincott-Raven, 1998:47–55.
15. King JW, Brelsford HJ, Tullos HS. Analysis of the pitching arm of the professional baseball pitcher. *Clin Orthop* 1969;67:116–123.
16. Brown LP, Niehues SL, Harrah A, et al. Upper extremity range of motion and isokinetic strength of the internal and external shoulder rotators in major league baseball players. *Am J Sports Med* 1988;6:577–585.
17. Bigliani LU, Codd TP, Connor PM, et al. Shoulder motion and laxity in the professional baseball player. *Am J Sports Med* 1997; 25:609–613.
18. Crockett HC, Gross LB, Wilk KE, et al. Osseous adaptation and range of motion at the glenohumeral joint in professional baseball pitchers. *Am J Sports Med* 2002;30:20–26.
19. Osbahr DC, Cannon DL, Speer KP. Retroversion of the humerus

in the throwing shoulder of college baseball pitchers. *Am J Sports Med* 2002;30:347–353.
20. Reagan KM, Meister K, Horodyski MB, et al. Humeral retroversion and its relationship to glenohumeral rotation in the shoulder of college baseball players. *Am J Sports Med* 2002;30:354–360.
21. Gillogly SD, Andrews JR. History and physical examination of the throwing shoulder. In: Andrews JR, Zarins B, Wilk KE, eds. *Injuries in baseball.* Philadelphia: Lippincott-Raven, 1998:57–74.
22. Pappas AM, Zawacki RM, McCarthy CF. Rehabilitation of the pitching shoulder. *Am J Sports Med* 1985;13:223–235.
23. Moseley JB Jr, Jobe FW, Pink M, et al. EMG analysis of the scapular muscles during a shoulder rehabilitation program. *Am J Sports Med* 1992;20:128–134.
24. Townsend H, Jobe FW, Pink M, et al. Electromyographic analysis of the glenohumeral muscles during a baseball rehabilitation program. *Am J Sports Med* 1991;19:264–272.
25. Matsen FA, Harryman DT. Mechanics of glenohumeral instability. *Clin Sports Med* 1991;10:783–788.
26. O'Brien SJ, Neves MC, Arnoczky SP, et al. The anatomy and histology of the inferior glenohumeral ligament complex of the shoulder. *Am J Sports Med* 1990;18:449–456.
27. Bigliani LU, Pollock RG, Soslowsky LJ, et al. Tensile properties of the inferior glenohumeral ligament. *J Orthop Res* 1992;10:187–197.
28. Warren RF, Kornblatt IB, Marchand R. Static factors affecting posterior shoulder stability. *Orthop Trans* 1984;8:89.
29. Rowe CR, Zarins B. Recurrent transient subluxation of the shoulder. *J Bone Joint Surg (Am)* 1981;63:863–872.
30. Andrews JR, Satterwhite YE. Anatomic capsular shift. *J Orthop Tech* 1993;1:151–160.
31. Andrews JR, Angelo RL. Shoulder arthroscopy for the throwing athlete. *Tech Orthop* 1988;3:75–81.
32. Walch G, Boileau P, Noel E, et al. Impingement of the deep surface of the supraspinatus tendon on the posterosuperior glenoid rim: an arthroscopic study. *J Shoulder Elbow Surg* 1992;1:238–245.
33. Levitz CL, Dugas J, Andrews JR. The use of arthroscopic thermal capsulorrhaphy to treat internal impingement in baseball players. *Arthroscopy* 2001;17:573–577.
34. Kvitne RS, Jobe FW, Jobe CM. Shoulder instability in the overhand or throwing athlete. *Clin Sports Med* 1995;14:917–935.
35. Andrews JR, Carson WG Jr, McLeod WD. Glenoid labrum tears related to the long head of the biceps. *Am J Sports Med* 1985; 13:337–341.
36. Snyder SJ, Karzel RP, Del Pizzo W, et al. SLAP lesions of the shoulder. *Arthroscopy* 1990;6:274–279.
37. Burkhart SS, Morgan CD. The peel-back mechanism: its role in producing and extending posterior type II SLAP lesions and its effect on SLAP repair rehabilitation. *Arthroscopy* 1998;14:637–640.
38. Bennett GE. Shoulder and elbow lesions of the professional baseball pitcher. *J Am Med Assoc* 1941;117:510–514.
39. Yoneda M, Nakagawa S, Hayashida K, et al. Arthroscopic removal of symptomatic Bennett lesions in the shoulders of baseball players: arthroscopic Bennett-plasty. *Am J Sports Med* 2002; 30:728–736.
40. Meister K, Andrews JR, Batts J, et al. Symptomatic thrower's exostosis. Arthroscopic evaluation and treatment. *Am J Sports Med* 1999;27:133–136.
41. Ferrari JD, Ferrari DA, Coumas J, et al. Posterior ossification of the shoulder: the Bennett lesion. Etiology, diagnosis, and treatment. *Am J Sports Med* 1994;22:171–175.
42. Bennett GE. Elbow and shoulder lesions of baseball players. *Am J of Surg* 1959;98:484–492.

43. Wilburn AJ, Porter JM. Thoracic outlet syndromes. *Spine: State Art Rev* 1988;2:597–626.
44. Rayan GM. Lower trunk brachial plexus compression neuropathy due to cervical rib in young athletes. *Am J Sports Med* 1988;16:79.
45. DiFelice GS, Paletta GA Jr, Phillips BB, et al. Effort thrombosis in the elite throwing athlete. *Am J Sports Med* 2002;30:708–712.
46. Ferretti A, Cerullo G, Russo G. Suprascapular neuropathy in volleyball players. *J Bone Joint Surg (Am)* 1987;69:260–263.
47. Ogino T, Minami A, Kato H, et al. Entrapment neuropathy of the suprascapular nerve by a ganglion. A report of three cases. *J Bone Joint Surg (Am)* 1991;73:141—147.
48. Skirving AP, Kozak TKW, Davis SJ. Infraspinatus paralysis due to spinoglenoid notch ganglion. *J Bone Joint Surg (Br)* 1994;76:588–591.
49. Tirman P, Feller J, Janzen D, et al. Association of glenoid labral cysts with labral tears and glenohumeral instability. Radiologic findings and clinical significance. *Radiology* 1994;190:653–658.
50. Cahill BR, Palmer RE. Quadrilateral space syndrome. *J Hand Surg* 1983;8:65–69.
51. Weinstein SM, Herring SA. Neurologic and vascular problems about the shoulder. In: Andrews JR, Zarins B, Wilk KE, eds. *Injuries in baseball*. Philadelphia: Lippincott-Raven, 1998:125–136.
52. Adams JE. Little league shoulder: osteochondrosis of the proximal humeral epiphysis in boy baseball pitchers. *Calif Med* 1966;105:22-25.
53. Cahill BR, Tullos HS, Fain RH. Little league shoulder. *Sports Med* 1974;2:150-153.
54. Ireland ML, Satterwhite YE. Shoulder Injuries. In: Andrews JR, Zarins B, Wilk K, eds. *Injuries in Baseball*. Philadelphia: Lippincott-Raven, 1998;271-281.
55. Ireland ML, Andrews JR. Shoulder and elbow injuries in the young athlete. *Clin Sports Med* 1988;7:3.
56. Black GB, McPherson JA, Reed MH. Traumatic pseudodislocation of the acromioclavicular joint in children. *Am J Sports Med* 1991;19:644–646.
57. Liberson F. Os acromiale—a contested anomaly. *J Bone Joint Surg (Am)* 1937;19:683–689.
58. Lyman S, Fleisig GS, Andrews JR, et al. Effect of pitch type, pitch count, and pitching mechanics on risk of elbow and shoulder pain in youth baseball pitchers. *Am J Sports Med* 2002;30:463–468.
59. Andrews JR, Fleisig GS. How many pitches should I allow my child to throw? *USA Baseball News* 1996;5.

22

FOOTBALL

RUSSELL F. WARREN
BRYAN T. KELLY
RONNIE P. BARNES
JOHN W. POWELL

INTRODUCTION

Football throwers are at risk for shoulder injury secondary to both the throwing motion and the contact injury incurred by collision with another player or the ground (1–3). Although the incidence of shoulder injury in football throwers appears to be less frequent than in baseball pitchers, in our clinical experience with both professional and collegiate football athletes, we have encountered a unique spectrum of shoulder injuries including acromioclavicular (AC) and sternoclavicular (SC) joint separations, deltoid and rotator cuff contusions, shoulder dislocations and subluxations, fractures, pectoralis major injury, disorders of the biceps tendon, and overuse rotator cuff pathology (1,2,4). The risk for shoulder injury may be increased with the level of athlete (elite versus nonelite), the style of throwing (side arm versus overhead), the length of the throw, and the associated muscle fatigue that occurs throughout a game or practice. These injuries may be secondary to trauma (AC joint separation, SC joint separation, deltoid contusion, rotator cuff contusion, pectoralis major muscle injury) (1,5,6) or to chronic overuse (rotator cuff tendonitis, biceps tendonitis, impingement syndrome) (2,3).

KINEMATICS AND BIOMECHANICS

In the limited research looking at the kinematics of football throwing (7–9), there have been no reports on the muscle activation of rotator cuff muscles and shoulder synergists during the overhead football throw. Even though the football throw is similar in some respects to other overhead throwing motions, the increased weight of the football (0.42 kg versus 0.14 kg for the baseball) appears to affect shoulder position and stresses throughout the throwing motion (7,10,11). Because of the mechanical adjustments the shoulder must make to compensate for the heavier football, this throwing motion is likely to have different muscular activation patterns compared to those of other overhead throwing events. In addition, the injury patterns observed clinically are unique in this population of athletes and include traumatic injuries to the pectoralis major, AC joint, and SC joint, as well as disorders of the biceps tendon and more common rotator cuff pathology (1–3,5,6,10,11).

Phase definition and electromyographic (EMG) analysis has been thoroughly investigated for the baseball throw and relatively consistent definitions have been previously established (12–16). Fleisig and colleagues (17) have published one description of the phases of the football throw, but their description of the throwing motion used the same six phases that had been previously defined for baseball pitching with no regard for mechanical adjustments associated with the heavier ball. This description was made to simplify the interpretation of the results, because the purpose of the study was to compare the kinematics of the football throw and the baseball pitch (17).

We have used video analysis of professional football quarterbacks to critically describe the phases of the football throw (18) (Fig. 22-1). Four sequential phases of the football throw were consistently observed: (a) early cocking (rear foot plant to maximal shoulder abduction and internal rotation), (b) late cocking (maximal shoulder abduction and internal rotation to maximal shoulder external rotation), (c) acceleration (maximal shoulder external rotation to ball release), and (d) follow-through (ball release to maximal cross-body horizontal adduction). The defined phases were highly consistent among the National Football League (NFL) athletes analyzed by video review, as well as among the amateur subjects tested by EMG and motion analysis (18). These phases were similar to the phases described for the baseball pitch (12,14–16,19). The average total duration of the throw was similar to what has been previously reported in the literature (1.00 ± 0.22 seconds) (9,18). Since the phases described in this study were based on discrete, functionally based extremes of shoulder motion, we were able to accurately apply these phases to all the amateur

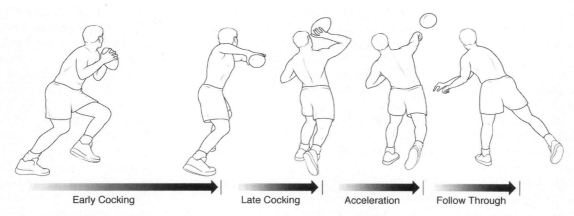

FIGURE 22-1. Four phases of the overhead football throw: early cocking, late cocking, acceleration, and follow-through. (From Kelly BT, Backus SI, Williams RJ, et al. Electromyographic analysis and phase definition of the overhead football throw. *Am J Sports Med* 2002;30:837–844, with permission.)

athletes that we tested. By simply identifying the point in the throw where each of the extremes was achieved, the events that marked the transitions between phases could be reproducibly identified in all of the subjects tested. We believe that such an objective measure of phase transitions is useful to help formulate relatively consistent definitions similar to those that have been previously established for the baseball throw.

We have also looked at the EMG activity of nine shoulder muscles and correlated muscle activation throughout the defined phases of the throw (18). Our findings demonstrated that the muscle activation patterns observed were also highly consistent among athletes, and changes in muscle activation throughout the throw correlated well with the defined phases.

In his EMG analysis of the baseball pitch, Gowan and colleagues (14), defined two types of muscle activity. He defined group I muscles as those that were more active during the early and late cocking stages than during acceleration and follow-through. The muscles included in this group were supraspinatus, infraspinatus, and biceps brachii. Group II muscles were more active in the acceleration stage than in the early and late cocking stages and their activity lasted into late follow-through. These muscles included the subscapularis and the latissimus dorsi. The three deltoid muscles were minimally to moderately active throughout all four phases with no clearly discernible phases of transition. The pectoralis, although active during acceleration and follow-through, was not included in the group II musculature because the peak activities for the baseball throw was during the late cocking phase at the period of maximal external rotation.

In comparing the football throw to the baseball throw, no muscles can be defined as group I muscles, using the definitions set forth by Gowan and colleagues (14). This defi-

nition of increased muscle activation during the early and late cocking phases as compared to the acceleration and follow-through phases was not appropriate for any of the muscles tested. There were, however, based on the firing patterns, two distinct groups of muscles for the football throw. We have defined group I muscles as stabilizers (18). These muscles demonstrated relatively static levels of activity throughout the throw and included the supraspinatus, the infraspinatus, all three deltoids, and the biceps. The supraspinatus and infraspinatus were further characterized as high-level stabilizers with moderate to maximal activity throughout all four phases. The three heads of the deltoid were characterized as moderate level stabilizers with moderate activity throughout all phases. The biceps was characterized as a low-level stabilizer with minimal activity throughout all four phases. We have defined group II muscles as accelerators (18). The group II muscles for the football throw were identical to the group II muscles identified during the baseball throw: more active in the acceleration phase than in the early and late cocking phases with activity present into late follow-through. The muscles included in this group were the subscapularis, the pectoralis major, and the latissimus dorsi. These muscles provided the majority of the force that was imparted into the football throw.

The presence of persistently high levels of activation of the three accelerator muscles into the follow-through phase may not be intuitively understood. All three of these muscles are internal rotators of the humerus and hence should not be expected to decelerate the internal rotation forces of the humerus as is required during the follow-through phase. However, two considerations may help to explain this phenomenon. With regard to the subscapularis, this muscle contributes to the normal co-contraction forces of the rotator cuff that are essential for maintaining the humeral head centered on the glenoid. Although the subscapularis functions as an accelerator during the acceleration phase, it has a dual role with the remainder of the rotator cuff as a co-contractor during the powerful joint distraction forces experienced during the follow-through phase. The latissimus dorsi and pectoralis major muscles may be recruited to provide additional co-contraction forces to reinforce the job that is routinely controlled by the rotator cuff musculature alone during less forceful activities. The high kinetic forces that are experienced across the shoulder joint during football throwing may not be adequately countered by the rotator cuff alone. Thus, during forceful overhead activities such as football throwing and baseball pitching, the latissimus dorsi and pectoralis major muscles may be required to control further distraction across the shoulder joint during the follow-through phase.

In comparing the kinematics and kinetics between the baseball pitch and the football pass, Fleisig and colleagues (7) demonstrated several differences between these two overhead activities. Most notably, during arm deceleration, pitchers produced greater forces and torques in the shoulder and elbow. They also demonstrated that higher arm speeds were generated in pitching. Shoulder internal rotation velocities were between 3 and 4.5 times faster during the baseball throw and elbow extension velocities were between 2 and 3 times faster during the baseball throw (7,9). In addition, greater degrees of shoulder abduction and external rotation were achieved during the baseball throw (B. Kelly, *unpublished data, 2003*). In further evaluating the baseball EMG work by Gowan and colleagues (14), it is notable that the accelerator muscle group demonstrated considerably more activity during the baseball throw compared to what was found during the football throw in this study. These findings are consistent with the theory that the accelerator muscles have a dual responsibility to provide additional co-contraction force during the follow-through phase to further stabilize the shoulder and prevent joint distraction. Since the baseball throw results in greater kinetic forces across the shoulder joint during deceleration (7), it is appropriate to see the greater levels of muscle activation in the accelerator group during baseball pitching compared to football throwing (14).

Clearly defining different types of muscle activation patterns has clinical implications. First, by knowing the manner in which different muscles fire during the throw, athletes can be given both sport- and muscle-specific conditioning protocols. The most effective training method for optimal conditioning of the stabilizer muscles should differ from the most effective conditioning of the accelerator muscles. Stabilizer muscles may benefit from more isotonic conditioning while accelerator muscles may be more effectively strengthened with plyometric and acceleration exercises. Knowledge of these two different muscle groups also provides insight into rehabilitation protocols. The goal of rehabilitation of injured muscles should be the return to sport-specific kinematics. If the mode of activation during the throw can be more accurately simulated during rehabilitation, we would anticipate a quicker return to full functional activity (20–23). Additional clinical correlation and investigation is warranted to confirm these hypotheses.

Ultimately, we seek to identify which anatomic structures are most important to the football throwing motion. Just as earlier EMG studies led to the development of sports-specific preventive and therapeutic protocols, EMG analysis of the shoulder musculature during the football throw will lead to a better understanding of throwing injuries associated with football throwing (12,23–25) and more specific rehabilitation and conditioning programs will be developed that might better protect quarterbacks from the development of shoulder conditions. By further identifying associated risk factors for shoulder injury, additional safety measures and precautions can be more intelligently exercised.

ETIOLOGY OF INJURY

We have accessed the NFL Injury Surveillance System (NFLISS) to identify all injuries to quarterbacks that have been reported to the NFL between 1980 and 2001. The injury data collected in the NFLISS is based on the primary clinical impression of the clinical diagnosis made by the medical staff involved. The data reflect only those cases reported during the season (training camp to Super Bowl) and that required the player to be restricted from playing for at least 2 days. Over 22 seasons, 1,534 quarterback injuries were reported to the NFLISS with a mean of 18.8 and a median of 6.0 days lost. Most of these injuries (83.8%) have occurred during a game, with slightly more occurring on grass (55.7%) compared to turf (44.3%). Passing plays are responsible for 77.4% of all quarterback-related injuries.

Of the 1,534 injuries reported, 233 (15.2%) involved the shoulder, including the glenohumeral joint, proximal humerus, scapula, clavicle, AC joint, SC joint, long head of the biceps tendon, rotator cuff, scapular stabilizers, deltoid, and pectoralis major muscles (Tables 22-1 and 22-2). Shoulder injuries were the second most common injury sustained by quarterbacks, following closely behind head injuries (15.4% of reported injuries). The most common mechanism of shoulder injury is related to direct trauma, either from contact with another player or with the ground (80.3%). Nearly 70% of shoulder injuries occurred while the quarterback was being tackled: 47.3% occurred while being tackled as the passer, 12.6% while being tackled as the ball carrier, and 9.6% while being tackled after the pass. Only 12.4% of injuries were reported as being secondary to the actual throwing motion.

Overall, the most common single shoulder injury identified was an AC joint sprain incurred while being tackled or during a collision with another player or the ground (39.6%). Of all AC joint sprains, 44% were type I, 24%

TABLE 22–1. INJURIES TO THE SHOULDER AND CHEST IN PROFESSIONAL QUARTERBACKS REPORTED TO THE NFLISS FROM 1980 TO PRESENT

Injuries to Shoulder and Chest	Overall	Tackled/Collision	Throwing	Other
Deltoid contusion	11.30%	10.90%	0%	0.40%
Rotator cuff contusion, sprain, tendonitis	18.10%	8.40%	6.10%	3.60%
Scapular, trapezius contusion	1.70%	1.70%	0%	0%
Anterior shoulder dislocation, subluxation, capsulolabral injury	8.40%	8.00%	0.40%	0.00%
Posterior shoulder dislocation, subluxation, capsulolabral injury	2.90%	2.50%	0.40%	0%
Synovitis, capsulitis	1.60%	0.00%	0.80%	0.80%
Nerve injury	0.40%	0.40%	0%	0%
Biceps tendinitis	4.30%	0.40%	3.50%	0.40%
Impingement, bursitis	2.90%	1.70%	0.40%	0.80%
Fracture (humerus or scapula)	1.20%	1.20%	0%	0.00%
Pectoralis major tear, sprain	1.20%	1.20%	0%	0%
	54.00%	**36.40%**	**12%**	**6%**

were type II, 20% were type III, and 12% were not specified. The second most common group of injuries was shoulder contusions from collisions or tackling and involved the deltoid (10.9%), rotator cuff (8.4%), and scapular stabilizers (1.7%). Other injuries reported as a result of direct trauma included anterior shoulder dislocations (8%), fractures of the proximal humerus, scapula, and clavicle (3.7%), posterior shoulder dislocations (2.5%), SC joint sprains (2.5%), impingement and bursitis (1.7%), pectoralis major injuries (1.2%), biceps tendonitis (0.4%), and axillary nerve injury (0.4%).

The most common injury identified as a result of the throwing motion itself was rotator cuff tendonitis (6.1%) followed by biceps tendonitis (3.5%). Other injuries reported as being associated with the throwing motion itself included synovitis and capsulitis (0.8%), anterior labral tear (0.4%), posterior capsular strain (0.4%), impingement (0.4%), and SC joint strain (0.4%). The clinical spectrum of injuries observed in the NFLISS are consistent with the kinematic and EMG findings reported previously (18). Compared to the baseball throw, the football throw is associated with significantly slower rotational velocities, decreased extremes of range of motion, and decreased electrical activity from the rotator cuff and surrounding shoulder musculature (7,9,14,18). Based on these biomechanical data, one would expect fewer problems with chronic

overuse types of injury such as those experienced much more commonly in baseball pitchers. This is, in fact, what is observed, with most shoulder injuries occurring as a result of trauma (80%) and less than 15% resulting from the actual throwing motion.

OVERVIEW OF SPECIFIC INJURIES

Acromioclavicular Joint Separation

Acute injuries to the AC joint are common in a variety of contact sports and are the most common isolated injury to the shoulder complex in quarterbacks (40% of reported shoulder injuries in the NFL). The typical mechanism for an acute traumatic injury is a fall onto the shoulder or a direct blow to the acromion while being tackled during or after passing. A shoulder separation occurs when there is sufficient energy to cause a partial or complete disruption of the AC or coracoclavicular (CC) ligaments. Acromioclavicular joint dislocations have been classified into six types based on the extent of ligament damage (26–30) (Fig. 22-2). Type I injuries involve a sprain of the AC ligament with intact AC and CC ligaments. Type II injuries are the result of more severe trauma, resulting in disruption of the AC ligaments but leaving the CC ligaments intact. Type III

TABLE 22–2. INJURIES TO THE CLAVICLE, AC JOINT, AND SC JOINT IN PROFESSIONAL QUARTERBACKS REPORTED TO THE NFLISS FROM 1980 TO THE PRESENT

Injuries to Clavicle/AC joint/SC joint	Overall	Tackled/Collision	Throwing	Other
AC Joint Sprain	40.00%	39.60%	0%	0.40%
SC Joint Sprain	3.40%	3%	0.40%	0%
Clavicle Fracture	2.50%	2.50%	0%	0%
	45.90%	**45.10%**	**0.40%**	**0.40%**

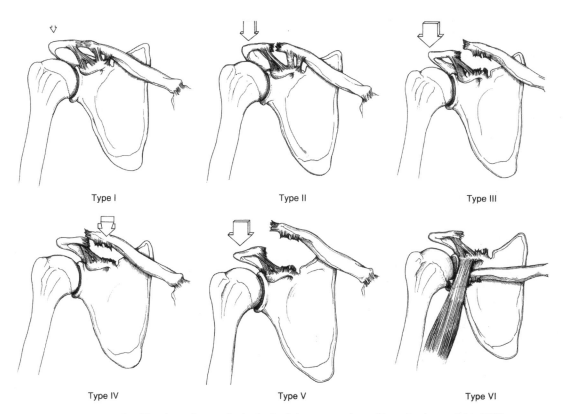

FIGURE 22-2. Classification of acromioclavicular joint separations. (From Rockwood CA, Williams GR, Young DC. Disorders of the acromioclavicular joint. In: Rockwood CA, Matsen FA, eds. *The shoulder,* 2nd ed. Philadelphia: WB Saunders, 1998:483–553, with permission.)

injuries involve disruption of both the AC and CC ligaments, which results in visible dislocation of the AC joint with displacement of 50% to 100%. Although there may be mild elevation of the distal clavicle, the more significant cause of the deformity is from depression of the dissociated shoulder girdle. Types IV, V, and VI injuries are the result of more violent forces leading to complete disruption of the surrounding ligaments and musculature. Type IV injuries involve posterior displacement and penetration of the trapezius muscle by the distal clavicle. Type V injuries are characterized by marked superior displacement with greater than 100% increase in CC distance. In type VI injuries, the distal clavicle dislocates to a subcoracoid position (28).

Patients with type I and II AC dislocations have pain and swelling over the superior shoulder, focal tenderness at the AC joint, and pain with cross-arm adduction. Type I injuries have no displacement of the clavicle, whereas in type II injuries, prominence of the joint is present with a radiographic displacement of up to 50%. Type I and II AC separations generally require only symptomatic care. Strengthening programs, including range-of-motion exercises, can usually be initiated within 1 to 2 weeks after the acute pain has subsided. Athletic participation can usually be resumed within 3 to 4 weeks, once normal strength and

range of motion has returned (27). Nonsurgical treatment of types I and II injuries leads to good results in more than 90% of cases, although posttraumatic degenerative joint disease may sometimes develop secondary to meniscus or articular cartilage damage at the time of injury. If pain persists, it is reasonable to perform a Mumford procedure with expectation of a good result and ultimate return to full preinjury level of activity (31).

The management of type III injuries remains somewhat controversial (11). In 1974, Powers and Bach (32) reported that 92% of 116 type III injuries were managed operatively. Seventeen years later, Cox (33) reported that most surgeons (72% of residency chairmen and 86% of team physicians) were managing type III injuries nonoperatively (34). Currently, there is much support in the literature for the nonoperative treatment of type III injuries in nearly all patients (34–37). However, disagreement remains regarding the appropriate management of the elite throwing athlete (11,35,37,38). McFarland and co-workers (35) surveyed 42 orthopedic surgeons representing 28 major league baseball teams concerning treatment of type III AC separations in professional throwing athletes. In this survey, 31% of the surgeons recommended immediate operative intervention and 69% believed that nonoperative management would be more appropriate. Twenty-five of the orthopedists surveyed had actually treated type III AC separations in throwing athletes and reported that 80% of the patients treated non-operatively regained normal function and achieved complete relief of pain, and 90% had normal range of motion after treatment. Of those treated operatively, 92% regained normal function, achieved complete relief of pain, and had normal range of motion after surgery. Absolute treatment guidelines for the elite throwing athlete cannot be made based on the available literature in that operative and non-operative treatment appear to give similar results (35), although some authors maintain that type III AC joint sprains may result in an alteration in throwing mechanics that can manifest as subacromial impingement and should therefore be addressed surgically (34).

As has been previously explained, the football throwing athlete must be considered differently than the baseball throwing athlete because their associated injuries are more commonly caused by traumatic force than by overuse. Cardone and colleagues (39) reviewed 14 Australian Rules Football (ARF) players who were seen consecutively by a single surgeon with grade III AC joint injuries. Treatment of this group may be more analogous to the situation encountered with quarterbacks. In this group, eight players elected for nonoperative management and six for operative management. Two players in the nonoperative group subsequently underwent surgical reconstruction after failure of nonoperative treatment. The mean return time to noncontact training was 2.4 weeks (range 1 to 4, SD 1.52) in the nonoperative group and 6.3 weeks (range 3.5 to 10, SD 2.99) in the operative group. However, return to sports-specific training (contact training) was at a mean of 20.8 weeks (range 10 to 32, SD 8.56) in the nonoperative group and 13.6 weeks (range 6 to 24, SD 7.06) in the operative group. Although limited by the small numbers, the results show a trend toward faster return to ARF and a more satisfactory outcome for patients undergoing surgery compared to their nonoperative cohorts.

Initial surgical intervention is usually indicated for the treatment of type IV, V, and VI injuries because of the severe displacement of the clavicle. Popular operative techniques described for reduction of the AC joint include fixation across the AC joint, dynamic muscle transfer, and fixation between the clavicle and the coracoid (34). Reconstruction of the ligament can be performed using the modified Weaver-Dunn procedure, which involves limited distal clavicle resection, transfer of the coracoacromial ligament, and stabilization of the coracoclavicular interval with suture, soft tissue, or hardware. The postoperative regimen often requires up to 6 weeks in a sling, followed by motion and strengthening exercises (27). The modified Weaver-Dunn has had favorable results in reducing pain and improving function in athletes with symptomatic type III, IV, and V acromioclavicular dislocations (40).

Verhaven and co-workers (41) prospectively followed 18 consecutive athletes with an acute type V AC sprain treated with a coracoclavicular repair using a double velour Dacron graft. All patients were reviewed after a mean follow-up period of 6 years (range 2 to 9 years). At follow-up, 12 patients (66.7%) showed a good or excellent result according to the Imatani evaluation system, and six patients (33.3%) demonstrated a fair or poor result according to the same system. Loss of reduction was encountered in eight shoulders (44.4%) despite an initial anatomic reduction. No correlation was seen between the overall scores at follow-up and the degree of residual dislocation, between the overall scores and the presence of coracoclavicular calcifications or ossifications, between the overall scores and the development of posttraumatic arthritic changes, or between the overall scores and the presence of osteolysis of the distal clavicle. These authors concluded that surgical treatment for acute type V AC separations in athletes provides fewer good results than similar treatment for type III lesions. However, in this series, all patients returned to the same level of sport activity as before injury (41).

Authors' Preferred Approach

Grade I and II injuries, as noted, are treated nonoperatively with a progressive rehabilitation program. Similarly, after initial protection with a sling, most grade III injuries in athletes are placed in a rehabilitation program and observed. Surgery has rarely been necessary: there is little in the literature to support early repair even in a quarterback. Taft (42) previously reported that about 10% of nonoperative AC joint injuries go on to need surgical care. In addition, most strength studies have failed to show significant deficits with nonoperative treatment in throwers. We have treated several NFL quarterbacks nonoperatively with a grade III separation who returned to play at 5 or 6 weeks.

In contrast, grade IV, V, and VI injuries need surgical treatment. With gross displacement as in a grade V injury, the standard Weaver-Dunn procedures appear to be inadequate in some patients. It appears that the instability is not only inferior but that the acromion migrates medially, which places excess stress on a simple coracoclavicular graft. Thus, we have preferred to use an autograft or allograft to reconstruct both the coracoclavicular ligament and the acromioclavicular ligaments (Fig. 22-3). In addition, when the joint has been fractured, we prefer to excise the distal clavicle and repair the ligaments and muscular attachments. This may be sufficient in acute cases but if the tissue is poor or the injury is old, then a reconstruction of the acromioclavicular as well as the coracoclavicular ligaments is indicated. In a limited number of these cases, we have noted improved maintenance of stability.

Rehabilitation Pearls

Acute AC sprains involving all classifications can be painful. Early immobilization is prescribed for most type III

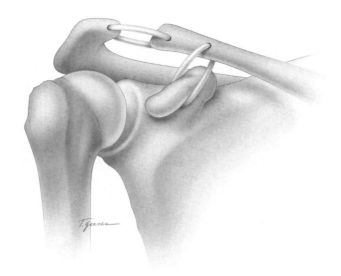

FIGURE 22-3. Autograft or allograft reconstruction of the coracoclavicular and acromioclavicular ligaments.

injuries. Acute nonsurgical management of these conditions includes pain management, reduction of swelling, and maintaining shoulder function and overall range of motion. Pain and swelling are the primary inhibitors to increased motion and initiation of progressive resistive exercises. Frequent applications of ice packs are helpful in pain control. Strengthening programs should include specific exercises for the deltoid muscles. Forward elevation to beyond 90 degrees or more is encouraged. Throwers with AC injuries to the shoulder progress in rehabilitation from Codman's and pendulum activities to more aggressive range-of-motion exercises as pain and swelling permits. Focus on strength, endurance, proprioception, and neural control can be achieved only as pain and swelling decreases. Functional activities involving throwing are performed only in the final phases of rehabilitation. Return to throwing in sports must be based on pain-free range of motion and healing of the joint with normal mechanics. Athletes who return to play with some lingering point tenderness may need a bridged hard shell protective pad to protect the area from direct impact while playing.

Sternoclavicular Joint Separation

Injury to the SC joint in quarterbacks is much less common than AC joint injuries, accounting for less than 3% of all reported shoulder girdle injuries in the NFLISS. The decreased incidence is related to the medial location of the joint, although indirect forces can be transmitted through the shoulder girdle, resulting in sprains, fractures, or dislocations (43). Difficulty in diagnosis is related to the relative rarity of the injury as well as limitations of standard radiographic views. Radiographic examination should include

standard anteroposterior (AP) and lateral chest radiograph looking for asymmetry of the SC joint compared to the contralateral side (43). Rockwood (44) described the "serendipity view" obtained with a 40-degree cephalic tilt, which reveals a true caudocephalic view of both SC joints and the medial clavicles. In an anterior dislocation, the affected clavicle appears superior and in a posterior dislocation it appears inferior (44). Acute sprains of the SC joint are classified as type I, type II, or type III, depending on the degree of injury to the supporting ligaments and joint capsule (43). In a type I injury, there is a partial disruption of the ligaments but the clavicle remains in its anatomic position with respect to its medial articulation. In type II injuries, there is an incomplete disruption of the ligaments and some degree of subluxation can occur in either the anterior posterior direction. Symptomatic treatment, consisting of local modalities, analgesics, and short-term immobilization, is preferred for type I and II injuries (45).

A type III sprain or dislocation results from a higher energy injury and produces a complete disruption of the supporting ligamentous structures. Most traumatic SC dislocations are anterior in direction, resulting from a posteriorly directed force to the anterolateral aspect of the shoulder. Clinically, localized pain and prominence over the medial end of the clavicle are present, and CT scans are useful in further evaluating the direction of the injury and the proximity of the injury to surrounding neurovascular structures (27). Closed reductions may be attempted, but are often difficult to maintain with immediate redisplacement of the medial clavicle, and sling immobilization is usually required for a minimum of 2 to 3 weeks (27,43). Nonsurgical management results in good functional outcomes in most cases (46), and open reduction of anterior dislocations is rarely indicated (43).

Because of the strong forces involved and the proximity of the joint to the great vessels and other mediastinal structures, posterior sternoclavicular injuries can be serious and potentially life threatening (47–49). The injury is typically a result of a direct blow to the anteromedial aspect of the clavicle or of an anteriorly directed force to the posterolateral aspect of the shoulder. Signs of dyspnea, dysphagia, venous congestion, or hemodynamic instability indicate possible compression or compromise of nearby mediastinal structures and require emergent reduction (47,48). Marker (50) reviewed the reported cases of posterior dislocation of the sternoclavicular joint and found only 100 cases since 1824. In reviewing the published reports, he found that this injury is seen particularly in connection with American football and that there is often a delay in diagnosis with potentially serious complications. Closed reduction of these injuries should be performed within 7 days by abduction and extension of the shoulder and manual manipulation of the clavicle. Rockwood (44) described a technique of reduction under general anesthesia in which the clavicle is percutaneously grasped with a towel clip to facilitate reduction. If closed reduction fails, the reduction is not stable, or the dislocation is greater than 7 days old, open reduction and stabilization is indicated (43).

Authors' Preferred Approach

Generally anterior dislocations are managed nonoperatively, whereas reduction is performed for posterior dislocations. Occasionally in teenagers, we encounter a voluntary type of anterior instability that is more commonly seen in females. Anterior instability is generally asymptomatic, but we have seen patients in whom recurrent pain with athletics requires treatment for anterior dislocation. The options include resection with stabilization of the clavicle to the first rib or attempted reduction. Recently we have performed reduction with ligament repair using biodegradable anchors to repair the anterior sternoclavicular ligament. Postoperatively, we placed the arm in an adducted position to decrease the deforming forces for approximately 6 weeks. If the joint is arthritic, then resection and clavicular stabilization is indicated.

In chronic cases of posterior dislocation, resection of the medial clavicle is required. Preoperatively, we obtain an MR angiogram to evaluate any vasculature structures that may be compromised by the displaced clavicle. A vascular surgeon should be available in these cases. Occasionally, the injury is not a complete dislocation but is at the growth plate in a teenager. The epiphysis on the medial end of the clavicle is the last to close and does not unite with the clavicle until the 23rd to 25th year of life. In these cases, observation is indicated because the remodeling process decreases or eliminates any bone deformity or displacement and allows for correction of the deformity.

Rehabilitation Pearls

Sternoclavicular sprains characteristically range from slight pain and point tenderness to the joint to a painful displaced joint requiring immobilization. Pain, swelling, point tenderness, and an inability to abduct the shoulder in full range of motion or the inability to bring the arm across the chest (horizontal adduction) limit the rehabilitation phases. Isometric exercises to the shoulder may be initiated if the injury requires immobilization. Pain and swelling management are important factors in the rehabilitation progression. Frequent application of ice packs is helpful in pain control. Reestablishing nonpainful range of motion, retardation of shoulder muscle atrophy, and neuromuscular control can only be achieved after the acute pain phase has been managed. Rehabilitation of sternoclavicular sprains should begin with pain-free dependent mobilization of the shoulder joint. The next phase includes more aggressive range-of-motion and strengthening exercises. Codman's and pendulum exercises may be used as the patient progresses to a sports cord program for the shoulder. Upper body bicycle ergometer and active and passive flexibility exercises should be performed as tolerated. Return to throwing is based on pain-free range of motion and adequate strength, power, endurance, and neuromuscular control. A graduated program of tosses and throws to a full throwing regimen with normal mechanics should be implemented.

Deltoid Contusion

Traumatic contusions to the shoulder account for the second most common group of shoulder injuries in quarterbacks resulting from being tackled or other collisions with the ground or another athlete. Contusions to the deltoid occur most frequently (10.9%), followed by the rotator cuff (8.4%) and scapular stabilizers (1.7%). Deltoid contusions resulting from a direct blow to the deltoid result in pain and weakness and may be associated with axillary nerve injury. Deltoid contusions without axillary nerve involvement should be treated symptomatically. Perlmutter (51) reports that axillary nerve injuries secondary to a direct blow to the deltoid muscle are amongst the most common peripheral nerve injuries in athletes who participate in contact sports. The injury results in deltoid muscle paralysis secondary to nerve trauma. The diagnosis may be difficult to distinguish from the so-called burner syndrome, which is also associated with muscle weakness and pain (52,53); however, it is most likely a separate entity with a different mechanism of injury and prognosis for neurologic recovery (53).

Perlmutter and co-workers (53) performed a long-term follow-up (31 to 276 months) of 11 contact athletes who had sustained isolated injuries to their axillary nerves during athletic competition with no known shoulder dislocations. Ten of the 11 patients had EMG confirmation of clinically defined injuries confined to their axillary nerves. All injuries were the result of direct trauma with another player or a collision during tackling or with the ground. Seven of the athletes sustained a direct blow to the anterior lateral deltoid muscle. Contralateral neck flexion and ipsilateral shoulder depression injuries occurred simultaneously in four patients. At follow-up, all patients had residual deficits of axillary sensory and motor nerve function with moderate to no improvement in five patients and major improvement in six patients. However, shoulder function remained excellent, in that all athletes maintained full range of motion with good to excellent motor strength and 10 of 11 athletes returned to their preinjury levels of sports activities, including professional athletics. Axillary nerve exploration and neurolysis in four patients did not significantly affect the outcomes (53). We have had a similar case in our 20 years of NFL care with an All-Pro linebacker who sustained a direct blow to his right shoulder early in his career, before our involvement with the team. However, the player paid little attention to his complete deltoid loss since his cuff had hypertrophied greatly. Clinical testing noted excellent motion and only mild weakness with elevation (Fig. 22-4).

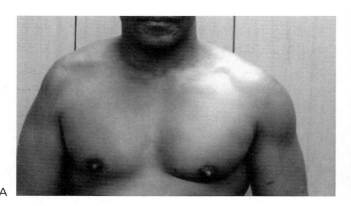

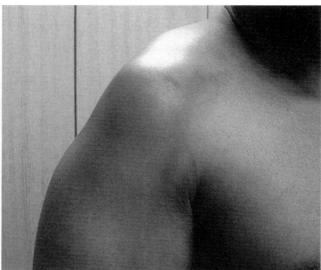

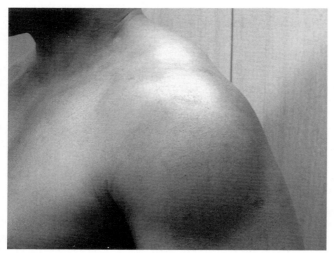

FIGURE 22-4. A: Complete axillary nerve palsy with subsequent deltoid atrophy in a professional football athlete. The right deltoid demonstrates significant muscle atrophy **(B)** compared with the left **(C)**.

A clinically suspected axillary nerve injury associated with deltoid muscle contusion should be confirmed by electrophysiologic testing, including EMG and nerve conduction studies. The athlete should be rested during the acute phase of injury and any associated ligamentous or bony injury should be treated as indicated. Rehabilitation should emphasize active and passive range of motion as well as strengthening of the rotator cuff and the deltoid and periscapular musculature. Loss of shoulder mobility should be avoided because this may ultimately affect functional outcome despite a return of axillary nerve function. If no axillary nerve recovery is observed by 3 to 4 months following injury, some authors recommend surgical exploration (51). Occasionally, an epineural hematoma develops in a nerve. If an injury leads to rapidly progressive pain, paresthesia, and weakness, then a magnetic resonance imaging (MRI) scan should be obtained to evaluate the nerve and early surgical decompression of the nerve should be seri-

ously considered. Athletes who sustain injury to the axillary nerve typically have good to excellent return of shoulder function, although nerve recovery has a variable prognosis. Return to contact sport participation is safe after the athlete achieves full active range of motion of the shoulder and when shoulder strength is documented to be good to excellent by isometric or manual muscle testing (51).

Rehabilitation Pearls

Recovery from deltoid contusions involves pain management and reduction of edema in the muscles. Frequent application of ice packs is helpful in the control of swelling. Early motion using an upper body ergometer, light dumbbells, and passive and active motion can be initiated. Manual resistance exercises to the shoulder and sports cord shoulder training should be initiated as tolerated. Shoulder stretches and massage may also be helpful. Resistive exercises requiring the deltoid muscles to contract establishes strength and endurance that allows early return to play. An isolated pad or an elongated epaulet on the shoulder pads may prevent a second impact to the area that may be painful and possibly precipitate a myositis ossificans.

Rotator Cuff Injury

Injuries to the rotator cuff in quarterbacks result from two discrete mechanisms. The first mechanism is from traumatic injury after an acute episode of macrotrauma to the shoulder and represents the third most common shoulder injury experienced by quarterbacks (8.4%). The second mechanism is chronic, repetitive overuse from the throwing motion itself and represents 6.1% of the injuries reported to the NFLISS. Although rotator cuff injury as a result of a single traumatic event is generally thought to be rare in young athletic patients, a recent report describing rotator cuff tears in 18 patients younger than age 40 years documented that approximately 90% could recall a specific traumatic event heralding the onset of their symptoms (54). Blevins and colleagues (1) retrospectively reviewed 10 male contact athletes with rotator cuff injuries related to trauma during football who underwent surgery after failure of nonoperative management. The spectrum of injury in these 10 patients included two isolated contusions, five partial-thickness tears, and three full-thickness tears. Indications for surgery in this group included physical examination findings consistent with rotator cuff injury and no improvement with nonoperative treatment consisting of rest, antiinflammatory medications, modalities, gentle range of motion, and progressive cuff strengthening exercises (1). The two cuff contusions and three of the partial thickness tears were treated with arthroscopic debridement. One full thickness and two partial thickness tears were repaired using a miniopen technique. The two remaining full thickness tears were treated with a formal open repair technique. At an average follow-up of 21 months, 9 of the 10 athletes had returned to active participation in football, seven at their preinjury level.

In another report on treatment of partial rotator cuff tears in young athletes, Payne and colleagues (55) reviewed cases of 43 athletes younger than age 40 years with partial rotator cuff tears, more than half of whom were collegiate or professional, who were treated arthroscopically and observed for a minimum of 24 months. They identified two main groups based on history and mechanism of injury. Group A had acute, traumatic injuries and group B were overhead athletes with insidious, atraumatic shoulder pain. Patients with traumatic causes and evidence of subacromial impingement achieved both excellent pain relief and frequent return to sports after an arthroscopic debridement and subacromial decompression. Overall satisfaction in this group was 86% with a return to sport rate of 64%. Most tears were articular sided, which suggests that direct com-

pression of the cuff into the undersurface of the acromion may produce a cuff contusion with subsequent tendon degeneration in the critical area of decreased vascular supply (55,56). The diagnosis of traumatic rotator cuff injury should be considered in a contact athlete who has persistent shoulder pain, impingement signs, weakness, and a positive shrug sign. In the setting of failure of nonoperative management, arthroscopic debridement of the subacromial space followed by debridement or repair of rotator cuff tears, likely results in marked improvement in function and rapid return to sport for these patients.

Rotator cuff injury and impingement resulting from repetitive overhead activities and chronic overuse from throwing in quarterbacks occurred in 6.1% of the shoulder injury cases reported to the NFLISS. This injury pattern appears to be significantly less problematic in quarterbacks than in other overhead athletes such as baseball pitchers, tennis athletes, swimmers, and volleyball players. The cause of shoulder pain associated with rotator cuff overuse is not universally agreed upon and is likely multifactorial. Important factors include extrinsic tendon impingement (impingement syndrome as originally described by Neer [57,58]), intrinsic tendon disease or tension tendinopathy (4,26), and intraarticular or internal impingement (59–61). Neer's description of the impingement syndrome emphasizes progressive degeneration of the supraspinatus tendon resulting from external compression from the anterior acromion and the coracoacromial arch and describes a continuum of disease from chronic bursitis and partial thickness damage to complete tears of the cuff (26,57,58). It is also possible, however, that the rotator cuff tendons undergo fatigue failure from excessive tension and repetitive use and the actual impingement is a secondary phenomenon (4). Throwers are even further at risk for cuff injury in that the position of the arm during the throwing motion may have a compressive effect on the already relatively avascular area at the insertion of the supraspinatus and intraarticular portion of the biceps tendon. Repetitive microscopic injury in this area may have decreased healing potential due to the compromised blood supply (4,56).

Quarterbacks appear to be less susceptible to chronic overuse injuries to the cuff for a variety of reasons. First, the kinetics of the football throw require slower rotational velocities and subsequently decreased rotator cuff and shoulder girdle muscle activation (7,18). Second, kinematic evaluation of the football throw demonstrates that the maximal shoulder and elbow excursions are less than those required during the baseball throw (7). Third, the distance, velocity and style of throwing have significant variation throughout a game or practice compared with the baseball throw. The subsequent variations in the position of the arm result in an overall decreased repetitive load to a single area of the shoulder and cuff. Finally, the total number of high-velocity throws required by quarterbacks is less than is required for pitchers (number of throws per game, number of games per season).

Nonetheless, overuse injuries can occur in quarterbacks and should be treated similarly to overuse injuries in other overhead athletes. The majority will respond to conservative treatment of rest, antiinflammatory medication, injections, and physical therapy (4). Surgical intervention may be considered when these conservative modalities fail. Tibone and colleagues (4) evaluated 45 athletes with either a partial or a complete tear of the rotator cuff secondary to chronic overuse and impingement. All athletes failed conservative management and subsequently were treated with anterior acromioplasty and repair of the tear. Postoperatively, 87% reported overall improvement; 76% reported significant decrease in their pain; 56% rated their result as good and were able to return to their former competitive level without significant pain; 41% of the 29 throwing athletes were able to return to the same level of play; only 32% of the 22 professional or collegiate athletes were able to return to their same competitive level. These authors concluded that surgical repair of the cuff and acromioplasty in a young active population does provide satisfactory pain relief, but does not guarantee the ability to return to the same level of competitive play.

Similarly, Payne and colleagues (55) found that young overhead athletes with partial rotator cuff tears of insidious onset demonstrated good pain relief from an arthroscopic debridement of the tear but many failed to return to their preinjury level of sports. In this study, patients with cuff tears from chronic overuse and insidious onset, normal-appearing subacromial spaces, increased anterior glenohumeral translation, and posterior labral injury produced the worst study results. Conversely, arthroscopic debridement of cuff tears resulting from acute trauma combined with subacromial decompression and stabilization or debridement of the labral injury provided excellent pain relief and a high rate of return to sports (55).

Authors' Preferred Approach

Rotator cuff injury varies from contusion to complete tear. Cuff contusions occur generally from a direct blow and clinically mimic a complete tear with pain, weakness in elevation, and a shrug sign. Physical therapy may restore normal function but if this fails after 4 to 6 months, arthroscopy is indicated. An early MRI study demonstrates cuff thickening and bleeding into the subacromial space. At times, cracks in the tuberosity are noted that are not visible on plain x-ray film. Cuff debridement and removal of soft tissue scarring around the acromion combined with a bursectomy restore range of motion and alleviate the pain. Rehabilitation is generally relatively rapid.

If there is a partial tear of the cuff that is less than one-third thickness, then debridement alone is performed. However, if the tear is greater in depth in a throwing athlete, a primary arthroscopic repair is performed. Generally, we prefer to complete the tear and insert two anchors from medial to lateral to anatomically restore the footprint of the supraspinatus. Full thickness tears may be associated with instability, and in these players both issues are addressed with arthroscopic repairs. If a full thickness tear is noted, an arthroscopic repair is performed using anchors and nonabsorbable sutures. An acromioplasty is combined only if it is a type III acromion and the etiology is atraumatic or if the space seems narrow on arthroscopic evaluation.

Rehabilitation Pearls

Rotator cuff rehabilitation protocols have been well defined in the literature. Established criteria have been described to avoid overstress on healing tissue. Most rotator cuff injuries respond well to a complete and comprehensive rehabilitation program. Postoperative patients follow the same routine as nonoperative patients except during the immediate postsurgical protection and healing phase. Repaired chronic or large tears require more caution with active range-of-motion and resistive exercises. Timing and speed of advancement through range-of-motion parameters is dependent upon the size and location of the repaired tear, as well as on the quality of the tissue. Generally cuff repairs require protection for 6 weeks during the healing phase of the injury, followed by 6 weeks of increasing motion and strength as healing matures. The final 6 weeks is a period of building power in the periscapular muscles. Subsequently, a toss program is initiated starting with 30 throws at 30 feet and at half speed and progressing over 6 weeks to full velocity.

Repairs to the rotator cuff involving more than one tendon require more effort in achieving range of motion postoperatively. Early passive range of motion postoperatively is essential to prevent capsular adhesions and fibrosis. General goals include pain management, regaining upper extremity strength and endurance, pain-free range of motion, and proprioception. Codman's and pendulums, ball or putty squeezing, progressing to shoulder mobilizations, proprioceptive neuromuscular facilitation (PNF) patterns and strengthening with sports cords, and graduated light weights should be included in the general program. Capsular stretching, plyoball tosses, rhythmic stabilization, and heavy weights can be initiated in the latter phases of the program. Precaution should be used with all shoulder programs to prevent impingement. Patients should not perform military presses behind the head or bench-pressing too soon. Behind the head lateral pull-downs, exercises above the head, dips, and lateral raises above shoulder level can be detrimental to the rehabilitation program if initiated early in the rehabilitation process. A complete rehabilitation program should focus on the subscapularis, serratus anterior, anterior and posterior deltoids and rhomboids, supraspinatus, pectorals, biceps, and triceps muscles. Exercises that include horizontal abduction and shoulder shrugs are beneficial. Attention to scapular motion and strength should not be neglected. Return to throwing may be initiated when all rehabilitation goals have been met and the athlete can throw pain-free with normal mechanics.

Fractures (Proximal Humerus, Scapula, Clavicle)

Fractures around the shoulder represented 3.7% of the injuries reported to the NFLISS. The clavicle was the most commonly affected (2.5%), followed by simple fractures of the greater tuberosity (.8%) and least commonly fractures of the scapula (.4%). All fractures occurred after the athlete was tackled or after collisions with another player or the ground. Management of these fractures in quarterbacks follows the principles of traditional fracture management.

Clavicle fractures are classified by location of the injury. Group I fractures involve the middle third, group II fractures involve the distal third, and group III fractures involve the medial third (62). Group II fractures of the distal third are further subdivided based on the location of the coracoclavicular ligaments relative to the fracture fragments. Type I fractures are interligamentous with minimal displacement. Type II fractures are displaced secondary to a fracture medial to the coracoclavicular ligaments (Fig. 22-5). In type IIA fractures, both the conoid and trapezoid are attached to the distal fragment, and the proximal fragment is displaced superiorly. In type IIB fractures, the conoid is torn, and the trapezoid remains attached to the distal fragment. Careful

evaluation of the associated soft tissue disruption, particularly of the coracoclavicular ligaments, should be performed because the type II injuries have numerous forces acting on the fracture fragments that may impair healing and contribute to the reported high incidence of nonunion in this pattern of injury (62). Most clavicle fractures can be treated nonoperatively with simple sling support or more involved reduction splinting (figure-of-eight bandage, plaster reinforcement, or shoulder spica casts). Surgical management is indicated for open fractures, skin tenting with the potential for skin compromise, significantly displaced type II distal third fractures, and nonunions. A variety of surgical techniques has been popularized including cerclage sutures, intramedullary devices, plate fixation, or external fixation (62).

Fractures of the proximal humerus occurred in 0.8% of the reported cases and in all instances involved simple greater tuberosity fractures. The Neer classification of proximal humerus fractures is based on four anatomic parts including the greater tuberosity, lesser tuberosity, surgical neck, and anatomic neck (63). When any of the four major segments is displaced greater than 1 cm or angulated more than 45 degrees, the fracture is considered displaced (64). A basic trauma radiograph series is required in all cases of suspected proximal humerus fractures, including AP, scapular Y view, and axillary view. Computed tomography (CT) scan may be required to realize the extent of bony injury.

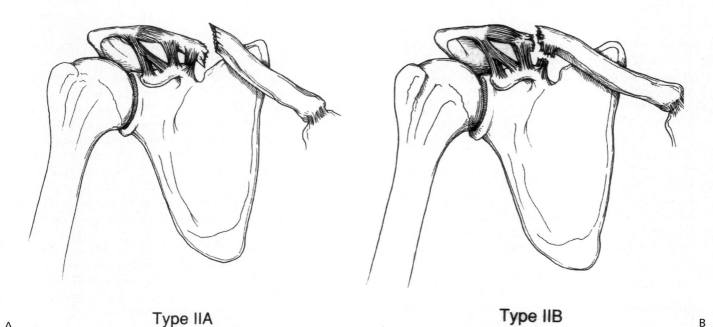

A Type IIA   Type IIB B

FIGURE 22-5. Type II distal clavicle fractures. Type IIa fractures **(A)** have an intact conoid and trapezoid ligament attached to the distal fragment, whereas Type IIb fractures **(B)** have an intact trapezoid but ruptured conoid. In both situations, the distal fragment is held by the ligamentous attachment while the proximal fragment is displaced superiorly. (From Craig EV. Fractures of the clavicle. In: Rockwood CA, Matsen FA, eds. *The shoulder,* 2nd ed. Philadelphia: WB Saunders, 1998:428–465, with permission.)

Fracture-dislocations involving the greater tuberosity typically result in disruption of the anterior capsulolabral complex and oftentimes are associated with a rotator cuff tear (65). Appropriate treatment is based on the number of parts involved and the degree of displacement and angulation. Greater tuberosity fractures may have associated rotator cuff compromise, and careful consideration of anatomic reconstruction should be made in the throwing athlete.

Fractures of the scapula are uncommon in quarterbacks, but were reported in 0.4% of the cases of shoulder injuries in the NFL. Fractures can involve the body, glenoid neck or rim, coracoid, and acromion, and are usually associated with additional injuries. As in cases of suspected proximal humerus fractures, a basic trauma radiograph series should be obtained to avoid missing these lesions. Anterior or anteroinferior glenoid rim fractures are typically the result of bony Bankart lesions associated with traumatic anterior dislocation and instability. Acromion fractures result from direct blows to the shoulder and can best be seen radiographically with the West Point or axillary view. Isolated coracoid process fractures are uncommon and are best detected with either the axillary view or a 30-degree cephalic tilt view. This injury produces pain anteriorly that worsens with deep inspiration, and pain can be recreated with resisted arm flexion and forearm supination (65). Management of these injuries must be addressed on a case by case basis.

Authors' Preferred Approach

Displaced mid third clavicle fractures in quarterbacks should probably be treated more aggressively than has been traditionally advocated. A recent paper by Hill and colleagues (66) noted a 15% nonunion rate and 31% incidence of overall dissatisfaction with markedly displaced mid third fractures of the clavicle. Fractures that go on to nonunion will likely endanger a thrower's future, thus early ORIF of these fractures may be the more conservative approach.

Fractures of the distal third of the clavicle may be significantly displaced as noted. Nonunion rates appear to be about 50% although many patients do not complain of this sequelae. Nonetheless, we believe that early ORIF is more advisable in the throwing athlete to remove some of the unpredictability associated with nonoperative treatment.

Rehabilitation Pearls

Rehabilitation following fractures to the humerus, scapula, or clavicle cannot begin until the fracture heals. Ball and putty squeezing may be the only exercise used during the fracture-healing phase. When the fracture is healed, a complete upper body program can begin with focus on the shoulder musculature of the affected side. Because of immobilization stiffness, restoring range of motion

becomes the primary objective, followed by strengthening of the upper body using isometric and isotonic exercises. An aggressive program using the upper body ergometer, dumbbells, and sports cords may be initiated shortly after immobilization is complete. Scapular fractures require particular attention and should include scapular mobilization. PNF patterns, T-bar, and flexibility exercises should be performed. A goal of restoration of normal scapulothoracic rhythm is essential. Return to weightlifting can begin after the fracture appears both radiographically and clinically healed. For clavicle fractures, this is usually a minimum of 8 weeks. Earlier return to play in football may result in refracture.

Shoulder Instability

Glenohumeral instability is generally described based on the direction of dislocation or subluxation (anterior, posterior, or multidirectional), the mechanism of injury (traumatic or atraumatic), and the timing of injury (acute, chronic, or recurrent). Unlike instability problems in other overhead throwing athletes (microinstability and internal impingement), quarterbacks typically suffer from macroscopic instability from frank dislocations that occur after being tackled. Anterior shoulder dislocations or subluxations account for 8% of all quarterback shoulder injuries, and posterior dislocations or subluxations account for 2.5% of the reported shoulder injuries. Of the 25 injuries resulting in damage to the anterior capsulolabral complex of the shoulder reported to the NFLISS, there was only one injury to the anterior labrum that was associated with the throwing motion itself rather than from trauma from direct impact to the shoulder.

Anterior GH dislocation is most commonly the result of a traumatic blow to the shoulder while it is in the abducted and externally rotated position. When traumatic anterior dislocations occur, detachment of the inferior glenohumeral ligament (IGHL) complex from the anterior glenoid is the most common defect noted (67,68). This injury has been referred to as the Bankart lesion (69,70); however, a spectrum of lesions may render the IGHL complex incompetent, including anterior periosteal sleeve avulsions (ALPSA) (71) and humeral avulsions of the glenohumeral ligament (HAGL) (72).

Taylor and Arciero (68) treated a series of first-time traumatic anterior shoulder dislocations with either early arthroscopic surgery or nonoperative treatment. The population was young (average age 19.6 years) and athletic (military cadets). Fifty-three patients chose nonoperative treatment and 63 patients elected to have arthroscopic procedures. Sixty-one of 63 (97%) patients treated surgically had complete detachment of the capsuloligamentous complex from the glenoid rim and neck (Bankart lesion) with no gross evidence of intracapsular injury. Of the other two patients, one had a HAGL lesion and one had an interstitial capsular tear adjacent to the intact glenoid labrum. Fifty-seven patients had Hill-Sachs lesions, none of which were large. Recurrent instability was present in 90% of the patients in the nonoperative group. They concluded that, in this population, the anterior capsulolabral avulsion appeared to be the primary gross pathologic lesion after a first-time dislocation and that there was a strong association between recurrent instability and the presence of an unrepaired Bankart lesion.

Initial management of athletes with traumatic anterior dislocations includes immediate reduction, immobilization, and standard radiographic examination (AP, scapular Y, West Point axillary). The Stryker's notch view is useful for evaluating the presence and size of an associated Hill-Sachs lesion. Whereas conservative treatment may be successful in older individuals, young athletic patients usually require surgical intervention to adequately stabilize their shoulder and prevent recurrence (68,73–79). Numerous studies have shown that conventional, nonoperative management of shoulder dislocations in young athletes, including a short period of immobilization followed by rehabilitation, has resulted in recurrent instability rates ranging from 17% to 96% (68,73–78,80–84). The level of activity a patient resumes after an initial shoulder dislocation may determine the risk for reinjury (76,85,86).

Because of this high rate of recurrence in young athletic patients, there have been several investigations looking at the role of early arthroscopic treatment of patients after shoulder dislocation (73–78,84,87). From these studies, it appears that early arthroscopic stabilization of traumatic first-time anterior shoulder dislocations is an effective and safe treatment that significantly reduces the recurrence rate of shoulder dislocations in young athletes, improves outcome, and avoids the frequent necessity of open reconstructive procedures to treat recurrent instability.

It has been reported that American football players are at high risk for postoperative instability even after arthroscopic stabilization of anterior shoulder instability (83,85,86,88–90). Although some authors have recommended open methods of stabilization in athletes who play contact sports, there are few data in the literature showing more favorable results with use of an open technique. Pagnani and co-workers (85) reviewed the results of an open technique of anterior shoulder stabilization in 58 American football players after a minimum of 2 years of follow-up. Ninety-five percent of the patients had a good or excellent result. The average ASES (91) postoperative shoulder score was 97.0 points (range 70 to 100 points). The Rowe and Zarins shoulder instability score (92) ranged from 49 to 100 points, with an average of 93.6 points. No patient lost more than 15 degrees of external rotation compared with the value on the contralateral side and 84% had a range of flexion and external rotation within 5 degrees of those of the contralateral shoulder. Ninety percent returned to full participation in American football for at least 1 year. These authors concluded that open stabilization is a predictable method of restoring shoulder stability in American football players and that motion and function need not be sacrificed in exchange for stability. They suggest that their results appear to be superior to those reported after arthroscopic stabilization in a similar population.

Yoneda and colleagues (93) have further suggested augmentation of the open Bankart repair with coracoid transfer for treatment of traumatic anterior shoulder instability in athletes playing contact sports. Their rationale is that athletes playing collision sports have a higher rate of recurrent subluxation even after open Bankart procedures performed alone due to the extreme forces that are repeatedly placed on the shoulder joint. Contact athletes with anterior shoulder instability often have severe bony defects of the anterior glenoid rim and the humerus (Hill-Sachs lesion) in addition to extensive soft tissue damage to the anterior glenohumeral ligaments and labrum. The researchers followed up 83 athletes (85 joints) with traumatic anterior shoulder instability who underwent this combined procedure (coracoid transfer and open Bankart repair) for a mean follow-up period of 5.8 years (range 2 to 12). They had an overall success rate of 93% with a complete return to contact sports in 73 of the 83 patients (88%). They reported an average loss of external rotation of 15 degrees with the arm at the side and 7 degrees with the arm in 90 degrees of abduction. They concluded that the combined procedure achieved a good clinical outcome for contact athletes with traumatic anterior shoulder instability but the loss of external rotation may interfere with throwing or dominant arm overhead activity and may not be appropriate for contact athletes who require this type of activity.

The timing of surgical intervention for quarterbacks with traumatic anterior dislocations depends on the severity of symptoms, the involved arm (throwing versus nonthrowing arm), and the time of the season. In athletes who have resolving symptoms early in the season, it is reasonable to attempt protected return to play with delayed surgical intervention at the completion of the season. Some athletes may not be able to perform with more severe injuries and would therefore benefit from more immediate surgical intervention with a plan for return to play the following season. The choice between arthroscopic and open stabilization remains controversial and should balance the issues of increased risk for recurrent instability after arthroscopic stabilization in the contact athlete with the potential for increased loss of external rotation after open stabilization in the overhead throwing athlete.

Posterior shoulder instability is less common than anterior injury, accounting for 2.5% of the shoulder injuries reported to the NFLISS. Of the six reported posterior capsular lesions, three were considered acute subluxations and three were considered posterior capsular sprains. Posterior shoulder injuries generally occur with the arm adducted and internally rotated. In general, posterior instability responds more favorably to nonoperative treatment (27) with generally poor results from operative intervention (94).

Structurally, posterior stability of the shoulder in flexion, internal rotation, and adduction depends on the integrity of various anatomic structures (95), including the posteroinferior aspect of the capsule and the posterior band of the inferior glenohumeral ligament complex (96–99). Cadaveric models (100) have demonstrated that forces causing posterior dislocation of the shoulder result in injury to the posteroinferior aspect of the capsule. Additional studies have demonstrated that elongation of the posteroinferior capsulolabral complex appears to result in clinical instability (96,101). In general, lesions of the posterior part of the labrum or so-called posterior Bankart lesions in patients with posterior laxity have been rarely reported (95). However, Fuchs and colleagues (95) found unequivocal abnormality of the posterior aspect of the labrum in 13 of 26 shoulders (50%) that they operated on for posterior shoulder capsular laxity. Seven (27%) of these labral injuries were true detachments that needed repair even though 80% of the patients in their series did not have any history of major trauma.

Mair and colleagues (102) reported on posterior labral injuries in nine contact athletes (seven football offensive linemen, one defensive lineman, and one lacrosse player) who were found at arthroscopy to have posterior labral detachment from the glenoid. The researchers thought that posterior labral detachment was the result of repeated exposure to posteriorly directed shear forces to the shoulder and could be considered a type of occupational hazard of contact athletics. They reported consistently good results with posterior labral reattachment, allowing for full return to competition. Weinberg and co-workers (103) reported on a college football player who sustained a posterior capsular avulsion after a posteriorly directed force to his shoulder. After failure of nonoperative management, arthroscopic examination was performed and revealed a large defect in the posterior capsule that was avulsed from the humeral side of the joint. The avulsed capsule was reattached to the humerus through a posterior arthrotomy and the patient was able to return to his previous level of competitive football 8 months after surgery.

We were unable to find any reports in the literature dealing with posterior capsulolabral complex injuries in competitive quarterbacks. The reported cases from the NFLISS all resulted from being tackled either as the ball carrier or as the passer with a subsequent posteriorly directed force to the glenohumeral joint. Management of these injuries should initially be conservative. MRI helps further delineate the extent of posterior capsulolabral injury. Persistent symptoms of pain or instability in the presence of soft tissue injury should be addressed surgically. Arthroscopic Suretac repair of detached labral tissue in the absence of instability on examination under anesthesia has reportedly good results in contact athletes (102) and is appropriate for quarterbacks. In the presence of posterior instability, open posteroinferior capsular shift may be required to fully address the pathology (95).

Authors' Preferred Approach

Anterior instability in a thrower often precludes return to play because of the forces applied to the joint during the late cocking phase. Thus, an early MRI study should be obtained. If there is only capsular injury noted on MRI, then a period of rest followed by attempted return is warranted, but, if the labrum is completely torn and displaced or if there is an associated cuff tear, then early repair is advisable to facilitate subsequent return the following year. An arthroscopic approach in a quarterback is indicated to allow full restoration of motion. A careful examination under anesthesia (EUA) is important and if there is anterior instability without significant inferior instability then suture stabilization using suture anchors with nonabsorbable suture is performed (Fig. 22-6).

Posterior instability in football players is usually associated with a significant labral injury. An MRI scan should be obtained in throwing athletes with suspected posterior shoulder injury to further delineate the extent of the pathology. Often these shoulders "quiet down," allowing some athletes to return to play with nonoperative treatment; however, residual pain with follow-through may be noted. Stabilization is generally performed arthroscopically. The technique requires a posterior labral portal to approach the posterior inferior labrum, which is generally detached (104,105) (Fig. 22-7). Repair with a Suretac anchor at the site of labral injury has been easy and reliable. However, if there is associated capsular laxity, then a suture anchor is used to facilitate labral repair and capsular plication. Postoperatively the shoulder is protected for 5 to 6 weeks with a sling and pillow. Rehabilitation avoiding adduction is important in the early phases. Generally it requires 4 to 5 months to resume activity.

Rehabilitation Pearls

Rehabilitation following shoulder dislocation and capsulolabral injury is important for both conservative and surgical management. Immobilization may be used in both cases. Ball and putty squeezing and pendulum exercises, when directed by the physician, can achieve retardation of muscular atrophy during immobilization. Isometric exercises are often permitted while immobilized in the protected position of shoulder internal rotation. The goals of tissue healing, reduction of pain and swelling, and reestablishment of range of motion and neuromuscular control of the arm are critical to recovery in surgical and nonsurgical rehabilitation. Application of ice and massage to the region controls pain and increases circulation in the region to promote

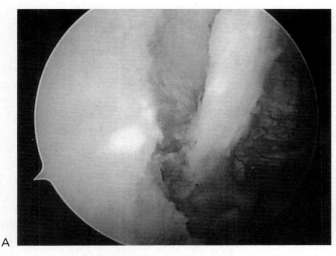 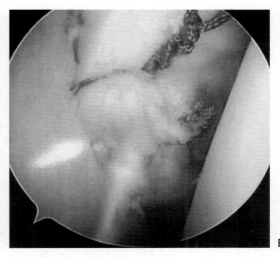

FIGURE 22-6. Arthroscopic view of a detached labrum **(A)** with subsequent suture anchor stabilization **(B)**.

healing. Following immobilization, motion can generally be initiated after 1 month. Although specific postoperative motion criteria are dependent upon the type and quality of the surgical repair, general guidelines can be followed. Active flexion between 120 and 150 degrees can generally be achieved by the 1-month period. External rotation is limited to 30 degrees for 1 to 4 weeks, followed by progressive restoration of full motion by week 8 in a thrower. Each

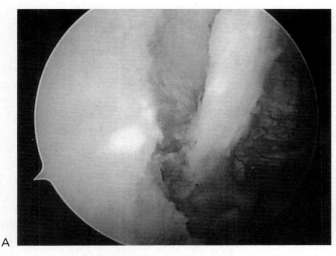

FIGURE 22-7. Posterior inferior portal used for repair of posterior labral injuries. (From Davidson PA, Rivenburgh DW. The 7-o'clock posteroinferior portal for shoulder arthroscopy. *Am J Sports Med* 2002;30:693–696, with permission.)

rehabilitation case may be slightly different depending on pain, swelling, and extent of injury. Progression to active assisted and active resistive exercise, followed by a well-established rotator cuff program is essential. Functional progression is based on rehabilitation goals that include strength, endurance, flexibility, and neuromuscular control. Scapular muscle control should not be ignored. Return to throwing activities should be based on a progression of tosses and throws in a graduated manner until full throwing mechanics with speed and velocity is attained. In posterior instability, adduction is avoided for 8 to 10 weeks and strengthening in the plane of the scapula is emphasized.

Pectoralis Major Injury

Injuries to the pectoralis major represented 1.2% of the reported shoulder injuries in the NFLISS. These injuries included partial tears and strains as well as complete ruptures. In all cases, they resulted from direct trauma during the throwing motion. Our biomechanical and kinematic data demonstrated a rapid increase in accelerator muscle activation (subscapularis, pectoralis major, and latissimus dorsi muscles) seen during the acceleration and follow-through phases of the football throwing motion (18). These findings suggest an etiology for the incidence of pectoralis major injuries that has been observed in our clinical experience and was identified through review of the NFLISS. The pectoralis major muscle may be predisposed to injury if an abduction and external rotation contact force is applied to the athlete's upper extremity during the latter two phases of the football throw (18).

Although rupture of the pectoralis major muscle was regarded as uncommon until the late 1970s, in the past 20 years there has been a significant increase in the number of reported cases (6). Most cases have been associated with participation in athletic endeavors, in particular the bench-press exercise (106–109). There have been several reports of pectoralis major muscle ruptures in football players (5,109,110); however, we were unable to find any reports on pectoralis major injuries in competitive quarterbacks.

In acute pectoralis major muscle ruptures, athletes present with loss of the anterior axillary fold, swelling, ecchymosis of the anterior chest wall and upper arm, and typically report pain and a sensation of tearing at the time of injury (106,111). Significant swelling may accompany the rupture and can make an accurate diagnosis difficult without additional imaging studies. Radiographic studies obtained shortly after injury show soft tissue swelling and loss of the pectoralis muscle shadow, but cannot accurately determine the extent of the injury. MRI allows accurate evaluation of the extent of muscle injury and enables identification of patients who would benefit from surgical repair if the focus of the study is on the insertion site of the pectoralis major tendon and not the shoulder (112).

Appropriate management of these injuries depends on the extent of the rupture and the disability it causes. Although the patient may be able to recover some power in internal rotation, flexion, and adduction with simple immobilization, it is likely necessary to surgically repair a complete rupture to allow an athletic patient to return to competitive sport, especially high demand sports such as football. Schepsis and colleagues (6) retrospectively reviewed 17 cases of complete distal pectoralis major muscle rupture to compare the results of repair in acute and chronic injuries and to compare operative and nonoperative treatment. Overall their reported subjective ratings were 96% in the acute group, 93% in the chronic group, and only 51% in the nonoperative group. Isokinetic testing showed that acute repair resulted in the highest adduction strength (102% of the opposite side) compared with repair of chronic injuries (94%) or nonoperative treatment (71%). Based on their results, they concluded patients treated operatively fared significantly better subjectively and objectively than those treated nonoperatively; however, delayed repair did not significantly compromise the subjective or objective results of surgery.

Partial rupture of the pectoralis major muscle was more common than complete rupture in the NFL quarterbacks reviewed. Appropriate management of partial ruptures is not as well agreed upon. Roi (108) evaluated the effect of conservative nonsurgical treatment in three athletes (two body builders and one shot putter) who sustained partial ruptures while bench-pressing. Functional recovery was evaluated between 4 and 7 years after injury with isokinetic dynamometer testing evaluating maximal shoulder adduction and abduction torques at different angular speeds (60, 180, and 300 degrees per second). They compared the results with those of five healthy athletes practicing either body building or weightlifting and concluded that nonoperative treatment of partial ruptures of the pectoralis major muscle produced almost complete functional recovery.

Authors' Preferred Approach

In evaluation of injury to the pectoralis major, it is important to determine whether the site of injury is in the tendon, the muscle tendon junction, or the muscle only. It appears that tears in the muscle may scar, and surgery, if performed, can be delayed until some scarring is present. In contrast, early repair of complete ruptures of the pectoralis major tendon insertion site is more appropriate. However, depending on a player's position and the time of the season, delayed repair may be discussed and surgery performed only if function is significantly compromised. Occasionally there are partial ruptures of the tendon that may heal with a period of rest and conservative management. However, too early return to play in these cases may result in a completion of the rupture. Nonoperative treatment of partial ruptures in quarterbacks has been effective in the clinical experience of these authors.

Rehabilitation Pearls

Rehabilitation to the pectoralis major muscle injury is dependent upon conservative or surgical management of the rupture. Postsurgical pectoralis major injuries are immobilized. Gentle shoulder elevation, internal rotation, and pendulum exercises are initiated postsurgically. Isometric contractions and ball and putty squeezing may be initiated as pain decreases. Assisted movements are begun when prescribed by the surgeon. These exercises are often begun a week or more after surgery. At about 1 month, more aggressive elevation and internal rotation, along with external rotation to neutral may be initiated. At 6 weeks, active exercises are begun, progressing to closely monitored internal rotation concentric and eccentric strength exercises. Following the immobilization period and for operative and nonoperative cases, the goal is to restore overall muscle strength, shoulder mobility and function, and neuromuscular control. Stretching, external rotation, and eccentric loading may be initiated at the appropriate later stage of rehabilitation. Functional activities involving throwing generally begin gradually at the 3- to 4-month period.

Biceps Tendonitis, Instability, and SLAP Lesions

Bicipital tendonitis represented 3.5% of the reported shoulder injuries to the NFLISS. This was the second most common injury resulting from the throwing motion itself and is, in all likelihood, secondary to chronic overuse. The functional role of the biceps tendon at the shoulder remains unclear. Several EMG studies have attempted to delineate the muscle activation patterns of the biceps with isolated shoulder motion (113,114), and have demonstrated that the long head of the biceps is not active in isolated shoulder motion when the elbow and forearm are controlled. These studies conclude that any hypothesis on bicipital function at the shoulder must be based on either a passive role of the tendon or tension in association with elbow and forearm activity. Other investigators have proposed that the long head of the biceps functions as a humeral head depressor and stabilizer (115–119). Although some authors have suggested that in many overhead sports the biceps helps to accelerate and decelerate the arm (120), our kinematic and EMG analysis of the overhead football throw demonstrated markedly low levels of muscle activation of the biceps throughout all four phases of the throwing motion (18).

Although relatively uncommon, quarterbacks do appear to be at risk for the development of biceps tendonitis. These patients typically have anterior shoulder pain that is exacerbated with continued overhead activities (27). It has been suggested that improper training or fatigue can place inordinate stresses on the biceps as it attempts to compensate for other muscles (120,121). These stresses can lead to attrition and failure, either within the tendon substance or at its origin, and can result in an important source of persistent shoulder pain when not specifically addressed. Some authors have suggested that persistent pain from the long head of the biceps is likely to have more negative functional consequences than loss of the tendon itself (121).

Overuse related bicipital problems in throwing athletes may occur in conjunction with other types of shoulder disorders, including subacromial impingement and glenohumeral instability, and can make determination of the role and degree of biceps involvement difficult (120). Physical examination demonstrates marked pain to palpation at the bicipital groove and positive provocative tests including the Yergason and Speed tests (122). Conditions affecting the biceps tendon in athletes can be generally classified as degeneration, instability, and disorders of the origin, and a thorough evaluation is essential to both identify the likely source as well as to rule out potential associated abnormalities (120). The initial treatment is directed at eliminating the inflammation and impingement symptoms through the judicious use of rest, physical therapy, and antiinflammatory medications. Refractory cases may require corticosteroid injection into the bicipital sheath. Oftentimes treatment of bicipital problems in athletes requires the additional treatment of associated shoulder conditions. Surgical options for recalcitrant symptoms include tendon debridement, release, or tenodesis (27,121).

Authors' Preferred Approach

Biceps tendonitis in older patients is generally a component of impingement and thus decompression with an acromioplasty is usually sufficient. In younger patients, direct trauma or fracture at the bicipital groove may result in localized injury. Tenodesis within the groove either arthroscopically or open manages the complaints.

Symptomatic subluxation of the biceps tendon is generally associated with tears (partial or complete) of the sub-scapularis. These tend to occur with violent external rotation and the biceps subluxes medially, producing a click that the patient and examiner may conclude represents instability of the glenohumeral joint. Weakness on the lift-off test (Fig. 22-8) and increased external rotation of the arm at the side are diagnostic of subscapularis ruptures (123). An MRI scan demonstrates the degree of subscapularis tearing and displacement. Complete tears require early operative treatment. In this setting, an arthroscopic approach allows direct reattachment of the subscapularis tendon with reduction of the biceps into its groove. If there is gross degeneration of the biceps (more than 50%), then a tenodesis is performed.

Lesions of the biceps anchor may occur, particularly in quarterbacks because the arm is forcefully abducted and externally rotated. SLAP lesions vary in severity from type I to IV, with type II being the most common. We have had experience with an All-Pro quarterback with a type II SLAP lesion and a compression fracture of the proximal humeral head from a forced abduction injury. He was able to throw well but had significant pain with horizontal adduction. He underwent labral stabilization at the conclusion of the season with a return to throwing pain-free at 4 months. Others may sustain a SLAP tear in association with a Bankart lesion during a subluxation or dislocation event. Subsequent arthroscopic repair of the Bankart lesion and labral repair of the type II SLAP or excision of the type III SLAP have allowed a full return to the NFL.

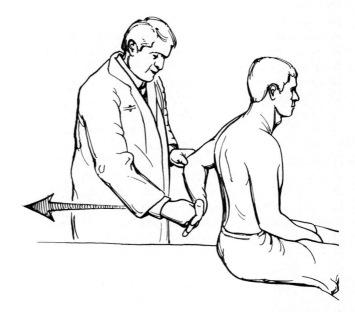

FIGURE 22-8. Lift-off test for evaluation of subscapularis integrity. (From Gerber C, Krushell RJ. Isolated rupture of the tendon of the subscapularis muscle. Clinical features in 16 cases. *J Bone Joint Surg (Br)* 1991;73:389–394; and Kelly BT, Kadrmas WR, Speer KP. The manual muscle examination for rotator cuff strength. An electromyographic investigation. *Am J Sports Med* 1996;24:581–588, with permission.)

Rehabilitation Pearls

Biceps tendonitis can be best treated by not ignoring the symptoms of a sore shoulder. After proper orthopedic evaluation and diagnosis, a rehabilitation program can be initiated. Avoiding overuse activities is important. Beginning specific exercises in a gradual manner to restore muscular strength, endurance, flexibility, and proprioception is beneficial. An early motion program with protection is ideal in the acute phase. Active and active assisted range-of-motion exercises should be initiated. A goal of pain-free activities and no pain at rest is important. Avoiding painful arcs and reducing inflammation and swelling are essential to the rehabilitation progression. Modalities including ice may allow the athlete to progress to upper body ergometer, PNF, gentle capsular stretching, and joint mobilization. A complete rotator cuff program can be initiated after the pain and protection phase has been mastered. Progressive ball tossing, plyoballs, sports cords, and weight training can all be initiated at the proper phase. Return to throwing should not begin until there is proper strength and the athlete is pain-free.

CONCLUSION

Like other overhead athletes, quarterbacks are at risk for shoulder injury. However, the spectrum of injury is unique and is more commonly related to trauma than to chronic overuse. Shoulder injuries are the second most common type of injury suffered by quarterbacks next to head injuries. The most common injury to the shoulder is AC joint separation, followed by shoulder contusions to the deltoid and the rotator cuff, traumatic dislocations, fractures, SC joint separations, and pectoralis major injuries. Chronic overuse type injuries represent less than 15% of the reported injuries and include rotator cuff tendonitis, cuff tears, impingement, and biceps tendonitis.

Kinematic and EMG analyses of the football throwing motion is important for understanding injury patterns and potential rehabilitation protocols. Four phases of the football throwing motion include early cocking, late cocking, acceleration, and follow-through (18). Muscle activation patterns during the football throw can be grouped into two categories. Group I muscles are stabilizer muscles. The supraspinatus and infraspinatus are high-level stabilizers; the deltoid muscles are moderate-level stabilizers; the biceps muscles are low-level stabilizers. Group II muscles are accelerator muscles (subscapularis, latissimus dorsi, and pectoralis major). The accelerator muscles have demonstrated persistently high activation levels during the follow-through phase, which suggests a secondary role in the prevention of joint distraction during the powerful deceleration forces across the shoulder. Muscle activity was greatest during the follow-through phase for all muscles except the anterior deltoid and the pectoralis major.

The observed shoulder muscle activation and throwing kinematics during the football throw have specific implications for the clinical patterns of injury documented through the NFLISS. First, the difference in the spectrum of injuries seen in the overhead football throw compared with the baseball pitch may be secondary to differences in firing patterns seen throughout the four phases of the throw. Overall lower levels of activation, as well as slower angular velocities and decreased extremes of the throwing motion, place the quarterback's shoulder at lower risk for chronic overuse types of injury compared with traumatic injury. Second, the maximal activation documented during the follow-through phase in all muscles tested suggests a potential mechanism of muscle injury as well as a period of high risk for shoulder injury during the football throw. Third, the rapid increase in accelerator muscle activation seen during the acceleration and follow-through phases suggests a potential etiology for pectoralis major injury, which has been observed in our clinical experience with this throwing population. The pectoralis major muscle may be predisposed to injury if an abduction and external rotation contact force is applied to the athlete's upper extremity during the latter two phases of the football throw. Fourth, that the biceps brachii has less than 50% activation of the other stabilizer muscles brings into question its functional role during the football throw as well as the etiology of the 3.5% incidence of biceps tendonitis seen in this population of professional athletes. Finally, the demonstration of two distinct patterns of muscle activation (stabilizers and accelerators) may have implications for changes in training and rehabilitation protocols. As future work incorporates joint kinematics and kinetics with EMG testing and as further analysis of injury patterns in both professional and amateur quarterbacks is performed, team physicians and trainers will gain further insight into the mechanism, prevention, and rehabilitation of quarterback-related shoulder injuries.

ACKNOWLEDGMENT

The authors gratefully acknowledge and appreciate the athletic trainers in the NFL for their dedication in maintaining the NFLISS for 22 years, without whom we would not have data for this chapter.

REFERENCES

1. Blevins FT, Hayes WM, Warren RF. Rotator cuff injury in contact athletes. *Am J Sports Med* 1996;24:263–267.
2. Hawkins RJ, Kennedy JC. Impingement syndrome in athletes. *Am J Sports Med* 1980;8:151–158.
3. Jobe FW, Jobe CM. Painful athletic injuries of the shoulder. *Clin Orthop Rel Res* 1983;173:117–124.
4. Tibone JE, Elrod B, Jobe FW, et al. Surgical treatment of tears

of the rotator cuff in athletes. *J Bone Joint Surg (Am)* 1986;68: 887–891.

5. Miller MD, Johnson DL, Fu FH, et al. Rupture of the pectoralis major muscle in a collegiate football player. Use of magnetic resonance imaging in early diagnosis. *Am J Sports Med* 1993;21:475–477.

6. Schepsis AA, Grafe MW, Jones HP, et al. Rupture of the pectoralis major muscle. Outcome after repair of acute and chronic injuries. *Am J Sports Med* 2000;28:9–15.

7. Fleisig GS, Escamilla RF, Andrews JR, et al. Kinematic and kinetic comparison between baseball pitching and football passing. *J Appl Biomech* 1996;12:207–224.

8. Rash GS, Shapiro R. A three-dimensional dynamic analysis of the quarterback's throwing motion in American football. *J Appl Biomech* 1995;11:443–459.

9. Wick H, Dillman CJ, Werner S. A kinematic comparison between baseball pitching and football passing. *Sports Med Update* 1991;6:13–16.

10. Meister K. Injuries to the shoulder in the throwing athlete. Part one: Biomechanics/pathophysiology/classification of injury. *Am J Sports Med* 2000;28:265–275.

11. Meister K. Injuries to the shoulder in the throwing athlete. Part two: evaluation/treatment. *Am J Sports Med* 2000;28: 587–601.

12. DiGiovine NM, Jobe FW, Pink M. An electromyographic analysis of the upper extremity in pitching. *J Shoulder Elbow Surg* 1992;1:15–25.

13. Dillman CJ, Fleisig GS, Andrews JR. Biomechanics of pitching with emphasis upon shoulder kinematics. *J Orthop Sports Phys Ther* 1993;18:402–408.

14. Gowan ID, Jobe FW, Tibone JE, et al. A comparative electromyographic analysis of the shoulder during pitching: professional versus amateur pitchers. *Am J Sports Med* 1987;15: 586–590.

15. Jobe FW, Moynes DR, Tibone JE, et al. An EMG analysis of the shoulder in pitching: a second report. *Am J Sports Med* 1984;12: 218–220.

16. Jobe FW, Tibone JE, Perry A, et al. An EMG analysis of the shoulder in throwing and pitching: a preliminary report. *Am J Sports Med* 1983;11:3–5.

17. Fleisig GS, Barrentine SW, Escamilla RF, et al. Biomechanics of overhand throwing with implications for injuries. *Sports Med* 1996;21: 421–437.

18. Kelly BT, Backus SI, Williams RJ, et al. Electromyographic analysis and phase definition of the overhead football throw. *Am J Sports Med* 2002;30:837–844.

19. Glousman R. Electromyographic analysis and its role in the athletic shoulder. *Clin Orthop Rel Res* 1993;288:27–34.

20. Ballantyne BT, O'Hare SJ, Paschall JL. Electromyographic activity of selected shoulder muscles in commonly used therapeutic exercises. *Phys Ther* 1993;73:668–682.

21. Clarys JP, Cabri J. Electromyography and the study of sports movement: a review. *J Sports Science* 1993;11:379–448.

22. Jobe FW, Moynes DR. Delineation of diagnostic criteria and a rehabilitation program for rotator cuff injuries. *Am J Sports Med* 1982;10:336–339.

23. Townsend H, Jobe FW, Pink M, et al. Electromyographic analysis of the glenohumeral muscles during a baseball rehabilitation program. *Am J Sports Med* 1991;19:264–272.

24. Maffet MW, Jobe FW, Pink MM, et al. Shoulder muscle firing patterns during the windmill softball pitch. *Am J Sports Med* 1997;25:369–374.

25. Wilk KE. Current concepts in the rehabilitation of athletic shoulder injuries. In: Andrews JR, ed. *The athlete's shoulder.* New York: Churchill Livingstone, 1994:335–354.

26. Hulstyn MJ, Fadale PD. Shoulder injuries in the athlete. *Clin Sports Med* 1997;16:663–679.

27. Ong BC, Sekiya JK, Rodosky MW. Shoulder injuries in the athlete. *Curr Opin Rheumatol* 2002;14:150–159.

28. Rockwood CA, Williams GR, Young DC. Disorders of the acromioclavicular joint. In: Rockwood CA, Matsen FA, eds. *The shoulder,* 2nd ed. Philadelphia: WB Saunders, 1998: 483–553.

29. VanFleet TA, Bach B Jr. Injuries to the acromioclavicular joint. Diagnosis and management. *Orthop Rev* 1994;23:123–129.

30. Woodward TW, Best TM. The painful shoulder: part II. Acute and chronic disorders. *Am Fam Phys* 2000;61:3291–3300.

31. Cook FF, Tibone JE. The Mumford procedure in athletes: an objective analysis of function. *Am J Sports Med* 1988;16: 97–100.

32. Powers JA, Bach PJ. Acromioclavicular separations. Closed or open treatment? *Clin Orthop* 1974;0:213–223.

33. Cox JS. Current method of treatment of acromioclavicular joint dislocations. *Orthopedics* 1992;15:1041–1044.

34. Lemos MJ. The evaluation and treatment of the injured acromioclavicular joint in athletes. *Am J Sports Med* 1998;26: 137–144.

35. McFarland EG, Blivin SJ, Doehring CB, et al. Treatment of grade III acromioclavicular separations in professional throwing athletes: results of a survey. *Am J Orthop* 1977;26:771–774.

36. Rawes ML, Dias JJ.: Long-term results of conservative treatment for acromioclavicular dislocation. *J Bone Joint Surg (Am)* 1996;78B:410–412.

37. Wojtys EM, Nelson G. Conservative treatment of Grade III acromioclavicular dislocations. *Clin Orthop* 1991:112–119.

38. Bannister GC, Wallace WA, Stableforth PG, et al. The management of acute acromioclavicular dislocation. A randomized prospective controlled trial. *J Bone Joint Surg (Br)* 1989;71: 848–850.

39. Cardone D, Brown JN, Roberts SN, et al. Grade III acromioclavicular joint injury in Australian Rules Football. *J Sci Med Sport* 2002;5:143–148.

40. Bradley JP, Tibone JE. Open treatment of complete acromioclavicular dislocations. *Oper Tech Sports Med* 1997;5:88–92.

41. Verhaven E, DeBoeck H, Haentjens P, et al. Surgical treatment of acute type-V acromioclavicular injuries in athletes. *Arch Orthop Trauma Surg* 1993;112:189–192.

42. Taft TN, Wilson FC, Oglesby JW. Dislocation of the acromioclavicular joint. An end-result study. *J Bone Joint Surg (Am)* 1987;69:1045–1051.

43. Medvecky MJ, Zuckerman JD. Sternoclavicular joint injuries and disorders. *Instr Course Lect* 2000;49:397–406.

44. Rockwood CA. Dislocations of the sternoclavicular joint. In Evans EB, ed. *American Academy of Orthopaedic Surgeons Instructional Course Lectures XXIV.* St. Louis: Mosby, 1975.

45. Rockwood CA, Wirth MA. Disorders of the sternoclavicular joint. In Rockwood CA, Matsen FA, eds. *The shoulder,* 2nd ed. Philadelphia: WB Saunders, 1998:555–601.

46. De Jong KP, Sukul DM. Anterior sternoclavicular dislocation: a long-term follow-up study. *J Orthop Trauma* 1990;4:420–423.

47. Jougon JB, Lepront DJ, Dromer CE. Posterior dislocation of the sternoclavicular joint leading to mediastinal compression. *Ann Thorac Surg* 1996;61:711–713.

48. Ono K, Inagawa H, Kiyota K, et al. Posterior dislocation of the sternoclavicular joint with obstruction of the innominate vein: case report. *J Trauma* 1998;44:381–383.

49. Yeh GL, Williams GR Jr. Conservative management of sternoclavicular injuries. *Orthop Clin North Am* 2000;31:189–203.

50. Marker LB, Klareskov B. Posterior sternoclavicular dislocation: an American football injury. *Br J Sports Med* 1996;30:71–72.

51. Perlmutter GS, Apruzzese W. Axillary nerve injuries in contact sports: recommendations for treatment and rehabilitation. *Sports Med* 1998;26:351–361.

52. Clancy WG, Brand RL, Bergfeld JA. Upper trunk brachial plexus injuries in contact sports. *Am J Sports Med* 1977;5: 209–216.

53. Perlmutter GS, Leffert RD, Zarins B. Direct injury to the axillary nerve in athletes playing contact sports. *Am J Sports Med* 1997;25:65–68.

54. Hawkins RJ, Morin WD, Bonutti PM. Surgical treatment of full-thickness rotator cuff tears in patients 40 years of age and younger. *Orthop Trans* 1993;17:1024.

55. Payne LZ, Altchek DW, Craig EV, et al. Arthroscopic treatment of partial rotator cuff tears in young athletes. A preliminary report. *Am J Sports Med* 1997;25:299–305.

56. Rathbun JB, MacNib I. The microvascular pattern of the rotator cuff. *J Bone Joint Surg (Br)* 1970;52:540–553.

57. Neer CS 2nd. Anterior acromioplasty for the chronic impingement syndrome in the shoulder: a preliminary report. *J Bone Joint Surg (Am)* 1972;54:41–50.

58. Neer CS 2nd. Impingement lesions. *Clin Orthop* 1983:70–77.

59. Edelson G, Teitz C. Internal impingement in the shoulder. *J Shoulder Elbow Surg* 2000;9:308–315.

60. McFarland EG, Hsu CY, Neira C, et al. Internal impingement of the shoulder: a clinical and arthroscopic analysis. *J Shoulder Elbow Surg* 1999;8:458–460.

61. Meister K. Internal impingement in the shoulder of the overhand athlete: pathophysiology, diagnosis, and treatment. *Am J Orthop* 2000;29:433–438.

62. Craig EV. Fractures of the clavicle. In: Rockwood CA, Matsen FA, eds. *The shoulder,* 2nd ed. Philadelphia: WB Saunders, 1998:428–465.

63. Neer CS 2nd. Displaced proximal humeral fractures. I. Classification and evaluation. *J Bone Joint Surg (Am)* 1970;52: 1077–1089.

64. Bigliani LU, Flatow EL, Pollock RG. Fractures of the proximal humerus. In: Rockwood CA, Matsen FA, eds. *The shoulder,* 2nd ed. Philadelphia: WB Saunders, 1998:337–374.

65. Owens S, Itamura JM. Differential diagnosis of shoulder injuries in sports. *Oper Tech Sports Med* 2000;8:253–257.

66. Hill JM, McGuire MH, Crosby LA. Closed treatment of displaced middle-third fractures of the clavicle gives poor results. *J Bone Joint Surg (Br)* 1997;79:537–539.

67. Lintner SA, Speer KP. Traumatic anterior glenohumeral instability: the role of arthroscopy. *J Am Acad Orthop Surg* 1997;5: 233–239.

68. Taylor DC, Arciero RA. Pathologic changes associated with shoulder dislocations. Arthroscopic and physical examination findings in first-time, traumatic anterior dislocations. *Am J Sports Med* 1997;25:306–311.

69. Bankart AS, Cantab MC. Recurrent or habitual dislocation of the shoulder-joint. *Clin Orthop* 1993:3–6.

70. Speer KP, Deng X, Borrero S, et al. Biomechanical evaluation of a simulated Bankart lesion. *J Bone Joint Surg (Am)* 1994;76: 1819–1826.

71. Neviaser TJ. The anterior labroligamentous periosteal sleeve avulsion lesion: a cause of anterior instability of the shoulder. *Arthroscopy* 1993;9:17–21.

72. Wolf EM, Cheng JC, Dickson K. Humeral avulsion of glenohumeral ligaments as a cause of anterior shoulder instability. *Arthroscopy* 1995;11:600–607.

73. Arciero RA, St. Pierre P. Acute shoulder dislocation. Indications and techniques for operative management. *Clin Sports Med* 1995;14:937–953.

74. Arciero RA, Taylor DC, Snyder RJ, et al. Arthroscopic bioab-

75. sorbable tack stabilization of initial anterior shoulder dislocations: a preliminary report. *Arthroscopy* 1995;11:410–417.

75. Arciero RA, Wheeler JH, Ryan JB, et al. Arthroscopic Bankart repair versus nonoperative treatment for acute, initial anterior shoulder dislocations. *Am J Sports Med* 1994;22:589–594.

76. Bottoni CR, Wilckens JH, DeBerardino TM, et al. A prospective, randomized evaluation of arthroscopic stabilization versus nonoperative treatment in patients with acute, traumatic, first-time shoulder dislocations. *Am J Sports Med* 2002;30:576–580.

77. DeBerardino TM, Arciero RA, Taylor DC. Arthroscopic stabilization of acute initial anterior shoulder dislocation: the West Point experience. *J South Orthop Assoc* 1996;5:263–271.

78. DeBerardino TM, Arciero RA, Taylor DC, et al. Prospective evaluation of arthroscopic stabilization of acute, initial anterior shoulder dislocations in young athletes. Two- to five-year follow-up. *Am J Sports Med* 2001;29:586–592.

79. Hovelius L. The natural history of primary anterior dislocation of the shoulder in the young. *J Orthop Sci* 1999;4:307–317.

80. Hoelen MA, Burgers AM, Rozing PM. Prognosis of primary anterior shoulder dislocation in young adults. *Arch Orthop Trauma Surg* 1990;110:51–54.

81. Hovelius L. Anterior dislocation of the shoulder in teen-agers and young adults. Five-year prognosis. *J Bone Joint Surg (Am)* 1987;69:393–399.

82. Hovelius L, Augustini BG, Fredin H, et al. Primary anterior dislocation of the shoulder in young patients. A ten-year prospective study. *J Bone Joint Surg (Am)* 1996;78:1677–1684.

83. O'Neill DB. Arthroscopic Bankart repair of anterior detachments of the glenoid labrum. A prospective study. *J Bone Joint Surg (Am)* 1999;81:1357–1366.

84. Wheeler JH, Ryan JB, Arciero RA, et al. Arthroscopic versus nonoperative treatment of acute shoulder dislocations in young athletes. *Arthroscopy* 1989;5:213–217.

85. Pagnani MJ, Dome DC. Surgical treatment of traumatic anterior shoulder instability in American football players. *J Bone Joint Surg (Am)* 2002;84:711—715.

86. Uhorchak JM, Arciero RA, Huggard D, et al. Recurrent shoulder instability after open reconstruction in athletes involved in collision and contact sports. *Am J Sports Med* 2000;28: 794–799.

87. Kirkley A, Griffin S, Richards C, et al. Prospective randomized clinical trial comparing the effectiveness of immediate arthroscopic stabilization versus immobilization and rehabilitation in first traumatic anterior dislocations of the shoulder. *Arthroscopy* 1999;15:507–514.

88. Cole BJ, L'Insalata J, Irrgang J, et al. Comparison of arthroscopic and open anterior shoulder stabilization. A two to six-year follow-up study. *J Bone Joint Surg (Am)* 2000;82: 1108–1114.

89. Cole BJ, Warner JJ. Arthroscopic versus open Bankart repair for traumatic anterior shoulder instability. *Clin Sports Med* 2000; 19:19–48.

90. Speer KP, Warren RF, Pagnani M, et al. An arthroscopic technique for anterior stabilization of the shoulder with a bioabsorbable tack. *J Bone Joint Surg (Am)* 1996;78:1801–1807.

91. Richards RR, Bigliani L, Gartsman GM, et al. A standardized method for the assessment of shoulder function. *J Shoulder Elbow Surg* 1994;3:347–352.

92. Rowe CR, Zarins B. Recurrent transient subluxation of the shoulder. *J Bone Joint Surg (Am)* 1981;63:863–872.

93. Yoneda M, Hayashida K, Wakitani S, et al. Bankart procedure augmented by coracoid transfer for contact athletes with traumatic anterior shoulder instability. *Am J Sports Med* 1999;27: 21–26.

94. Hawkins RJ, Koppert G, Johnston G. Recurrent posterior

instability (subluxation) of the shoulder. *J Bone Joint Surg (Am)* 1984;66:169–174.

95. Fuchs B, Jost B, Gerber C. Posterior-inferior capsular shift for the treatment of recurrent, voluntary posterior subluxation of the shoulder. *J Bone Joint Surg (Am)* 2000;82:16–25.

96. Blasier RB, Soslowsky LJ, Malicky DM, et al. Posterior glenohumeral subluxation: active and passive stabilization in a biomechanical model. *J Bone Joint Surg (Am)* 1997;79:433–440.

97. O'Brien SJ, Neves MC, Arnoczky SP, et al. The anatomy and histology of the inferior glenohumeral ligament complex of the shoulder. *Am J Sports Med* 1990;18:449–456.

98. O'Brien SJ, Schwartz RS, Warren RF, et al. Capsular restraints to anterior-posterior motion of the abducted shoulder: a biomechanical study. *J Shoulder Elbow Surg* 1995;4:298–308.

99. Terry GC, Hammon D, France P, et al. The stabilizing function of passive shoulder restraints. *Am J Sports Med* 1991;19:26–34.

100. Weber SC, Caspari RB. A biochemical evaluation of the restraints to posterior shoulder dislocation. *Arthroscopy* 1989;5:115–121.

101. Warner JJ, Micheli LJ, Arslanian LE, et al. Patterns of flexibility, laxity, and strength in normal shoulders and shoulders with instability and impingement. *Am J Sports Med* 1990;18:366–375.

102. Mair SD, Zarzour RH, Speer KP. Posterior labral injury in contact athletes. *Am J Sports Med* 1998;26:753–758.

103. Weinberg J, McFarland EG. Posterior capsular avulsion in a college football player. *Am J Sports Med* 1999;27:235–237.

104. Davidson PA, Rivenburgh DW. The 7-o'clock posteroinferior portal for shoulder arthroscopy. *Am J Sports Med* 2002;30:693–696.

105. DiFelice GS, Williams RJ 3rd, Cohen MS, et al. The accessory posterior portal for shoulder arthroscopy: description of technique and cadaveric study. *Arthroscopy* 2001;17:888–891.

106. Kretzler HH Jr, Richardson AB. Rupture of the pectoralis major muscle. *Am J Sports Med* 1989;17:453–458.

107. Orava S, Sorasto A, Aalto K, et al. Total rupture of pectoralis major muscle in athletes. *Int J Sports Med* 1984;5:272–274.

108. Roi GS, Respizzi S, Dworzak F. Partial rupture of the pectoralis major muscle in athletes. *Int J Sports Med* 1990;11:85–87.

109. Zeman SC, Rosenfeld RT, Lipscomb PR. Tears of the pectoralis major muscle. *Am J Sports Med* 1979;7:343–347.

110. Goriganti MR, Bodack MP, Nagler W. Pectoralis major rupture during gait training: case report. *Arch Phys Med Rehabil* 1999;80:115–117.

111. Anbari A, Kelly JD, Moyer RA. Delayed repair of a ruptured pectoralis major muscle. A case report. *Am J Sports Med* 2000;28:254–256.

112. Connell DA, Potter HG, Sherman MF, et al. Injuries of the pectoralis major muscle: evaluation with MR imaging. *Radiology* 1999;210:785–791.

113. Levy AS, Kelly BT, Lintner SA, et al. Function of the long head of the biceps at the shoulder: electromyographic analysis. *J Shoulder Elbow Surg* 2001;10:250–255.

114. Yamaguchi K, Riew KD, Galatz LM, et al. Biceps activity during shoulder motion: an electromyographic analysis. *Clin Orthop Rel Res* 1997:122–129.

115. Healey JH, Barton S, Noble P, et al. Biomechanical evaluation of the origin of the long head of the biceps tendon. *Arthroscopy* 2001;17:378–382.

116. Itoi E, Kuechle DK, Newman SR, et al. Stabilizing function of the biceps in stable and unstable shoulders. *J Bone Joint Surg (Br)* 1993;75:546–550.

117. Kumar VP, Satku K, Balasubramaniam P. The role of the long head of biceps brachii in the stabilization of the head of the humerus. *Clin Orthop* 1989:172–175.

118. Pagnani MJ, Deng XH, Warren RF, et al. Role of the long head of the biceps brachii in glenohumeral stability: a biomechanical study in cadavera. *J Shoulder Elbow Surg* 1996;5:255–262.

119. Warner JJ, McMahon PJ. The role of the long head of the biceps brachii in superior stability of the glenohumeral joint. *J Bone Joint Surg (Am)* 1995;77:366–372.

120. Eakin CL, Faber KJ, Hawkins RJ, et al. Biceps tendon disorders in athletes. *J Am Acad Orthop Surg* 1999;7:300–310.

121. Sethi N, Wright R, Yamaguchi K. Disorders of the long head of the biceps tendon. *J Shoulder Elbow Surg* 1999;8:644–654.

122. Yergason RM. Supination sign. *J Bone Joint Surg (Am)* 1931;13:160.

123. Gerber C, Krushell RJ. Isolated rupture of the tendon of the subscapularis muscle. Clinical features in 16 cases. *J Bone Joint Surg (Br)* 1991;73:389–394.

23

TENNIS

DAVID W. ALTCHEK
DANIEL E. WEILAND

HISTORICAL OVERVIEW

The tennis athlete is exposed to repetitive overhead activity and is predisposed to overuse injuries about the shoulder (Fig. 23-1). Twenty-four percent of tennis players between 12 and 19 years of age complain of shoulder pain; among middle-aged players, the incidence of shoulder pain increases to 50% (1). In the tennis player, the shoulder girdle is susceptible to injury because it is responsible for both rapidly accelerating and decelerating the upper extremity while both controlling arm rotation and providing a stable scapular platform to enable the player to have precise control of the racquet for effective ball striking. The weight of the tennis racquet creates a lever arm that adds power to the tennis stroke, but it also increases stresses around the shoulder. The tennis player must be able to harness the high forces required at ball strike while maintaining control and shoulder stability. Although shoulder injuries in the tennis athlete are fairly common, most are easily reversible. Decreasing playing time and carefully prescribed rehabilitation exercises can alleviate most injuries and return tennis athletes of all abilities to their previous levels of play. However, if neglected, certain tendon and ligamentous injuries that initially present as benign can become complex.

Shoulder injuries can develop from muscle fatigue, eccentric overload, instability, and secondary impingement. Repetitive microtrauma initially causes inflammation and tendonitis, which leads to tissue breakdown and progression of altered shoulder mechanics. Because tennis is a highly repetitive sport requiring extensive practice and playing time, minor injuries can become exacerbated by a change in stroke production by a tennis athlete in order to compensate and play through pain and or injury. Eventually, these maladaptions diminish a player's ability and worsen the original injury. Maladaption is more common in tennis than in other overhead sports such as volleyball or baseball. For one reason, tennis is an individual sport, and for professional athletes, increased injury time directly affects monetary compensation. A second reason lies in the nature of the game of tennis. An experienced player who has sustained a shoulder injury may alter stroke mechanics or even match strategy to compensate for certain deficiencies. Maladaption allows the player to continue to participate, but decreases maximal performance level and eventually exacerbates the original injury.

Areas of injury to the shoulder in the tennis player include soft tissue structures such as ligaments, tendons, and capsulolabral complexes, as well as bone and articular cartilage. Location and severity of injury is most often dependent on player age, but can be related to skill level. Tennis is a sport with an age range of players that spans from adolescents to senior citizens; it is important to consider the age of the patient when developing the diagnosis and comprehensive plan for treatment. This chapter identifies common shoulder injuries specific to the tennis athlete and details critically important nonoperative, as well as operative measures necessary for the care of these patients.

ANATOMY AND BIOMECHANICS

The glenohumeral joint is a ball and plate construct requiring both static and dynamic stabilizers. The static components consist of the bony architecture of the humeral head and the glenoid, along with the labrum and the glenohumeral ligaments. The congruent surfaces of the humeral head in contact with the glenoid and labrum create a suction effect that increases the stability of the shoulder. This glenohumeral stability is maximized with anatomic positioning. The dynamic stabilizers consist of the rotator cuff muscles and the deltoid and the periscapular musculature. The rotator cuff is a four-muscle tendon complex that works to stabilize the humeral head in the glenoid fossa. The largest segment, the subscapularis, is innervated by the subscapular nerves and inserts on the lesser tuberosity. The supraspinatus, infraspinatus, and teres minor assist in arm elevation and externally rotate the humerus. The rotator cuff muscles center the humeral head on the glenoid during motion. Fatigue of this complex network results in loss of normal concavity compression. The resultant increased

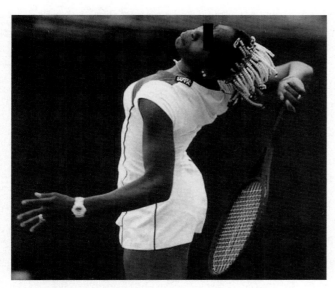

FIGURE 23-1. The five stages of a tennis serve. Stage 1: preparation. Stage 2: early cocking. Stage 3: late cocking. Stage 4: acceleration. Stage 5: follow-through. (From Morris M, Jobe FW, et al. Electromyographic analysis of elbow function in tennis players. *Am J Sports Med* 1989;17:241–247, with permission.)

translation of the humeral head on the glenoid can lead to plastic deformation of the static stabilizers.

The elite tennis player generates exceptional forces and rotational velocities around the shoulder during play. Ball speed during overhead serve routinely travels between 100 and 120 miles per hour (mph). Rotational velocities as fast as 1,500 degrees/second are achieved in the overhead serve, and 895 and 387 degrees/second have been demonstrated in the backhand and forehand, respectively (2). As a result of these shoulder velocities, hand speed at ball impact has been measured at 47 mph during service, 33 mph during backhand, and 37 mph during forehand strokes (2). Although one does not expect most recreational players to generate such high velocities, the short duration and high intensity forces that must continually be generated from a near static position create extreme stresses across the shoulder joint. As in most sports, the increase in efficiency of force transfer leads to increased performance. Ineffective stabilization of scapulothoracic motion or the glenohumeral joint at ball strike results in compromised efficiency, muscle fatigue, and increased mechanical stresses on the shoulder.

Understanding the mechanics of the common tennis strokes can be helpful in identifying pathology and developing a treatment program. The tennis serve can be broken down into four stages: (a) wind-up, (b) cocking, (c) acceleration, and (d) deceleration/follow-through (3). During the cocking phase of the serve, the subscapularis helps accelerate the arm in internal rotation and adds anterior stability to the humeral head. At overhead ball strike, stability is largely dependent on the labrum and the capsular liga-

ments. These static stabilizers are at most risk for injury during periods of muscle fatigue and decreased efficiency. During the deceleration phase, stress is then transferred to the supraspinatus. The ground strokes in tennis consist of both the forehand and the backhand. They are the strokes most commonly used and are less likely to directly cause overhead injury, but they do contribute to periscapular muscle fatigue. The ground strokes can be broken down into three phases: (a) racquet preparation, (b) acceleration, and (c) follow-through (4). Studies using electromyographic (EMG) activity have correlated muscle activation with each stage. During the serve and the forehand, the subscapularis, the pectoralis major, and the serratus anterior demonstrate the greatest muscle activation. The backhand uses mostly middle deltoid, supraspinatus, and infraspinatus muscles (4).

During a tennis match, or even a practice, several repetitive motions are performed, each requiring synchronous firing of muscle activity. Multiple force couples constrain glenohumeral translation. An example of a force couple routinely used is between the deltoid, a continual humeral head elevator, working in conjunction with the supraspinatus and the infraspinatus, which are humeral head compressors. Asynchronous firing of injured or fatigued muscles can result in either humeral head elevation or scapular winging evidenced by poor retraction and protraction. The trapezius, serratus anterior, rhomboids, and levator scapularis are all subject to eccentric overload failure. Once the dynamic musculotendinous constraints of the shoulder lose effectiveness, the ligamentous constraints become the primary restraints to excessive humeral head translation.

COMMON TENNIS INJURIES

In the adult tennis player, shoulder injury can occur in a variety of anatomic locations. Although the tennis athlete may present with multiple injuries, the most common injuries are presented here.

Rotator Cuff Injuries

Most tennis injuries are secondary to overuse and result from eccentric loading of the rotator cuff muscles. Fatigue and weakness of the rotator cuff musculature from overhead activity allows the humeral head to migrate superiorly due to the pull of the deltoid muscle. Subtle joint laxity can cause internal impingement, which is a result of the posterosuperior glenoid rubbing on the undersurface of the rotator cuff muscles (Fig. 23-2). Subacromial impingement is the result of the greater tuberosity rubbing the undersurface of the anterolateral acromion. Impingement may present as a broad spectrum of disease that ranges from cuff tendinopathy to massive rotator cuff tears. Tears of the sub-

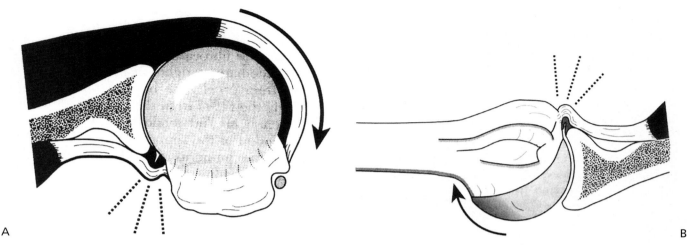

FIGURE 23-2. Illustration of internal impingement showing posterior **(A)** and superior **(B)** glenoid rubbing on the undersurface of the rotator cuff.

scapularis during tennis have been reported, but they rarely occur from repetitive microtrauma. The usual cause of subscapularis tear is a high energy trauma in a position of humeral external rotation.

Acromioclavicular Joint

Acromioclavicular (AC) joint arthritis may also accompany impingement syndrome and can produce severe symptoms in the tennis player during backhand shots, which require arm adduction across the body. Isolated AC joint arthritis may also present as a result of previous trauma.

Instability

Shoulder instability in the adult tennis player is a pathologic increase in glenohumeral translation after injury, either a single traumatic event or repetitive microtrauma. Multidirectional instability (MDI) is not usually caused by a single traumatic episode and can be associated with generalized laxity. An athlete with MDI frequently complains of unilateral instability, but may demonstrate bilateral shoulder laxity. MDI may be related to an imbalance in the dynamic stabilizers of the shoulder. Unidirectional instability usually follows a single traumatic episode. Instability most often behaves in either the anterior or posterior direction (most often anterior) and is commonly associated with a Bankart lesion. The acceleration phase of the serve is typically symptomatic in patients with anterior instability, whereas the follow-through phase is symptomatic in patients with posterior instability. Subtle instability is a form of instability that is seen more commonly in tennis players. Often there is no history of trauma and the injury presents as internal impingement, which describes the collision of the posterior superior labrum with the posterior rotator cuff. Internal impingement is typically present when

a player experiences repeated pain during the cocking phase of the serve.

Suprascapular Neuropathy

Compression neuropathy of the suprascapular nerve resulting in paralysis of the infraspinatus muscle is a rare, but well described clinical entity in the overhead athlete that can result in posterior shoulder pain and localized wasting of the infraspinatus muscle. Suprascapular nerve injuries can result from traction injuries at the level of the transverse scapular ligament or the spinoglenoid ligament. The resulting muscle paralysis caused by injury to the suprascapular nerve is dependent upon the location of injury as the nerve travels from proximal to distal. Injuries occurring at or proximal to the suprascapular notch causes paralysis of both the supraspinatus and infraspinatus muscles, whereas more distal lesions in the spinoglenoid notch only affect the infraspinatus. Another mechanism of injury is compression of the suprascapular nerve by ganglion cysts, which act as space-occupying lesions occurring in the vicinity of the suprascapular notch (5). Although their cause is not known, ganglia may be associated with labral tears. Most commonly, suprascapular nerve paralysis is caused by isolated injury to the inferior branch of the suprascapular nerve as it courses laterally and inferiorly around the spinoglenoid notch.

PRESENTATION AND PHYSICAL EXAMINATION

Successful treatment of shoulder problems in any athlete is dependent on accurate diagnosis, the first step in either developing an appropriate rehabilitation program or planning a reparative surgical procedure. Most tennis players with shoulder injuries present with pain. After obtaining a detailed history, the physical examination should begin with inspection of the standing patient. Both shoulders should be evaluated for scapular asymmetry and muscular atrophy. Depression of the dominant shoulder with the appearance of scoliosis is a posture frequently seen in tennis players and has been termed *tennis shoulder* (6). Tennis shoulder, however, has not yet been correlated with any specific injury. Elite tennis players may also present with atrophy of the biceps and triceps, with hypertrophy of the forearm musculature (1).

Systematic palpation of the cervical spine, shoulder, and upper extremity should follow inspection. The authors recommend beginning with the cervical spine and finishing with the fingertips. It is essential to evaluate range of motion of the cervical spine as well as assess for radiculopathy or myelopathy. A thorough examination includes palpation of the sternoclavicular joint, the clavicle, the AC joint, and the scapula. Shrugging of the scapula is due to weakness of the periscapular stabilizers. This may also be evidenced by a loss of protraction, retraction, or scapular winging (Fig. 23-3). If AC joint tenderness is present, the examiner should assess for tenderness with the arm adducted in a horizontal position. This helps maximize the pressure on the AC joint and exacerbates any potential symptoms (7). The presence of AC joint tenderness could also suggest a possible os acromiale, an unfused acromial epiphysis, and follow-up radiographic studies are needed for corroboration. Depending on the associated pathology, tenderness may be elicited from the long head of the biceps, the deltoid insertion, or the greater tuberosity. Speed's and Yergason's tests can be used to evaluate the biceps as a potential cause of pain. Speed's test is performed by having the patient attempt flexion of the arm with the elbow flexed at 30 degrees and the forearm held in supination. The test is positive if it elicits pain in the bicipital groove. Yergason's test is considered positive if pain is elicited by resisted supination of the forearm with the elbow flexed.

Both active and passive range of motion in all planes should be evaluated in both shoulders. Studies have shown decreased internal rotation in the dominant shoulder of elite tennis players (8,9) (Fig. 23-4). Loss of dominant shoulder internal rotation has been associated with both age and years of play (9). It has been postulated that decreased range of motion can be corrected with vigorous stretching exercises to avoid injury from altered stroke mechanics. The remainder of the examination should test motor function of all muscle groups, dermatomal sensation, and vascular status of both upper extremities. Positive physical findings should be noted and the examination can be focused accordingly.

Patients with rotator cuff injuries can present with shoulder pain of varying locations, depending on the location of tendon injury. Appropriate impingement tests should be performed whenever suspecting rotator cuff pathology. As a general rule, anterior shoulder pain is usually elicited from an injury to the subscapularis or the anterior supraspinatus. Lateral pain is usually caused by injury to the supraspinatus and anterior infraspinatus, and posterior pain can be referred to the infraspinatus and teres minor. Players with rotator cuff pathology often complain of intermittent shoulder pain that is exacerbated with overhead activity. Ground strokes in these patients are usually not painful. In cases of cuff tendinopathy, shoulder pain occasionally improves with moderate use, but always worsens with excessive or vigorous play. Symptomatic shoulders with rotator cuff injuries demonstrate limited internal rotation and patients can complain of weakness or clicking in the shoulder. Weakness is noted particularly during backhand or backhand volley, and is even more pronounced in players who use a one-handed backhand. In tennis players younger than age 30 years, rotator cuff injuries are often found in conjunction with tears of either the capsular ligaments or labrum. Radiographs are almost always normal in these patients and suspected injuries can be confirmed with magnetic resonance imaging (MRI).

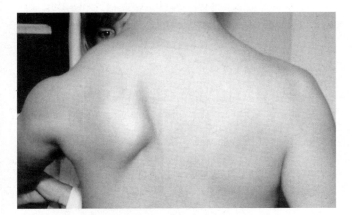

FIGURE 23-3. Photo demonstrating scapular winging resulting from periscapular muscle weakness.

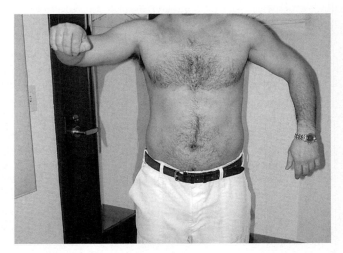

FIGURE 23-4. Photo of patient demonstrating loss of dominant arm internal rotation.

ROTATOR CUFF INJURIES

Rotator cuff injuries are defined as primary or secondary based on the presence of glenohumeral instability and as tensile or compressive based on the mechanism of failure of the cuff fibers (31). Primary tensile cuff disease (PTCD) results from the large repetitive loads placed on the rotator cuff as it acts to decelerate the shoulder during the deceleration phase of the throwing motion in a stable shoulder. This injury is manifested as a partial undersurface tear of the supraspinatus or infraspinatus. Primary compressive cuff disease (PCCD) is found on the bursal surface of the rotator cuff in throwers with stable shoulders. This process occurs secondary to the inability of the rotator cuff to produce sufficient adduction torques and inferior forces during the deceleration phase of throwing motion. Processes that decrease the subacromial space such as acromial spurs, os acromiale, coracoacromial ligament hypertrophy, or acromioclavicular joint hypertrophy increase the risk for PCCD. Poor scapulothoracic coordination leading to an improperly positioned glenoid during the throwing motion may also contribute to PCCD.

Baseball players with secondary tensile cuff disease (STCD) and secondary compressive cuff disease (SCCD) have underlying glenohumeral instability. This instability places increased demands on the rotator cuff because it must function not only to decelerate the arm following ball release but also to stabilize the glenohumeral joint against the anterior force, which can equal body weight, that produces anterior translation of the humeral head on the glenoid. The underlying cuff pathology seen in STCD is similar to that in PTCD with partial thickness tearing of the infraspinatus and supraspinatus. Patients with SCCD may exhibit either bursal or articular surface cuff injury. The site of injury to the cuff in SCCD depends on whether the abnormal glenohumeral translation leads to impingement of the rotator cuff against the coracoacromial arch, producing bursal cuff injuries, referred to as *external impingement*, or impingement of the cuff against the posterosuperior glenoid, producing articular cuff injuries, referred to as *internal impingement*.

Since first described by Walch and colleagues (32), internal impingement has been found to be a common cause of disability in the overhead athlete. Although Walch and colleagues did not find any instability in their initial subset of patients, it appears that, in baseball players, excessive anterior translation of the glenohumeral joint, coupled with excessive external rotation seen in these athletes, predisposes the rotator cuff to impingement against the glenoid labrum (33). As the shoulder reaches maximal external rotation in the cocking phase and the humeral head subluxes anteriorly on the glenoid with occult instability, the posterior cuff contacts the posterior glenoid labrum. This may produce a partial thickness tear over time. It is important that the underlying laxity of the glenohumeral joint be addressed at the time of treatment for an internal impingement lesion in order to prevent recurrence of the lesion.

Treatment of most rotator cuff injuries in baseball players begins with a period of active rest and rehabilitation. Because overuse and fatigue are the primary causes of most rotator cuff injuries, it is important to give these tissues time to heal and resolve the inflammatory stage. Once the inflammatory stage has resolved, a structured rehabilitation program specifically designed for overhead athletes is begun. This program is focused on improving the strength of the rotator cuff muscles and the coordination of the shoulder girdle. After this period of active rest and shoulder-specific rehabilitation, an interval throwing program is begun to allow the thrower to phase into full throwing activities over a period of time. Only if the athlete fails this nonoperative treatment protocol is surgery considered. We often consider surgery only after an athlete continues to have symptoms consistent with rotator cuff disease despite 3 months of active rest and shoulder-specific rehabilitation.

The surgical treatment of the rotator cuff in baseball players is dictated by the underlying cause of the rotator cuff injury. Primary compressive disease is a common source of symptoms in older patients; however, it is an uncommon cause of rotator cuff injuries in young overhead athletes and is commonly misdiagnosed (32,34). Before diagnosing PCCD in an athlete, the examiner must make certain that no underlying instability exists in the affected shoulder that must be addressed at the time of surgery. If PCCD is diagnosed, the surgical treatment is an arthroscopic subacromial decompression. For PTCD, the surgical treatment is an arthroscopic debridement of the partial thickness rotator cuff tear. This is followed by a prolonged period of rehabilitation of up to 6 months. For both secondary tensile and compressive cuff diseases, the underlying instability must be addressed at the time of surgery. We address this instability with thermal capsulorrhaphy. For articular surface SCCD (internal impingement) or STCD, we perform an arthroscopic debridement of the partial thickness rotator cuff tear followed by a thermal capsular shrinkage. It is important to know that return to competition following arthroscopic debridement of a partial thickness rotator cuff tear coupled with thermal capsulorrhaphy takes approximately 8 months.

We recently reviewed our results of surgical debridement of partial thickness rotator cuff tears consistent with internal impingement lesions in a population restricted to baseball players to determine whether TACS would improve the results of arthroscopic treatment of this injury (33). Our results showed that, at 24 months after surgery, 64% of those patients treated without TACS were still competing compared with 93% of those treated with TACS. Thus, the addition of TACS improved results of treatment of internal impingement lesions by approximately 25%.

A specific question that arises when addressing partial thickness rotator cuff tears is when to "take down" the par-

Tennis players with posterior pain in the region of the scapula should be inspected visually. Isolated atrophy of the infraspinatus muscle usually represents a suprascapular neuropathy. With a traction injury, pain usually subsides over a 2- to 3-week period, but weakness and atrophy may progress. Suspected injuries of the suprascapular nerve should be evaluated with an MRI scan to rule out compressive lesions such as ganglion cysts.

Tennis athletes with instability most often present with pain in the afflicted shoulder, but pain may also be associated with weakness, description of a "dead arm," or even frank instability with a history of multiple dislocations. It is essential to obtain a complete history and physical examination to determine which activities or motions produce symptoms. During the acceleration phase of the serve, the anterior capsule and the subscapularis are stressed with significant tension and can cause symptoms in patients with anterior instability. As the service motion continues, energy is transferred to the posterior shoulder structures during follow-through. Patients with posterior instability or posterior labral tears complain of instability only elicited during follow-through. As previously described, internal impingement produces pain during the maximal cocking phase of the serve or overhead volley.

When evaluating any patient with instability, it is important to document any evidence of generalized laxity. The patient should be evaluated for elbow and metacarpophalangeal (MCP) joint hyperextension as well as thumb to forearm distance. Although laxity does not always equate with instability, shoulder laxity should be evaluated in three planes and two positions. Glenohumeral translation can be documented with manual testing in the inferior, anterior, and posterior directions. Inferior laxity is measured pulling downward traction on the humerus when it is adducted. The inferior displacement of the humeral head is reflected by the size of the "sulcus" that can be visualized below the lateral margin of the acromion (Fig. 23-5). An abnormally large sulcus is one that is greater than 2 cm. Anterior and posterior displacement is described by the position of the humeral head relative to the glenoid: 1+ to the glenoid rim, 2+ over the glenoid rim but spontaneously reduces when the applied force is withdrawn, and 3+ completely dislocated with locking over the glenoid rim. Anterior and posterior displacement should then be tested more precisely in two functional positions: (a) with the humerus adducted and (b) at 90 degrees of abduction. Anterior and posterior testing is easier to perform when the patient is lying supine. With the patient in this position, the apprehension test can be performed by abducting and externally rotating the humerus while placing an anteriorly direct force on the humeral head. A positive test reproduces the pain and sensation of impending dislocation with anterior instability. The relocation test is positive when apprehension is relieved and greater external rotation is achievable with a posteriorly directed force on the humeral head. The relocation maneu-

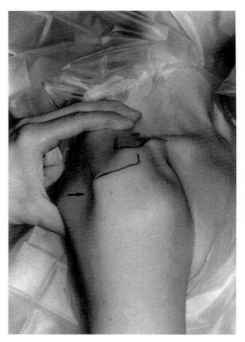

FIGURE 23-5. Physical examination demonstrating a sulcus sign.

ver can also test for subtle anterior instability and internal impingement, which is likely present if posterior joint line pain is relieved (10).

RADIOGRAPHIC AND DIAGNOSTIC EVALUATION

Routine radiographic evaluation of a tennis player with shoulder pain should include standard anteroposterior (AP) and lateral views of the scapula, and an axillary view. Further radiographic studies can then be ordered when clinically indicated. In patients with impingement and rotator cuff symptoms, a 30-degree caudal tilt view and a supraspinatus outlet view can both be effective for visualizing subacromial spurs. If a Bankart lesion is suspected in an athlete with instability, a West Point view allows visualization of the anteroinferior glenoid rim. MRI has rapidly evolved into a powerful adjunct in the evaluation of soft tissues and cartilage, and can illustrate capsular ligament, labral, and rotator cuff tears that cannot be visualized on plain film radiography. Occasionally, gadolinium contrast may be used to enhance labral pathology.

NONOPERATIVE TREATMENT, REHABILITATION, AND RESULTS

Most tennis players with shoulder dysfunction have some form of overuse injury and present to the sports physician with complaints of pain. Injuries in tennis athletes typically progress from a loss of internal rotation with obligate anterosuperior migration of the humeral head. Continuing play under these conditions can easily cause instability, subacromial impingement, or labral tears to develop. After early diagnosis, the cornerstone of treatment is rehabilitation exercises, with the goal being a quick return to pain-free function and maximal peak performance. Tennis players who are asymptomatic can increase their level of play as well as prevent injury by adopting modified rehabilitation programs. The initial goal in the treatment of any overuse injury is to alleviate pain and inflammation by eliminating stress and protecting the extremity. Occasionally, complete cessation of overhead activity may be required, but players should continue concurrent core strengthening and cardiovascular conditioning. After the acute phase of injury turns quiescent, the first step in recovery is to restore functional range of motion. In the shoulder, functional motion is in or anterior to the scapular plane. Motion in the coronal plane should be avoided because it is not functional and may increase stresses on rotator cuff musculature and exacerbate symptoms of impingement.

After full passive and active range of motion has been restored, submaximal resistive exercises for the rotator cuff and periscapular muscles can be initiated. Periscapular muscle strengthening is essential in obtaining a stable platform at the shoulder. Exercises using short lever arms are recommended early. Concurrent core strength and cardiovascular fitness exercises should be maintained. A successful tennis shot requires concentric contraction from the larger lower extremity and torso muscles to be coordinated with eccentric control of the shoulder musculature. Shoulder shrugs are effective in conditioning the trapezius muscle, and wide grip seated rows help strengthen the rhomboids, levator scapulae, and serratus anterior muscles. Wide grip pull-downs are excellent strengthening exercises for the biceps brachii and latissimus dorsi, which help protect the shoulder.

The next step in shoulder rehabilitation involves gaining eccentric control of the rotator cuff muscles. The force couple of the compressive and caudal force role of the rotator cuff opposing the superior force of the deltoid muscle predicates the importance of rotator cuff strengthening in shoulder rehabilitation. Differential patterns of rotator cuff muscles showing high relative activation on EMG analysis have helped the authors develop recommendations for specific exercises helpful for rotator cuff strengthening (11,12). Elevation of the humerus with thumbs pointed down in the scapular plane, side lying external rotation, and prone extension and abduction exercises with the thumb pointed up should be initiated with low resistance and high repetition. Exercises that exacerbate shoulder pain should be discontinued. Rehabilitation can then proceed to tennis-specific actions that can be individualized to the athletes need. Initially, overhead exercises should be performed under close supervision with a keen focus on proper mechanics.

In any sport, developing and adhering to an appropriate warm-up and stretching routine are essential. For elite tennis players to stay competitive, flexibility is necessary and helps decrease the incidence of injury. Elite tennis players are often limited in internal rotation and frequently demonstrate tight posterior capsule structures (8,9). Stretch programs designed for the tennis athlete focus on maintaining posterior shoulder flexibility (13). Stressing cross-arm adduction and full internal rotation is effective for posterior capsule stretching. To isolate the posterior inferior capsule, elevate the arm overhead with the elbow flexed, pulling the arm behind the head. This maneuver simulates the overhead smash. Care should be taken when prescribing a flexibility program to avoid some stretches that can be counterproductive. Stretching the arm in abduction and external rotation might exacerbate symptoms when excess external rotation or anterior instability is already present.

In tennis athletes with rotator cuff injuries, treatment depends on the extent of the injury as well as the activity and age of the athlete. Initially, antiinflammatory medication, ice, and a reduction of overhead activity reduce pain. Muscular rehabilitation should focus initially on strengthening the scapular stabilizers, which could exhibit significant weakness even before injury as a result of guarding. Direct strengthening of the rotator cuff begins always with light resistance and should not be painful. Specific exercises for the rotator cuff can gradually increase in intensity. The athlete should be informed that timeframe for maximal rehabilitation is variable, but usually falls between 3 and 6 months.

Nonoperative treatment of instability in the tennis player can be variable in its effectiveness. Instability is a spectrum of disease, and depending on the extent of the injury, operative treatment may be the only solution. In most tennis players, however, instability is due to repetitive trauma and responds to more conservative treatments. The foundation of rehabilitation involves shoulder girdle strengthening and the development of proprioception to allow for compensation and protection of the soft tissue injury by sharing forces dissipated by the shoulder. This process can be quite extensive, requiring time and patient compliance in conjunction with a skilled physical therapist. Patients who fail to improve with shoulder girdle and rotator cuff strengthening are candidates for surgical repair of the capsulolabral complex.

OPERATIVE TREATMENT, REHABILITATION, AND RESULTS

Surgical treatment of shoulder injuries in tennis players is reserved for athletes who have failed conservative treatment and should be viewed as a means to allow appropriate rehabilitation and strengthening to allow the player to return to a level of peak performance. The surgeon identifies whether the shoulder pathology is reparable and must be confident that the athlete can participate in a possibly painful and lengthy recovery program.

Operative repair of rotator cuff injuries in tennis players is indicated when the athlete desires a return to tennis and has failed a rehabilitation program. An intrascalene block is generally used for anesthesia. Examination under anesthesia is then performed in the same manner as the preoperative examination. This examination is essential because it can alter the proposed surgical plan. Subtle instability that can be masked with involuntary guarding can sometimes be discerned. Diagnostic arthroscopy is then performed with the patient in the beach chair position (14). The entire glenohumeral joint and subacromial space should be visualized before proceeding with the procedure. Generally, tendon tears are debrided and assessed for completeness of tear. If the depth of tear is less than 50% of thickness, debridement alone is performed. Full thickness tears as well as tears approaching full thickness are repaired arthroscopically. Concurrent labral detachments are repaired, and capsular attenuation with associated subluxation is treated with capsular plication.

After addressing glenohumeral pathology, the subacromial space should always be evaluated for evidence of subacromial impingement. When subacromial impingement is present, the bursa appears thickened and inflamed, and the coracoacromial ligament is often thickened and abraded. Subacromial spurs should be resected if present. Depending on preoperative history, physical examination, and intraoperative findings, the AC joint can be addressed when pathology is present. Large spurs on the undersurface of the distal clavicle adding to the impingement warrant AC joint resection. When performed, the AC joint debridement should measure 12 mm wide (Fig. 23-6).

Postoperative rehabilitation is similar to conservative treatment programs. Initially, it is important to maintain range of motion while minimizing pain and swelling, which

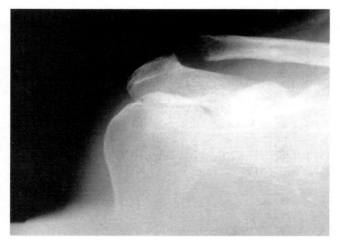

FIGURE 23-6. Postoperative radiograph of a distal clavicle resection.

can contribute to the formation of adhesions. Next, active range-of-motion exercises should follow before the initiation of balanced shoulder strengthening. Playing and practicing can commence gradually in conjunction with tennis-specific exercises. Return to preinjury level after rotator cuff repair is variable and can depend on the age of the tennis player, as well as on the severity of the tear. A recent study by Sonnery-Cottet and colleagues has shown that, after surgical treatment, 80% of middle-aged tennis players with rotator cuff injuries were able to return to participation, with the majority playing at preinjury level (15).

Operative treatment in tennis players with suprascapular neuropathy can be successful when a compression lesion is acutely identified and addressed. When the lesion has been present for more than 6 months, operative treatment may help in pain reduction, but is unlikely to result in return of muscle function. Compression of the suprascapular nerve is usually caused by a ganglion cyst in the spinoglenoid notch. If the ganglion is accessible arthroscopically, it can be decompressed under direct visualization. Yellow or mucoid cystic fluid confirms decompression, and entrance into the cyst should be attempted to break up any loculations. The labrum should then be inspected for pathology, and any detachment should be debrided and repaired if possible. If the ganglion cyst cannot be reached arthroscopically, an open procedure should be performed.

Surgical treatment of instability in the tennis athlete is rarely necessary and is reserved for players who fail conservative treatment. In the elite tennis player, acute surgical treatment of instability is reserved for athletes with anatomic lesions that are identifiable and repairable. The player must also demonstrate the ability to participate in a lengthy, painful recovery process with strict compliance to rehabilitation protocol. Surgery is usually performed with an intrascalene block, and a complete examination under anesthesia is compared with the preoperative stability examination. The patient's history, activity level, and athletic requirements are all important pieces of information to consider. Glenohumeral stability should be assessed in the anterior, posterior, and inferior directions. "Normal" stability for a tennis player demonstrates a 2+ posterior laxity and 1+ anterior laxity with a 1 to 2+ sulcus. Increased laxity in either the anterior or posterior direction should raise concern whether capsulolabral repair is required.

Diagnostic arthroscopy is then performed before finalizing the surgical plan. Beginning with the arthroscope in the posterior portal, the biceps and biceps anchor can be visualized. In overhead athletes, this area of the labrum can be meniscoid in shape and can have recessed attachment. Next the anterior superior labrum is evaluated. The surgeon should be aware that two variations exist in the attachment of the superior and middle glenohumeral ligaments. The first is a bandlike middle glenohumeral ligament that is usually accompanied by a complete lack of anterosuperior labral tissue. The second is a defect in the anterosuperior labrum occurring below the attachment site of the middle gleno-humeral ligament. If these normal variations are not recognized, attempted repair will result in overtightening of the middle glenohumeral ligament and an external rotation contracture will develop. A true labral detachment is usually evidenced by fraying or visualization of a direct tear (Fig. 23-7).

Arthroscopic evaluation can then proceed to the anteroinferior labrum, which, if detached, requires repair. The inferior glenohumeral ligament can be difficult to evaluate because direct tears rarely occur. It has been described as a distinct structure that is tensioned as the arm is externally rotated, and injury occurs if it fails to tighten (16). Another indication of a ligamentous laxity is a positive drive-through sign, which occurs with shoulder laxity. The supraspinatus should then be evaluated, and any undersurface tears should be debrided. The arthroscope can then be switched to the anterior portal to evaluate the infraspinatus tendon and the posterior labrum. From this view, it is possible to diagnose internal impingement that is evident by fraying and partial tearing of the infraspinatus tendon without detachment of the posterosuperior labrum. All frayed tissue should be debrided to properly evaluate the integrity of the remaining tendon and labrum. In cases of internal impingement, simple debridement is adequate treatment as long as subtle anterior instability does not coexist. A recent case series reported by Sonnery-Connet and colleagues of 28 young tennis players (average age 26.9 years) with posterior shoulder pain resulting from internal impingement treated with arthroscopic debridement demonstrated 50% of players returning to equal or superior level play (17). Posterior labral detachment is uncommon but should be debrided and repaired when evident after probing. Finally, the arthroscope is switched to the subacromial space, and the bursa is evaluated. Normally, a large bursal sac is present, and the coracoacromial ligament is easily visualized. If

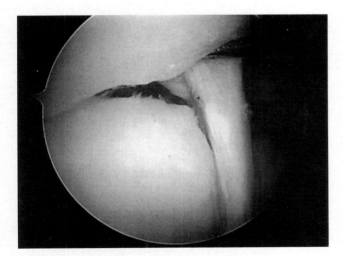

FIGURE 23-7. Intraoperative photo of a SLAP tear of the superior labrum.

impingement is present, the thickened bursal tissue can be debrided, and subacromial spurs can be removed if present.

Postoperative rehabilitation after instability repair should focus on restoration of range of motion, and passive motion exercises can begin immediately. Full forward flexion with 90 degrees of external rotation should be restored at 8 weeks. Strengthening begins with periscapular musculature and progresses to rotator cuff muscles. Simultaneous cardiovascular training and core strengthening exercises expedite return to peak maximal performance. Hitting can commence when full motion and 80% of shoulder strength has been obtained. Ground strokes are progressed gradually over a period of months until the player is ready to return to competitive tennis. This timeframe is lengthy and can last 6 months for minor surgery and 12 months for major surgery.

SHOULDER INJURY IN THE ADOLESCENT TENNIS PLAYER

The etiology of shoulder injuries in young or adolescent tennis players are different from injury patterns in adults. Injuries in the adolescent tennis player are rare, but they do occur. Typically they are self-limited and resolve with rest. In cases of refractory pain, it is important to consider the possibility of injury to the proximal humeral physis. The cartilage zone of hypertrophy is the weakest layer of the physis and can be susceptible to chronic stresses associated with overhead activity. Patients with growth plate injuries typically present with chronic anterolateral shoulder pain with no history of trauma. Pain is reproduced with rotator cuff resistance and no impingement signs. AP radiographs of the proximal humerus demonstrate widening of the physis compared with that in the contralateral shoulder. Treatment consists of rest from all overhead activities for 6 weeks or until complete absence of symptoms.

A second shoulder problem affecting the adolescent tennis player is instability. Typically, a player complains that the shoulder is occasionally slipping in or out of the joint during serve or while hitting an overhead volley. A history of frank dislocation is rare, but, if present, it is usually preceded by significant trauma. Most players complaining of shoulder instability also reveal some evidence of generalized ligamentous laxity. It has been shown that shoulder laxity peaks during adolescence (18). Shoulder examination usually demonstrates MDI with no apprehension; in contrast, patients with instability caused by traumatic dislocation usually demonstrate apprehension with provocative maneuvers. A complete physical examination is necessary, and it is important to check for hyperextension of the elbow or hand MCP joints. Patients with generalized laxity can touch their thumb to their forearm. The mainstay of treatment for instability secondary to generalized ligamentous laxity is strengthening exercises that focus on the shoulder girdle and the rotator cuff muscles. As the patient ages, the laxity usually resolves.

AUTHORS' PREFERRED TREATMENT, ALGORITHMS AND TECHNIQUES

The following list should provide a guide for the *surgical* treatment of instability in the tennis player.

Type 1: Athlete complains of shoulder pain with no discernible symptoms of true instability and is refractory to rehabilitation.

I-A: Minor rotator cuff injury, subacromial bursitis with or without a thickened coracoacromial ligament. In this case, minor "dynamic" rotator cuff instability occurs because of chronic rotator cuff dysfunction. Surgical treatment consists of debridement of undersurface cuff tear and arthroscopic subacromial decompression.

I-B: Rotator cuff injury is severe (greater than 50% of tendon thickness), and the anterior capsule and labrum are intact. Arthroscopic repair is performed on the torn portion of the rotator cuff.

I-C: Internal impingement. Posterior pain is reproduced by the position of abduction and external rotation. Arthroscopy reveals typical lesion of internal impingement. This is treated with debridement of the undersurface of the rotator cuff and careful evaluation for capsular laxity.

I-D: SLAP lesion. Athletes have joint line pain and an MRI scan that confirms a SLAP lesion. Surgical treatment involves debridement or repair of the labrum depending on whether the labrum is torn or detached.

Type II: Athletes with anterior instability. Symptomatically, they complain primarily of pain but may, if questioned, admit that the shoulder feels excessively loose and that the shoulder "comes apart" during the acceleration phase of serving. Examination under anesthesia reveals 2 to 3+ anterior laxity and arthroscopy reveals a loose anterior capsule with a large drive-through "signs."

II-A: Capsular laxity without rotator cuff tear. The surgeon's goal in this type of patient is to tighten the anterior capsule such that the humeral head remains centered on the glenoid during the act of serving. The difficulty in the usual method of capsular plication is that errors in capsular tensioning, even slight, lead to restriction of motion and cause significant disability in the overhead athlete.

II-B: Capsular laxity with rotator cuff tear. In this patient, both issues must be addressed surgically. The rotator cuff is assessed as described previously in this chapter. If the tear is thought to extend more than 50% of the tendon thickness, it is repaired arthroscopically. Concomitant subacromial decompression is completed only if distinct arthroscopic evidence of subacromial impingement is present. We have found that subacromial decompression is rarely helpful in this group of patients who have distinct instability.

II-C: Capsular tear with or without rotator cuff tear: Capsular tears rarely occur in tennis players. Such injuries usually involve the anterior portion of the anteroinferior glenohumeral ligament. Surgical repair is indicated for definitive treatment.

CONCLUSION

Shoulder injuries in the tennis player are common and are most often due to overuse. The best treatment is prevention, which requires careful attention to proper stroke mechanics and moderation of playing time. Total body conditioning with adequate time reserved for shoulder strengthening and flexibility may help reduce the stress imparted on soft tissue structures. Appropriate diagnosis, rest, and rehabilitation can cure most injuries, but in certain circumstances, operative intervention may be necessary.

REFERENCES

1. Lehman RC. Shoulder pain in the competitive tennis player. *Clin Sports Med* 1988;7(2):309–327.
2. Kibler WB. Biomechanical analysis of the shoulder during tennis activities. *Clin Sports Med* 1995;14(1):79–85.
3. Morris M, et al. Electromyographic analysis of elbow function in tennis players. *Am J Sports Med* 1989;17(2):241–247.
4. Ryu RK, et al. An electromyographic analysis of shoulder function in tennis players. *Am J Sports Med* 1988;16(5):481–485.
5. Romeo AA, Rotenberg DD, Bach BR Jr. Suprascapular neuropathy. *J Am Acad Orthop Surg* 1999;7(6):358–367.
6. Priest JD, Nagel DA. Tennis shoulder. *Am J Sports Med* 1976;4(1):28–42.
7. O'Brien SJ, et al. The active compression test: a new and effective test for diagnosing labral tears and acromioclavicular joint abnormality. *Am J Sports Med* 1998;26(5):610–613.
8. Ellenbecker TS, et al. Glenohumeral joint internal and external rotation range of motion in elite junior tennis players. *J Orthop Sports Phys Ther* 1996;24(6):336–341.
9. Kibler WB, et al. Shoulder range of motion in elite tennis players. Effect of age and years of tournament play. *Am J Sports Med* 1996;24(3): 279–285.
10. Jobe FW, Kvitne RS, Giangarra CE. Shoulder pain in the overhand or throwing athlete. The relationship of anterior instability and rotator cuff impingement. *Orthop Rev* 1989;18(9): 963–975.
11. Townsend H, et al. Electromyographic analysis of the glenohumeral muscles during a baseball rehabilitation program. *Am J Sports Med* 1991;19(3):264–272.
12. Ellenbecker TS. Rehabilitation of shoulder and elbow injuries in tennis players. *Clin Sports Med* 1995;14(1):87–110.
13. Plancher KD, Litchfield R, Hawkins RJ. Rehabilitation of the shoulder in tennis players. *Clin Sports Med* 1995;14(1): 111–137.
14. Skyhar MJ, et al. Shoulder arthroscopy with the patient in the beach-chair position. *Arthroscopy* 1988;4(4):256–259.
15. Sonnery-Cottet B, et al. Rotator cuff tears in middle-aged tennis players: results of surgical treatment. *Am J Sports Med* 2002;30(4):558–564.
16. O'Brien SJ, et al. The anatomy and histology of the inferior glenohumeral ligament complex of the shoulder. *Am J Sports Med* 1990;18(5):449–456.
17. Sonnery-Cottet B, et al. Results of arthroscopic treatment of posterosuperior glenoid impingement in tennis players. *Am J Sports Med* 2002;30(2):227–232.
18. Emery RJ, Mullaji AB. Glenohumeral joint instability in normal adolescents. Incidence and significance. *J Bone Joint Surg (Br)* 1991;73(3):406–408.

24

SWIMMING

SCOTT A. RODEO

INTRODUCTION

Shoulder pain and injuries are common in swimming because more than 90% of the propulsive power in swimming comes from the upper extremity (1). Competitive swimming is known for its long and arduous training sessions. Swimmers at the elite level practice 20 to 30 hours per week and may swim up to 15,000 yards (9 miles) per day. During one practice season, the average competitive swimmer performs nearly 500,000 stroke revolutions per arm (2). This repetitive arm action, over the course of many years, is believed to be the main etiologic factor in the overuse syndrome known as "swimmer's shoulder."

Kennedy (3) used the term *swimmer's shoulder* in the 1970s to describe anterior shoulder pain in swimmers during and after workouts. Originally this pain was attributed to impingement and tendonitis of the rotator cuff and biceps tendon complex. As investigations of shoulder pain in swimmers continues, it is becoming increasingly evident that swimmer's shoulder represents a spectrum of maladies, including impingement and glenohumeral instability, which result in shoulder pain. The common factor is repetitive microtrauma from overuse.

Shoulder pain is the most common orthopedic complaint in swimmers. The incidence of shoulder pain ranges from 40% to 70% in competitive swimmers. Although rarely seen in children younger than 10 years of age (4), the incidence of pain increases with time participating in the sport (5). At the elite level, more than half the athletes report a history of significant, interfering shoulder pain. Approximately 15% of swimmers report bilateral shoulder pain (2). Shoulder pain is reported in all four strokes, in both distance swimmers and sprinters, and no gender difference has been reported.

This chapter reviews the mechanics of the swimming stroke and its relationship to overuse injury, the patterns of muscle activation in the normal and the painful shoulder, and the etiology of shoulder pain. This information is then used to discuss rehabilitation of the injured shoulder, the role of surgical management, and strategies for prevention.

The overriding theme is to describe the relationship between muscle overuse and fatigue, subtle glenohumeral laxity, and impingement.

ETIOLOGY OF SHOULDER PAIN IN SWIMMERS

Competitive swimmers perform nearly a half-million shoulder revolutions per arm per year. It is generally agreed that repetitive overuse is a major contributor to shoulder pain. Contributing factors for swimmer's shoulder are thought to include (a) overuse and subsequent fatigue of the muscles around the shoulder, scapula, and upper back, (b) glenohumeral laxity, and (c) the mechanics of the swimming stroke, in which impingement can occur in various positions during the swimming stroke. Other associated findings include muscle imbalances and inflexibility, such as tightness of the pectoral muscles, and sometimes inflexibility of the posterior rotator cuff and posterior capsule. The incidence of pain and injury appears to be greater in swimmers who use poor technique. The use of hand paddles to increase resistance while swimming to build strength also contributes to muscle overload and fatigue.

Although muscle fatigue and shoulder instability with excessive glenohumeral translation can by themselves cause pain, it is likely that some element of impingement and subsequent rotator cuff tendinitis is the final common pathway causing shoulder pain in swimmers. Impingement may be caused by the particular mechanics of the swimming stroke as well as altered glenohumeral kinematics resulting from muscle fatigue or glenohumeral laxity. Although shoulder pain in swimmers has a varied and often confusing presentation, it is likely that a combination of impingement, instability, and muscle overuse and fatigue is the underlying cause in the majority of cases. The variable presentation may just represent different stages along this spectrum. Each of these etiologic factors is considered in detail.

Impingement During the Swimming Stroke

Swimmers usually have a nonoutlet type of impingement, in which altered kinematics rather than subacromial pathologic changes (acromial osteophyte or coracoacromial ligament abnormalities) results in abnormal contact. Impingement can occur in various positions during the swimming stroke. Such impingement may be subacromial (the bursal surface of the rotator cuff against the anteroinferior acromion) or intraarticular (the articular surface of the rotator cuff or biceps tendon impinging on the anterosuperior glenoid and labrum). During the recovery phase of the stroke, the glenohumeral joint goes into forward flexion and internal rotation, which is a classic position for subacromial impingement (Fig. 24-1). At the end of the pull-through phase of the stroke, the arm goes into hyperextension, which pushes the humeral head anteriorly, also exacerbating impingement. Yanai and colleagues used a video analysis system to document impingement during the freestyle stroke. They reported that impingement occurred when the hand entered the water and in the middle of the recovery phase (6). The mean duration of impingement was nearly 25% of the total stroke time: 14.4% of the stroke time while the arm was in the water and 10.4% while the arm was recovering above the surface. These authors reported that impingement was most likely in swimmers using the following stroke characteristics: (a) a large amount of internal rotation during the pulling phase, (b) delayed initiation of external rotation of the arm during the recovery phase, and (c) decreased upward scapular rotation (7).

Hydrodynamic forces exerted by the water may also exacerbate impingement. At the point when the hand enters the water, the hydrodynamic force exerted on the hand generates a large moment about the shoulder joint due to the long moment arm in this position. This moment forcibly elevates the arm, possibly increasing impingement (6).

Alternatively, a form of intraarticular impingement may occur during the swimming stroke. The articular surface of the rotator cuff may impinge against the anterosuperior labrum adjacent to the biceps attachment as the arm is placed into forward flexion and internal rotation. This may account for the frequent localization of pain in swimmers around the biceps tendon. Coracoid impingement may also occur in swimmers. The position of forward elevation, adduction, and internal rotation may result in impingement of the coracoid process on the lesser tuberosity and subscapularis tendon. The author has documented this cause of pain in a swimmer using a lidocaine injection around the tip of the coracoid process.

Muscle Fatigue and Dysfunction

The repetitive overhead activity in the swimming stroke may lead to overuse and subsequent fatigue of the muscles around the shoulder, scapula, and upper back. Shoulder function is highly dependent on the coordinated function of many muscle groups. These include the muscles around the shoulder, those that control the scapula, and those in the upper and lower back, as well as abdominal and pelvic muscles. The shoulder does not act in isolation during swimming; rather, muscles of the back, trunk, and legs help stabilize the body and help in the pulling movement. Because the shoulder is an inherently unstable joint, muscle forces are critical for maintaining stability, proper motion, and painless function. The repetitive overhead activity of the swimming stroke can result in fatigue of these muscles.

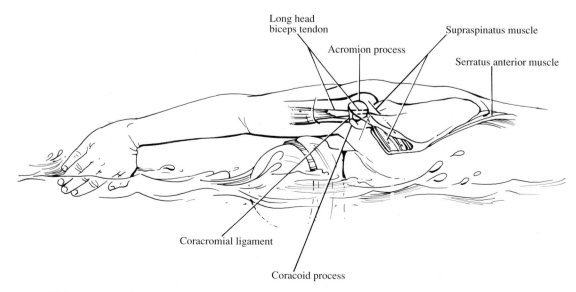

FIGURE 24-1. The recovery phase of the freestyle stroke places the shoulder in a position that is typical for subacromial impingement.

Most of the forward propulsive force in swimming is generated by adduction and internal rotation of the upper extremity. The stronger the internal rotators of the shoulder, the faster the swimmer can move through the water (8). Therefore, it is not surprising that competitive swimmers have greater adduction and internal rotation strength compared to abduction and external rotation strength (9). While providing a competitive advantage, these imbalances may also result in abnormal glenohumeral kinematics and subsequent instability. In fact, swimmers who complain of a painful shoulder are likely to have greater strength imbalances around the shoulder (10,11).

Competitive swimming is comprised of four basic strokes: (a) freestyle, (b) butterfly, (c) backstroke, and (d) breaststroke. Three of these strokes (freestyle, butterfly, and backstroke) involve repetitive overhead activity (12–14). Regardless of the stroke performed in competition, swimmers spend a considerable amount of their training time swimming freestyle. The swimming stroke is divided into two phases: the pull-through phase and the recovery phase (2) (Fig. 24-2). The pull-through is the underwater portion of the swimming stroke and has been further subdivided into hand entry, mid pull-through, and late pull-through (15,16). The pull-through phase is the longest portion of the stroke, accounting for 65% to 70% of the time spent in the freestyle stroke (14). As the hand and arm pull in this phase, they follow an S-shaped pattern (16). This pattern is believed to provide an additional forward lift (17), while at the same time placing the arm and shoulder in the most efficient position for generating power. Muscles around the shoulder girdle generate the propulsive power during the stroke.

Pink and co-workers have contributed greatly to current knowledge of muscle function around the shoulder and scapula during swimming. They have demonstrated that performance of the swimming stroke requires a highly coordinated pattern of muscles firing at precisely the right time to provide the most efficient and powerful stroke. This group has used electromyography (EMG) to define muscle firing patterns during the different phases of the various swimming strokes (12). They then went on to define differences in muscle firing patterns in swimmers with painful shoulders (10,13).

Muscle Activity in the Normal Shoulder: Pull-Through Phase

The hand enters the water forward of and lateral to the head. The elbow is slightly flexed and pointing upward, so that the fingers are the first to break the water with the palm facing outward (15). This has been referred to as the "high" elbow position (16). At the time of hand entry, this places the shoulder in an abducted, flexed, and internally rotated position. Phasic muscle activity is predominantly seen in the upper trapezius, rhomboids, supraspinatus, and anterior and middle deltoids (12). The serratus anterior also shows an increase in activity as it upwardly rotates and protracts the scapula (12). These muscle actions position the glenoid fossa for the humeral head as the arm is flexed and abducted to achieve hand entry. The position of the arm at hand entry essentially reproduces the Hawkins impingement test, illustrating the propensity for subacromial impingement during swimming (18).

Once the hand enters the water, there is a brief period of reaching and gliding, which serves as a transition between recovery and actual pulling. At this point, an upward force by the water further flexes the shoulder into a position that may cause subacromial impingement (6). The hand and arm then begin a sequential sweeping motion: out, down, in, and up (15) as the hand follows an S-shaped curve during the pulling phase. The in-sweep, although briefest in duration, creates

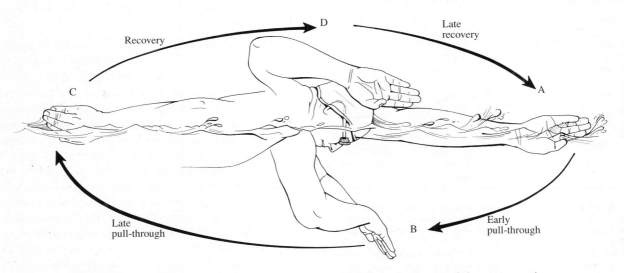

FIGURE 24-2. The swimming stroke is divided into the pull-through phase and the recovery phase.

the highest muscular activity (19). The predominant muscles that provide this intense pulling activity are the pectoralis major and the latissimus dorsi (12,14). They powerfully adduct the humerus, causing the hand to sweep under the chest before passing laterally to the pelvis (15).

The pectoralis major fires first and is responsible for the initial powerful adduction and extension (12). When the hand reaches its deepest point in the water, mid pull-through begins. Here the shoulder is at 90 degrees abduction with neutral rotation and body roll is maximal at 40 to 60 degrees from horizontal (2). As the pectoralis major continues to contract during mid pull-through, the shoulder internally rotates with a flexed elbow. The teres minor simultaneously fires to provide an antagonistic external rotation force to this internal rotation (12). This force couple between the teres minor and the pectoralis major serves to balance the humeral head on the glenoid.

As the humerus crosses the point where it is perpendicular to the body, the late pull-through phase begins. In late pull-through, the latissimus dorsi has the mechanical advantage. It begins to fire and, along with the subscapularis, continues the pull by forcefully extending the internally rotated arm. Active pulling stops as the palm approaches the thigh, as opposed to when the hand exits the water (12). This results in a fully adducted and internally rotated shoulder at the end of the pull. Activity in the posterior deltoid continues to extend the arm as it nears the thigh; this is followed by activity of the middle and anterior deltoid, respectively, as the hand proceeds to exit. The serratus anterior and the other muscle involved in hand entry are also active as the hand exits the water in preparation for recovery.

The serratus anterior and subscapularis are active throughout the entire swimming stroke (12,14) (Fig. 24-3).

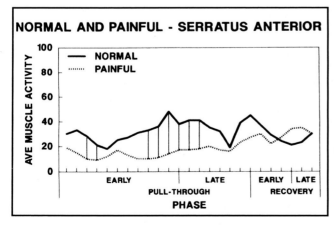

FIGURE 24-3. The serratus anterior muscle continuously fires at a high rate during the swimming stroke and is thus susceptible to fatigue. There is significantly diminished serratus anterior muscle activity in the painful swimmer's shoulder. (From Scovazzo ML, et al. The painful shoulder during freestyle swimming. An electromyographic cinematographic analysis of twelve muscles. *Am J Sports Med* 1991;19(6):577–582).

By helping to position the scapula, the serratus anterior is able to maintain glenohumeral joint congruency during the entire pull-through phase. In a similar manner, it assists in preventing impingement of the coracoid process or acromion on the humerus at hand exit. Finally, by providing a stable scapula, the serratus anterior allows the body to move over the arm as it is pulled through the water by the pectoralis major and latissimus dorsi. The subscapularis is continually active due to its function as a powerful internal rotator. Because of their continuous activity during the swimming stroke, the serratus anterior and subscapularis are susceptible to fatigue (12).

Muscle Activity in the Normal Shoulder: Recovery Phase

The recovery phase refers to the part of the swimming stroke wherein the hand is above water. This phase can be subdivided in to three parts: (a) elbow lift, (b) mid recovery, and (c) hand entry (2). This phase is shorter than the pull-through phase, accounting for 30% to 35% of the freestyle stroke (12,14). As the elbow lifts out of the water, the arm and hand are internally rotated, thus reducing drag (15). The shoulder then proceeds to follow a sequence of extending, abducting, and internally rotating, as the scapula is retracting to accomplish recovery. The muscles involved in this sequence include the middle deltoid, supraspinatus, subscapularis, and rhomboids (12). Another muscle of primary importance from mid recovery to hand entry is the infraspinatus. The infraspinatus serves as a humeral head depressor and provides a stabilizing force for the strong pull of the antagonizing subscapularis (12). The subscapularis and infraspinatus form another important force couple to control glenohumeral kinematics. Following these movements, the hand is again in position for entry into the water.

Muscle Activity in the Painful Swimmer's Shoulder

EMG analysis in competitive swimmers with clinically confirmed shoulder pain has provided insight into alterations in muscle firing patterns in the painful shoulder (10). Abnormal muscle firing may be a cause of shoulder pain by leading to altered kinematics or, alternatively, it may represent a compensatory attempt to avoid painful positions. Swimmers with painful shoulders exhibit a different pattern of hand entry than do those with normal shoulders. There is a decrease in activity of the anterior and middle deltoid, rhomboids, and upper trapezius. The hand enters further away from the midline with the elbow lower to the water (10), referred to as *dropped elbow* (16). Assuming this position at hand entry avoids the classic impingement position of flexion and internal rotation of the humerus described by Hawkins (18), but it places the arm in a less powerful and less efficient externally rotated posture.

Swimmers with painful shoulders show significant differences in muscle activity during pulling. There is markedly less activity seen in the serratus anterior (10) (see Fig. 24-3). To compensate for loss of serratus anterior function, increased activity of the rhomboids attempt to stabilize the scapula. However, the rhomboids function antagonistically to the serratus, resulting in retraction and downward rotation of the scapula, which are opposite movements to those normally done by the serratus anterior. The loss of normal scapular rotation is likely to increase the propensity for impingement. In these swimmers, the hand often exits early before the palm passes the thigh, with the elbow bent (10). This early hand exit is associated with decreased activity of the anterior and middle deltoid. Early hand exit allows the swimmer to avoid the extreme internal rotation and hyperextension positions that can cause impingement. Thus, such subtle stroke alterations are likely an attempt to avoid impingement positions.

As the elbow leaves the water at the end of pull-through, another abnormal muscle action is seen. The infraspinatus shows significantly increased muscle activity in the painful shoulder as it externally rotates the humerus (10). At the same time, there is decreased subscapularis activity. This may be an attempt to avoid painful internal rotation. The anterior deltoid is the only muscle to show significantly reduced activity during the recovery phase in painful shoulders, as abduction and forward flexion of the humerus is decreased (10). Once again, the arm assumes the dropped elbow position to prevent impingement.

Abnormal muscle firing patterns even occur in the painful shoulder during breaststroke swimming, in which there is not as much overhead activity because the arms largely stay in the water during the recovery phase. During the pull-through phase, there is increased activity in the subscapularis and a concomitant decrease in teres minor activity (20). This would result in a relative increase in internal rotation, which predisposes to impingement in the forward flexed position. Like with other strokes, there is decreased serratus anterior activity in the painful shoulder with increased activity of the upper trapezius, likely an attempt to compensate for loss of serratus function.

During the recovery phase breaststroke swimmers with painful shoulders have decreased activity in the supraspinatus and upper trapezius and concomitant increased activity in the infraspinatus and latissimus dorsi. The abnormal supraspinatus activity disrupts the normal force couple with the deltoid, leading to proximal humeral migration during recovery and increasing the propensity for impingement. The normal rotator cuff functions to stabilize the glenohumeral joint and acts as a humeral head depressor, preventing subacromial impingement. It is well established that loss of the humeral head depressor function of the rotator cuff results in superior migration of the humeral head and increases the risk of impingement (21). The latissimus dorsi may increase activity to depress the humeral head to compensate for the loss of the humeral head depressor function of the supraspinatus. Increased activity of the infraspinatus may be a response to the increased internal rotation in swimmers with painful shoulders. Decreased upper trapezius activity contributes to impingement by decreasing scapular elevation. Overall, the serratus anterior and teres minor muscles fire at a high level throughout the breaststroke and are thus susceptible to fatigue.

In summary, muscle fatigue with subsequent altered muscle firing patterns can predispose to impingement by adversely affecting glenohumeral kinematics. The altered firing patterns discussed previously would increase impingement by (a) leading to a relative increase in internal rotation, (b) loss of humeral head depressor function of the rotator cuff, and (c) loss of upward rotation and elevation of the scapula. Loss of the stabilizing effect of muscles may be especially problematic in swimmers with associated shoulder laxity (discussed later). Fatigue of the abdominal and pelvic muscles may also contribute by affecting scapular kinematics and body position in the water.

Role of Laxity in Swimmer's Shoulder

Many competitive swimmers have an element of shoulder laxity (22,23). In fact, a certain degree of laxity may be advantageous by allowing a swimmer to achieve both a body position that reduces drag and a longer sweep during the pull-through phase. Like for other overhead athletes, there is a fine line between physiologic laxity and pathologic instability. Normal laxity may increase over time as a result of repetitive overuse and eventually may become pathologic. Shoulder stability is controlled by static (glenohumeral ligaments) and dynamic (rotator cuff muscles) factors. Loss of the static component (glenohumeral capsular laxity) requires a greater contribution from the rotator cuff, which can result in muscle overload and eventual muscle fatigue, as described earlier. The challenge for the medical practitioner is to distinguish between normal laxity and abnormal instability.

Previous studies have documented the presence of increased joint laxity and glenohumeral instability in swimmers. McMaster and Troup reported "recognizable looseness" in 15% of elite female swimmers (5). Bak and Faunl reported that 37 of 49 competitive swimmers had increased humeral head translation with associated apprehension (24). Furthermore, McMaster and colleagues found a significant correlation between shoulder laxity and shoulder pain in a group of 40 elite level swimmers (25). The presence of underlying generalized joint hypermobility was reported by Zemek and Magee (23). These authors reported both increased glenohumeral laxity and increased generalized joint hypermobility in elite swimmers compared to recreational swimmers. Taken together, these studies suggest that a combination of acquired and inherent factors contribute to shoulder laxity in swimmers.

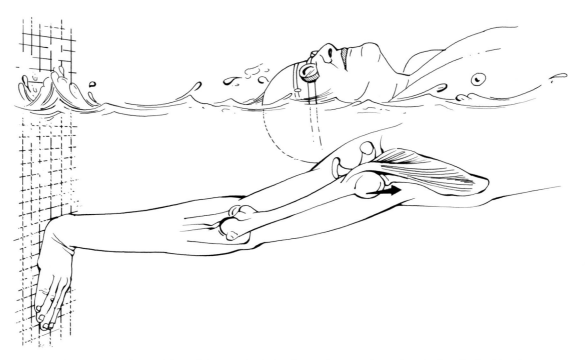

FIGURE 24-4. The position of the arm in abduction and external rotation during the backstroke can predispose to anterior instability.

The most common pattern of instability is anteroinferior, but there is often a component of multidirectional instability. Posterior instability symptoms, although less common, may be exacerbated by the position of the arm in flexion, adduction, and internal rotation. Distinct subluxation can occur during the backstroke, in that the arm is in full abduction and is externally rotated as the hand enters the water while the swimmer is on his or her back (Fig. 24-4). The risk of subluxation is increased in backstroke if the hand contacts the wall for the turn with the arm in this position of abduction and external rotation. However, current rules allow the swimmer to turn over onto the stomach one stroke before the turn in backstroke, obviating this position of hand contact on the wall.

DIAGNOSTIC EVALUATION

The typical complaint is pain localized around the front of the shoulder, often described as being over the biceps tendon. Although some swimmers may describe a sense that the shoulder slips or feels loose (similar to other overhead athletes), the usual complaint is pain rather than distinct instability. As in any injury, an accurate diagnosis begins with a careful history and examination. A comprehensive examination is performed with specific attention to glenohumeral laxity, strength of the rotator cuff and periscapular muscles, impingement signs, localizing tenderness, labral

signs, and signs indicative of acromioclavicular joint pathology. The office examination is often normal with few localizing findings. There is often a degree of glenohumeral laxity, as described earlier. Significant motion or strength deficits are uncommon. Scapulohumeral rhythm should be carefully examined and compared with the contralateral side to detect subtle asymmetry. The cervical spine and acromioclavicular joint should also be examined, especially in the older swimmer.

Insight into the cause of pain may be gained from careful analysis of the swimming stroke. Similar to altered throwing mechanics seen in a pitcher with shoulder pain, subtle stroke alterations may be seen in the swimmer with a painful shoulder. These include a dropped elbow (this position avoids internal rotation), a wider hand entry (avoids impingement due to forward flexion), an early hand exit during pull-through (avoids hyperextension position), and excessive body roll (allows less hyperextension). Such stroke alterations may be causing shoulder pain or, alternatively, may be compensatory changes to relieve or avoid painful positions.

A thorough evaluation should include a standard series of plain radiographs. Bone or soft tissue lesions, although uncommon, can present in the young patient as sports-related pain. However, plain radiographs generally have limited value in the evaluation of nontraumatic glenohumeral instability and rarely show spurring of the anterior acromion or abnormal anatomy that may suggest impingement. Magnetic resonance imaging (MRI) provides further information, especially if a frank labral tear is suspected. Although ancillary studies such as MRI have traditionally not been thought to be beneficial, high-resolution MRI may demonstrate thickening of the capsule (supporting evidence of previous instability episodes) and signal change in the rotator cuff consistent with tendinosis (suggestive of tendon overload). Full thickness tendon tears or significant partial thickness tears are rare. However, labral tears are seen in swimmers (26). Anterior labral damage may be most likely in backstrokers as a result of the repetitive positioning of the arm in full abduction and external rotation (1).

Diagnostic injection may be helpful to confirm the source of pain. Such injection may be performed around the biceps tendon, acromioclavicular joint, subacromial space, or coracoid process. For example, the diagnosis of coracoid impingement is made by a positive response to lidocaine injection. Dynamic EMG recordings using intramuscular needle electrodes may also help evaluate painful shoulders in swimmers. EMG studies may reveal altered firing patterns of the rotator cuff muscles and scapular stabilizers. This information can provide the clinician with evidence of the underlying etiology of the shoulder pain and help in the formulation of a specific therapy protocol to restore normal kinematics. However, this modality is rarely used because the diagnosis is made on clinical grounds. Finally, examination under anesthesia and arthroscopy are recommended in patients who fail extensive conservative management and when glenohumeral instability is suspected (discussed later).

CLASSIFICATION OF INJURY

No classification schemes specific for the swimmer's shoulder have been described. Jobe and Glousman have described four different groups along the spectrum of instability and impingement for the injured shoulder in overhead athletes (27). Group I patients have pure impingement with no instability. Group II patients have anterior instability resulting from labral or capsular trauma and associated secondary impingement. Group III patients have atraumatic anterior instability resulting from capsular laxity and have associated secondary impingement. Finally, group IV patients have pure anterior instability and no impingement signs (28). A study of competitive swimmers using this classification system found most swimmers with shoulder pain to fall into group II (24). This system may be useful for guiding treatment of the painful swimmer's shoulder. An alternative classification scheme has been proposed that divides swimmer's shoulder into four phases based on the severity of symptoms (29—31) (Table 24-1). Most swimmers who present for evaluation fall into group III in this system. Such a system is also helpful in guiding treatment.

TABLE 24–1. CLASSIFICATION SCHEME THAT DIVIDES SWIMMER'S SHOULDER INTO FOUR PHASES BASED ON SEVERITY OF SYMPTOMS

I. Pain only during workout; does not interfere with performance.
II. Pain during and after workout, which resolves with ice and rest, and does not affect performance.
III. Pain during and after workout, which affects performance.
IV. Pain severe enough to prevent competitive swimming.

DIFFERENTIAL DIAGNOSIS

Although most cases of swimmer's shoulder appear to be due to tendon overload or tendinitis with or without associated instability, other entities need to be considered in the differential diagnosis. Labral tears can occur in this group of athletes, from either underlying instability or intraarticular impingement of the anterosuperior labrum. Shoulder pain and injury may also result from other sports activities that the athlete is involved in outside of swimming. Frank rotator cuff tendon tear is uncommon but should be considered in the older athlete. Biceps tendon pathology often coexists with rotator cuff pathology but may represent the primary problem. As mentioned previously, coracoid impingement should be considered in the differential diagnosis. Thoracic outlet syndrome is another uncommon condition that may occur in this group of athletes. Thoracic outlet syndrome often causes paresthesias down the arm and may mimic the "dead arm" symptoms seen with instability. The kyphotic, forward shoulder posture that is often seen in swimmers has also been associated with thoracic outlet syndrome.

Several specific entities should also be considered in skeletally immature athletes. Coracoid apophysitis has been reported in an adolescent swimmer (Craig Ferrell, MD, *personal communication, 2002*). Traction injury to the acromial apophysis is another uncommon injury that has been reported in the skeletally immature overhead athlete (32). Specific diagnoses to consider in the older (Masters) swimmer include glenohumeral and acromioclavicular joint arthritis, cervical spine disease, and rotator cuff tear (33,34). Although it is important to include nonspecific causes of shoulder pain in the differential diagnosis, the majority of shoulder pain in swimmers is related to stroke mechanics and the demands specific to the sport.

AUTHOR'S PREFERRED TREATMENT, ALGORITHMS, AND TECHNIQUES

Treatment of swimmer's shoulder should be directed at the phase of pain. Because shoulder pain is so common in swimmers, the physician working with a swimming team should provide guidelines for the coach and trainer that will direct the initial management and help to determine when the athlete should be evaluated by the physician. I have used the following algorithm to guide initial management of shoulder pain in swimmers:

ALGORITHM FOR COACH'S INITIAL MANAGEMENT OF SHOULDER PAIN

The initial treatment for swimmers complaining of shoulder pain is to identify the strokes and positions that cause pain. These positions and strokes (typically butterfly and freestyle) should be avoided. The athlete should use ice on the shoulder. A long, slow warm-up should be done before training. Although absolute rest from swimming is often not necessary, swimmers should modify their training regimen. Distance, frequency, and intensity of training should all be reduced. The athlete should stop using hand paddles and stop doing pulling sets. Kicking sets should be performed (vertical kicking rather than using a kick board to avoid an impingement position). If the swimmer uses a kick board, he or she should hold the board with the arms flexed slightly at the elbows and shoulders to prevent shoulder impingement. Fins may be used to maintain good body position while decreasing upper body stress. Use of a pull-buoy may be helpful by changing the position of the shoulder in the water and thus decrease drag. Patients may take part in more breaststroke swimming if there is no pain. Dry land upper extremity exercises should also be stopped initially. Some swimmers have found use of a strap around the upper arm over the biceps muscle (counterforce strap) to be helpful. Use of such a strap was first described by Blatz (31). Similar to its use in lateral epicondylitis, a counterforce strap may work by diminishing stresses transmitted to the tendon.

After a period of rest, the athlete may gradually try to resume training. If there is recurrent pain upon resumption of more swimming activities, then the athlete should consider staying out of the water entirely for 3 days. Use of nonsteroidal antiinflammatory medication may be considered. After this 3-day period of rest, the athlete is reassessed. The athlete once again tries to begin a normal training regimen. If the shoulder pain recurs, then the athlete should be evaluated by a physician.

Subtle stroke alterations may be seen in the swimmer with a painful shoulder. Any obvious stroke abnormalities, such as dropped elbow, should be identified and corrected. For example, the coach or physician may suggest that the arm be held in less internal rotation during recovery, hand entry may be made more lateral to the midline at the entry phase, or body roll may be increased to the side of the painful shoulder during the recovery phase. However, stroke alterations should only be suggested in conjunction with careful discussion with the coach. The physician or trainer should *not* make technique suggestions without careful analysis of the individual swimmer's stroke.

Other factors that should prompt evaluation by a physician include pain that persists outside of swimming, pain that persists at night, or pain that is present during everyday activities or while at school. The swimmer should also be evaluated by a physician if he or she complains of a sense that the shoulder slips or feels loose, if there has been distinct trauma (e.g., a fall), if the athlete reports a new painful click inside the joint, or if there has been recurrent periods of missed training due to shoulder pain over several seasons.

NONOPERATIVE TREATMENT AND REHABILITATION

Like for other overhead athletes, conservative management is the mainstay of treatment. In the acute phase of shoulder pain the principal goal is to reduce pain and inflammation. This begins with relative rest, as described previously. Most swimmers who are treated by the physician, therapist, or trainer have already had a trial of relative rest. Physical modalities are often beneficial in the early treatment of shoulder pain. Icing the shoulder for 20 to 30 minutes can reduce pain and inflammation. In all phases of swimmer's shoulder, a short course (7 to 10 days) of high-dose nonsteroidal antiinflammatory medication may be effective (29). However, nonsteroidal medications should not be taken for extended periods of time or for chronic shoulder pain, and they should not be taken to allow the athlete to train through the pain. Use of an oral steroid dose pack may be considered for athletes with significant pain and inflammation, but steroids are rarely used. Corticosteroid injection is also rarely used, but may be considered in the older athlete with recalcitrant pain caused by subacromial inflammation and impingement. Injection may also be useful for diagnostic purposes.

An integral part of the treatment program involves the physical therapist. It is important to have a therapist who understands the demands of the sport and who has experience with shoulder injuries in overhead athletes. Modalities such as electrical stimulation and ultrasound are useful to control pain and inflammation in the initial treatment phase. Manual therapy, such as friction massage, may also be beneficial in the subacute stage of swimmer's shoulder. Deeper heat modalities such as ultrasound can be used in the intermediate and late stages of rehabilitation as the pain resolves and the patient is able to perform isometric exercises pain-free.

The most important part of the rehabilitation program is identification of any deficits in muscle strength, endurance, balance, and flexibility. This is where an experienced therapist is valuable. An individual approach is required. Each individual swimmer should be assessed to determine that individual's strength, endurance, and flexibility deficits. This allows precise, effective rehabilitation prescription. The treating therapist or physician should have an understanding of the muscles that are most susceptible to fatigue and overuse injury, as described earlier. For example, it is well established that the serratus anterior, subscapularis, and teres minor muscles continually fire at a high level during the swimming stroke and are thus susceptible to fatigue. A well-structured rehabilitation program should focus on improving strength and, in particular, endurance of these muscles. The therapist should be able to discern subtle abnormalities in function of the scapular stabilizing muscles and be able to design an appropriate rehabilitation program. Deficits in flexibility are uncommon, but gentle stretching of the pectoralis major muscle and posterior capsule may be required. Gentle stretching of the rotator cuff and periscapular muscles is reasonable, but aggressive stretching is usually not necessary. In particular, swimmers should generally avoid positions that stretch the anterior capsule. Such stretches can exacerbate shoulder laxity. Rehabilitation and strengthening exercises should be performed after swimming training or several hours before practice. These exercises should not be performed right before swimming training because this may fatigue these muscles before swimming.

An exercise program typically begins with isometric exercises that are carried out below the level of the shoulder, to avoid positions that may aggravate subacromial impingement. This can then proceed to variable-resistance exercises using Thera-Band, and then advance to isotonics and isokinetics as the rehabilitation program progresses (35). The program should focus on the rotator cuff and periscapular muscles described above. The primary goal is to develop muscle endurance. Attention should also be focused on restoration of normal proprioception, because deficits in proprioception may occur with capsular injury (36). Furthermore, proprioceptive deficits are more likely with muscle fatigue. For athletes with distinct abnormalities in scapulohumeral kinematics, taping the scapula may allow for more effective strengthening and may improve proprioceptive awareness. Specific exercises are discussed later in the section on injury prevention. When the swimmer has no pain, adequate strength and range of motion, a gradual return to swimming may begin.

OPERATIVE TREATMENT, REHABILITATION, AND RESULTS

Like for shoulder injury in other repetitive overhead sports, operative management is generally indicated only after a comprehensive course of conservative treatment. Exceptions include injuries such as an unstable labral tear, in which early operative repair is often indicated. Surgical intervention is most commonly required to address instability and secondary impingement. Given the atraumatic nature of the instability, frank labral pathology is uncommon although it does occur. Traditionally, open capsular tightening procedures, such as capsular shift, have been used in this group of athletes (37). More recently, arthroscopic techniques for capsular tightening have been developed and are being used with greater frequency by the author. Whether an arthroscopic or open technique is used, the principal factor is to address the underlying pathology.

Surgery is begun with a careful examination under anesthesia to document the degree and direction of laxity. A thorough arthroscopic inspection of the glenohumeral joint as well as the subacromial space is then performed. The posterior aspect of the glenohumeral joint should be examined via the anterior portal. Signs of capsular laxity, such as a positive drive-through sign, are noted. The biceps tendon and labral attachment are carefully examined. Distinct rotator cuff pathology is uncommon in this group, but may be present in the older athlete. There is often a thickened, inflamed subacromial bursa. The coracoacromial ligament is inspected for signs of wear, which is indicative of secondary impingement. The results of the examination under anesthesia, arthroscopic inspection, and the preoperative examination and imaging findings are all considered together to determine the treatment required.

Subacromial bursectomy is carried out using standard arthroscopic techniques. The coracoacromial ligament is recessed from its acromial attachment. Acromioplasty is only performed if there is an anteroinferior acromial osteophyte, which is uncommon in the young athlete with a diagnosis of primary instability. Labral debridement or repair is performed arthroscopically. I favor use of suture anchors with arthroscopic knot tying for labral fixation, but fixators such as the Suretac device have been used successfully. Capsular tightening is then addressed by either arthroscopic or open technique.

Open Capsular Repair

Open capsular shift allows the ability to selectively address capsular laxity. The most common direction of instability is anteroinferior; thus a standard anterior approach is used. Some athletes have a multidirectional component of instability; if there is similar laxity in both anterior and posterior directions, an anterior approach is recommended. If laxity is clearly greater in the posterior direction and the clinical examination is supportive of posterior instability, a posterior approach is used. With an anterior approach, I favor using a subscapularis split rather than subscapularis tenotomy, given the important role of the subscapularis muscle in the swimming stroke. The exception is when there is a large sulcus sign, which is often associated with a defect in the rotator interval capsule. In that setting, I use a subscapularis tenotomy if an open approach is being used, because this allows identification and closure of a rotator interval capsular defect. Rotator interval closure cannot be reliably performed through a subscapularis split through a deltopectoral approach. More recently, I have performed arthroscopic closure of the rotator interval capsule (described later).

If a posterior approach is used (uncommon), the infraspinatus tendon is split horizontally (analogous to a subscapularis split). This approach leaves the tendon attachment intact and the axillary nerve is at minimal risk in that the teres minor muscle lies between the nerve and the surgical exposure. The posterior capsule is dissected off of the infraspinatus muscle. A Gelpie retractor is used to spread the split in the infraspinatus and expose the underlying capsule. The humeral attachment of the infraspinatus tendon is left intact. The capsule is opened transversely in its mid aspect and then dissected from its glenoid attachment. A glenoid-based capsular shift is then performed by shifting the inferior capsular flap superiorly and medially, and then the superior capsular flap is shifted inferiorly and medially. The superior capsular flap partially overlaps the inferior flap, providing a two-layer repair. The capsule is repaired to the glenoid with suture anchors. The arm is maintained in neutral rotation and 30 degrees of abduction for the capsular repair. The infraspinatus tendon can be used to augment the repair if necessary by detaching the tendon from the infraspinatus muscle and suturing the tendon to the posterior capsule. This is rarely required in this group of athletes, and I favor maintaining the integrity of the infraspinatus muscle and tendon unit.

Arthroscopic Capsular Repair

In recent years, arthroscopic techniques for capsular tightening have been developed and are being used increasingly by the author. With an arthroscopic approach, the subscapularis can be left intact. I currently favor using sutures to plicate the capsule. The synovium overlying the capsule is lightly abraded to provide a bleeding surface to encourage healing. Arthroscopic suture passing instruments (e.g., Spectrum suture passer) are used to imbricate the capsule (Fig. 24-5). If there labral repair is also undertaken, the labral sutures can be passed through a "bite" of capsule, thereby advancing the capsule toward the glenoid. This also aids in recreating more of a "bumper" at the labral edge. If the labrum is well attached, as is typical in atraumatic instability, a bite of capsule is simply advanced up to the labral edge and sutured into the native labrum. This also aids in recreating a labral bumper. This is performed with the arm in adduction and neutral rotation with the patient in the beach chair position. The amount of capsular imbrication (size of the capsular bite) is determined by the degree of capsular laxity, as judged by the examination under anesthesia and the arthroscopic inspection. The capsule is usually imbricated by approximately 8 to 10 mm. The suturing is begun inferiorly (at approximately the 5-o'clock position in a right shoulder) in the inferior glenohumeral ligament. Care is taken to avoid taking an excessively large bite of capsule to minimize the risk of injury to the axillary nerve. Successive sutures are placed more superiorly. Typically, three such sutures are passed, followed by arthroscopic knot tying. Mobilization and advancement of the capsule may be facilitated by dissecting the capsule from the undersurface of the subscapularis tendon. This is done using a small elevator (such as a freer elevator) to first develop the interval between the middle glenohumeral ligament and subscapularis tendon, and then proceeding inferiorly to the inferior glenohumeral ligament. If this is done, a rotator interval capsular closure is often also performed (described later). The posterior capsule can be imbricated in a similar fashion. Further study is needed to determine the degree of capsular tightening that can be achieved with this arthroscopic technique. Basic science studies are also required to define the time required for adequate healing of a capsular imbrication performed in this manner.

Thermal capsulorrhaphy has also been used in swimmers. With this technique, heat energy (provided by laser or a radiofrequency device) is used to shorten the capsule. The improvement in stability appears to be due primarily to thickening and fibrosis of the capsule that occurs following the heat-induced injury, in addition to the shortening of the capsule achieved at the time of surgery. It is important to note that, following the heat treatment, the capsule has diminished stiffness compared to normal capsule and thus may be stretched out even beyond its initial length if not adequately protected from excessive loads (38). In my opinion, the principal drawback of thermal techniques is the unpredictability in capsular healing. Furthermore, higher failure rates have been reported for thermal treatment of the posterior capsule (39).

In patients with a large sulcus sign, which suggests a defect in the rotator interval capsule, this area of the capsule is also repaired. This is performed arthroscopically by passing an 18-gauge spinal needle through the superior capsule at the anterior edge of the supraspinatus tendon. A suture is passed through the spinal needle into the joint. An arthroscopic suture grasper (such as the Arthrex Penetrator) is

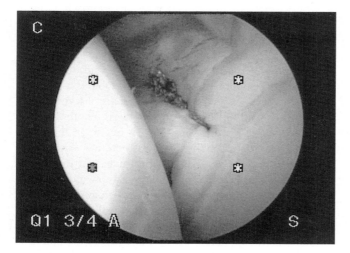

FIGURE 24-5. Imbricating sutures passed through the capsule using arthroscopic techniques.

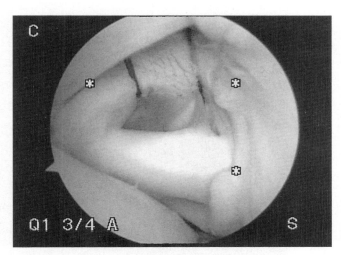

FIGURE 24-6. Sutures passed arthroscopically for closure/tightening of the rotator interval capsule.

then passed through the upper edge of the middle glenohumeral ligament via the lower anterior skin portal. This grasper retrieves the suture, which is then pulled out the anterior portal. Three such sets of sutures are passed, beginning laterally and working medially (Fig. 24-6). After all the sutures have been passed, they are tied on the bursal side of the rotator cuff. This can be done by placing the arthroscope into the subacromial space and retrieving the sutures. The inferior sutures can be difficult to retrieve with the arm at the side in neutral rotation. External rotation of the arm brings these sutures into view, but excessive external rotation should be avoided after suture plication of the anterior capsule. If there is difficulty tying the sutures arthroscopically in the subacromial space, then I have simplified this part of the procedure by enlarging the anterosuperior portal, directly retrieving the sutures with a finger in the subacromial space, and tying the sutures under direct vision.

Alternative methods to arthroscopically suture the rotator interval capsule have also been described. The rotator interval capsule can be plicated directly from the subacromial space. This is facilitated by placing the arm in forward elevation. The bursa is removed to allow visualization of the interval capsule. Care must be taken to avoid injuring the biceps tendon. Another technique has been described in which rotator interval suture placement and suture tying is performed all inside the joint by withdrawing the cannula just outside of the joint and then tying the sutures in a somewhat "blind" fashion (40). I have no experience with that technique.

Postoperative Rehabilitation

The overall rehabilitation framework is similar whether the capsular repair is performed via an open or an arthroscopic technique, because the capsule must be allowed to heal. A sling is used for 4 to 6 weeks. Gentle scapular plane elevation may be started within the first week within safe limits

as determined intraoperatively. Safe limits of external rotation (following anterior repair) and internal rotation (following posterior capsular plication) are determined intraoperatively. Cross-body adduction is avoided for the first 4 to 6 weeks after posterior capsular plication. In general, motion is limited for the first 3 to 4 weeks following capsular repair in swimmers. A slightly more aggressive program may be followed for the older athlete, whereas a more conservative program may be indicated for the younger swimmer with multidirectional instability. The goal is to establish full range of motion by 12 weeks postoperatively.

Gentle isometric exercises are begun within the first week of surgery. A progressive strengthening program with emphasis on the rotator cuff and scapular stabilizers is followed. Particular attention is paid to the serratus anterior, subscapularis, and teres minor muscles because of their importance in the swimming stroke (12). A well-structured rehabilitation program should focus on improving strength and, in particular, endurance of these muscles. The rehabilitation program typically begins with isometric exercises and then proceeds to variable-resistance exercises using Thera-Band. The program then advances to isotonic and isokinetic exercises (35). The primary goal is to develop muscle endurance. Attention should also be focused on restoration of normal proprioception.

The swimmer may get in the water at approximately 8 to 12 weeks postoperatively. At that time, some gentle sculling motions with the arms may be performed. Vertical kicking may also be performed. This helps the athlete begin to regain the "feel" for the water. No attempt is made to begin the freestyle stroke until there is full range of motion, which is usually around 12 weeks. Swimming training may gradually progress as the athlete develops increasing strength and endurance. It is important to have open communication between the coach, athlete, therapist, and physician during the return to swimming phase. Like after shoulder surgery in other sports, return to full function can take up to 1 year.

Results of Operative Treatment

There are no published series of the results of surgical treatment of shoulder problems in swimmers. Swimmers have been included in outcome studies of the surgical treatment of instability, labral pathology, and impingement in athletes, but no studies have focused exclusively on swimmers. Surgical treatment of other overhead athletes has been associated with variable rates of return to high level overhead activity. It is well recognized that not all athletes can return to their preoperative performance level after surgery. Older studies demonstrated poor results with respect to return to activities (41). However, some patients in these studies may have had undiagnosed microinstability that was not treated, accounting for the high failure rates. More recent studies of similar groups of athletes report higher rates of return to athletics (42). For example, McMaster reported successful results in swimmers undergoing surgery for labral injury (26). The implications of labral pathology and conditions such as internal impingement were not recognized in the past and may have accounted for the higher failure rates in previous studies. Accurate diagnosis and surgery directed at the pathology is expected to result in higher rates of success. Further studies are required to identify the factors that govern the return to high level, repetitive overhead activity in swimmers and other overhead athletes.

PREVENTION AND REHABILITATION

The information reviewed in this chapter makes it clear that a comprehensive program to develop strength, endurance, balance, and flexibility of the muscles is the most important way to prevent swimmer's shoulder. These exercises address three important areas: (a) the rotator cuff, (b) the muscles that stabilize the scapula, and (c) the muscles of the low back, abdomen, and pelvis that make up the "core" of the body. A comprehensive program for the shoulder and periscapular muscles is required, with emphasis placed on endurance training and strengthening for the serratus anterior, rhomboids, lower trapezius, and subscapularis (12). Each swimmer should be assessed to determine any strength, endurance, or flexibility deficit. This allows precise, effective exercise prescription. Strengthening exercises should be performed after swimming training or several hours before practice. These exercises should not be performed right before swimming training because this may fatigue these muscles before swimming.

The exercises that follow are recommended as a comprehensive program that the swimmer can perform with minimal equipment (43). For all of these exercises, the goal is to perform three sets of 2 minutes, with 30 seconds of rest

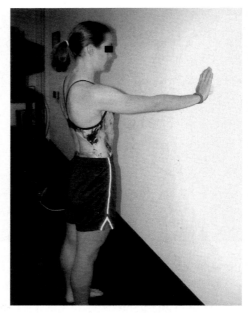

FIGURE 24-8. The "ball on the wall" exercise strengthens muscles that stabilize the scapula as well as the rotator cuff.

between sets. Initially, the athlete may fatigue before the 2-minute point.

Primary Rotator Cuff Exercises

1. External rotation using Thera-Bands. This is performed using a looped band to allow strengthening of both sides. The exercise is performed in a standing position. The scapulae should be maintained in retraction (the shoulders roll forward as the athlete fatigues).
2. "Full can" scaption (straight arm lifts) (Fig. 24-7). This exercise emphasizes the supraspinatus.
3. Ball on the wall (Fig. 24-8). This exercise strengthens muscles that stabilize the scapula as well as the rotator cuff.

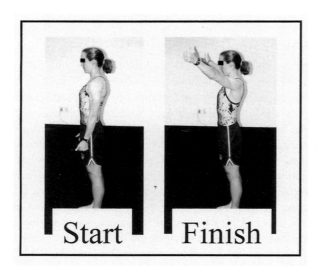

FIGURE 24-7. Straight arm lift exercises for the supraspinatus.

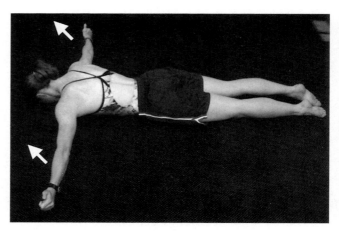

FIGURE 24-9. The "hitchhiker" exercise for the scapular stabilizers.

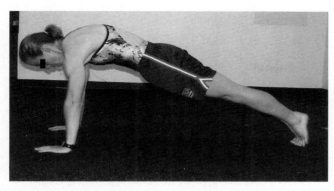

FIGURE 24-10. Push-ups with a plus. This exercise emphasizes the serratus anterior muscle.

Scapular Muscle Exercises

1. Seated rows using Thera-Band. A loop of Thera-Band is used. Emphasis is placed on maintaining scapular retraction.
2. Hitchhiker (Fig. 24-9). This exercise is performed lying on the stomach. Initially only the weight of the arm is used; as strength develops, 1- or 2-pound weights may be used.
3. Push-ups with a plus (Fig. 24-10). This exercise emphasizes the serratus anterior muscle. There is a progression to this exercise. It is first performed against a wall while standing, then on the knees, and finally in a traditional push-up position.

Abdominal and Lower Back Exercises

1. "Dead bug" exercise (Fig. 24-11). This exercise strengthens the abdominal muscles. The athlete lies on his or her back with hands under the pelvis. The back must be kept flat on the floor during this exercise. The athlete first performs a light "flutter kick" with the legs and can progress to a similar motion with the arms.
2. "Quadruped" (Fig. 24-12). This exercise emphasizes the lower back muscles. It is important to keep the back flat.

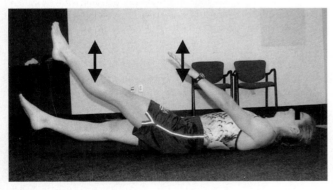

FIGURE 24-11. The "dead bug" exercise to strengthen the abdominal muscles.

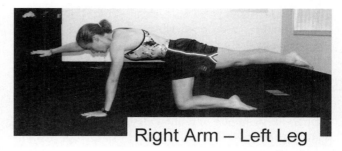

Right Arm – Left Leg

FIGURE 24-12. The "quadruped" exercise for the lower back.

The right arm and left leg are lifted and held for 1 second, and then the left arm and right leg are lifted. This alternating pattern is performed for 2 minutes or until the athlete fatigues. As strength develops, the exercise can be performed with the eyes closed, which emphasizes use of the postural muscles to a greater degree to develop balance and stability.

Stretching Exercises

Gentle stretching of the rotator cuff and periscapular muscles is reasonable, but aggressive stretching is usually not necessary. In particular, swimmers should generally avoid positions that stretch the anterior capsule. Such stretches can exacerbate shoulder laxity. Gentle stretching of the pectoralis major muscle and posterior capsule may be required. The hamstrings should also be stretched, because this muscle group plays an important role in controlling the position of the pelvis, which impacts body position and balance in the water. The upper trapezius muscle is often tight in swimmers; thus stretching of this muscle is incorporated into the flexibility program. In each of these exercises, the stretched position should be held for 30 seconds, with two or three repetitions performed.

FUTURE STUDY

There is a need for further study of the anatomic and pathologic basis of shoulder pain in swimmers. Current understanding of shoulder pain will be aided by identification of the relationship between shoulder pain and physical characteristics such as posture, glenohumeral laxity, scapular kinematics, and sternoclavicular joint and ribcage kinematics. Further study is needed to explore the relationship of shoulder pain to pathology in other areas. For example, further studies may define the relationship between back and shoulder injury and the role of sternoclavicular joint mobility and ribcage mechanics in swimmers with and without shoulder pain. We need to define the exact stroke mechanics that may lead to impingement and pain. This will aid in identification of the anatomic source of pain.

Further study should also explore the relationship of stroke alterations (e.g., a dropped elbow) with scapular motion and stretch of the anterior capsule. Because muscle overuse and resultant fatigue is associated with shoulder pain, there is a need to develop objective measures of muscle fatigue immediately after intense swimming. Further information in these areas will improve current understanding of shoulder pain in swimmers and allow design of improved rehabilitation and prevention programs, as well as improved surgical treatment.

REFERENCES

1. Pink MM, Tibone JE. The painful shoulder in the swimming athlete. *Orthop Clin North Am* 2000;31(2):247–261.
2. Richardson AB, Jobe FW, Collins HR. The shoulder in competitive swimming. *Am J Sports Med* 1980;8(3):159–163.
3. Kennedy JC, Hawkins R, Krissoff WB. Orthopaedic manifestations of swimming. *Am J Sports Med* 1978;6(6):309–322.
4. Dominguez R. Shoulder pain in age group swimmers. In: Erickson BFB, ed. *Swimming medicine IV.* Baltimore: University Park Press, 1978:105–109.
5. McMaster, WC, Troup J. A survey of interfering shoulder pain in United States competitive swimmers. *Am J Sports Med* 1993;21(1):67–70.
6. Yanai T, Hay JG, Miller GF. Shoulder impingement in front-crawl swimming: I. A method to identify impingement. *Med Sci Sports Exerc* 2000;32(1):21–29.
7. Yanai T, Hay JG. Shoulder impingement in front-crawl swimming: II. Analysis of stroking technique. *Med Sci Sports Exerc* 2000;32(1):30–40.
8. Magnusson SP, et al. Strength profiles and performance in Masters' level swimmers. *Am J Sports Med* 1995;23(5):626–631.
9. McMaster WC, Long SC, Caiozzo VJ. Shoulder torque changes in the swimming athlete. *Am J Sports Med* 1992;20(3):323–327.
10. Scovazzo ML, et al. The painful shoulder during freestyle swimming. An electromyographic cinematographic analysis of twelve muscles. *Am J Sports Med* 1991;19(6):577–582.
11. Bak K, Magnusson SP. Shoulder strength and range of motion in symptomatic and pain-free elite swimmers. *Am J Sports Med* 1997;25(4):454–459.
12. Pink M, et al. The normal shoulder during freestyle swimming. An electromyographic and cinematographic analysis of twelve muscles. *Am J Sports Med* 1991;19(6):569–576.
13. Pink M, et al. The painful shoulder during the butterfly stroke. An electromyographic and cinematographic analysis of twelve muscles. *Clin Orthop* 1993(288):60–72.
14. Nuber GW, et al. Fine wire electromyography analysis of muscles of the shoulder during swimming. *Am J Sports Med* 1986;14(1):7–11.
15. Maglischo E. *Swimming faster.* Mountain View, CA: Mayfield Publishing, 1982:53–99.
16. Richardson AR. The biomechanics of swimming: the shoulder and knee. *Clin Sports Med* 1986;5(1):103–113.
17. Schleihauf R Jr. A biomechanical analysis of freestyle. *Swim. Tech* 1974(11):89–96.
18. Hawkins RJ, Kennedy JC. Impingement syndrome in athletes. *Am J Sports Med* 1980;8(3):151–158.
19. Clarys JP, Rouard AH. The frontcrawl downsweep: shoulder protection and/or performance inhibition. *J Sports Med Phys Fitness* 1996;36(2):121–126.
20. Ruwe PA, et al. The normal and the painful shoulders during the breaststroke. Electromyographic and cinematographic analysis of twelve muscles. *Am J Sports Med* 1994;22(6):789–796.
21. Paletta GA Jr, et al. Shoulder kinematics with two-plane x-ray evaluation in patients with anterior instability or rotator cuff tearing. *J Shoulder Elbow Surg* 1997;6(6):516–527.
22. Rupp S, Berninger K, Hopf T. Shoulder problems in high level swimmers—impingement, anterior instability, muscular imbalance? *Int J Sports Med* 1995;16(8):557–562.
23. Zemek MJ, Magee DJ. Comparison of glenohumeral joint laxity in elite and recreational swimmers. *Clin J Sport Med* 1996;6(1):40–47.
24. Bak K, Faunl P. Clinical findings in competitive swimmers with shoulder pain. *Am J Sports Med* 1997;25(2):254–260.
25. McMaster WC, Roberts A, Stoddard T. A correlation between shoulder laxity and interfering pain in competitive swimmers. *Am J Sports Med* 1998;26(1):83–86.
26. McMaster WC. Anterior glenoid labrum damage: a painful lesion in swimmers. *Am J Sports Med* 1986;14(5):383–387.
27. Jobe FW, et al. An EMG analysis of the shoulder in throwing and pitching. A preliminary report. *Am J Sports Med* 1983;11(1):3–5.
28. Jobe FWG, et al. *Rotator cuff dysfunction and associated glenohumeral instability in the throwing athlete.* In: Paulos T, ed. *Operative techniques in shoulder surgery.* Gaithersburg, MD: Aspen, 1991.
29. Johnson JE, Sim FH, Scott SG. Musculoskeletal injuries in competitive swimmers. *Mayo Clin Proc* 1987;62(4):289–304.
30. Richardson AB. Orthopedic aspects of competitive swimming. *Clin Sports Med* 1987;6(3):639–645.
31. Blatz D. Upper arm strap. In: *Swimming world.* 1985:43–44.
32. Richardson AB. Overuse syndromes in baseball, tennis, gymnastics, and swimming. *Clin Sports Med* 1983;2(2):379–390.
33. McMaster WC. Shoulder injuries in competitive swimmers. *Clin Sports Med* 1999;18(2):349–359, vii.
34. Richardson AB. Thoracic outlet syndrome in aquatic athletes. *Clin Sports Med* 1999;18(2):361–378.
35. Scott SG. Current concepts in the rehabilitation of the injured athlete. *Mayo Clin Proc* 1984;59(2): 83–90.
36. Swanik KA, et al. The effects of shoulder plyometric training on proprioception and selected muscle performance characteristics. *J Shoulder Elbow Surg* 2002;11(6):579–586.
37. Neer CS 2nd, Foster CR. Inferior capsular shift for involuntary inferior and multidirectional instability of the shoulder. A preliminary report. *J Bone Joint Surg (Am)* 1980;62(6):897–908.
38. Schaefer SL, et al. Tissue shrinkage with the holmium:yttrium aluminum garnet laser. A postoperative assessment of tissue length, stiffness, and structure. *Am J Sports Med* 1997;25(6):841–848.
39. Hawkins RJ, Karas SG. Arthroscopic stabilization plus thermal capsulorrhaphy for anterior instability with and without Bankart lesions: the role of rehabilitation and immobilization. Instr Course Lect 2001;50:13–15.
40. Gartsman GM, Taverna E, Hammerman SM. Arthroscopic rotator interval repair in glenohumeral instability: description of an operative technique. *Arthroscopy* 1999;15(3):330–332.
41. Tibone JE, et al. Shoulder impingement syndrome in athletes treated by an anterior acromioplasty. *Clin Orthop* 1985(198):134–140.
42. Levitz CL, Dugas J, Andrews JR. The use of arthroscopic thermal capsulorrhaphy to treat internal impingement in baseball players. *Arthroscopy* 2001;17(6):573–577.
43. Rodeo S. Shoulder injury prevention: a series of exercises for the un-injured swimmer. *Coaches Q* 2002:2–18.

APPENDIX

Thrower's Ten Exercise Program

The Thrower's Ten Program is designed to exercise the major muscles necessary for throwing. The Program's goal is to be an organized and concise exercise program. In addition, all exercises included are specific to the thrower and are designed to improve strength, power and endurance of the shoulder complex musculature.

1A. **Diagonal Pattern D2 Extension:** Involved hand will grip tubing handle overhead and out to the side. Pull tubing down and across your body to the opposite side of leg. During the motion, lead with your thumb. Perform _____ sets of _____ repetitions _____ daily.

1B. **Diagonal Pattern D2 Flexion:** Gripping tubing handle in hand of involved arm, begin with arm out from side 45° and palm facing backward. After turning palm forward, proceed to flex elbow and bring arm up and over involved shoulder. Turn palm down and reverse to take arm to starting position. Exercise should be performed _____ sets of _____ repetitions _____ daily.

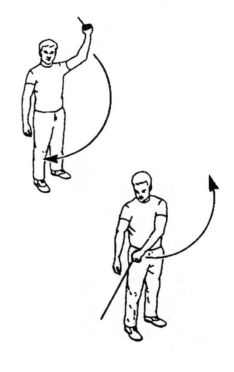

2A. **External Rotation at 0° Abduction:** Stand with involved elbow fixed at side, elbow at 90° and involved arm across front of body. Grip tubing handle while the other end of tubing is fixed. Pull out arm, keeping elbow at side. Return tubing slowly and controlled. Perform _____ sets of _____ repetitions _____ times daily.

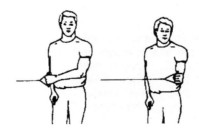

2B. **Internal Rotation at 0° Abduction:** Standing with elbow at side fixed at 90° and shoulder rotated out. Grip tubing handle while other end of tubing is fixed. Pull arm across body keeping elbow at side. Return tubing slowly and controlled. Perform _____ sets of _____ repetitions _____ times daily.

A

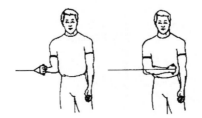

APPENDIX 7-1. Thrower's Ten-Exercise Program referred to in Chapter 7.

2C. (Optional) **External Rotation at 90°
Abduction:** Stand with shoulder abducted
90°. Grip tubing handle while the other end
is fixed straight ahead, slightly lower than
the shoulder. Keeping shoulder abducted,
rotate shoulder back keeping elbow at 90°.
Return tubing and hand to start position.
I. Slow Speed Sets: (Slow and Controlled)
Perform _____ sets of _____ repetitions
_____ times daily.
II. Fast Speed Sets: Perform _____ sets of
_____ repetitions _____ times daily.

2D. (Optional) **Internal Rotation at 90°
Abduction:** Stand with shoulder abducted
to 90°, externally rotated 90° and elbow bent
to 90°. Keeping shoulder abducted, rotate
shoulder forward, keeping elbow bent at 90°.
Return tubing and hand to start position.
I. Slow Speed Sets: (Slow and Controlled)
Perform _____ sets of _____ repetitions
_____ times daily.
II. Fast Speed Sets: Perform _____ sets of
_____ repetitions _____ times daily.

3. Shoulder Abduction to 90°: Stand with
arm at side, elbow straight, and palm
against side. Raise arm to the side, palm
down, until arm reaches 90° (shoulder level).
Perform _____ sets of _____ repetitions
_____ times daily.

4. Scaption, External Rotation: Stand
with elbow straight and thumb up. Raise
arm to shoulder level at 30° angle in front of
body. Do not go above shoulder height.
Hold 2 seconds and lower slowly. Perform
_____ sets of _____ repetitions _____ times
daily.

5. Sidelying External Rotation: Lie on
uninvolved side, with involved arm at side of
body and elbow bent to 90°. Keeping the
elbow of involved arm fixed to side, raise
arm. Hold seconds and lower slowly.
Perform _____ sets of _____ repetitions
_____ times daily.

APPENDIX 7-1. *(continued)*

6A.   Prone Horizontal Abduction (Neutral): Lie on table, face down, with involved arm hanging straight to the floor, and palm facing down. Raise arm out to the side, parallel to the floor. Hold 2 seconds and lower slowly. Perform _____ sets of _____ repetitions _____ times daily.

6B. Prone Horizontal Abduction (Full ER, 100° ABD): Lie on table face down, with involved arm hanging straight to the floor, and thumb rotated up (hitchhiker). Raise arm out to the side with arm slightly in front of shoulder, parallel to the floor. Hold 2 seconds and lower slowly. Perform _____ sets of _____ repetitions _____ times daily.

6C. Prone Rowing: Lying on your stomach with your involved arm hanging over the side of the table, dumbbell in hand and elbow straight. Slowly raise arm, bending elbow, and bring dumbbell as high as possible. Hold at the top for 2 seconds, then slowly lower. Perform _____ sets of _____ repetitions _____ times daily.

6D.   Prone Rowing into External Rotation: Lying on your stomach with your involved arm hanging over the side of the table, dumbbell in hand and elbow straight. Slowly raise arm, bending elbow, up to the level of the table. Pause one second. Then rotate shoulder upward until dumbbell is even with the table, keeping elbow at 90°. Hold at the top for 2 seconds, then slowly lower taking 2 – 3 seconds. Perform _____ sets of _____ repetitions _____ times daily.

7. Press-ups: Seated on a chair or table, place both hands firmly on the sides of the chair or table, palm down and fingers pointed outward. Hands should be placed equal with shoulders. Slowly push downward through the hands to elevate your body. Hold the elevated position for 2 seconds and lower body slowly. Perform _____ sets of _____ repetitions _____ times daily.

APPENDIX 7-1. *(continued)*

8. **Push-ups:** Start in the down position with arms in a comfortable position. Place hands no more than shoulder width apart. Push up as high as possible, rolling shoulders forward after elbows are straight. Start with a push-up into wall. Gradually progress to table top and eventually to floor as tolerable. Perform _____ sets of _____ repetitions _____ times daily.

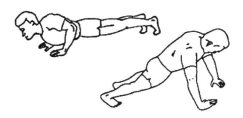

9A. **Elbow Flexion:** Standing with arm against side and palm facing inward, bend elbow upward turning palm up as you progress. Hold 2 seconds and lower slowly. Perform _____ sets of _____ repetitions _____ times daily.

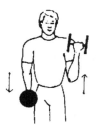

9B. **Elbow Extension (Abduction):** Raise involved arm overhead. Provide support at elbow from uninvolved hand. Straighten arm overhead. Hold 2 seconds and lower slowly. Perform _____ sets of _____ repetitions _____ times daily.

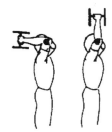

10A. **Wrist Extension:** Supporting the forearm and with palm facing downward, raise weight in hand as far as possible. Hold 2 seconds and lower slowly. Perform _____ sets of _____ repetitions _____ times daily.

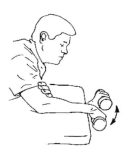

10B. **Wrist Flexion:** Supproting the forearm and with palm facing upward, lower a weight in hand as far as possible and then curl it up as high as possible. Hold for 2 seconds and lower slowly.

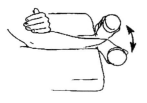

APPENDIX 7-1. *(continued)*

10C. **Supination:** Forearm supported on table with wrist in neutral position. Using a weight or hammer, roll wrist taking palm up. Hold for a 2 count and return to starting position. Perform _____ sets of _____ repetitions _____ times daily.

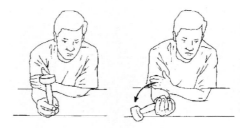

10D. **Pronation:** Forearm should be supported on a table with wrist in neutral position. Using a weight or hammer, roll wrist taking palm down. Hold for a 2 count and return to starting position. Perform _____ sets of _____ repetitions _____ times daily.

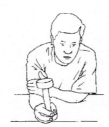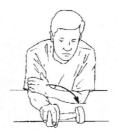

APPENDIX 7-1. *(continued)*

INDEX

Page numbers in *italics* indicate figures. Those followed by "t" indicate tables.

A

Abdominal exercises for swimmer, 361, *361*
Abduction arc sign, painful, *30*
Abduction test, resisted, 44
Acromioclavicular compression test, 32
Acromioclavicular distraction test, 32
Acromioclavicular joint disorders, 209–221
  acromioclavicular arthrosis, *216*
  acute injuries, 217, *217*
  anatomy, 209, *209*
  biomechanics, 210
  chronic injuries, 217–218
    operative technique, 218, *219*
  classification, 211
  coracoclavicular screw fixation, grade III
    injury, *217*
  degenerative disease, 218–220
  gracilis graft, suture placement, *219*
  grade II acromioclavicular injury,
    radiographic appearance, *213*
  grade III acromioclavicular injury, *213*
    deformity seen with, *213*
  grade V acromioclavicular joint injury,
    radiographic appearance of, *214*
  mechanism of injury, *210*, 210–211
  nonoperative treatment, 214–215
  operative treatment, 215–217
    arthroscopic distal clavicle excision,
      215, *215, 216*
    distal clavicle stabilization, 215–217
    technique, 217
  outstretched hand, fall on, injury from,
    210
  in pediatric athlete, 289, *289*
  physical examination, 211, *213*
  postoperative care, 217
  presentation, 211, *213*
  reconstructed joint, *219*
  separation, in football, 321–324, *322*
    authors' preferred approach, 323, *324*
    classification of, *322*
    rehabilitation, 323–324
  synovitis, imaging, *54*
  tenderness, 29
  in tennis, 342
  testing, 32
    acromioclavicular compression test,
      32
    acromioclavicular distraction test, 32
    active compression test, 32–33, *33*
  treatment, 214–217
  type IV, *290*
Acromioclavicular joint injection, 39, *39*

Acromioclavicular ligament, in football,
    autograft, allograft reconstruction, *324*
Acromion
  tenderness of, 29
  types of, *150*
Active compression test
  for acromioclavicular joint testing,
    32–33, *33,* 34
  throwing shoulder, 304
Adson's maneuver, 46, *46*
AMBRI, multidirectional instability, 186
American Orthopaedic Society for Sports
  Medicine, 8
American Shoulder and Elbow Surgeons, 8
  Standardized Shoulder Assessment and
    Shoulder Score Index of, 71–72
Anatomy of shoulder, 10–19
  acromioclavicular, with motion, 13
  capsuloligamentous, *12*, 12–13
  glenohumeral, with motion, 10–12
  injured shoulder, 16
  labral, *12*, 12–13
  normal shoulder, 14–16
  overhead athletics, 10–14
  pitching, throwing motion, stages of,
    14–16, *15*
  scapulothoracic, with motion, 13
  sternoclavicular, with motion, 13
  tennis, stages of, *18*, 18–19
Anterior capsular shift, multidirectional
  instability, *190*
Anterior capsulolabral reconstruction, *170*
Anterior instability, unidirectional, 163–185
  algorithm, treatment, 173t
  anatomy, 163–164, *164*
  anterior capsulolabral reconstruction, *170*
  biomechanics, 163–164, *164*
  capsular repair, with no labral
    detachment, technique, *171*
  classification of, 167–168, 168t
  complications, 172
  coracohumeral ligament, 163
  diagnostic evaluation, 166–167, *167*
  etiology of injury, 165
  historical review, 163–164
  inferior glenohumeral labral, 163
  middle glenohumeral ligament, 163
  nonoperative treatment, rehabilitation,
    results, 168, 168–169
  operative treatment, rehabilitation,
    results, 169–172, *170, 171,*
    172–175, 173t, *174*
  physical examination, 165, *166*

  pitch, muscle activity during stages of,
    164
  pitching baseball, phases of, *164*
  presentation, 165, *166*
  radiographic evaluation, 166–167, *167*
  relocation test, provocative component
    of, *166*
  superior glenohumeral ligament, 163
  throw, muscle activity during stages of,
    164
Anterior instability tests, throwing shoulder,
  304
Anterior labral tear, after intravenous
  gadolinium, *52*
Anterior tests, 41–43, *42*
  apprehension test, 41, *42*
  load and shift test, *42*, 42–43
  relocation test for instability, 41–42, *42*
  slide test, 34
Anteroposterior labrum injuries, in baseball,
  311
Apprehension test, *42*
Arc sign, painful abduction, 30, *30*
Archery, repetitive stressing of posterior
  capsule with, 177
Arm acceleration phase, pitching mechanics,
  301–302
Arm cocking phase, pitching mechanics,
  301
Arm deceleration phase, pitching
  mechanics, 302
Arthritis Impact Measurement Scale, 69
Arthroscopic debridement
  internal impingement, 130–131, *131*
  for internal impingement, 130–131, *131*
Arthroscopic distal clavicle excision, 215,
    215, 216
  acromioclavicular joint injury, 215, *215,
    216*
Arthroscopic evaluation of biceps tendon,
  200–202, *201*
Arthroscopic posterior, posterosuperior
  labral repair, 8
Arthroscopic rotator cuff repair, full
    thickness rotator cuff tears, 156–158,
    157
  patient positioning, *155*
Arthroscopic treatments
  multidirectional instability, 187–188,
    193, *193*
    historical overview, 187–188
  rotator cuff tears, full thickness rotator
    cuff tear, 156–158, *157*

Arthroscopic view of SLAP repair,
    completed repair, *8*
Arthroscopy
    capsular repair, swimming injury, *358,*
        358–359, *359*
    capsular shift, *193*
        multidirectional instability, *193*
    diagnostic
        full thickness rotator cuff tears, 155,
            156
        rotator cuff tears, full thickness, 155,
            156
    posterior, posterosuperior labral repair, *8*
Assessment of outcomes for treatment. *See*
    Outcome assessment
Athlete, overhead
    acromioclavicular joint disorders,
        209–221
    anatomy, 10–22
    axillary nerve injury, 270–272
    in baseball, 301–317
    biceps tendon disorders, 196–208
    biomechanics, during overhead motions,
        10–22
    clinical examination, 23–49
    decision-making in care of, 3–9
    in football, 318–339
    fractures, 236–266
    general population, contrasted, *3*
    imaging, 50–64
    instability of shoulder
        multidirectional, 186–195
        unidirectional anterior, 163–185
        unidirectional posterior, 177–185
    internal impingement, 125–134
    pathologic dilemma, 6, *6*
    pediatric, 284–298
    resistance training, 82–94
    rotator cuff tear
        full thickness, 146–162
        partial thickness, 135–145
    scapulothoracic problems, 222–235
    serratus anterior palsy, 275–277
    subacromial impingement, 146–162
    suprascapular neuropathy, 267–270
    in swimming, 349–362
    in tennis, 340–348
    throwing
        exercises for, 95–114
        interval program, 115–121
    trapezius dysfunction, 277–299
    treatment outcome assessment, 65–81
    vascular injury, 272–275
Athlete's Shoulder Assessment Tool, 79–80
Athletic Shoulder Outcome Rating Scale,
    77–78
Axillary artery, patent branches of, *271*
Axillary nerve injury, 270–272
    anatomy, 270
    authors' preferred method, 272
    diagnostic studies, 271, *271*
    etiology, 270
    historical overview, 270
    history, 270
    nonoperative management, 271
    operative management, 271–272

physical examination, 270
Axillary nerve palsy, in football, with deltoid
    atrophy, *326*

B
Backhand, in tennis, *18*
Backhand throw for distance, in testing of
    athlete, 92
Backstroke, abduction, external rotation
    during, *354*
"Bad cop" test. *See* Acromioclavicular
    distraction test
"Ball on wall" exercise, *360*
Bankart lesion
    glenohumeral instability, 60–61, *61*
    multidirectional instability, 186
Baseball, 301–317
    anterior instability tests, throwing
        shoulder, 304
    Bennett's lesion, *311*
    crank test, throwing shoulder, 304
    glenohumeral instability, 305–307, *307*
    history, 303t, 303–304, 304t
        in throwing shoulder, 303t
    internal impingement test, throwing
        shoulder, 304
    interval hitting program, 305t
    labrum injuries, 309
        anteroposterior labrum injuries, 311
        SLAP lesions, *309,* 309–311
        classification of, *310*
    Lemak test, throwing shoulder, 304
    Mimori test, throwing shoulder, 304
    neurovascular pathology, 312
        adolescent injuries, *314,* 314–315
        long thoracic nerve palsy, 314
        quadrilateral space syndrome, *313,*
            313–314
        suprascapular nerve entrapment, 313
        thoracic outlet syndrome, *312,* 312t,
            312–313
    O'Brien's test, throwing shoulder, 304
    physical examination, 303t, 303–304,
        304t
    pitching mechanics, 301–302, *302*
        arm acceleration phase, 301–302
        arm cocking phase, 301
        arm deceleration phase, 302
        stride, 301
        wind-up phase, 301
    pitching pathophysiology, 302–303,
        303t, 304t
    posterior glenoid exostosis, 311, *311*
    posterior instability test, throwing
        shoulder, 304
    rehabilitation, 304–305, 305t
    rotator cuff injuries, 308–309, *309*
    SLAP test, throwing shoulder, 304
    stability test, throwing shoulder, 304
    throwing shoulder, physical exam, 304t
    young baseball players, pitch limits in,
        315
Baseball pitch, phases of, *15*
Batting, repetitive stressing of posterior
    capsule with, 177
Belly-press test for weakness, 31, *32*

Bennett's lesion, *311*
    throwing shoulder, 110–111
Biceps tendon, 196–208
    arthroscopic evaluation, 200–202, *201*
    bicipital tenosynovitis, 201–203
    clinical evaluation, 197–198
    degenerative changes, 199–200, *200*
    degenerative lesions, 201–203
    dislocation, imaging, *59*
    imaging, 198–199
    inflammation, 199–200, *200*
    instability, *203,* 203–204, 204t
        subtle, vicious cycle in overhead
            throwers with, *201*
        treatment, 204
    long head
        anatomy, 196–197, *197*
        dislocation, types of, 204t
        function, 196–197, *197*
    Ludington's test, 33, *34*
    nonoperative treatment, 200
    pathophysiology of injuries, 199
    physical examination, 198
    sheath injection, 39, *39*
    SLAP lesions, 204, 204t
        treatment, 205–206, *206*
    Speed's test, 33, *33*
    surgical treatment, 200–203
    tear, *59*
    tenderness, 29
    Yergason's test, 33, *34*
Biceps tendonitis, in football, 334–336
    authors' preferred approach, 335, *335*
Bicipital tenosynovitis, 201–203
Biomechanics
    acromioclavicular, 13
    glenohumeral, 10–12
    of injuries in overhead athletes, 19
        instability, 19
        SLAP lesions, 19
    during overhead motions, 10–22
    pitching
        stages of, 14–16, *15*
        throwing motion, stages of, 14–16, *15*
    scapulothoracic, 13
        with motion, 13
    sternoclavicular, 13
        with motion, 13
    swimming motion, stages of, *17,* 17–18
    tennis, stages of, *18,* 18–19
    throwing motion, stages of, 14–16, *15*
Blade plate, AO, *255*
Boxing, repetitive stressing of posterior
    capsule with, 177
Brachial neuritis, 37, 45–46
Burners, 37
    brachial neuritis, 37
    thoracic outlet syndrome, 37

C
Calcific tendonitis, *57*
    imaging, *57*
Capsular repair, swimming injury,
    357–358
Capsulolabral reconstruction, for internal
    impingement, *131,* 131–132

Capsulorraphy, thermal, for internal impingement, 132
"Catching," as chief complaint, 46–47
Cervical spine pathology, pain secondary to, 35–36
  compression tests, 36
  distraction tests, 36
  "Neer relief" test, 36
  provocative tests, 36
  Spurling's test, 36, *36*
  Valsalva maneuver, 36
Clavicle, distal, osteolysis, in pediatric athlete, 289
Clavicle fracture, 240–243, *244*, 261–262, *329*, 329–330
  anatomy, 237
  distal, 25–258, *257*
    algorithms for treatment, 263
    classification of, *244*
    type II, *257, 329*
  midshaft, 2358
    algorithms for treatment, 263
  nonoperative shoulder conditioning therapy, 245t
  nonoperative treatment, rehabilitation, 246–247
  in pediatric athlete, 287–288, *288*
  postoperative shoulder conditioning, 259t
Clavicle resection, distal, tennis injury, *346*
Clinical examination, 23–49
  abduction test, resisted, 44
  acromioclavicular joint, 29
    as site of tenderness, 29
    tenderness, 29
    testing of, 32
      acromioclavicular compression test, 32
      acromioclavicular distraction test, 32
      active compression test, 32–33, *33*
  acromion, as site of tenderness, 29
  anterior tests, 41–43, *42*
    apprehension test, 41, *42*
    load and shift test, *42*, 42–43
    relocation test for instability, 41–42, *42*
  belly-press test for weakness, 31, *32*
  biceps tendon
    pathology (non-anchor related), 33–34
      Ludington's test, 33, *34*
      Speed's test, 33, *33*
      Yergason's test, 33, *34*
    as site of tenderness, 29
  brachial neuritis, 45–46
  burners, 37
    brachial neuritis, 37
    thoracic outlet syndrome, 37
  "catching," as chief complaint, 46–47
  cervical spine pathology, pain secondary to, 35–36
    compression and distraction tests, 36
    "Neer relief" test, 36
    provocative tests, 36
    Spurling's test, 36, *36*
    Valsalva maneuver, 36
  chief complaint, 25–27
  clinical course, 26–27

"clunking," as chief complaint, 46–47
Codman's point, *30*
"coming out of joint," as chief complaint, 40–41
  questions for patient, 26
coracoantecubital distance, for measurement of posterior capsular tightness, *48*
coracoid
  pain at, 35
  as site of tenderness, 29
degree of disability, 27
direct inspection of shoulder, *28*
elbow extension test, resisted, 44
elbow flexion test, resisted, 44
Erb's point, 29
  as site of tenderness, 29
external rotation, resisted, 31, *31*
finger abduction test, resisted, 44
forearm supination test, resisted, 44
full can test for weakness, 31, *31*
greater tuberosity tenderness, 29
Hawkins' sign, 30, *30*
"heaviness," as chief complaint, 44–46
injection tests, 38–40
  acromioclavicular joint injection, 39, *39*
  biceps tendon sheath injection, 39, *39*
  intraarticular glenohumeral joint injection, 40
  subacromial injection, 39, *39*
  subscapular injection, 40
  suprascapular nerve injection, 40
instability, 40–41
  examination of shoulder for, 41
  pain secondary to, 35
  pertinent questions, 41
internal rotation resisted strength test, 38
Jobe's test for weakness, 30–31, *31*
lag signs for weakness, 30
laxity, examination of shoulder for, 41
lesser tuberosity tenderness, 29
lift-off test for weakness, 31, *31*
"looseness," as chief complaint, 40–41
loss of control, 47–48
multidirectional instability, tests for, 43–44
muscle tests, shoulder, 44t
Neer impingement test, *25*
Neer's sign, 29–30, *30*
neurologic conditions, pain secondary to, 36–37
  suprascapular nerve compression, 37
neurologic levels in upper extremity, 45t
"noise," as chief complaint, 47
numbness, 46
of overhead athlete, 4
pain, 28–40, 29t
  common causes for, 29t
  common sites of, 29t
  descriptions of, 29t
  palpation to reproduce, 29, 29t, *30*
  provocative tests to reproduce, 29–32
  of uncertain origin, 38
painful abduction arc sign, 30, *30*
paresthesias, 46

past medical history, 27
patient history, principles of, 25–27
physical examination, principles of, 27–28, *28*
posterior capsule tenderness, 29
posterior tests, 43, *43*
  Jahnke test, 43, *44*
  push-pull test, 43, *43*
present injury, history of, 26–27
relocation test for pain, 35, *35*
  inferior sulcus test for pain, 35, *36*
  sulcus sign, *36*
rent test for weakness, 32
review of systems in, 27
scapular dyskinesia, pain in presence of, *37*, 37–38
  scapular stabilization test, 38, *38*
  scapular winging, *37*
shrug test, 44
SLAP tears, 34
  active compression test, *33*, 34
  anterior slide test, 34
  biceps load test, 34
  O'Driscoll's SLAP test, 34
  "SLAP" prehension test, 34
"slipping," 40–41
"stiffness," as chief complaint, 48, *48*
subacromial impingement, maneuvers producing, 29–30
subcoracoid impingement, 35
suprascapular nerve, 45
systems review, in clinical examination, 27
tenderness, common sites of, 29t
thoracic outlet syndrome, provocative maneuvers, 46
  Adson's maneuver, 46, *46*
  hyperabduction syndrome test, 46
  modified Adson's maneuver, *46*
  Wright's test, 46
tingling, as chief complaint, 46
"tiredness," as chief complaint, 44–46
velocity, loss of, as chief complaint, 47–48
weakness
  as chief complaint, 44–46
    muscle sources, 44, 44t
    scapular dyskinesia, 44–45
  neurologic sources of, 45, 45t
  tests for, 30–32, *31*
wrist extension test, resisted, 44
wrist flexion test, resisted, 44
Closed kinetic chain exercises, throwing shoulder, 99
Cloverleaf plate, modified, *254*
"Clunking," as chief complaint, 46–47
Coach's initial management of pain, algorithms for, 356
Codman's point, *30*. *See also* Greater tuberosity
"Coming out of joint," as chief complaint, 40–41
  questions for patient, 26
Communication with overhead athlete, 7
Contrast imaging, 52, *52*

Control of shoulder, loss of, 47–48
  as chief complaint, 47–48
Coracoantecubital distance, for
    measurement of posterior capsular
    tightness, *48*
Coracoclavicular ligament, autograft,
    allograft reconstruction, *324*
Coracoclavicular screw fixation, grade III
    injury, *217*
Coracohumeral ligament, 163
Coracoid, pain at, 29, 35
Core strength, modalities of, 88
Core strengthening, 82–94
  backhand throw for distance, in testing of
    athlete, 92
  bridging with knee extension, 90
  current concepts, 85–86, 86t
  "dead bug" progression, 90
  designing, 88–91
  elongation of muscle spindles, 91
  forehand throw for distance, in testing of
    athlete, 92
  global stabilizers, 89–90
    exercises for, 90, *90, 91*
  hamstring stretch, 83, *83*
  historical background, *83*, 83–85, *84, 85,*
    86
  "hooklying" position, *83*
  kinetic chain, 82
  knee-to-chest, 83
  local stabilizers, 89
    exercises for, 89, *89*
  lunges, 83
  McKenzie, Robin, MD, 84
    movements proposed by, 84–85
  medicine ball exercises for, *92*, 92–93, *93*
    backward throws, 93
    chest pass toss, 92
    double pump, 93
    power drops, 93
    pullover tosses, 92
    side tosses, 93
    sit-up toss, 92
    superman tosses, 93
  medicine ball weights, based on age,
    91t
  modalities of core strength, 88
  multifidus, assessing, facilitating, *87*,
    87–88
  object of core strengthening, 86–88
  overhead throw for distance, in testing of
    athlete, 92
  partial sit-up, 83, 90
  plyometric exercise, 91
  program of, 84–85, *85*
  progressive extension with pillows,
    85, *85*
  prone lying, 85, *85*
  prone press-ups, 85, *85*
  seated flexion, 83, *84*
  side-lying bridge, 90
  sport-specific, 91t, 91–94
  squat, 83
  stabilizing system, of local musculature,
    global stabilizing system of spine,
    differentiating, 85

stabilizing systems, muscular, 86t
standing extension, 85, *86*
standing lat pull-down, 90
strength, defined, 86
tennis player, testing, sample procedure,
    92
testing overhead athlete, sample
    procedure, 92
transversus abdominis, assessing,
    facilitating, 87
Williams, Paul, MD, 83
Williams Flexion Exercises, 83, 84
  lunges, *84*
  partial sit-up, *83*
  squat, *84*
Crank test, throwing shoulder, 304
"Crow hop" technique, throwing, with
    follow-through, *118*

D

"Dead bug" exercise, 90, 361
Deltoid contusion, in football, 325–327,
    326
  rehabilitation, 326–327
Differential directed approach to clinical
    examination, 23–49
  rationale for, 24–25, *25*
Direct inspection of shoulder, *28*
Disability, degree of, 27
Disease-specific outcome assessment tools,
    73–76
Dislocation of long head, biceps tendon,
    types of, 204t
Distal clavicle stabilization,
    acromioclavicular joint, 215–217
Distal clavicular edema, imaging, 55
Distance
  forehand throw for, in testing of athlete,
    92
  overhead throw for, in testing of athlete,
    92
Dyskinesis, scapular, 44–45
  bony posture, injury, 223
  classification of, 224–225, *225*
  clinical symptoms around scapula, 226
  effect of, 225–226
  elevation control, loss of, 225–226
  evaluation of, 226–228, *227, 228*
  factors creating, 223–224
  kinetic chain function, loss of, 226
  lateral scapular slide, *228*
  muscular alterations, 223–224
  one-leg stability series, *227*
  pain in presence of, *37*, 37–38
    scapular stabilization test, 38, *38*
    scapular winging, *37*
  protraction control, loss of, 225
  rehabilitation, 29–234, 230t, *231, 232,*
    233
  retraction control, loss of, 225
  scapular assistance test, *227*
  scapular retraction test, *227*
  soft tissue inflexibility, 224
  stable base, loss of, 226
  treatment, 228–229
  type I dyskinesis, *224*

type II dyskinesis, *225*
type III dyskinesis, *225*

E

Edema, distal clavicular, 55
Effect size, in assessment tools, 66
Elbow extension test, resisted, 44
Elbow flexion test, resisted, 44
Elongation of muscle spindles, 91
Ender rods, open reduction, internal
    fixation of fracture, *253*
Enders nail, *254*
Erb's point, as site of tenderness, 29
Evaluation of athlete's shoulder. *See* Clinical
    examination
Examination. *See* Clinical examination
Exostosis, thrower's. *See* Bennett's lesion
External rotation, resisted, 31, *31*

F

Finger abduction test, resisted, 44
First aid exercises. *See* Williams Flexion
    Exercises
Football, 318–339
  acromioclavicular joint separation,
    321–324, *322*
    authors' preferred approach, 323, *324*
    classification of, *322*
    rehabilitation, 323–324
  acromioclavicular ligament, autograft,
    allograft reconstruction, *324*
  axillary nerve palsy, with deltoid atrophy,
    326
  biceps tendonitis, 334–336
    authors' preferred approach, 335, *335*
  biomechanics, 318–320, *319*
  clavicle fracture, distal, type II, *329*
  coracoclavicular ligament, autograft,
    allograft reconstruction, *324*
  deltoid contusion, 325–327, *326*
    rehabilitation, 326–327
  etiology of injury, 320–321, 321t
  fractures, 330
    authors' preferred approach, 330
    proximal humerus, scapula, clavicle,
    329, 329–330
    rehabilitation, 330
  injuries, 321–336
  instability, biceps, 334–336
  kinematics, 318–320, *319*
  labrum, detached
    posterior inferior portal for repair of,
    333
    with suture anchor stabilization, *333*
  overhead football throw, phases of, *319*
  pectoralis major injury, 333–334
    authors' preferred approach, 334
  professional quarterbacks
    acromioclavicular joint injury, 321t
    clavicle injury, 321t
    injuries to shoulder, chest, 321t
  repetitive stressing of posterior capsule
    with, 177
  rotator cuff injury, 327–329
    authors' preferred approach, 328
    rehabilitation, 328–329

shoulder instability, 330–333
    authors' preferred approach, 332,
        333
    SLAP lesions, 334–336
    sternoclavicular joint separation,
        324–325
    authors' preferred approach, 325
    rehabilitation, 325
    subscapularis integrity, lift-off test, *335*
Forearm supination test, resisted, 44
Forehand, tennis, *18*
Forehand throw for distance, in testing of
    athlete, 92
Fractures, 236–266
    algorithms for treatment, 262–265
        distal clavicle fractures, 263
        humeral shaft fractures, 263–265, *265*
        midshaft clavicle fractures, 263
        proximal humerus fractures, *262*,
            262–263, *264*
    anatomy, 236–237
    biomechanics, 236–237
    blade plate, AO, *255*
    classification of injury, 240–243
    clavicle, 240–243, *244*, 261–262
        anatomy, 237
        biomechanics, 237
        distal, 25–258, *257*
            classification of, *244*
            type II, *257*
        midshaft, 2358
        nonoperative shoulder conditioning
            therapy, 245t
        postoperative shoulder conditioning,
            259t
    cloverleaf plate, modified, *254*
    complications, 260–262
        humerus fractures, proximal, 260–261
    diagnosis, 238–239, *239–240*
    Enders nail, *254*
    etiology of injury, 237–238
    in football, 330
    humerus, proximal, 240, *241*, 242–243,
        245
        anatomy, 236–237
        AO/ASIF classification, *242–243*
        closed reduction, *262*
        four-part valgus impacted, *243*
        Neer classification, *241*
        ORIF, postoperative shoulder
            conditioning, 260t
        percutaneous pinning, postoperative
            shoulder conditioning, 260t
    nonoperative treatment, rehabilitation,
        244–247, 245t, 246t
        clavicle fractures, 246–247
        humerus fractures, proximal, 246
        spiral humerus shaft fractures, 247
    open reduction, internal fixation, with
        modified Ender rods, *253*
    operative treatment, rehabilitation,
        247–258
        humerus fractures, proximal, 2
            47–257
            intramedullary nailing techniques,
                255–257, *256*

open reduction, internal fixation
    techniques, 250–255, *251*, *252*,
    253, *254*, *255*
percutaneous fixation techniques,
    248, 248–249, *249*, *250*
percutaneous fixation, using terminally
    threaded AO pins, *248*
physical examination, 238
Polarus nail, *256*
postoperative rehabilitation, 258–260,
    259t, 260t
presentation, 238
radiographic evaluation, 238–239,
    239–240
    axillary views, *239*
shoulder girdle fractures, three-phase
    shoulder conditioning, 259t
spiral humeral shaft, 258
    fracture bracing, *265*
stable, nondisplaced shoulder fractures,
    nonoperative shoulder conditioning
    therapy for, 246t
tension band technique, *252*
valgus-impacted four-part fracture, open
    reduction, internal fixation, *251*
Freestyle stroke
    pull-through phase of, stages of, *17*
    recovery phase of, *350*
Full can test for weakness, 31, *31*
Full thickness rotator cuff tears, 56–58, *57*,
    146–162
    algorithms for treatment, 154–161
    classification system, 152, 152t
    nonoperative treatment, 154
    operative treatment, 153–154, 154–158
        arthroscopic, 156–157, *157*, 158
        diagnostic arthroscopy, 155, *156*
        patient positioning for arthroscopic
            surgery, *155*
        portal placement, 154–155
        preoperative preparation, 154, *155*
        surgical procedure, 155–156, *156*
    rehabilitation, 157t, 158t, 158–161, *159*,
        159t, 161t
        phase 1, 158t
        phase 2, 159t
        phase 3, 161t
    rotator cuff disease, classification of, 152t
    Snyder classification of rotator cuff tears,
        152t
    treatment techniques, 154–161

G
Gadolinium, intravenous, anterior labral
    tear after, *52*
General health assessment scale, 66–69
    Arthritis Impact Measurement Scale, 69
    Nottingham Health Profile, 69
    Sickness Impact Profile, 69
    Standard Form 36 Questionnaire, 66–69
General population shoulder, shoulder of
    athlete, contrasted, *3*
GLAD lesions, glenolabral articular
    disruption, 61
Glenohumeral capsule, 285
Glenohumeral dislocation, anterior, *293*

Glenohumeral injection, intraarticular, 40
Glenohumeral instability
    in baseball, 305–307, *307*
    imaging, 60–62
        anatomic lesions of instability, 60–62
        anatomy, 60
        Bankart lesions, 60–61, *61*
        GLAD lesions, glenolabral articular
            disruption, 61
        HAGL lesions, 61
        Hill-Sachs lesions, 61
        Perthes lesions, 61, *61*
        posterior lesions, 61–62, *62*
    in pediatric athlete, 292–293, *293*
Glenohumeral ligament, inferior, humeral
    avulsion of, imaging, 61
Glenoid exostosis, posterior, in baseball,
    311, *311*
Glenoid impingement, posterosuperior,
    throwing shoulder, 108
Glenoid (internal) impingement, posterior
    superior, *55*
Global shoulder assessment tools, 69t,
    69–73, 70t
    American Shoulder and Elbow Surgeons
        Standardized Shoulder Assessment
        and Shoulder Score Index, 71–72
Global stabilizers, 89–90
    exercises for, 90, *90*, *91*
    spine, local musculature, differentiating,
        85
Golf, repetitive stressing of posterior capsule
    with, 177
Gracilis graft, suture placement,
    acromioclavicular joint, *219*
Greater tuberosity tenderness, 29
Ground strokes, tennis, *18*
"Gunslinger" brace, *183*
Gymnastics, repetitive stressing of posterior
    capsule with, 177

H
HAGL lesions, 61
Hamstring stretch, 83
Hand, outstretched, fall on,
    acromioclavicular joint injury, *210*
Hawkins' sign, 30, *30*
Hawkins test for impingement, *147*
"Heaviness," as chief complaint, 44–46
Hill-Sachs lesions, 61
Hitchhiker exercise, 361
"Hooklying" position, *83*
"Hornblower's sign." *See* Signe de clarion
Humeral avulsion, inferior glenohumeral
    ligament, 61
Humeral physis, proximal, *285*
Humerus
    fracture, *329*, 329–330
        in pediatric athlete, *291*
        proximal, fracture, 240, *241*, *242–243*,
            245, 247–257, 260–261, *262*,
            262–263, *264*, *329*, 329–330
            anatomy, biomechanics, 236–237
            AO/ASIF classification, *242–243*
            closed reduction, *262*
            four-part valgus impacted, *243*

Humerus, proximal, fracture (*contd.*)
  intramedullary nailing techniques,
      255–257, *256*
  Neer classification, *241*
  nonoperative treatment, rehabilitation,
      246
  open reduction, internal fixation
      techniques, 250–255, *251, 252,
      253, 254, 255*
  ORIF, postoperative shoulder
      conditioning, 260t
  percutaneous fixation techniques, *248,*
      248–249, *249, 250*
  percutaneous pinning, postoperative
      shoulder conditioning, 260t
  shaft, fracture
      algorithms for treatment, 263–265,
          265
      spiral, 258
          bracing, *265*
          nonoperative treatment,
              rehabilitation, 247
Hyperabduction syndrome test, 46
Hyperangulation during overhead throwing
    motion, *96*

I

Imaging, 50–64
  acromioclavicular joint synovitis, *54*
  biceps tendon dislocation, *59*
  calcific tendonitis, *57*
  contrast imaging, 52, *52*
  distal clavicular edema, *55*
  gadolinium, intravenous, anterior labral
      tear after, *52*
  glenohumeral instability, 60–62
      anatomic lesions of instability, 60–62
      anatomy, 60
      Bankart lesions, 60–61, *61*
      GLAD lesions, glenolabral articular
          disruption, 61
      HAGL lesions, 61
      Hill-Sachs lesions, 61
      Perthes lesions, 61, *61*
      posterior lesions, 61–62, *62*
  inferior glenohumeral ligament, humeral
      avulsion of, 61
  labral capsular disruption, 62
  labral tears, acute, chronic, *61*
  latissimus dorsi injury, 63
  long biceps tendon tear, *59*
  microinstability, 63
      peel-back SLAP lesions, 63
      SLAC lesion, 63
  MR arthrography, 52, *52*
  MRI
      general, 51
      specific, 51–52
  osseous acromial outlet, *53,* 53–54, *54, 55*
  of overhead athlete, 5
  partial articular surface supraspinatus
      tendon tear, *57*
  posterior labral tear, *62*
  posterior superior glenoid (internal)
      impingement, *55*
  posterolateral rotator cuff tear, *57*
  radiographic evaluation, 50–51
  reverse Bankart, 62
  reverse Hill-Sachs, 62
  rotator cuff, 54–58
      full thickness tears, 56–58, *57*
      impingement syndromes, 54–56, *55*
      partial thickness tears, 56, *57*
      posterolateral, tendinosis of, *56*
      tendinosis, 56, *56, 57*
  rotator interval, 58–60
      injuries to, *58,* 58–60, *59*
  SLAP lesion, *62,* 62–63
      paralabral cyst, 63, *63*
          with denervation changes, *63*
  subscapularis tendon tear, *59*
Impingement, 125–134
  conservative treatment, 129–130
  differential diagnosis, 127–128
  etiology, *126,* 126–127
  history, 128–129
  initial treatment, 129–130
  outcome analysis following surgery,
      grading scale, 139t
  physical examination, 128–129
  in pitcher
      professional, shoulder rotation, *125*
      throwing properly, *130*
  posterosuperior glenoid, throwing
      shoulder exercises, 108
  subacromial, 146–162, *147*
      acromion, types of, *150*
      classification of, 150, 150t
      diagnostic evaluation, *148,* 148–150,
          149, 150
      etiology of injury, 146
      Hawkins test for impingement, *147*
      lift-off test for subscapularis strength,
          148
      maneuvers producing, 29–30
      Neer classification, 150t
          phase 1 (protective), 151
          phase 2 (progressive strengthening),
              151
      nonoperative treatment of, 150–151
      operative treatment of, 151–152
      physical examination, 146–148, *147,*
          148
      presentation, 146–148, *147, 148*
      radiographic evaluation, *148,*
          148–150, *149, 150*
      signe de clarion, 147
      throwing shoulder exercises, 108–109,
          109
      treatment of, 150–152
  subcoracoid, 35
  surgical treatment, 130
      arthroscopic debridement, 130–131,
          131
      capsulolabral reconstruction, *131,*
          131–132
      rotational osteotomy, 132, *132,* 133
      subacromial decompression, 133
      thermal capsulorrhaphy, 132
  during swimming stroke, 350, *350*
  tennis injury, *342*
Impingement syndromes, 54–56, *55*
Impingement test, 304
  Neer, 25, *147*
  throwing shoulder, 304
Inferior sulcus test for pain, 35, *36*
Inflammation, biceps tendon, 199–200, *200*
Injection tests, 38–40
  acromioclavicular joint injection, 39, *39*
  biceps tendon sheath injection, 39, *39*
  intraarticular glenohumeral joint
      injection, 40
  subacromial injection, 39, *39*
  subscapular injection, 40
  suprascapular nerve injection, 40
Injections, in imaging, 5
Instability, 40–41
  biceps, 334–336
      tendon
          cycle in overhead throwers with, *201*
          treatment, 204
  diagnosis of, 4–5
  examination of shoulder for, 41
  in football, 330–333
      authors' preferred approach, 332, *333*
  multidirectional, 186–195
      AMBRI, 186
      Bankart lesion, 186
      diagnosis, 188–189
      historical overview, 187–188
          arthroscopic surgical treatment,
              187–188
          nonoperative treatment, 187
          open surgical treatment, 187–188
      postoperative care, 194, *194*
      prefabricated orthosis, *194*
      prognosis, 194
      surgical failures, 194–195
      surgical treatment, 189–193
          anterior capsular shift, *190*
          arthroscopic capsular shift, *193*
          arthroscopic techniques, 193, *193*
          open inferior capsular shift, *189,*
              189–191, *190, 191*
          posterior capsular shift, 191–193,
              192, 193
      TUBS, 186
  pertinent questions, 41
  posterior, unidirectional, 177–185
      algorithms for treatment, 180–183,
          181, 182, 183
      anatomy, 177–178
      biomechanics, 177–178
      capsular plication
          bumper effect, *181*
          pinch, tuck method, *182*
      classification, 178–179
      complications, 183–184
      diagnostic evaluation, 179–180
      etiology of injury, 178–179
      "gunslinger" brace, *183*
      historical overview, 177, 177t
      laxity, posterior capsular, *181*
      nonoperative treatment, rehabilitation,
          results, 180
      operative treatment, rehabilitation,
          results, 180
      physical examination, 179, *179*

plication, posterior capsular, with recreation of bumper effect, *181*
posterior capsule, athletic activities repetitively stressing, 177t
posterior portal closure, *182*
presentation, 179, *179*
radiographic evaluation, 179–180
voluntary posterior instability, *179*
relocation test for, 41–42, *42*
in tennis, 342
throwing shoulder, rehabilitation guidelines, 110
Internal rotation resisted strength test, 38
Interval hitting program, 305t
Interval throwing program, 115–121
criteria for entry into, 116, 116t
"crow hop" technique, with follow-through, *118*
exercise variables, controlling, 116–117, 117t
flat ground work, *119*
nonsurgical mound work, 120
nonsurgical *versus* postsurgical approach, 116
phase I, 100t
long toss, 117t, 117–119
phase II
flat ground work, 119
throwing off mound, 106t
phase III, progressive mound work, 119
phase IV, simulated game activity, 120
phase V, game progression, 120–121
phase VI, maintenance with return to play, 121
postsurgical mound work, 119–120, *120*
postsurgical positional throw, 120
problem-based modification of, 116t
progressive mound work, *120*
sequencing for rehabilitation program, 117t
time frames for initiation of, after surgical procedure, 115t
Intraarticular glenohumeral joint injection, 40
IRRST. *See* Internal Rotation Resisted Strength Test
Isokinetic shoulder strength criteria, 98t

J

Jahnke test, 43, *44*
Jerk test. *See* Jahnke test
Jobe's test for weakness, 30–31, *31*

K

Kinetic chain, 82

L

Labral capsular disruption, imaging, 62
Labral tear
acute, chronic, *61*
anterior, after intravenous gadolinium, *52*
posterior, *62*
Labrum
detached
posterior inferior portal for repair of, *333*

with suture anchor stabilization, *333*
superior, SLAP tear, in tennis, *347*
Labrum injuries in baseball, 309
anteroposterior labrum injuries, 311
SLAP lesions, *309*, 309–311
classification of, *310*
Lag signs for weakness, 32
Lateral scapular slide, *228*
Lateral tubing pull, scapulothoracic rehabilitation, *231*
Latissimus dorsi injury, imaging, 63
Laxity, 285–286, 286t
examination of shoulder for, 41
overhead athlete, 97
posterior capsular, *181*
Lemak test, throwing shoulder, 304
Lesions in overhead athlete, 122–298
acromioclavicular joint disorders, 209–221
anterior instability, unidirectional, 163–185
biceps tendon, disorders of, 196–208
fractures, 236–266
internal impingement, 125–134
multidirectional instability, 186–195
neurologic lesions, 267–283
pediatric athletes, 284–298
posterior instability, unidirectional, 177–185
rotator cuff tears
full thickness, 146–162
partial thickness, surgical treatment of, 135–145
scapulothoracic problems, 222–235
subacromial impingement, 146–162
vascular lesions, 267–283
Lesser tuberosity tenderness, 29
Lift-off test, 31, *31*, *148*
Little League shoulder, 289–290, *290*, *291*
Load and shift test, *42*, 42–43
Local musculature, stabilizing system of, global stabilizing system of spine, differentiating, 85
Local stabilizers, 89
exercises for, 89, *89*
Long biceps tendon tear, imaging, *59*
Long thoracic nerve palsy, in baseball, 314
"Looseness," as chief complaint, 40–41
Lower back exercises, for swimmer, 361, *361*
Ludington's test, 33, *34*

M

Magnetic resonance arthrography, use of, 52, *52*
McKenzie, Robin, MD, 84
movements proposed by, 84–85
Medicine ball exercises for core strengthening, *92*, 92–93, *93*
backward throws, 93
chest pass toss, 92
double pump, 93
power drops, 93
pullover tosses, 92
side tosses, 93
sit-up toss, 92

superman tosses, 93
Medicine ball weights, based on age, 91t
Microinstability, imaging, 63
peel-back SLAP lesions, 63
SLAC lesion, 63
Mimori test, throwing shoulder, 304
MRI
general, 51
specific, 51–52
Multidirectional instability, 186–195
AMBRI, 186
Bankart lesion, 186
diagnosis, 188–189
historical overview, 187–188
arthroscopic surgical treatment, 187–188
nonoperative treatment, 187
open surgical treatment, 187–188
postoperative care, 194, *194*
prefabricated orthosis, *194*
prognosis, 194
surgical failures, 194–195
surgical treatment, 189–193
anterior capsular shift, *190*
arthroscopic capsular shift, *193*
arthroscopic techniques, 193, *193*
open inferior capsular shift, *189*, 189–191, *190*, *191*
posterior capsular shift, 191–193, *192*, *193*
tests for, 43–44
TUBS, 186
Multifidus, assessing, facilitating, *87*, 87–88
Muscle spindles, elongation of, 91
Muscle tests, shoulder, 44t
Muscular stabilizing systems, 86t

N

Neer classification of subacromial impingement, 150t
phase 1 (protective), 151
phase 2 (progressive strengthening), 151
Neer impingement test, *25*, *147*
"Neer relief" test, 36
Neer's sign, 29–30, *30*
Neuritis, brachial, 37, 45–46
Neurologic conditions, pain secondary to, 36–37
suprascapular nerve compression, 37
Neurologic lesions, 267–283
Neurologic levels in upper extremity, 45t
Neurovascular pathology, in baseball, 312
adolescent injuries, *314*, 314–315
long thoracic nerve palsy, 314
quadrilateral space syndrome, *313*, 313–314
suprascapular nerve entrapment, 313
thoracic outlet syndrome, *312*, 312t, 312–313
"Noise," as chief complaint, 47
Nondisplaced shoulder fracture, nonoperative shoulder conditioning therapy for, 246t

Nottingham Health Profile, 69
Numbness, 46

O

O'Brien's test. *See* Active compression test
O'Driscoll's SLAP test, 34
One-leg stability series, with scapulothoracic
    problems, *227*
Open inferior capsular shift,
    multidirectional instability, *189*,
    189–191, *190, 191*
Os acromiale, in pediatric athlete, *294*
Osseous acromial outlet, imaging, *53*,
    53–54, *54, 55*
Osteolysis
    distal clavicle, in pediatric athlete, 289
Osteotomy, rotational, for internal
    impingement, 132, *132, 133*
Outcome assessment, 8, 65–81
    effect size, 66
    general health assessment scale, 66–69
        Arthritis Impact Measurement Scale,
            69
        Nottingham Health Profile, 69
        Sickness Impact Profile, 69
        Standard Form 36 Questionnaire,
            66–69
    global shoulder assessment tools, 69t,
        69–73, 70t
        American Shoulder and Elbow
            Surgeons Standardized Shoulder
            Assessment and Shoulder Score
            Index, 71–72
    overview, 65
    population/disease-specific assessment
        tools, 73–76
        Athlete's Shoulder Assessment Tool,
            79–80
        Athletic Shoulder Outcome Rating
            Scale, 77–78
        Rowe Score for Evaluating Bankart
            Operation, 73, 74
        Western Ontario Shoulder Instability
            Index, 73, 75–76
    relative efficiency, 66
    reliability of, 65–66
    responsiveness of, 65–66
    standard response mean, 66
    tools for, hierarchy of, 66, 66t
    validity of, 65–66
Outstretched hand, fall on, injury from,
    acromioclavicular joint, *210*
Overhead athlete
    acromioclavicular joint disorders,
        209–221
    anatomy, 10–22
    axillary nerve injury, 270–272
    in baseball, 301–317
    biceps tendon disorders, 196–208
    biomechanics, during overhead motions,
        10–22
    clinical examination, 23–49
    decision-making, in care of, 3–9
    in football, 318–339
    fractures, 236–266
    general population, contrasted, *3*

imaging, 50–64
instability of shoulder
    unidirectional anterior, 163–185
    unidirectional posterior, 177–185
    internal impingement, 125–134
    multidirectional instability, shoulder,
        186–195
    pathologic dilemma, 6, *6*
    pediatric, 284–298
    resistance training, 82–94
    rotator cuff tear
        full thickness, 146–162
        partial thickness, 135–145
    scapulothoracic problems, 222–235
    serratus anterior palsy, 275–277
    subacromial impingement, 146–162
    suprascapular neuropathy, 267–270
    in swimming, 349–362
    in tennis, 340–348
    throwing
        exercises for, 95–114
        interval program, 115–121
    trapezius dysfunction, 277–299
    treatment outcome assessment, 65–81
    vascular injury, 272–275
Overhead football throw, phases of, *319*
Overhead throw for distance, in testing of
    athlete, 92
Overuse syndrome tendinitis, throwing
    shoulder, 108–110

P

Pain, 28–40, 29t
    causes for, 29t
    common sites of, 29t
    descriptions of, 29t
    inferior sulcus test for, 35, *36*
    palpation to reproduce, 29, 29t, *30*
    provocative tests to reproduce, 29–32
    relocation test for
        inferior sulcus test for pain, 35, *36*
        sulcus sign, *36*
    secondary to cervical spine pathology,
        distraction tests, 36
    secondary to instability, 35
    secondary to neurologic conditions,
        36–37
    suprascapular nerve compression, 37
    sites of, 29t
    of uncertain origin, 38
Painful abduction arc sign, 30, *30*
PAINT lesions. *See* Posterior articular
    surface intratendinous rotator cuff
Palpation to reproduce pain, 29, 29t, *30*
Palsy
    axillary nerve, in football, with deltoid
        atrophy, *326*
    serratus anterior, 275–277
Paralabral cyst, with denervation changes,
    63
Paralabral cysts, 63, *63*
Paresthesias, 46
Posterior articular surface intratendinous
    rotator cuff lesions, 135–137, *136*
Partial articular surface supraspinatus
    tendon tear, imaging, *57*

Partial thickness rotator cuff tears, 56, *57*
    surgical treatment, 135–145
        articular-surface rotator cuff tears,
            treatment algorithm, *138*
        depth, width, delamination grading
            scale, for outcome analysis, 139t
        magnetic resonance imaging, 139, *139*
        multiply injured thrower's shoulder
            structures, treatment of, 140t
        posterior articular surface
            intratendinous rotator cuff lesions
            (PAINT lesions), 135–137, *136*
        pathomechanics, 135
        postoperative protocol, 143
        surgical technique, 139–143, *140*,
            140t, *141, 142, 143*
        treatment, 137–138, *138*, 139t
Past medical history, use of in clinical
    examination, 27
Pathologic dilemma, in overhead athlete, 6,
    6
Patient examination. *See* Clinical
    examination
Patient history, principles of, 25–27
Pectoralis major injury, in football, 333–334
    authors' preferred approach, 334
Pediatric athletes, 284–298
    acromioclavicular joint injury, 289, *289*
        type IV, *290*
    adolescent tennis player, 347
    baseball injuries, *314*, 314–315
    clavicle fracture, 287–288, *288*
    developmental anatomy, 284–286, *285*
    epidemiology, 286–287
    glenohumeral dislocation, anterior, *293*
    glenohumeral instability, 292–293, *293*
    glenohumeral joint capsule, *285*
    humeral physis, proximal, *285*
    humerus fracture, proximal, *291*,
        291–292, *292*
    injury patterns, 286–287
    laxity, 285–286, 286t
    Little League shoulder, 289–290, *290*,
        291
    maturation, 285–286, 286t
    os acromiale, *294*
    osteolysis of distal clavicle, 289
    prevention, 294–295
    rotator cuff injury, 294, *294*
    scapula, ossification centers of, *285*
    scapulothoracic dysfunction, 294
    sternoclavicular joint injury, 287, *287*
    Tanner staging classification, secondary
        sexual characteristics, 286t
    young baseball players, pitch limits in,
        315
Peel-back SLAP lesions, 63
Perthes lesions, 61, *61*
Physical characteristics of overhead athlete,
    96–98
    laxity, 97
    muscle strength, 97–98, 98t
    proprioception, 98
    range of motion, 96–97
Physical examination, principles of, 27–28,
    28

Physical signs, diagnosing, 5
Pillows, progressive extension with, 85, *85*
Pinch and tuck method, capsular plication, *182*
Pitch
  baseball, phases of, *15*
  muscle activity during stages of, *164*
  phases of, *164*
Pitch limits, in young baseball players, 315
Pitcher
  shoulder rotation, *125*
  throwing properly, *130*
Pitching, repetitive stressing of posterior capsule with, 177
Pitching mechanics, 301–302, *302*
  arm acceleration phase, 301–302
  arm cocking phase, 301
  arm deceleration phase, 302
  stride, 301
  wind-up phase, 301
Pitching motion, stages of, with electromyographic data, 14–16, *15*
Pitching pathophysiology, 302–303, 303t, 304t
Plication, posterior capsular, with recreation of bumper effect, *181*
Plyometric exercise, 91
Polarus nail, *256*
Population-specific assessment tools, 73–76
  Athlete's Shoulder Assessment Tool, 79–80
  Athletic Shoulder Outcome Rating Scale, 77–78
  Rowe Score for Evaluating Bankart Operation, 73, *74*
  Western Ontario Shoulder Instability Index, 73, 75–76
Posterior, posterosuperior labral repair, arthroscopic, *8*
Posterior capsular shift, multidirectional instability, 191–193, *192, 193*
Posterior capsular tightness, coracoantecubital distance, for measurement of, *48*
Posterior capsule, athletic activities repetitively stressing, 177t
Posterior capsule tenderness, 29
Posterior glenoid exostosis, in baseball, 311, *311*
Posterior instability, unidirectional, 177–185
  algorithms for treatment, 180–183, *181, 182, 183*
  anatomy, 177–178
  biomechanics, 177–178
  capsular plication
    bumper effect, *181*
    pinch, tuck method, *182*
  classification, 178–179
  complications, 183–184
  diagnostic evaluation, 179–180
  etiology of injury, 178–179
  "gunslinger" brace, *183*
  historical overview, 177, 177t
  laxity, posterior capsular, *181*

nonoperative treatment, rehabilitation, results, 180
operative treatment, rehabilitation, results, 180
physical examination, 179, *179*
plication, posterior capsular, with recreation of bumper effect, *181*
posterior capsule, athletic activities repetitively stressing, 177t
posterior portal closure, *182*
presentation, 179, *179*
radiographic evaluation, 179–180
voluntary posterior instability, *179*
Posterior instability test, throwing shoulder, 304
Posterior labral tear, imaging, *62*
Posterior rotator cuff musculature tendinitis, throwing shoulder, 110, *110*
Posterior superior glenoid (internal) impingement, imaging, *55*
Posterior tests, 43, *43*
  Jahnke test, 43, *44*
  push-pull test, 43, *43*
Posterolateral rotator cuff tear, imaging, *57*
Posterosuperior glenoid impingement, throwing shoulder, 108
Posterosuperior labral repair, arthroscopic, *8*
Prefabricated orthosis, for multidirectional instability, *194*
Present injury, history of, 26–27
Prevention, in overhead athlete, 6–7
Proprioception, overhead athlete, 98
Provocative tests to reproduce pain, 29–32
Proximal humerus fracture, 291–292, *292*
Pull-through phase, swimming, *351*, 351–352, *352*
  freestyle stroke, stages of, *17*
Push-pull test, 43, *43*
Push-ups with plus exercise, 361

Q

Quadrilateral space syndrome, in baseball, *313*, 313–314
"Quadruped" exercise, 361
Quarterbacks, professional. *See also* Football
  acromioclavicular joint injury, 321t
  clavicle injury, 321t
  injuries to shoulder, chest, 321t

R

Racquet sports, repetitive stressing of posterior capsule with, 177
Radiographic evaluation, 50–51
Range of motion, overhead athlete, 96–97
Recovery phase, swimming stroke, *351*, 352
Rehabilitation in overhead athlete, 6–7
  scapulothoracic, 230t
    lateral tubing pull, *231*
    rhythmic stabilization, *233*
    scapular clock exercises, *232*
    "shoulder dump" exercise, *231*
    slow row exercise, *233*
    sternal lift exercise, *232*
    wall slide exercise, *233*
Relative efficiency, in assessment tools, 66
Reliability of outcome assessments, 65–66

Relocation test for instability, 41–42
Relocation test for pain, 35, *35*
  inferior sulcus test for pain, 35, *36*
  sulcus sign, *36*
Rent test for weakness, 32
Resistance training, 82–94
  backhand throw for distance, in testing of athlete, 92
  current concepts, 85–86, 86t
  forehand throw for distance, in testing of athlete, 92
  hamstring stretch, 83, *83*
  historical background, 83, 83–85, *84, 85, 86*
  "hooklying" position, *83*
  kinetic chain, 82
  knee-to-chest, 83
  lunges, 83
  McKenzie, Robin, MD, 84
    movements proposed by, 84–85
  medicine ball exercises for core strengthening, *92*, 92–93, *93*
    backward throws, 93
    chest pass toss, 92
    double pump, 93
    power drops, 93
    pullover tosses, 92
    side tosses, 93
    sit-up toss, 92
    superman tosses, 93
  medicine ball weights, based on age, 91t
  modalities of core strength, 88
  multifidus, assessing, facilitating, *87*, 87–88
  object of core strengthening, 86–88
  overhead throw for distance, in testing of athlete, 92
  partial sit-up, 83
  program of core strengthening, 84–85, *85*, 91
    bridging with knee extension, 90
    "dead bug" progression, 90
    designing, 88–91
    elongation of muscle spindles, 91
    global stabilizers, 89–90
      exercises for, 90, *90, 91*
    local stabilizers, 89
      exercises for, 89, *89*
    partial sit-up, 90
    plyometric exercise, 91
    side-lying bridge, 90
    sport-specific, 91t, 91–94
    standing lat pull-down, 90
  progressive extension with pillows, 85, *85*
  prone lying, 85, *85*
  prone press-ups, 85, *85*
  seated flexion, 83, *84*
  squat, 83
  stabilizing system, muscular, 86t
    local, global stabilizing system of spine, differentiating, 85
  standing extension, 85, *86*
  strength, defined, 86
  tennis player, testing, sample procedure, 92

Resistance training (*contd.*)
testing overhead athlete, sample procedure, 92
transversus abdominis, assessing, facilitating, 87
Williams, Paul, MD, 83
Williams Flexion Exercises, 83, 84
lunges, *84*
partial sit-up, *83*
squat, *84*
Resisted abduction test, 44
Resisted elbow extension test, 44
Resisted elbow flexion test, 44
Resisted external rotation, 31, *31*
Resisted finger abduction test, 44
Resisted forearm supination test, 44
Resisted wrist extension test, 44
Resisted wrist flexion test, 44
Responsiveness of assessment tools, 65–66
Return to play, variables involved, 7
Reverse Bankart, imaging, 62
Reverse Hill-Sachs, imaging, 62
Review of systems in clinical examination, 27
Rotational osteotomy, for internal impingement, 132, *132*, 133
Rotator cuff
imaging, 54–58
full thickness tears, 56–58, *57*
impingement syndromes, 54–56, *55*
partial thickness tears, 56, *57*
tendinosis, 56, *56*, *57*
posterolateral, tendinosis of, *56*
Rotator cuff exercises, for swimmer, 360, *360*
Rotator cuff injury in baseball, 308–309, *309*
Rotator cuff injury in football, 327–329
authors' preferred approach, 328
rehabilitation, 328–329
Rotator cuff injury in pediatric athlete, 294, *294*
Rotator cuff injury in tennis, 341–342, *342*
Rotator cuff musculature tendinitis, throwing shoulder, 110, *110*
Rotator cuff tear
full thickness, 146–162
algorithms for treatment, 154–161
classification system, 152, 152t
nonoperative treatment, 154
operative treatment, 153–154, 154–158
arthroscopic assisted (miniopen) technique, *157*, 158
arthroscopic rotator cuff repair, 156–157, *157*
diagnostic arthroscopy, 155, *156*
patient positioning for arthroscopic surgery, *155*
portal placement, 154–155
preoperative preparation, 154, *155*
surgical procedure, 155–156, *156*
rehabilitation, 157t, 158t, 158–161, *159*, 159t, 161t
phase 1, 158t
phase 2, 159t

phase 3, 161t
rotator cuff disease, classification of, 152t
Snyder classification of rotator cuff tears, 152t
treatment techniques, 154–161
partial thickness, surgical treatment, 135–145
articular-surface rotator cuff tears, treatment algorithm, *138*
depth, width, delamination grading scale, for outcome analysis, 139t
magnetic resonance imaging, 139, *139*
multiply injured thrower's shoulder structures, treatment of, 140t
posterior articular surface intratendinous rotator cuff lesions (PAINT lesions), 135–137, *136*
pathomechanics, 135
postoperative protocol, 143
surgical technique, 139–143, *140*, 140t, *141*, *142*, *143*
treatment, 137–138, *138*, 139t
posterolateral, *57*
Rotator interval
imaging, 58–60
injuries to, *58*, 58–60, *59*
Rowe Score for Evaluating Bankart Operation, 73, 74

S
Scapula
fracture, *329*, 329–330
ossification centers of, *285*
in shoulder function, 222–223
Scapular assistance test, *227*
Scapular clock exercises, scapulothoracic rehabilitation, *232*
Scapular dyskinesia, 44–45
pain in presence of, *37*, 37–38
scapular stabilization test, 38, *38*
scapular winging, *37*
Scapular muscle exercises, for swimmer, 360, 361, *361*
Scapular muscle strength values, unilateral ratios, 98t
Scapular retraction test, *227*
Scapular stabilization test, 38, *38*
Scapular winging, *37*
from periscapular weakness, in tennis, *343*
Scapulothoracic dysfunction, 222–235, 294
biomechanics of, 222
dyskinesis, scapular
bony posture, injury, 223
classification of, 224–225, *225*
clinical symptoms around scapula, 226
effect of, 225–226
elevation control, loss of, 225–226
evaluation of, 226–228, *227*, *228*
factors creating, 223–224
kinetic chain function, loss of, 226
lateral scapular slide, *228*
muscular alterations, 223–224
one-leg stability series, *227*
protraction control, loss of, 225

rehabilitation, 29–234, 230t, *231*, *232*, *233*
retraction control, loss of, 225
scapular assistance test, *227*
scapular retraction test, *227*
soft tissue inflexibility, 224
stable base, loss of, 226
treatment, 228–229
type I dyskinesis, *224*
type II dyskinesis, *225*
type III dyskinesis, *225*
in pediatric athlete, 294
physiology of scapular motion, 222
rehabilitation, scapulothoracic, 230t
lateral tubing pull, *231*
rhythmic stabilization, *233*
scapular clock exercises, *232*
"shoulder dump" exercise, *231*
slow row exercise, *233*
sternal lift exercise, *232*
wall slide exercise, *233*
scapula in shoulder function, 222–223
Screw fixation, coracoclavicular, grade III injury, *217*
Serratus anterior palsy, 275–277
anatomy, 275
authors' preferred method, 279–280
diagnostic studies, 279
etiology, 275–276
history, 275, 279
nonoperative management, 279
operative management, 279
physical examination, 279
Serve, tennis, stages of, *341*
SF 36 Questionnaire. *See* Standard Form 36 Questionnaire
Shoulder
acromioclavicular joint disorders, 209–221
anatomy of, 10–22
of athlete, general population, contrasted, *3*
axillary nerve injury, 270–272
in baseball, 301–317
biceps tendon disorders, 196–208
biomechanics, during overhead motions, 10–22
clinical examination, 23–49
decision-making, in overhead athlete care, 3–9
in football, 318–339
fractures, 236–266
imaging of, 50–64
instability
unidirectional anterior, 163–185
unidirectional posterior, 177–185
internal impingement, 125–134
multidirectional instability, 186–195
pediatric athletes, 284–298
resistance training, 82–94
rotator cuff tear
full thickness, 146–162
partial thickness, 135–145
scapulothoracic problems, 222–235
serratus anterior palsy, 275–277
subacromial impingement, 146–162

suprascapular neuropathy, 267–270
  in swimming, 349–362
  in tennis, 340–348
  throwing
    exercises for, 95–114
    interval program, 115–121
  trapezius dysfunction, 277–299
  treatment outcome assessment, 65–81
  vascular injury, 272–275
"Shoulder dump" exercise, scapulothoracic
    rehabilitation, *231*
Shoulder girdle fractures, three-phase
    shoulder conditioning, 259t
Shrug test, 44
Sickness Impact Profile, 69
Signe de clarion, 147
SLAC lesion, 63
SLAP lesion, 3, 204, 204t. *See also* SLAP
    tear
  in baseball, *309,* 309–311
  in football, 334–336
  imaging, *62,* 62–63
    paralabral cyst, with denervation
        changes, *63*
    paralabral cysts, 63, *63*
    peel-back, 63
    throwing shoulder, rehabilitation, 111
    treatment, 205–206, *206*
"SLAP" prehension test, 34
SLAP tear, 34
  active compression test, *33,* 34
  anterior slide test, 34
  biceps load test, 34
  O'Driscoll's SLAP test, 34
  "SLAP" prehension test, 34
SLAP test, throwing shoulder, 304
"Slipping," as chief complaint, 40–41
Slow row exercise, scapulothoracic
    rehabilitation, *233*
Speed's test, 33, *33*
Spindles of muscle, elongation of, 91
Spine, global stabilizing system of,
    stabilizing system of local musculature,
    differentiating, 85
Spurling's test, 36, *36*
Stability test, throwing shoulder, 304
Stabilizers, local, 89
  exercises for, 89, *89*
Stabilizing system, of local musculature,
    global stabilizing system of spine,
    differentiating, 85
Stabilizing systems, muscular, 86t
Standard Form 36 Questionnaire, 66–69
Standard response mean, in assessment
    tools, 66
Sternal lift exercise, scapulothoracic
    rehabilitation, *232*
Sternoclavicular joint injury, 287, *287*
  in pediatric athlete, 287, *287*
  separation, in football, 324–325
    authors' preferred approach, 325
    rehabilitation, 325
"Stiffness," as chief complaint, 48, *48*
Stingers. *See* Burners
Strength, defined, 86
Stride, pitching mechanics, 301

Subacromial decompression, for internal
    impingement, 133
Subacromial impingement, 146–162
  acromion, types of, *150*
  classification of, 150, 150t
  diagnostic evaluation, *148,* 148–150,
    149, 150
  etiology of injury, 146
  Hawkins test for impingement, *147*
  lift-off test for subscapularis strength, *148*
  maneuvers producing, 29–30
  Neer classification of, 150t
    phase 1 (protective), 151
    phase 2 (progressive strengthening),
        151
  Neer test for impingement, *147*
  nonoperative treatment of, 150–151
  operative treatment of, 151–152
  physical examination, 146–148, *147, 148*
  presentation, 146–148, *147, 148*
  radiographic evaluation, *148,* 148–150,
    149, 150
  signe de clarion, 147
  throwing shoulder, 108–109, *109*
  treatment of, 150–152
Subacromial injection, 39, *39*
Subcoracoid impingement, 35
Subscapular injection, 40
Subscapularis integrity, lift-off test, *335*
Subscapularis strength, lift-off test for, *148*
Subscapularis tendon tear, imaging, *59*
Sulcus sign, *36*
  tennis injury, *344*
Superior labrum anterior-to-posterior
    lesions. *See* SLAP lesion
Suprascapular nerve, 45
  compression, 37
  entrapment, in baseball, 313
  injection, 40
Suprascapular neuropathy, 267–270
  anatomy, 267
  authors' preferred method, 269–270
  diagnostic studies, 268–269
  etiology of injury, 267–268
  historical overview, 267
  history, 268, *268*
  nonoperative management, 269
  operative intervention, 269
  physical examination, 268, *268*
  in tennis, 342
Supraspinatus, straight arm lift exercises for,
    360
Supraspinatus tendon tear, partial articular
    surface, *57*
Surgical decisions, overview of, 7–8, *8*
Swimming, 349–362, *359*
  abdominal exercises, 361, *361*
  algorithms for treatment, 355–356
  arthroscopic techniques, imbricating
    sutures through capsule, *358*
  backstroke, abduction, external rotation
    during, *354*
  "ball on wall" exercise, *360*
  classification of injury, 355, 355t
  coach's initial management of pain,
    algorithms for, 356

"dead bug" exercise, 361
diagnostic evaluation, 354–355
differential diagnosis, 355
freestyle stroke, recovery phase of, *350*
hitchhiker exercise, 361
impingement, during swimming stroke,
    350, *350*
laxity, 353–354, *354*
lower back exercises, 361, *361*
muscle fatigue, dysfunction, 350–353,
    351
nonoperative treatment, rehabilitation,
    356–357
operative treatment, rehabilitation,
    357–360
  arthroscopic capsular repair, *358,*
    358–359, *359*
  open capsular repair, 357–358
  postoperative rehabilitation, 359
  results of operative treatment, 359–360
painful swimmer's shoulder, muscle
    activity in, 352–353
prevention, 360–361
primary rotator cuff exercises, 360, *360*
pull-through phase, *351,* 351–352, *352*
push-ups with plus exercise, 361
"quadruped" exercise, 361
  stretching exercises, 361
recovery phase, *351, 352*
rehabilitation, 360–361
repetitive stressing of posterior capsule
    with, 177
scapular muscle exercises, 360, 361, *361*
shoulder pain in, etiology of, 349–354
supraspinatus, straight arm lift exercises
    for, *360*
Swimming motion, stages of, with
    electromyographic data, *17,* 17–18
Swimming stroke, freestyle, pull-through
    phase of, stages of, *17*
Synovitis, acromioclavicular joint, *54*
Systems review, in clinical examination, 27

T
Tanner staging classification, secondary
    sexual characteristics, 286t
Tenderness. *See* Pain
Tendinitis
  biceps, in football, 334–336
  calcific, *57*
  overuse syndrome, throwing shoulder,
    108–110
  posterior rotator cuff musculature,
    throwing shoulder, 110, *110*
Tendinosis, rotator cuff, 56, *56, 57*
Tennis, 340–348
  acromioclavicular joint, 342
  adolescent tennis player, 347
  algorithms for treatment, 348
  anatomy, 340–341
  biomechanics, 340–341
  clavicle resection, distal, *346*
  diagnostic evaluation, 344
  dominant arm internal rotation, loss of,
    343
  ground strokes, *18*

Tennis (*contd.*)
historical overview, 340, *341*
injuries, 341–342
instability, 342
internal impingement, *342*
labrum, superior, SLAP tear, *347*
nonoperative treatment, rehabilitation,
344–345
operative treatment, rehabilitation,
345–347, *346, 347*
physical examination, 342–344, *343, 344*
presentation, 342–344, *343, 344*
radiographic evaluation, 344
rotator cuff injuries, 341–342, *342*
scapular winging, from periscapular
weakness, *343*
serve, five stages of, *341*
stages of, with electromyographic data,
18, 18–19
sulcus sign, *344*
suprascapular neuropathy, 342
testing patient, sample procedure, 92
Tenosynovitis, bicipital, 201–203
Tension band technique, for fractures, *252*
Thermal capsulorraphy, for internal
impingement, 132
Thoracic outlet syndrome, 37
in baseball, *312*, 312t, 312–313
provocative maneuvers, 46
Adson's maneuver, 46, *46*
hyperabduction syndrome test, 46
modified Adson's maneuver, *46*
Wright's test, 46
Throw, muscle activity during stages of, *164*
Thrower's exostosis. *See* Bennett's lesion
Thrower's shoulder structures, multiply
injured, surgical treatment, 140t
Thrower's ten program, 99, 100t
Throwing athlete, interval program for,
115–121
criteria for entry into, 116, 116t
"crow hop" technique, with follow-
through, *118*
exercise variables, controlling, 116–117,
117t
flat ground work, *119*
nonsurgical mound work, 120
nonsurgical *versus* postsurgical approach,
116
phase I, long toss, 117t, 117–119
phase II, flat ground work, 119
phase III, progressive mound work, 119
phase IV, simulated game activity, 120
phase V, game progression, 120–121
phase VI, maintenance with return to
play, 121
postsurgical mound work, 119–120, *120*
postsurgical positional throw, 120
problem-based modification of throwing
program, 116t
progressive mound work, *120*
sequencing for rehabilitation program,
117t
time frames for initiation of, after surgical
procedure, 115t

Throwing motion, stages of, with
electromyographic data, 14–16, *15*
Throwing shoulder, physical exam, 304t
Throwing shoulder exercises, 95–114
core stabilization, 99
criteria to initiate throwing program,
106t, *107*, 107t, 107–108
dynamic stabilization, 99
hyperangulation, during overhead
throwing motion, *96*
interval throwing program
phase I, 100t
phase II, throwing off mound, 106t
isokinetic shoulder strength criteria,
overhead athletes, 98t
overhead athlete, physical characteristics
of, 96–98
laxity, 97
muscle strength, 97–98, 98t
proprioception, 98
range of motion, 96–97
overview, 95
plyometric exercises, 99–101
rehabilitation guidelines, 108–112
Bennett's lesion, 110–111
improper mechanics, 111–112
overuse syndrome tendinitis, 108–110
posterior rotator cuff musculature
tendinitis, 110, *110*
posterosuperior glenoid impingement,
108
primary instability, 110
SLAP lesions, 111
subacromial impingement, 108–109,
109
rehabilitation principles, 98–101
closed kinetic chain exercises, 99
core stabilization, 99
dynamic stabilization, 99
plyometric exercises, 99–101
thrower's ten program, 99, 100t
rehabilitation program, 101–107, 106t
acute phase, 101–102, *102*
advanced phase, 103–105, *104*
intermediate phase, 102–103, *103*
return to activity phase, *105*, 105–107,
106t, 107t
T scapular muscle strength values,
unilateral ratios, 98t
"Tingling," as chief complaint, 46
"Tiredness," as chief complaint, 44–46
Translation, diagnosis, 4–5
Transversus abdominis, assessing,
facilitating, 87
Trapezius dysfunction, 2799–279
anatomy, 277
authors' preferred method, 278–279
diagnostic studies, 278
etiology, 277–278
history, 277, 278
nonoperative management, 278
operative management, 278
physical examination, 278
TUBS, multidirectional instability,
186

U
Unidirectional anterior instability, 163–185
algorithm, treatment, 173t
anatomy, 163–164, *164*
anterior capsulolabral reconstruction, *170*
biomechanics, 163–164, *164*
capsular repair, with no labral
detachment, technique, *171*
classification of, 167–168, 168t
complications, 172
coracohumeral ligament, 163
diagnostic evaluation, 166–167, *167*
etiology of injury, 165
historical review, 163–164
inferior glenohumeral labral, 163
middle glenohumeral ligament, 163
nonoperative treatment, rehabilitation,
results, *168*, 168–169
operative treatment, rehabilitation,
results, 169–172, *170, 171*,
172–175, 173t, *174*
physical examination, 165, *166*
pitch, muscle activity during stages of,
164
pitching baseball, phases of, *164*
presentation, 165, *166*
radiographic evaluation, 166–167, *167*
relocation test, provocative component
of, *166*
superior glenohumeral ligament, 163
throw, muscle activity during stages of,
164
Unidirectional posterior instability,
177–185
algorithms for treatment, 180–183, *181*,
182, 183
anatomy, 177–178
biomechanics, 177–178
capsular plication
bumper effect, *181*
pinch, tuck method, *182*
classification, 178–179
complications, 183–184
diagnostic evaluation, 179–180
etiology of injury, 178–179
"gunslinger" brace, *183*
historical overview, 177, 177t
laxity, posterior capsular, *181*
nonoperative treatment, rehabilitation,
results, 180
operative treatment, rehabilitation,
results, 180
physical examination, 179, *179*
plication, posterior capsular, with
recreation of bumper effect, *181*
posterior capsule, athletic activities
repetitively stressing, 177t
posterior portal closure, *182*
presentation, 179, *179*
radiographic evaluation, 179–180
voluntary posterior instability, *179*

V
Valgus-impacted four-part fracture, open
reduction, internal fixation, *251*

Validity of outcome assessment tools, 65–66
Valsalva maneuver, 36
Vascular injuries, 272–275
    anatomy, 272
    authors' preferred method, 275
    diagnostic tests, 273–274
    etiology, 273
    history, 272, 273
    nonoperative management, 274
    operative management, 274–275
    physical examination, 273
Velocity, loss of, as chief complaint, 47–48
Volleyball, repetitive stressing of posterior
    capsule with, 177
Voluntary posterior instability, *179*

W
Wall slide exercise, scapulothoracic
    rehabilitation, *233*
Weakness
    as chief complaint, 44–46
        muscle sources, 44, 44t
        scapular dyskinesia, 44–45
    neurologic sources of, 45, 45t
    tests for, 30–32, *31*
Weight lifting, repetitive stressing of
    posterior capsule with, 177
Weights of medicine ball, based on age, 91t
Western Ontario Shoulder Instability Index,
    73, 75–76
Williams, Paul, MD, 83

Williams Flexion Exercises, 83, 84
    lunges, *84*
    partial sit-up, *83*
    squat, *84*
Wind-up phase, pitching mechanics,
    301
Winging, scapular, *37*
WOSI. *See* Western Ontario Shoulder
    Instability Index
Wright's test, 46
Wrist extension test, resisted, 44
Wrist flexion test, resisted, 44

Y
Yergason's test, 33, *34*